EMERGENCY MEDICATIONS

Albumin
Alphaprodine (Nisentil)
Aminophylline
Amobarbital
Ampicillin
Aromatic spirits of ammonia
Atropine
Calcium chloride
Calcium gluconate
Cefazolin
Clindamycin
Dexamethasone
Dextrose 50 percent
Diazepam (Valium)
Digoxin
Diphenhydramine (Benadryl)
Dopamine
Ephedrine
Epinephrine
Ergonovine
Furosemide
Gentamicin
Heparin
Hydralazine
Hydrocortisone
Isoproterenol
Lactated Ringer's Solution
Lidocaine
Mannitol
Magnesium sulfate 50 percent
Meperidine (Demerol)
Methylergonovine
Methylprednisolone
Morphine
Naloxone (Narcan)
Oxytocin
Penicillin
Pentobarbital
Phenobarbital
Phenytoin (Dilantin)
Plasma protein fraction
Potassium chloride
Probenecid
Promethazine (Phenergan)
Progesterone in oil
Sodium bicarbonate

MANUAL OF GYNECOLOGIC AND OBSTETRIC EMERGENCIES

BEN-ZION TABER, M.D.

Clinical Associate Professor of Gynecology and Obstetrics, Stanford University; Associate Director, Department of Obstetrics and Gynecology, Santa Clara Valley Medical Center, San Jose, California

1979

W. B. SAUNDERS COMPANY

Philadelphia / London / Toronto

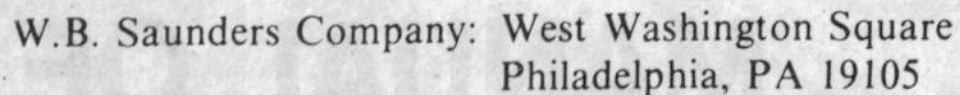

W.B. Saunders Company: West Washington Square
Philadelphia, PA 19105

1 St. Anne's Road
Eastbourne, East Sussex BN21 3UN, England

1 Goldthorne Avenue
Toronto, Ontario M8z 5T9, Canada

Library of Congress Cataloging in Publication Data

Taber, Ben-Zion, 1927-
Manual of gynecologic and obstetric emergencies.

1. Gynecology. 2. Pregnancy, Complications of. 3. Medical emergencies. I. Title. [DNLM: 1. Emergencies. 2. Gynecologic diseases. 3. Obstetrics. 4. Pregnancy complications. WP100 T123m]

RG103.T25 618 77-84692

ISBN 0-7216-8721-0

Manual of Gynecologic and Obstetric Emergencies ISBN 0-7216-8721-0

Last digit is the print number: 9 8 7 6 5 4 3 2 1

What has happened
  Will happen again.
What has been done
  We still must do.
Nothing under the sun
  Is entirely new.

ECCLESIASTES, Chapter one, verse nine

FOREWORD

Spontaneous abortion, pelvic infection, and venereal disease are the more common female reproductive tract problems seen in the Emergency Department. On reading Dr. Taber's manual, however, it becomes obvious that the potential for other obstetric and gynecologic emergencies to occur is quite significant.

It is possible that the renewed interest of the laity in do-it-yourself obstetrics will cause us to see complications and to have to cope with emergencies that are not within the scope of our past experience. Not many years need pass without one's being exposed to a rare emergency situation before one's clinical ability to handle such an emergency diminishes. This applies to the obstetrician and to the gynecologist, but it is especially applicable to the emergency physician, who must attempt to have up-to-date knowledge of how to handle *any* medical or surgical emergency.

For emergency physicians, and others with limited experience in handling obstetric and gynecologic emergencies, this manual has much to commend it. Dr. Taber covers all obstetric and gynecologic emergencies, rare and common, with clarity, detailing the least controversial approaches. His logical and consistent use of the SOAP (Subjective data, Objective data, Assessment, Plan) approach also makes this manual a useful reference for those physicians who see many obstetric and gynecologic emergencies and find themselves faced with difficulties in diagnosis or management. For those of this group who are not yet using ultrasonic B-scanning, the manual affords a good introduction to its use and advantages. This is especially important as patients grow increasingly concerned about the possible dangers of ionizing radiation.

Many problems and conditions that are associated with obstetric and gynecologic emergencies also occur in other groups of patients, male and female. All these problems are dealt with succinctly by Dr. Taber, so that the manual can be an excellent to-hand reference text for such problems as can be found in the interpretation of blood gases, electrolyte therapy, and the management of coagulation disorders, to give but a few examples.

No matter what one's interest is in the various fields of medicine, the chances are that a knowledge of obstetrics and gynecology will be necessary at some time or another. The psychiatric aspects of childbirth, stillbirth, and abortion cannot be fully understood without a knowledge of the physiology and pathology of these conditions. A dermatologist's patient can complicate his attempts at treatment by becoming pregnant or taking birth control pills. An orthopedist taking care of a fractured pelvis can have more on his hands than a cracked bony structure. The general surgeon may unexpectedly find any one of a number of disturbing obstetric and gynecologic conditions staring him in the face as the peritoneum is opened. Any physician, of any specialty, might ask himself, "Do I know enough about the most wondrous elements of the physiology of the female of our species? Should I know more about those abnormalities and catastrophes that might mar its perfection?"

This manual should fill many needs.

Edward L. McNeil, M.D.

Emergency Physician,
Northern Westchester
Hospital Center,
Mount Kisco, New York;
Past President, New York
Chapter, American College
of Emergency Physicians

PREFACE

Although women in the reproductive years are usually young and healthy, obstetric and gynecologic emergencies can occur suddenly and unexpectedly. Alarmed by profuse vaginal bleeding or acute pelvic pain, patients in great discomfort demand immediate medical care either from their personal physician or from a hospital emergency service.

Not every emergency visit involves a life-threatening crisis. From the patient's point of view, an emergency is any sudden, unexpected event that she feels is potentially serious and requires immediate medical attention. The physician faced with a frightened, distraught patient must act rapidly in order to assess the significance of the patient's symptoms and objective findings and must consider the following questions: Is hospitalization required or can the patient return to her home environment? Which laboratory tests or diagnostic procedures will be helpful in the assessment of the acute problem? Is surgery or medical therapy required? Careful assessment is even more difficult in obstetric emergencies, since they are complicated by the fact that two lives are involved. Concern for both must influence the management plan.

This manual has been prepared for all clinicians faced with gynecologic and obstetric emergency situations. Specific problems have been organized in the format of a problem-oriented medical record. The SOAP approach provides a concise outline of the problem-related data, assessment, and action plan.

S—*subjective* data—covers the patient's *current symptoms* as well as her essential *history*. Usually, this information is related by the patient herself, although under certain emergency situations, necessary history must be obtained from a family member or friend.

O—*objective* data—includes the findings derived from *physical examination* and preliminary *laboratory tests.*

A—*assessment*—provides a synthesis of the subjective and objective data base. This includes

1. Differential diagnosis—the diagnostic possibilities to be considered
2. Etiologic or predisposing factors that may be responsible for the clinical problem
3. Complications or associated problems that should be anticipated or considered in the formulation of diagnostic and therapeutic plans
4. An evaluation of the severity of the disease process or clinical syndrome

P—*plan*—is considered in three parts:

1. Additional diagnostic data include laboratory tests, x-rays, sonograms, and other diagnostic procedures that may elucidate the patient's problem and rule out other possible diagnoses.
2. Management program includes therapeutic goals: initial therapy, medications, surgery, diet, activity, and so forth.
3. Patient education highlights the information a patient should know in order to participate fully in her personal health care. This usually covers the physician's assessment of her problem and recommendations for management and follow-up care.

Patient education is an important component of the management plan, since the emotional impact of sudden illness may have as much potential for disability as the medical problem itself. Obstetric and gynecologic emergencies, in particular, not only interrupt a woman's usual activities and plans but also threaten her hopes for future childbearing and sexual expression.

Definitions of clinical entities are usually those recommended by the Committee on Terminology of the American College of Obstetricians and Gynecologists.*

Incidence figures quoted for the various problems have been gathered from reviews in the medical literature. It must be remembered that the incidence of all problems varies greatly from hospital to hospital, depending on the population served and the likelihood that unusual problems will be referred to a particular medical center.

---

*From Hughes ED (ed): Obstetric-Gynecologic Terminology. Philadelphia, F.A. Davis Company, 1972.

The procedures and programs recommended are those most commonly used in the obstetric and gynecologic service at the Santa Clara Valley Medical Center in California. Since there are many areas of clinical uncertainty and controversy in obstetrics and gynecology, the specific measures outlined are not necessarily the only proper methods. Other centers may emphasize alternative approaches.

References have been included to enable interested readers to pursue specific subjects in greater depth. For the most part, the references have been restricted to publications that have appeared within the past ten years.

Part I of the manual reviews general principles of gynecologic and obstetric evaluation.

Part II provides an outline of specific problems: subjective and objective data base; assessment relative to the problem; and plan (additional diagnostic data, management, and patient education). To facilitate rapid reference the subjects have been arranged in alphabetical order.

When the data base is initially incomplete and problems can be defined only in symptomatic terms (abdominal pain, vaginal bleeding, convulsive seizures, and so forth, the chapter outlines the diagnostic possibilities to be considered.

Many patients are discharged from the hospital a few days or even a few hours after delivery or surgery. Other patients may deliver their babies at home or en route to the hospital. Consequently, postpartum and postoperative complications are frequently dealt with in the Emergency Department. The interval between the recent delivery or surgery and the onset of symptoms alerts the physician to the probable relationship. The chapters on postoperative and postpartum complications suggest the diagnostic possibilities that should be considered.

Part III provides more detailed information on various procedures and therapy required for the assessment and management of gynecologic and obstetric emergency problems.

It is hoped that this manual will meet currently unfilled needs of emergency physicians, nurses, and assistants, family practitioners, and obstetrician-gynecologists faced with the emergency care of female reproductive and related problems.

Ben-Zion Taber, M.D.

The procedures and practices recommended are those most commonly used in the obstetric and gynecologic services at the Santa Clara Valley Medical Center in California. Since there are many areas of clinical uncertainty and controversy in obstetrics and gynecology, the specific measures outlined are not necessarily the only proper method. Other centers may prefer alternative approaches.

References have been included to enable interested readers to pursue specific subjects in greater depth. For the most part, the references have been restricted to publications that have appeared within the past ten years.

Part I of the manual reviews general principles of gynecologic and obstetric evaluation.

Part II provides an outline of specific problems: subjective and objective data base, assessments relative to the problem, and plans (additional diagnostic data, management, and patient education). To facilitate rapid reference, the subjects have been arranged in alphabetical order.

When the data base is initially incomplete and problems can be defined only as symptoms (in terms of abdominal pain, vaginal bleeding, convulsive seizures, and so forth), the chapter outlines the diagnostic possibilities to be considered.

Many patients are discharged from the hospital a few days or even a few hours after delivery or surgery. Other patients may deliver their babies at home or en route to the hospital. Consequently, postpartum and postoperative complications are frequently dealt with in the Emergency Department. The interval between the recent delivery or surgery and the onset of symptoms alerts the physician to the probable relationship. The chapters on postoperative and postpartum complications suggest the diagnostic possibilities that should be considered.

Part III provides more detailed information on emergency procedures and therapy required for the assessment and management of gynecologic and obstetric emergency problems.

It is hoped that this manual will meet currently unfilled needs of emergency physicians, nurses, and assistants, family practitioners, and obstetrician-gynecologists faced with the emergency care of female reproductive and related problems.

Ben-Zion Taber, M.D.

CONTENTS

PART ONE GENERAL PRINCIPLES

PART TWO SPECIFIC PROBLEMS

PART THREE PROCEDURES AND THERAPY

PART FOUR APPENDICES

PART I

GENERAL PRINCIPLES

1 EMERGENCY GYNECOLOGIC EVALUATION

GENERAL CONSIDERATIONS

IDENTIFICATION

Whenever emergency care is required, essential information must be obtained rapidly (see Table 1-1). Problems must be assessed expeditiously in order to formulate immediate action plans. When a woman arrives in the emergency room collapsed in shock with obvious intraabdominal or vaginal hemorrhage, resuscitative meaures (airway, oxygen, intravenous fluids, blood) must be instituted at the same time that the history is obtained and preparations are made for emergency surgery.

If the patient is confused, disoriented, or unconscious, identification information and essential history must be obtained from the people accompanying the patient.

The patient's age is always important, since different problems may be anticipated prior to puberty, during adolescence and the earlier reproductive years, during the later reproductive years, and after the cessation of childbearing.

Throughout the reproductive years, pregnancy complications and pelvic infection must always be expected. Dysfunctional anovulatory bleeding is more common during adolescence or the perimenopausal years than at other times. Neoplasia must always be considered during the advanced years.

TABLE 1-1. Emergency Gynecoiogic Evaluation

Identification
- Name, age

Subjective Data
- Chief complaint
- Current symptoms
  - Abdominal pain: Onset; location; quality; duration; aggravating and relieving factors; associated symptoms
  - Vaginal bleeding; Discharge: Quantity; duration
  - Menstrual symptoms: Last menstrual period (LMP), preceding menstrual period (PMP), menstrual pattern
  - Pregnancy symptoms: Nausea, vomiting, breast symptoms
  - Contraceptive methods
  - Fever, chills
  - Other symptoms: Cardiovascular, psychiatric, urinary
- Prior history
  - Reproductive history: Gravida, para
  - Pelvic disease
  - Surgery or hospitalizations

Objective Data
- Physical examination
  - General examination: Temperature, pulse, blood pressure, respiration, appearance
  - Breast examination: Inspection, palpation
  - Abdominal examination: Inspection, palpation, percussion, auscultation
  - Pelvic examination: Inspection, speculum, vaginal, bimanual, rectovaginal
- Laboratory tests
  - Complete blood count with blood smear
  - Urinalysis
  - Blood type and Rh

Assessment
- Differential diagnosis
- Etiologic or predisposing factors
- Complications or associated problems
- Severity of disease process

Plan
- Additional diagnostic data
- Management: Medical, surgical
- Patient education

SUBJECTIVE DATA

CHIEF COMPLAINT

The principal complaint, the basic reason why the patient is seeking emergency care, is described succinctly in the patient's own words.

CURRENT SYMPTOMS

Abdominal Pain: Abdominal pain and vaginal bleeding are the two most common symptoms of emergency gynecologic problems. Although these two symptoms in combination almost invariably suggest a primary process in the reproductive tract, a pathologic condition in the intestinal tract, urinary tract, heart, pleural cavity, or dorsal spine coexisting with normal menses or menstrual dysfunction must also be considered.

People vary greatly with respect to the amount of stimuli necessary to evoke a pain sensation. Even the same person under different conditions may react differently to a similar pain stimulus. The severity of pain perception depends on the person's pain threshold, preexistent inflammation, and any alterations in blood supply. Anxiety, inflammation, and ischemia heighten the sensitivity to painful stimuli.

Accurate evaluation of abdominal pain requires detailed information concerning its onset, location, quality, duration, aggravating and relieving factors, and associated symptoms.

Helpful questions include

1. Did the pain start suddenly or develop gradually? (The nature of onset may be elucidated by details of the patient's activities at the time the pain was first noted.)
2. Where is the pain located? Is it in one spot or is it diffuse? Has the pain moved from one site to another?
3. Is the pain cramping or steady?
4. How long has the pain been present?
5. What tends to aggravate or relieve the pain? Eating? Movement?
6. Are there associated symptoms? Anorexia, nausea, vomiting, syncope, dysuria, fever, chills, or others?

(See Abdominal Pain, p. 70)

Vaginal Bleeding and Vaginal Discharge: From infancy to advanced age, abnormal vaginal bleeding may occur at any time. During the reproductive years, cyclic menstrual bleeding is normal; before menarche and after menopause, however, vaginal bleeding has special significance, since uterine bleeding is not a normal occurrence during these phases of life.

Abnormal vaginal bleeding may be irregular and acyclic (metrorrhagia), excessive or prolonged menses (menorrhagia), or irregular excessive bleeding during menstruation and between the menstrual periods (menometrorrhagia). Accurate evaluation demands detailed information concerning the duration and quantity of bleeding, particularly the dates of bleeding, compared with the normal or expected menstrual flow. (See Vaginal Bleeding, p. 686).

Vaginal discharge, with or without pruritus, is a common gynecologic problem. The onset, duration, quantity, color, odor, and consistency aid in the diagnostic evaluation. A malodorous, purulent discharge that develops shortly after delivery or abortion is usually an indication of cervical and endometrial infection, particularly when the temperature is elevated and the white count is increased.

Vaginal discharge during childhood may be particularly disturbing to the patient and her parents. Although gonorrhea should be considered and excluded, it is a relatively infrequent cause of discharge in children. Much more common causes are intestinal parasites or foreign bodies inserted into the vagina.

Menstrual Symptoms: The menstrual history should include the age of onset of menstrual periods (*menarche*), the interval between the periods, the duration of flow, and the usual quantity of flow. A formula for recording menarche, interval between periods in days, and duration of flow is exemplified by "13 × 28 × 3", which signifies that menarche occurred at age 13, the first day of the period follows the first day of the preceding period by 28 days, and the duration of flow is three days.

The dates of the last menstrual period (LMP) and preceding menstrual period (PMP) are recorded. Whenever menses do not occur at the expected time or the last menstrual period is lighter than usual, pregnancy is a possibility. For this reason, the time interval between the onset of the patient's current symptoms and the onset of the last menstrual period is important diagnostic information. It is often helpful to ask whether the patient herself considered her last and next to last menstrual periods to be normal for her.

Knowledge of the patient's *menstrual pattern* (regularity of irregularity) aids in the interpretation of menstrual symptoms. Amenorrhea is not as diagnostic of pregnancy when the patient's previous menstrual cycles are characteristically irregular. The causes of secondary amenorrhea and the differential diagnosis of amenorrhea are outlined in Tables 1-2 and 1-3.

TABLE 1-2. Causes of Secondary Amenorrhea

Physiologic Causes
- Pregnancy
- Puerperium
- Menopause

Failure of Uterine Response
- Hysterectomy
- Cryptomenorrhea (due to acquired stenosis of cervix or vagina)
- Destruction of endometrium (Asherman's syndrome)
  - Tuberculosis
  - Traumatic

Ovarian Insufficiency
- Destruction (surgery, irradiation, infections)
- Neoplasms
- Premature menopause
- Polycystic ovary (Stein-Leventhal) syndrome

Central Nervous System Disorders
- Pituitary hypothalamic dysfunction
- Tumor
- Steroid hormones

Psychogenic Causes

Psychotropic drugs

Thyroid disease

Adrenal disease

Nutritional causes
- Anorexia nervosa
- Malnutrition
- Marked obesity

Chronic systemic disease

TABLE 1-3. Amenorrhea: Differential Diagnosis

Persistent estrogen and progesterone stimulation of endometrium
Pregnancy
Persistent corpus luteum
Persistent estrogenic stimulation of endometrium
Anovulation
Absent estrogen
Ovarian agenesis or dysgenesis
Surgical absence of ovaries
Hypothalamic or pituitary disorders
Uterine or vaginal abnormalities
Imperforate hymen
Vaginal agenesis
Absent uterus
Asherman's syndrome (endometrial destruction)
Testicular feminization

Pregnancy Symptoms: Pregnancy is always suspected when amenorrhea is accompanied by subjective symptoms of morning nausea, vomiting, breast fullness, breast tenderness, or urinary frequency. (See Pregnancy Diagnosis, p. 29.)

In some instances, the diagnosis of a pregnancy complication is immediately obvious. A patient with profuse vaginal bleeding, cramping pain, and a history of two missed periods is most likely aborting an intrauterine pregnancy. Speculum, vaginal, and bimanual examination confirm the initial suspicion.

Contraceptive Methods: Asssessment of the pregnancy possibility is aided by knowledge of the patient's use of contraceptive methods. Oral contraceptives are highly effective for pregnancy prevention as long as the patient has not missed taking any tablets. Intrauterine devices are less effective, and one or two pregnancies may be expected among 100 women over the course of a year. Furthermore, when pregnancy occurs with an intrauterine device *in situ*, the possibility of ectopic gestation must always be considered.

Contraceptive methods may also alter the menstrual cycle. Oral contraceptives may be responsible for oligomenorrhea or amenorrhea, whereas the intrauterine device may be associated with hypermenorrhea.

Fever, Chills: Fever and chills are common symptoms of systemic infection. Severe bilateral pelvic pain associated with fever and chills always suggests pelvic infection: endometritis, parametritis, or salpingitis or all three.

Other Symptoms:

Cardiovascular Symptoms: Syncope, lightheadedness, or orthostatic changes are frequently signs of blood loss.

Psychiatric Symptoms: Sexual assault and genital trauma are virtually always emergency problems. Under these circumstances, emotional symptoms assume great importance. Emergency evaluation must take into consideration the patient's psychosexual concerns.

Urinary Symptoms: Dysuria, hematuria, frequency, or costovertebral angle pain suggest a primary process in the kidney, ureter, or bladder. Urinalysis helps confirm the diagnosis of urinary tract disease.

PRIOR HISTORY

Reproductive History: Details of the patient's previous reproductive history often help one make an emergency gynecologic evaluation. At times, the patient may recognize similar symptoms and even offer the correct diagnosis. Women with repeat abortions or repeat ectopic pregnancies are particularly apt to be aware of the similarity of their current symptoms to the previous event.

The terminology of previous reproductive history is often abbreviated. *Gravida* refers to the number of pregnancies, and *para* refers to the number of births.* Parity is often expressed in four numbers: The first refers to the number of *term births*; the second, to the number of *premature deliveries*; the third, to the number of *abortions*; and the fourth, to the number of *living children*. For example, gravida 9, para $^{4-2-3-1}$ designates a woman who has been pregnant nine times with four term deliveries, two premature births, three abortions, and one living child.

Pelvic Pathologic Conditions: Knowledge of a prior pelvic pathologic condition, such as a preexisting ovarian cyst, endometriosis, or pelvic

---

*For the purpose of defining parity, a multiple birth is a single parous experience.

infection, may be particularly helpful in the evaluation of an emergency problem.

Surgery or Hospitalizations: Details of the patient's previous medical history, particularly surgical procedures and hospital care, can be helpful in sorting out complex diagnostic problems. In addition, emergency gynecologic problems may be complicated by preexisting medical diseases. Knowledge of previous events often facilitates diagnostic and therapeutic decisions.

OBJECTIVE DATA

PHYSICAL EXAMINATION

General Examination: The basic examination of every patient includes temperature, pulse, blood pressure, respiration, and evaluation of general appearance. Pallor of the skin, nail beds, and conjunctiva coupled with cold moist extremities portends the shock associated with internal or external hemorrhage. The patient's behavior is also significant. Patients with severe colic are likely to be restless, whereas patients with peritoneal irritation prefer to remain as motionless as possible. Patients who are unusually frightened, anxious, or tense are difficult to examine. These patients, in particular, require a calming atmosphere and adequate reassurance prior to examination.

Temperature: Temperature may be normal, subnormal, or elevated. In cases of severe hemorrhage, for example, the temperature may be subnormal. During the initial phase of acute appendicitis, the temperature is usually normal, but within a few hours the temperature may gradually rise to approximately 100 or 101°. If and when perforation occurs, the temperature will usually go higher. Temperatures up to 104° may be associated with acute pyelonephritis or septicemia.

Pulse: Tachycardia, or rapid pulse, is another sign of sepsis or shock. The correlation of pulse with blood pressure is particularly important in the evaluation of peripheral circulation and tissue perfusion. (See Shock, p. 612.)

Blood Pressure: Hypotension and hypertension are both potentially serious. Interpretation must take into consideration the total physical examination, as well as the appropriate laboratory tests.

Orthostatic hypotension is characterized by a fall of 20 mm Hg in both systolic and diastolic pressure when the patient stands. In addition, the patient feels dizzy, weak, and faint. Possible causes include depletion of intravascular volume due to hemorrhage.

Respiration: Increased respiratory rate is an index of the severity of the patient's problem. Pulmonary disease, hemorrhage, and metabolic acidosis cause tachypnea in order to compensate for decreased oxygenation or increased carbon dioxide.

Breast examination may be helpful in the evaluation of pregnancy probability. During early pregnancy many women become aware of slight changes in their breasts: increased tenderness, increased turgor, areolar pigmentation, or prominence of the follicles of Montgomery (see Fig. 1-1).) On palpation, any unusual tenderness, masses, or nipple discharge should be noted.

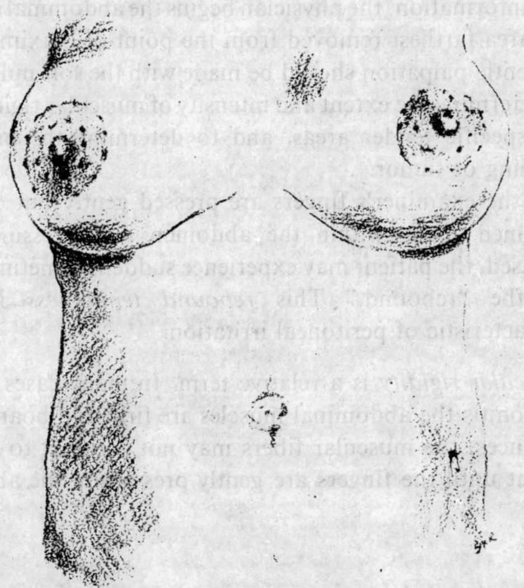

Figure 1-1. Nipples with prominent follicles of Montgomery.

Abdominal Examination:

Inspection: The abdominal *contour* should be carefully inspected for evidence of local or general distention, tumor, or uterine enlargement. It is always possible that a patient has not been aware of missing any periods and has not realized that she could be pregnant. The outline of the enlarged pregnant uterus may present the first clue to the patient's problem.

Respiratory movement of the abdominal wall should be noted, since limitation of respiratory movement may indicate rigidity of the diaphragm or abdominal muscles. When appendicitis is associated with local peritonitis, the right iliac area may appear immobile. In some cases of acute pancreatitis, the epigastric zone is motionless.

The presence of a *surgical scar* on the abdomen may be the first clue to intestinal obstruction associated with intraabdominal adhesions.

Palpation:

Tenderness: Prior to palpation the patient should be asked to point out with one finger the exact spot or area of maximal pain. Aware of this information, the physician begins the abdominal examination at the area farthest removed from the point of maximal pain.

Gentle palpation should be made with the soft pulp of the fingers to determine the extent and intensity of muscular rigidity, to identify the specific tender areas, and to determine the presence of any swelling or tumor.

If the examiner's fingers are pressed gently but deeply over an inflamed focus within the abdomen and pressure is suddenly released, the patient may experience sudden, sometimes severe, pain on the "rebound." This *rebound tenderness* is particularly characteristic of peritoneal irritation.

Muscular rigidity is a relative term. In many cases of generalized peritonitis the abdominal muscles are firm and boardlike. In other instances, the muscular fibers may not contract to any detectable extent until the fingers are gently pressed on the abdominal wall.

Muscular rigidity and resistance may be slight, even in the presence of severe peritonitis, if the abdominal wall is flabby and the abdominal muscles are thin and weak. This situation is frequently encountered in the postpartum patient.

Interpretation of abdominal wall rigidity is often difficult since the psychologic attitude of the patient can contribute to muscular guarding. Frightened adolescents often hold the abdominal wall very rigid, even with slight intraabdominal disease.

Masses: A palpable abdominal mass may be due to an enlarged uterus, ovarian cyst, tuboovarian abscess, or hematoma.

In cases of intrauterine pregnancy, fetal parts and fetal movements may be palpable. When fetal parts appear unusually close to the skin surface, the possibility of an abdominal pregnancy must be considered.

In the examination of a distended abdomen, *percussion* aids in the differentiation of an ovarian cyst from ascites. Dullness in the flanks with anterior tympany suggests ascites; tympany in the flanks with anterior dullness is associated with an ovarian cyst. In addition, shifting dullness is characteristic of ascites.

Auscultation is important for the assessment of bowel sounds and the identification of the fetal heart. With an ultrasound stethoscope the fetal heart may be heard at 12 to 14 weeks of gestation.

In cases of diffuse peritonitis, bowel sounds are absent or, at best, markedly hypoactive. In cases of localized peritonitis, intestinal sounds may be present but hypoactive. When gastroenteritis or early mechanical obstruction is present, the bowel sounds are hyperactive.

Pelvic Examination: Prior to pelvic examination the patient should be asked to void in order to provide a urine specimen for analysis and in order to facilitate the evaluation of the pelvic structures. The patient should be placed in the lithotomy position and appropriately draped on an examining table with stirrups (Fig. 1-2).

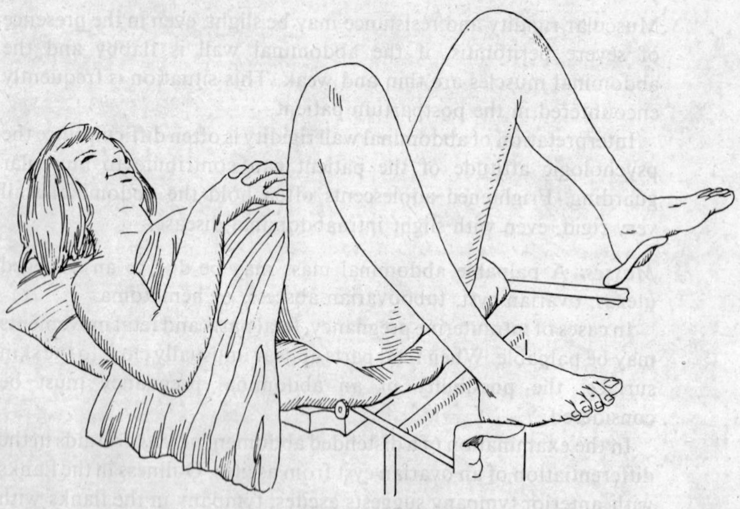

Figure 1-2. The patient is placed in lithotomy position and appropriately draped in preparation for pelvic examination.

Inspection: The external genitalia (Fig. 1-3) are inspected for any evidence of inflammation, hypertrophy, atrophy, or ulcerations. The vulva is carefully observed for lesions, and hair distribution is noted. The labia are separated and the clitoris and hymen examined. The urethral meatus is observed for redness and purulent exudate. Any evidence of vaginal discharge is noted.

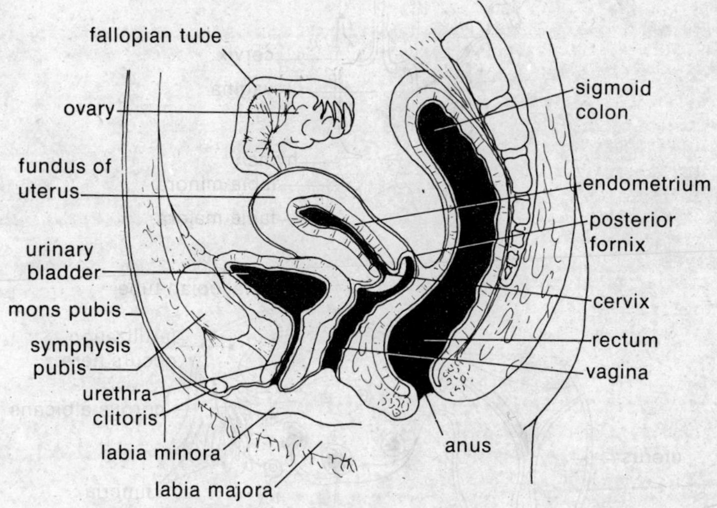

Figure 1-3. Female genitalia.

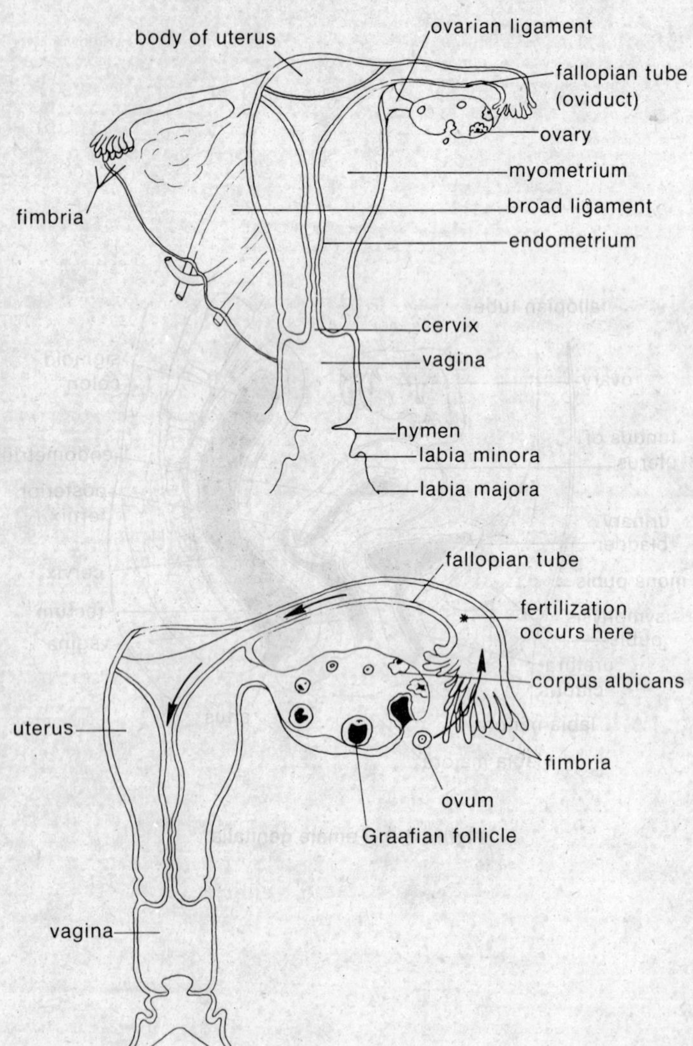

Figure 1-3 Continued.

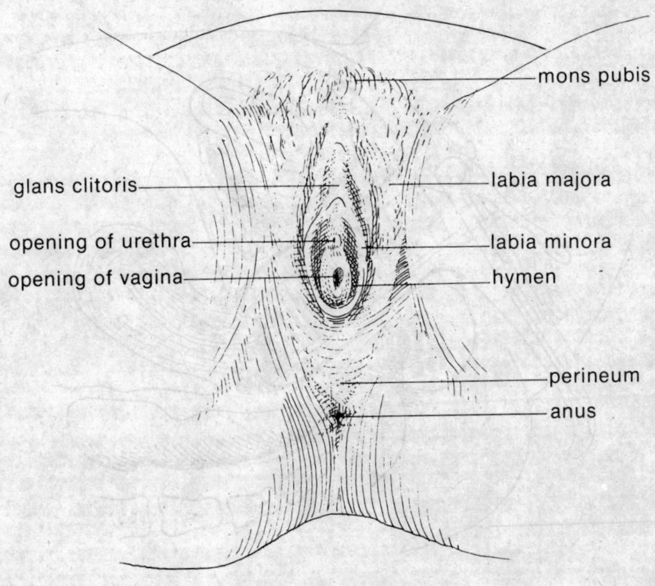

Figure 1-3 Continued.

Speculum Examination: Prior to digital examination, a speculum is inserted into the vagina in order to visualize the vagina and the cervix (Fig. 1-4). For the patient's comfort, the speculum should be moistened with warm water. Artificial lubrication is rarely necessary. When the speculum is inserted the patient is asked to relax while the labia are spread with the gloved fingers of one hand. The speculum should be inserted, with the blades closed, in such a way that it is directed downward and inward to avoid the urethra. A good light source is essential for adequate visualization of the cervix.

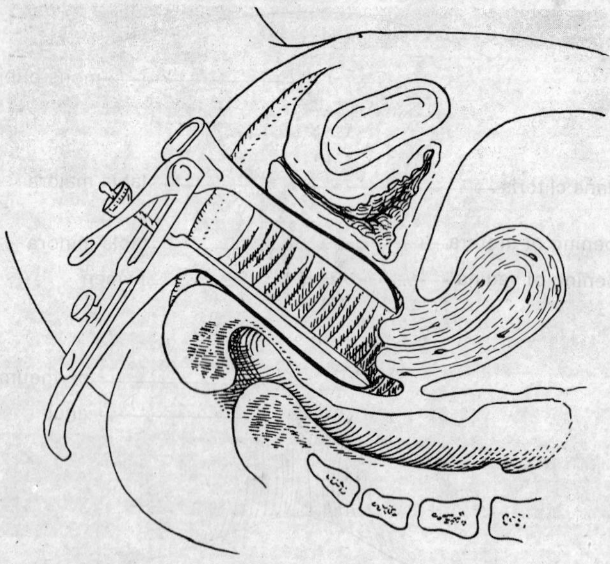

Figure 1-4. A speculum is inserted into the vagina in order to visualize the vagina and the cervix.

Vaginal and cervical secretions are noted. The cervical os is visualized in order to identify any discharge, particularly blood or purulent fluid. If the cervical os is dilated and fetal or placental tissue is visible, the patient is aborting an intrauterine pregnancy. Obvious placental tissue should be removed with a ring forceps and sent to the pathology laboratory. If a purulent discharge is observed, a swab of this discharge should be sent to the bacteriology laboratory for culture and gram stain.

Lesions of the cervix and vagina are noted, as well as the size, coloration, and position of the cervix. Displacement of the cervix may indicate adnexal disease. Unless contraindicated by an emergency situation or the presence of profuse bleeding, a *Pap smear* of the cervix is usually taken for cytologic evaluation.

While the speculum is being withdrawn the vaginal walls are inspected; the mucosal color, the presence or absence of rugae, and any abnormal ulceration or tumor are noted. Bluish discoloration of the vagina and cervix may be an early sign of pregnancy. *Trichomonas vaginalis* infection is suggested by the presence of a "strawberry" erythema of the vaginal walls with a frothy yellow-green discharge. Candidal (monilial) vaginitis is signaled by the presence of "cottage cheese" particles on the vaginal walls.

Vaginal Examination: When vaginal bleeding occurs during the latter half of pregnancy, vaginal examination is contraindicated because of the danger of placental previa unless the patient is prepared for immediate cesarean section. Under all other circumstances the gloved, lubricated index finger is inserted gently into the vagina with slight backward pressure applied at the fourchette to aid perineal relaxation. The insertion of one finger initially helps to determine the patient's apprehensiveness and allows the examiner to note whether the hymen is intact.

After a pause to enhance relaxation, unless the vagina is very painful and tight, the middle finger of the examining hand is inserted along with the forefinger. Tenderness, masses, and thickening of the introitus are noted. With the thumb outside and the palm turned downward, enlargement and sensitivity of Bartholin's glands can be palpated (Fig. 1-5). The urethra is then palpated for evidence of induration and to determine whether pus can be expressed from the urethral orifice or Skene's glands (Fig. 1-6).

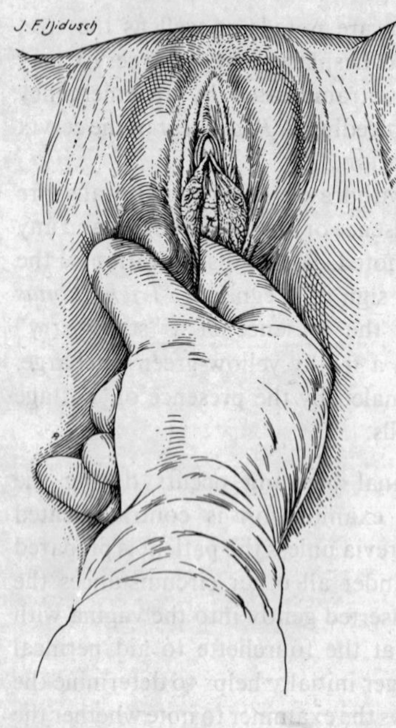

Figure 1-5. The method used to palpate a Bartholin's cyst. (From Dunphy JE, Botsford TW: Physical Examination of the Surgical Patient. Philadelphia, W.B. Saunders Company, 1975.)

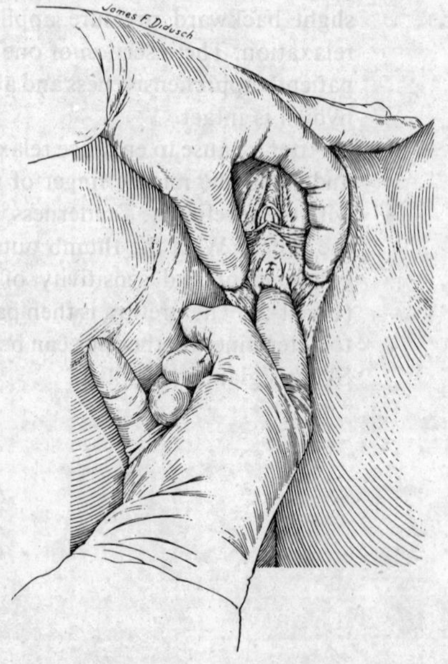

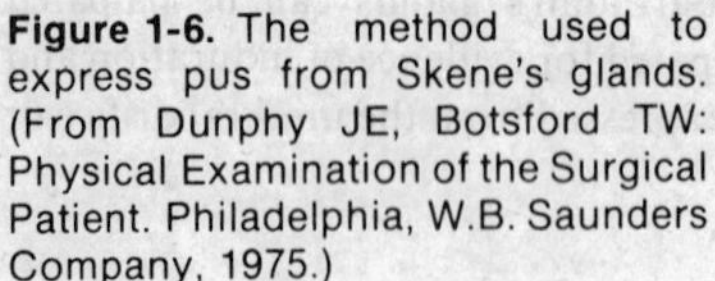

Figure 1-6. The method used to express pus from Skene's glands. (From Dunphy JE, Botsford TW: Physical Examination of the Surgical Patient. Philadelphia, W.B. Saunders Company, 1975.)

The cervix can be outlined with the fingers, and its size, position, contour, consistency, effacement, and dilatation determined. Cervical softening suggests pregnancy.

The cervix is moved about in order to stretch the uterosacral and transverse cervical ligaments. This motion reveals the degree of freedom of the cervix and signals the presence of unusual pelvic tenderness. The fornices are explored for mass, tenderness, or distortion.

When the cervix is deviated from its normal position, an extrauterine mass should be suspected.

Bimanual Examination: Digital examination of the vagina combined with lower abdominal palpation, bimanual examination, is of prime importance in the evaluation of pelvic disease. While performing the digital examination described above the examiner places the other hand on the lower abdomen in order to palpate the deeper structures of the pelvis. The abdominal hand is held palm down with the fingers together but slightly flexed. The fingers are then pressed firmly against the abdominal wall to displace the lower abdominal pelvic organs toward the fingers in the vagina (Fig. 1-7).

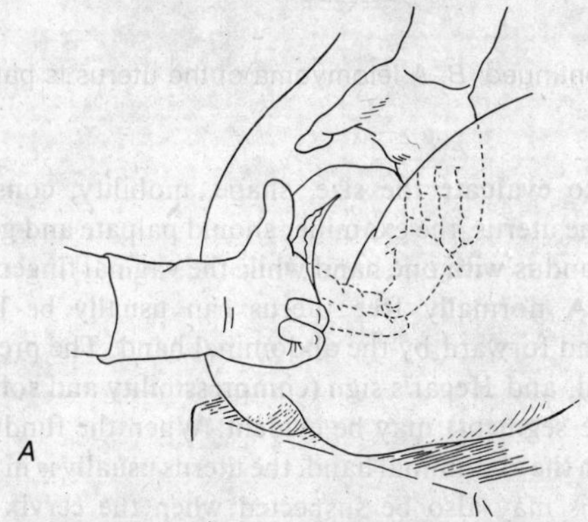

Figure 1-7. Bimanual examination. *A*, While performing digital examination the examiner places the other hand on the patient's abdomen in order to palpate the deeper pelvic structures. The abdominal hand is held palm down with fingers together and slightly flexed. The fingers are then pressed firmly against the abdominal wall to displace the lower abdominal pelvic organs toward the fingers in the vagina.

Figure continued on following page.

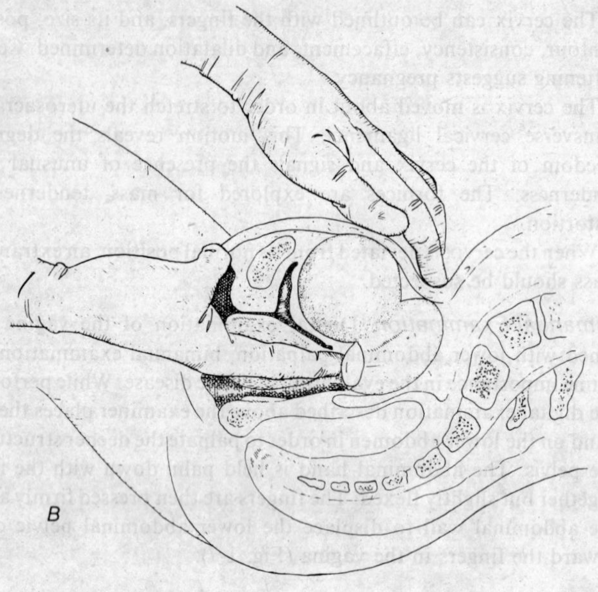

Figure 1-7 Continued. *B*, A leiomyoma of the uterus is palpated.

In order to evaluate the size, shape, mobility, consistency, and position of the uterus, the examiner should palpate and gently depress the uterine fundus with one hand while the vaginal fingers rest against the cervix. A normally free uterus can usually be brought well downward and forward by the abdominal hand. The pregnant uterus feels enlarged, and Hegar's sign (compressibility and softening of the lower uterine segment) may be evident. When the fundus cannot be palpated with the abdominal hand, the uterus usually is in a retroverted position. This may also be suspected when the cervix is displaced anteriorly behind the symphysis pubis.

For a diagram of uterine positions, see Figure 1-8.

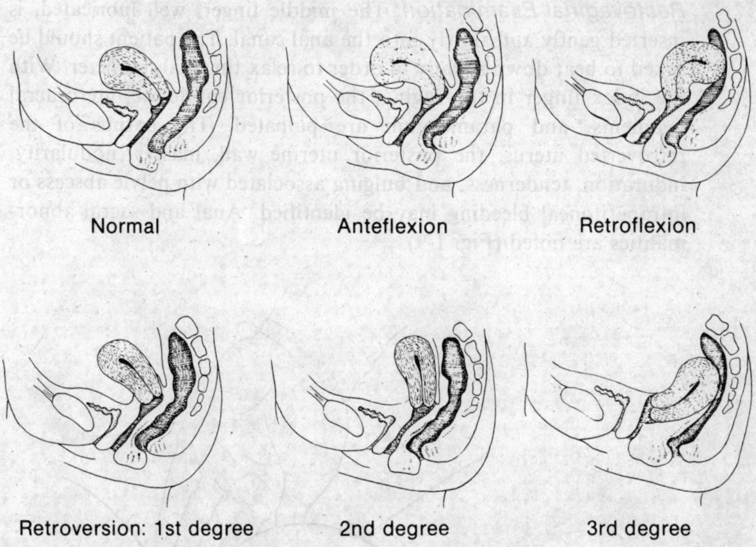

Figure 1-8. The positions of the uterus in sagittal section. (From Dunphy JE, Botsford TW: Physical Examination of the Surgical Patient. Philadelphia, W.B. Saunders Company, 1975.)

In order to palpate the adnexa, the vaginal examining fingers are placed into the lateral fornix. The abdominal examining hand is then swept downward over the fingers in the vagina in order to trap the ovary and tube between the two hands. Normally, the ovary lies just lateral to the uterus near its midportion. If the ovary and tube are not felt initially, they may be lying in the cul-de-sac or displaced into the space anterior to the uterus.

The normal ovary is slightly tender. This helps distinguish it from nontender masses such as fecal material within the bowel. The fallopian tube, however, is not ordinarily sensitive, and not palpable unless a pathologic condition is present.

Rectovaginal Examination: The middle finger, well lubricated, is inserted gently and slowly into the anal canal. The patient should be asked to bear down slightly in order to relax the anal sphincter. With the index finger in the vagina, the posterior cul-de-sac, uterosacral ligaments, and parametrium are palpated. The corpus of the retroverted uterus, the posterior uterine wall, masses, nodularity, induration, tenderness, and bulging associated with pelvic abscess or intraperitoneal bleeding may be identified. Anal and sacral abnormalities are noted (Fig. 1-9).

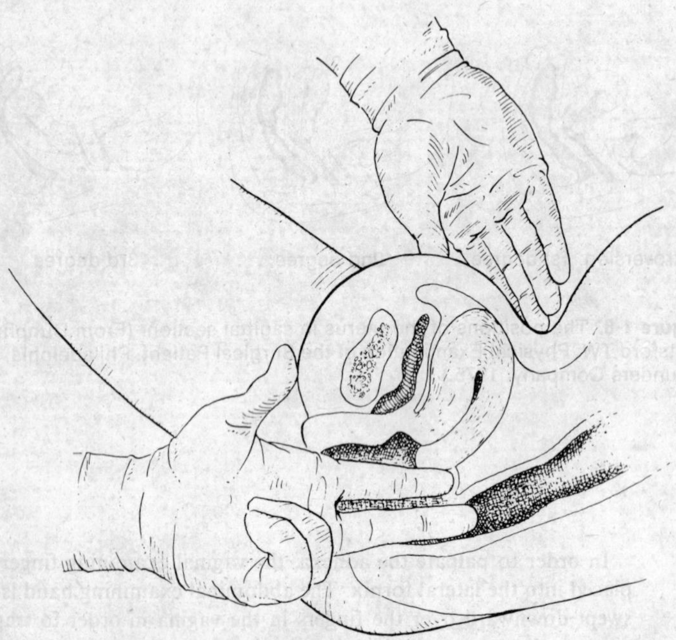

Figure 1-9. Bimanual rectovaginal examination. (From Dunphy JE, Botsford TW: Physical Examination of the Surgical Patient. Philadelphia, W.B. Saunders Company, 1975.)

Finally, reaching with the tips of both vaginal and rectal fingers as high as possible, the examiner palpates the lower abdomen bimanually.

During rectal examination attention is directed to hemorrhoids, fistulas, fissures, anorectal polyps and tumors, and condylomas. As the rectal finger is withdrawn the glove is inspected for blood or mucus.

Rectovaginal examination of children and older women—patients with a small vaginal introitus—is particularly valuable. In addition, rectovaginal examination may be more informative than the two-finger vaginal examination in patients with vaginal stricture, pelvic abscess, acute pelvic tenderness, or other disorders that interfere with vaginal examination.

LABORATORY TESTS

Although the choice of laboratory tests and supplementary procedures depends on the nature of the chief complaint and is usually part of the diagnostic plan, a *complete blood count with blood smear, urinalysis,* and *blood type and Rh* are three basic tests that provide crucial objective data for virtually every emergency gynecologic evaluation.

Complete Blood Count with Blood Smear: Hemoglobin or hematocrit determinations are essential for the evaluation of bleeding. Serial values are particularly helpful for assessment of concealed bleeding.

Elevation of the white blood count suggests systemic infection.

The blood smear provides a differential white cell count, details of red cell form and structure, and an estimate of the blood platelets. Leukocytosis with increased neutrophils and a shift to the left signifies systemic infection. Abnormal red cell form and structure suggest pre-existing anemia or an active hemolytic process. Deficient blood platelets may be the first clue to a coagulation disorder.

Interpretation of the blood count and blood smear is aided by comparison with previously known values for the individual patient.

Urinalysis is an essential aid in the diagnosis of a urinary tract pathologic condition. Protein, sugar, blood, or cells in the urine may indicate the disease entity responsible for the emergency problem.

Blood Type and Rh: Whenever there is any evidence of active bleeding, anemia, or hypovolemia, 10 ml of blood should be sent to the blood bank for type, Rh determination, and antibody screen. If blood replacement is anticipated, 2 to 4 units of whole blood or packed red cells should be cross-matched.

ASSESSMENT

DIFFERENTIAL DIAGNOSIS

Gynecologic evaluation aims to distinguish abnormalities of the reproductive tract from other pathologic processes. Synthesizing the subjective and objective data, the physician must consider all the diagnostic possibilities.

Often the findings are so specific that the diagnosis is obvious. For example, the patient with vaginal bleeding and placental tissue visible in the dilated cervical os obviously has an incomplete abortion.

Other times the diagnosis is obscure. Multiple diagnostic possibilities require additional laboratory tests and procedures for evaluation.

The differential diagnosis includes all the diagnostic possibilities that must be considered in order to prepare an appropriate therapeutic plan.

ETIOLOGIC FACTORS

Reproductive tract disorders may be caused by infection, neoplasms, pregnancy complications, or hormonal disturbances. In addition, metabolic abnormalities and psychologic and social factors, as well as prior medical or surgical problems, may affect the patient's resistance or susceptibility to a pathogenic stimulus.

Recognition of multiple factors contributing to specific problems provides the basis for a comprehensive therapeutic plan.

COMPLICATIONS AND ASSOCIATED PROBLEMS

When making an emergency evaluation one must always consider the possible complications as well as the associated problems that may contribute to the patient's disability.

SEVERITY OF DISEASE PROCESS

The necessity for hospitalization, as opposed to out-patient care, is based on the severity of the disease process and the potential for temporary or permanent disability.

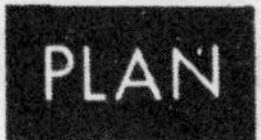

ADDITIONAL DIAGNOSTIC DATA

Laboratory Tests: Under specific circumstances one or more of the following supplementary laboratory tests may be helpful:

Pregnancy Test for Chorionic Gonadotropin (HCG): During the reproductive years, pregnancy complications are an important cause of emergency problems. Consequently, a pregnancy test for the presence of chorionic gonadotropin can be a valuable aid in the diagnosis of early pregnancy.

Erythrocyte Sedimentation Rate (ESR): Differentiation of acute from chronic pathologic processes may be aided by determination of the sedimentation rate. Acute exacerbations of chronic pelvic inflammatory disease tend to be associated with an elevated sedimentation rate, whereas patients with acute appendicitis or ectopic pregnancy usually have a normal sedimentation rate. From the third month of pregnancy to approximately three weeks after delivery the sedimentation rate is increased and rarely of diagnostic value.

Bacteriologic Culture and Gram Stain: Whenever bacterial infection is suspected, gram stain can be helpful. Visualization of gram-negative intracellular diplococci, for example, points to the diagnosis of gonorrhea. Bacteriologic cultures and antibiotic sensitivity studies are essential for the identification of specific organisms and knowledge of appropriate antibiotic sensitivities.

Specimens from an anaerobic site, such as an abscess cavity, or from the blood stream should be sent to the laboratory for both aerobic and anaerobic cultures, since anaerobic organisms are frequently responsible for gynecologic infections.

Cytologic Smear (Pap Smear): A cytologic smear from the cervix is always indicated when there is any suspicion of cervical malignancy. Cytologic smears may also be helpful with the diagnosis of herpes genitalis.

Serologic Test for Syphilis (VDRL): Although syphilis has become relatively uncommon, blood for a diagnostic serologic test is drawn routinely by many physicians. A serologic test for syphilis is always indicated for any victim of a sexual assault.

Other Blood Tests: Blood chemistries, electrolytes, and coagulation studies may be indicated, depending on the specific problem. Studies of arterial blood gases are helpful whenever there is any evidence of impaired ventilation or inadequate tissue perfusion.

Diagnostic Procedures:

X-rays: The decision to use x-rays for the diagnosis of gynecologic problems must always depend upon the condition of the individual patient. Whenever intrauterine pregnancy is suspected, x-rays should be avoided if possible. When they are essential, appropriate shielding is advisable.

Ultrasound B-Scan: Diagnostic ultrasound has become widely available and increasingly useful for the evaluation of various obstetric and gynecologic problems.

Culdocentesis is often indicated for the diagnosis of intraperitoneal bleeding or peritoneal infection. (See Culdocentesis, p. 772.)

MANAGEMENT

An effective therapeutic plan must consider the general goals of therapy, as well as the specific measures required to achieve those goals.

Medical Procedures: In many emergency situations therapy must be initiated even before a specific diagnosis is established. Airway patency must be assured for adequate ventilation. Intravenous fluids are initiated for circulatory support. A central venous line is valuable for monitoring central venous pressure and administering large volume infusions if necessary. Since impaired ventilation leads to hypoxemia, asphyxia, and brain damage, any airway obstruction must be relieved. If foreign material, blood, mucus, or vomitus is discovered in the mouth or oropharynx, suctioning should be performed immediately. The head should be tilted backward so that the jaw is pointing upward, thereby relieving obstruction in the airway by moving the base of the tongue away from the back of the throat.

Circulatory insufficiency may be caused by hypovolemia secondary to blood loss or by cardiac arrest. Victims of the latter require external cardiac massage in order to restore the circulation immediately. Since circulation without ventilation is useless, the treatment of circulatory arrest involves restoration of both ventilation and circulation. Hypovolemia is treated by the rapid administration of electrolyte solutions until blood is available.

Surgical Procedures: In the management of emergency gynecologic problems, curettage, colpotomy, laparoscopy, or exploratory laparotomy may be indicated. These procedures are usually performed in a hospital operating room. Curettage and procedures that require limited local anesthesia or no anesthesia, however, may be carried out in a properly equipped office or emergency room.

Preoperative Orders: The following orders are appropriate for virtually all patients prior to surgery:

1. A complete blood count is taken, and urinalysis is done.
2. The patient may have nothing to eat or drink orally.
3. Blood is sent to the blood bank for determination of type, Rh, and antibody screen. Cross-matched blood is prepared if transfusion is anticipated.
4. Perineal (or abdominal) preparation (shave) is done.
5. Preoperative medication is usually prescribed by the anesthesiologist. Often, meperidine, 50 to 75 mg I.M., or morphine, 6 to 10 mg subcut., is given for sedation to allay apprehension. If the patient is to receive a general anesthetic, 0.4 mg of atropine or scopolamine may be given to help lessen respiratory tract secretions and possibly minimize undesirable reflex activity in response to anesthesia and surgery.
6. Consent for the proposed procedure is obtained. (See Informed Consent, p. 52.)

PATIENT EDUCATION

Patient education is an essential aspect of health care. Since unspoken fears and attitudes toward sudden illness can influence symptoms as well as responses, the patient should be informed of diagnostic possibilities, procedures, and therapeutic measures. In addition, members of the immediate family should be advised of the doctor's assessment and recommendations. The information imparted to the patient is included in the medical record in order to assist others involved in the patient's care, as well as for future reference.

Patients should always be advised of the importance of follow-up care including cervicovaginal cytologic (Pap) smear at regular intervals.

If emergency surgery may result in future sterility, the patient should be provided appropriate counseling and emotional support.

2 PREGNANCY DIAGNOSIS

GENERAL CONSIDERATIONS

Often the diagnosis of pregnancy is obvious and the patient herself is aware of being pregnant even before she consults a physician. At other times, the diagnosis is ambiguous and difficult, requiring the most careful interpretation of subjective symptoms, objective findings, and laboratory tests.

For a summary of the following diagnostic features of pregnancy, see Table 2-1.

TABLE 2-1. A Summary of the Diagnostic Features of Pregnancy

First Trimester		
SUBJECTIVE	Amenorrhea	Presumptive
	Nausea	Presumptive
OBJECTIVE	Breast changes	Presumptive
	Chadwick's sign	Presumptive
	Cervical softening	Presumptive
	Hegar's sign	Probable
	Uterine enlargement and softening	Probable
	Positive HCG test	95 to 98 per cent certain
	Ultrasonic confirmation	Certain
Second Trimester		
SUBJECTIVE	Amenorrhea	Presumptive
	Abdominal enlargement	Presumptive
	Quickening	Presumptive
OBJECTIVE	Uterine contractions	Probable
	Fetal movements	Certain
	Fetal palpation	Certain
	Fetal heart tones	Certain
	X-ray of fetal skeleton	Certain

SUBJECTIVE DATA

CURRENT SYMPTOMS

Amenorrhea: The most reliable subjective symptom of pregnancy is the abrupt cessation of menstruation in a healthy woman who has previously menstruated regularly. Under these circumstances the absence of a second period provides an even stronger probability that the patient is pregnant.

Nausea (with or without vomiting): During the first trimester of pregnancy many women note gastric upset ranging from anorexia to nausea and even vomiting, which most often occur in the morning.

Urinary Frequency: During the first few months of pregnancy urinary frequency may be caused by pressure on the bladder from the enlarging uterus. This symptom frequently reappears near term.

Breast Fullness and Tenderness: In early pregnancy many women become aware of an increased vascularity and sensation of heaviness in the breasts. The nipple and surrounding area may appear to be more pigmented. As pregnancy progresses the breasts tend to increase in size and become nodular as a result of hypertrophy of the mammary alveoli. After the first few months a thick yellowish fluid, colostrum, may often be expressed from the breasts by gentle massage.

Fatigue and Lethargy: Although fatigue and lethargy are nonspecific symptoms, some women are able to self-diagnose pregnancy by these subjective sensations.

Abdominal Enlargement: Many patients become aware of abdominal enlargement after the third gestational month, when formerly well-fitting clothing begins to feel tight.

Fetal Movements: Women usually become aware of the fetal movements, or "quickening," between the sixteenth and eighteenth weeks of gestation.

OBJECTIVE DATA

PHYSICAL EXAMINATION

Breast Examination: During pregnancy the breasts increase in size and tend to become nodular. Delicate veins may be visible just beneath the skin. The nipples become larger and more deeply pigmented. The areolae are also more deeply pigmented and contain numerous small elevations representing hypertrophic sebaceous glands, the glands (follicles) of Montgomery.

Abdominal Examination: The uterus may be palpable through the abdominal wall by the twelfth week of gestation. At 16 weeks the fundus is usually palpable midway between the symphysis and the umbilicus.

As pregnancy progresses the height of the fundus provides an approximate estimate of the duration of pregnancy (Fig. 2-1). Between 20 and 22 weeks' gestation the fundus is palpable at the umbilicus. After this time the duration of the pregnancy in lunar months may be calculated by dividing the fundal height in centimeters by 3.5. The fundal height is measured with a centimeter tape from the symphysis pubis, following the contour of the abdominal wall. One hand is placed at the highest part of the fundus and held perpendicular to the long axis of the body while the tape is held against the middle finger by the thumb. The usual height of the uterus at term is 35 centimeters (McDonald's rule) (Fig. 2-2).

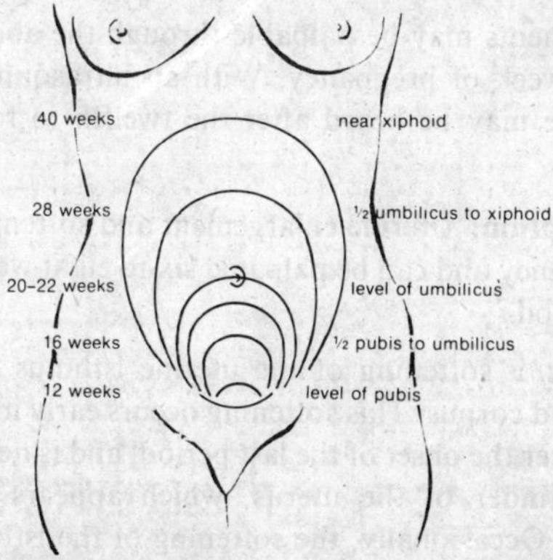

Figure 2-1. The relative level of the uterine fundus during pregnancy.

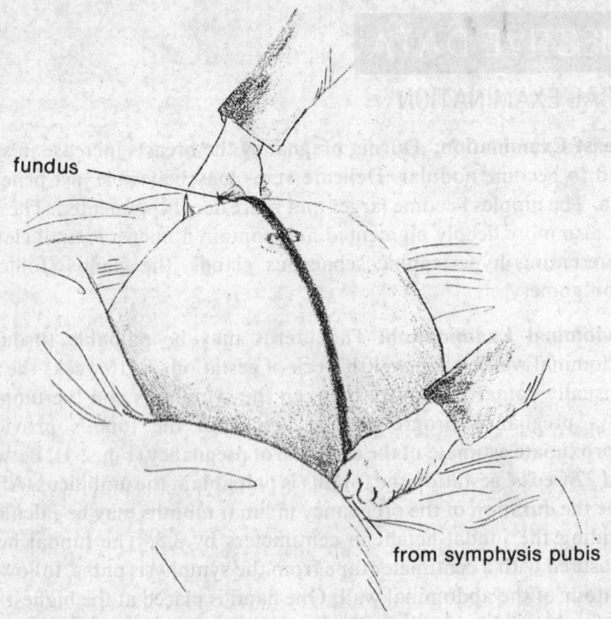

Figure 2-2. Measuring the length of the fetus by McDonald's rule.

Fetal movements may be palpable through the abdominal wall after the sixteenth week of pregnancy. With an ultrasound stethoscope the fetal heart rate may be heard after the twelfth to fourteenth week of pregnancy.

Pelvic Examination: Uterine enlargement and softening are the earliest signs of pregnancy and can be palpated six to eight weeks after the onset of the last period.

Hegar's sign is softening of the uterine isthmus at the junction of the cervix and corpus. This softening occurs early in pregnancy, about six weeks after the onset of the last period, and is notable as a contrast to the remainder of the uterus, which appears to have a firmer consistency. Occasionally, the softening of the isthmus is so marked that the cervix and corpus appear to be separate. (See Fig. 2-3.)

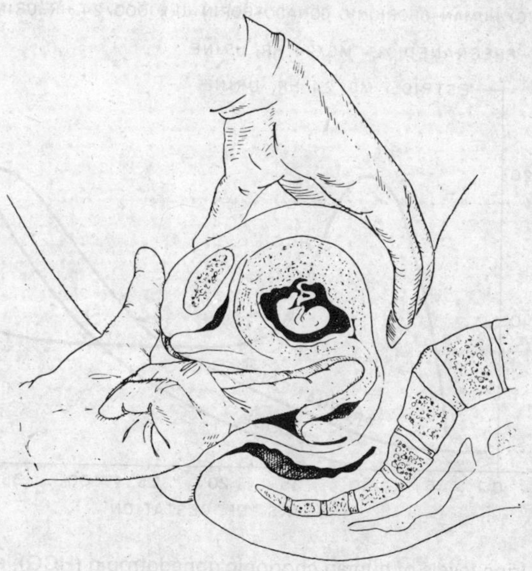

Figure 2-3. The bimanual method for detecting Hegar's sign in pregnancy.

Chadwick's sign is a bluish discoloration of the vagina, which may be noted on speculum examination.

LABORATORY TESTS

Chorionic Gonadotropin (HCG) in Maternal Urine (Fig. 2-4): Three types of tests are commonly used: latex-inhibition slide test, latex-agglutination slide test, and hemagglutination-inhibition tube test. The last is the most sensitive with minimal detectable levels of 750 to 1000 international units of HCG per liter of urine. Although the hemagglutination-inhibition test requires one or two hours' incubation, it usually becomes positive 36 days or more after the first day of the last menstrual period in approximately 95 per cent of intrauterine pregnancies. The more rapid slide tests tend to become positive three to five days later. With ectopic pregnancy, however, the level of HCG is often insufficient to give a positive test.

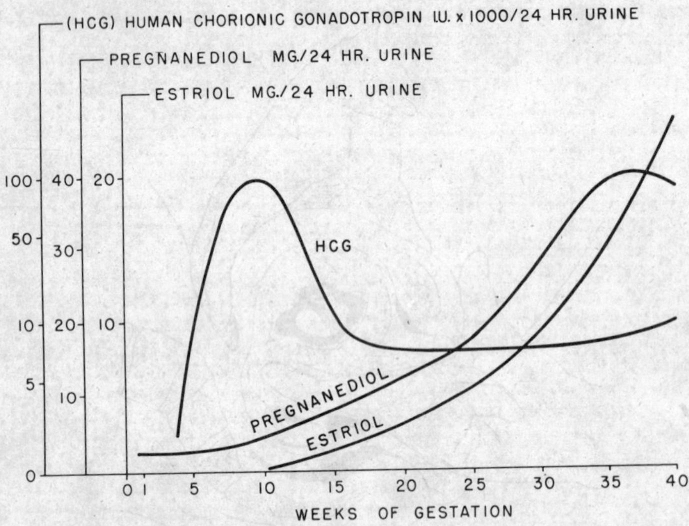

Figure 2-4. Urine levels of human chorionic gonadotropin (HCG), estriol, and pregnanediol during pregnancy. (From Davidsohn I, Henry JB: Clinical Diagnosis by Laboratory Methods. Philadelphia, W.B. Saunders Company, 1974.)

False positive pregnancy tests may be caused by the ingestion of drugs such as methadone, chlorpromazine, promethazine hydrochloride, haloperidol, and thioridazine hydrochloride. In addition, proteinuria in excess of 1 gm per 24 hours and grossly bloody urine are also associated with false positive tests.

False negative tests may occur when the urine specimen is of low specific gravity or the pregnancy test is performed too early in gestation. The stage of pregnancy has a marked influence on the incidence of false negatives even if a very sensitive assay is used. Between the seventh and thirteenth weeks following the last menstrual period even a relatively insensitive assay tends to be almost 100 per cent positive. The first voided morning urine is preferred, since this sample tends to be more concentrated than a random specimen.

The most specific test for chorionic gonadotropin assays the beta subunit and does not cross-react with luteinizing hormone (LH). With this test, pregnancy hormone can be demonstrated as early as one week prior to the time of the anticipated menses in a fertile cycle. Since this test is not readily available at the present time, however, it is used only for the follow-up care of patients with molar pregnancy.

DIAGNOSTIC PROCEDURES

Ultrasound B-Scan: Five weeks after the previous menstrual period, a normal intrauterine pregnancy can be demonstrated with the B-scan. A small white ring in the uterine fundus represents the gestational sac and can be observed between five and ten weeks of gestation. After the ninth week, the placenta can be demonstrated; by the fourteenth week the fetal head can usually be identified. Measurements of the biparietal diameter provide an estimate of gestational age.

Radiology: Radiologic identification of the fetal skeleton provides a positive diagnosis of pregnancy. However, possible radiation risks preclude the use of x-ray, whenever possible, during the early stages of pregnancy. Furthermore, the fetal skeleton usually cannot be visualized until 16 to 20 weeks of gestation.

3 EMERGENCY EVALUATION OF THE OBSTETRIC PATIENT

GENERAL CONSIDERATIONS

Emergency problems during pregnancy may be due to specific pregnancy complications or coexisting medical or surgical diseases. The fact that two lives are involved must always be considered in the formulation of diagnostic and therapeutic plans.

The patient's age and previous obstetric history provide important identifying information. The information necessary for the emergency evaluation of the obstetric patient is summarized in Table 3-1.

DEFINITIONS

Gravida—a woman who is pregnant.

Primigravida (G 1)—one pregnant for the first time.
Nulligravida (G 0)—one who has never been pregnant.
Multigravida—one who has been pregnant several times.
Gravidity—a pregnancy, regardless of its duration.

Para—the number of pregnancies that have continued to viability. For the purpose of defining parity, a multiple birth is a single parous experience.

Primipara (P 1)—a woman who has given birth one time to a viable infant, regardless of whether the child was living at birth and regardless of whether the birth was single or multiple.
Nullipara (P 0)—a woman who has never given birth to a viable infant.
Multipara—a woman who has given birth two or more times.

The past obstetric history may also be designated by a series of four numbers, for example, 5-3-1-4. The first digit refers to the number of full-term births; the second, to the number of premature births; the third, to the number

TABLE 3-1. Emergency Evaluation of the Obstetric Patient (Patient Known to be Pregnant)

Identification
- Name, age, gravida, para

Subjective Data
- Chief complaint
- Current symptoms
  - Last menstrual period (LMP) and Estimated date confinement (EDC)
  - Abdominal pain: Onset, nature
  - Vaginal bleeding: Quantity
  - Bag of waters: Intact; ruptured
  - Other: Convulsions, coma, dyspnea, fever, headache, nausea, vomiting, weight gain
- Prior history
  - Prenatal complications
  - Prior reproductive history
  - Prior medical and surgical history or hospitalizations

Objective Data
- Physical examination
  - General examination: Temperature, pulse, blood pressure, respiration, appearance, weight
  - Abdominal examination: Palpation for uterine size, contractions, fetal presentation; Auscultation for fetal heart sounds, bowel sounds
  - Vaginal speculum examination
  - Vaginal digital examination
- Laboratory tests
  - Complete blood count with blood smear
  - Urinalysis
  - Blood type and Rh
  - Serology (VDRL)

Assessment
- Diagnosis or differential diagnosis
- Etiologic or predisposing factors
- Complications or associated problems
- Severity of disease process

Plan
- Additional diagnostic data
- Management: Medical, obstetric, surgical
- Patient education

of abortions; and the fourth, to the number of living children. Gravida 9 Para 5-3-1-4 designates a woman who has been pregnant nine times, with five full-term births, three premature births, one abortion, and four living children.

SUBJECTIVE DATA

CURRENT SYMPTOMS

Last Menstrual Period: The dates of the last menstrual period (LMP) provide an approximate estimate of the date of confinement (EDC). On the average, a pregnancy is at term 40 weeks after the first day of the last menstrual period (LMP). When a problem arises prior to term, the gestational age provides an estimate of fetal size and probable viability.

Abdominal Pain: Uterine contractions account for most periodic, cramping abdominal pain during pregnancy. Prior to 20 weeks of pregnancy, painful uterine contractions usually signify abortion (threatened, inevitable, or incomplete). After the twentieth week of gestation, increasingly painful uterine contractions usually denote labor (premature or at-term).

Irregular, brief pains in the lower abdomen or groin tend to be symptomatic of threatened abortion or false labor. In contrast, the pain of inevitable abortion or true labor generally occurs at regular intervals and is felt in the abdomen and back. As labor proceeds, the interval between contractions decreases, whereas the duration and intensity of the contractions increase. When uterine contractions are palpated abdominally, the patient's perception of maximal pain coincides with the acme of the contraction. Progressive effacement and dilatation of the cervix confirm the progress of labor.

Pain that does not coincide with uterine contractions, particularly *steady* pain, may be due to a number of pathologic processes, both intrinsic and extrinsic to the reproductive tract. During the first trimester of pregnancy, ectopic pregnancy must always be considered. During the latter half of pregnancy, constant, persistent abdominal pain can be caused by premature placental separation (abruptio), uterine rupture, abdominal pregnancy, a twisted ovarian cyst, or a degenerative leiomyoma.

Accurate diagnosis of abdominal pain during pregnancy is critical, since initial symptoms of an acute surgical problem must be distinguished from infection or the "normal" discomfort of uterine muscular contraction and fetal activity.

Epigastric pain during the latter half of pregnancy is a potentially ominous symptom, since it may be associated with *severe preeclampsia.* **Determination of the patient's blood pressure is mandatory.**

Vaginal bleeding or spotting during pregnancy may come from the placenta, the genital tract, or the fetus. The quantity is significant, since profuse bleeding is a life-threatening emergency. (See Vaginal Bleeding, Late Pregnancy, p. 699.)

Bag of Waters (Intact or Ruptured): Every obstetric patient should be questioned concerning leakage of amniotic fluid. Most patients are aware of the exact time that membranes rupture and whether the rupture is associated with uterine contractions. Once the amniotic membranes have ruptured, the risk of intrauterine infection increases markedly. (See Premature Rupture of the Membranes, p. 562.)

Other Symptoms: In addition to the diseases specific to pregnancy, an obstetric patient may have the same medical or surgical disorders as her nonpregnant sister. Coexisting and coincidental medical and surgical problems must always be considered.

Convulsions or coma during the latter half of pregnancy is among the most serious obstetric emergencies. Although eclampsia must always be suspected when a previously healthy teenaged nullipara has a sudden convulsive seizure, other diagnostic possibilities must also be considered. (See Convulsive Seizures in Pregnancy, p. 268 and Coma in Pregnancy, p. 234.)

Dyspnea during pregnancy may be an early symptom of cardiac failure, severe anemia, or pulmonary disease. (See Dyspnea during Pregnancy, p. 298.)

Fever is another common emergency symptom and may represent infection in any part of the body. Since the urinary tract is the most common site of bacterial infection during pregnancy, urinalysis is essential and often diagnostic. When the urine is negative, a careful search must be made for other potential sites of infection.

Headache should always be considered a *potential* symptom of severe preeclampsia and even a forerunner of an eclamptic convulsion. For this reason every patient with a severe headache *must* have a blood pressure determination and urinalysis for protein.

Visual Disturbances: Blurred vision or double vision may be caused by retinal edema associated with severe preeclampsia.

Weight Gain: Any sudden increase in body weight almost invariably signifies fluid retention. In and of itself the symptom may not be serious. When associated with hypertension and proteinuria, however, it can denote preeclampsia.

Nausea and vomiting are so common during the first trimester of pregnancy that these symptoms (particularly "morning sickness") are often considered an aid in the diagnosis of early pregnancy. Nevertheless, pathologic causes (pyelonephritis, pancreatitis, intestinal obstruction, and so forth) must be considered when vomiting is severe and persistent or develops suddenly during the second or third trimester.

PRIOR HISTORY

Prenatal complications (heart disease, diabetes, urinary tract infections, and so forth) often explain the nature of emergency symptoms.

Reproductive history may provide clues to the diagnosis of current problems. A patient with a history of multiple abortions may be aborting again; a patient with a history of premature placental separation may be having a recurrence of the same pathologic condition. The patient with a history of previous cesarean section is at greater risk of uterine rupture.

Medical and Surgical History:

Hospitalizations: Details of a patient's previous medical and surgical history can be extremely helpful when the diagnosis is obscure. Important questions to be asked include the following: Has the patient ever had diabetes, cardiac disease, hypertension, bleeding disorders, and so forth? Is the patient taking any drugs or medications currently? Is she allergic to any medicines? Is there a history of previous appendectomy or other surgery? (Although intestinal obstruction during pregnancy is rare, the possibility must be considered when a patient with a previous abdominal scar suddenly experiences distention and abdominal pain.)

Since most serious illnesses will have required prior hospital care, the patient should always be questioned concerning previous hospitalizations.

OBJECTIVE DATA

PHYSICAL EXAMINATION

General Examination:

Temperature: The basal body temperature during the first half of pregnancy is essentially the same as during the luteal phase of the menstrual cycle.

Pulse: The resting pulse rate typically increases about 10 to 15 beats per minute during pregnancy.

Blood Pressure: Arterial blood pressure decreases somewhat during midpregnancy only to return to the original level during the third trimester. Any rise of 30 mm systolic or 15 mm diastolic under basal conditions is indicative of pregnancy-induced hypertension.

Respiration: The respiratory rate is increased only slightly by pregnancy. However, the tidal volume, minute ventilatory volume, and minute oxygen uptake increase appreciably as pregnancy advances. An increased awareness of breathing is common during pregnancy. The increased tidal volume normally lowers the blood pCO_2 slightly, causing mild respiratory alkalosis, which is well compensated.

Weight: Any sudden increase in body weight usually signifies fluid retention. Puffiness of the face and tightness of finger rings indicate facial and digital edema. Blood pressure determination and urinalysis are mandatory to evaluate the possibility of preeclampsia.

Abdominal Examination:

Palpation: By the third gestational month the uterus usually can be felt through the abdominal wall. By 20 to 22 weeks the fundus is palpable at the umbilicus, and as pregnancy progresses the fundal height increases. (See Pregnancy Diagnosis, p. 29.)

Emergency evaluation includes a measurement of fundal height as an estimate of gestational age. Palpation of the uterus determines the resting tone and the presence of uterine contractions. If contractions are present, their frequency and intensity should be determined.

Uterine palpation assesses fetal size and presentation and the presence of fetal movements. The following are questions to be answered through uterine palpation: Is the presenting part cephalic or breech? Is the fetal presentation longitudinal, oblique, or transverse? Is the presenting part engaged in the pelvic brim? Is multiple pregnancy a possibility?

Auscultation: With an ultrasound stethoscope fetal heart tones can be detected as early as the twelfth to fourteenth week of gestation. Electronic amplification facilitates auscultation of the fetal heart rate at any gestational age.

Abdominal auscultation may detect the uterine souffle and evaluate maternal bowel sounds.

Pelvic Examination:

Speculum Examination: Whenever the patient reports a vaginal discharge, ruptured bag of water, leakage of amniotic fluid, or slight bleeding, the vagina and cervix are usually visualized with a speculum. Nitrazine paper is commonly used to determine the pH of the vaginal fluid. Amniotic fluid is alkaline (pH 7.0 to 7.5), whereas vaginal secretions are usually acid (pH 4.5 to 5.5). If the nitrazine test paper turns deep blue (pH 7.5), ruptured membranes are likely. However, if the pH remains 6.0 or less, the diagnosis of ruptured membranes is virtually excluded.

In cases of slight bleeding, the speculum examination may reveal the bleeding site. If fetal bleeding is suspected, the blood should be sent to the clinical laboratory for a determination of fetal hemoglobin.

Digital Examination: Any patient with *vaginal bleeding* during the latter half of pregnancy should never have a vaginal examination unless blood is ready for transfusion and the patient is in an operating room prepared for immediate cesarean section. Even the gentlest examination could cause torrential hemorrhage from a placenta previa. (See Placenta Previa, p. 510.)

Otherwise, vaginal examination is essential for evaluation of the cervix (consistency, dilatation, effacement, position) and the fetal presenting part, including the station of the presenting part in relation to the ischial spines.

During early pregnancy, bimanual examination provides an assessment of uterine size, position, and tenderness.

If the patient is in active labor, vaginal examination includes an assessment of the pelvic architecture: the diagonal conjugate, ischial spines, pelvic sidewalls, sacral curve, intertuberous diameter, and subpubic angle.

The *diagonal conjugate*—the distance from the lower margin of the symphysis pubis to the sacral promontory—provides an estimate of the *pelvic inlet.* When two fingers are inserted into the vagina, the anterior surface of the sacrum can be palpated. In normal pelves, only the last three sacral vertebrae can be felt without indenting the perineum; usually the sacral promontory cannot be reached. In the case of a contracted pelvis, the entire anterior surface of the sacrum may be palpated. When the sacral promontory is reached by the tip of the middle finger, the vaginal hand is elevated and the point where the index finger touches the symphysis pubis is noted. After the hand is withdrawn, the distance between the latter point and the tip of the middle finger is measured, determining the diagonal conjugate. Pelvic inlet contracture is unlikely whenever the diagonal conjugate is greater than 11.5 cm.

For evaluation of the midpelvis, the distance between the ischial spines—the interspinous diameter—is estimated. A measurement of 10 cm or more usually indicates ample room for the average baby.

The *sacral contour* is also important. A sacrum with a gently curving shape is usual and provides maximal pelvic room. A flat sacrum or one that juts anteriorly diminishes the pelvic capacity and is frequently associated with abnormal labor.

The *pelvic outlet* is evaluated by estimating the *subpubic angle* and measuring the *intertuberous diameter*. The shape of the pubic arch is determined by external palpation of the inferior rami of the pubis, with both thumbs placed along these structures and pointed toward the symphysis. The intertuberous diameter is measured with an instrument or by apposing the clenched fist to the perineum in order to obtain an estimate of the diameter. The mobility of the coccyx can be determined best by rectal examination. An adequate outlet is characterized by a wide, well-rounded subpubic arch, widely spaced ischial tuberosities (9 cm or more), and a mobile coccyx.

Four basic pelvic types have been described on the basis of the pelvic inlet. The *gynecoid* pelvis has a rounded or oval shape, with a well-rounded anterior and posterior segment. It represents the normal female pelvis and is found in 45 per cent of women. The *android* pelvis is wedge- or heart-shaped, with the transverse diameter of the inlet approximately equal to the anteroposterior diameter, but with the widest transverse diameter closer to the sacrum. The posterior segment of the android pelvis is short and flattened, and the anterior segment is narrowed. This type of pelvis is found in approximately 15 per cent of women. The *anthropoid* pelvis has an elongated anteroposterior diameter. It is found in approximately 35 per cent of women. The *platypelloid* pelvis has marked flattening of the anteroposterior dimension, with relative widening of the transverse. It is the least common, occurring in less than 5 per cent of women.

LABORATORY TESTS

The following tests provide basic essential objective data that should be known about every obstetric patient:

Complete Blood Count with Blood Smear: The hemoglobin and hematocrit determinations provide evidence of anemia, hypovolemia, and hemoconcentration. The white count and differential count are of value when infection is suspected.

Urinalysis: Tests for sugar and albumin are performed on every patient. Additional tests may be required, depending on the patient's symptoms.

Blood Type and Rh: This information is crucial whenever a patient is bleeding actively. In addition, Rh-negative unsensitized patients require Rh-immune globulin prophylaxis whenever there is any possibility that fetal Rh-positive cells may have entered the maternal circulation. (See Rh Immune Globulin Prophylaxis, p. 853.)

If there is any possibility that blood transfusion will be required, 10 ml of blood are sent to the blood bank to be cross-matched.

Serologic Test for Syphilis (VDRL): This test is performed routinely on all pregnant patients and may not be necessary at the time of an emergency visit as long as the results of a prior prenatal determination are available.

ASSESSMENT

DIAGNOSIS OR DIFFERENTIAL DIAGNOSIS

The subjective and objective data provide the basis for emergency diagnosis or differential diagnosis:

Obstetric Problems: Is the patient in labor? Is there an obstetric complication—preeclampsia, placenta previa, placental separation, or other?

Preexisting Medical Conditions Aggravated by Pregnancy: Is there evidence of diabetes, cardiac disease, or other medical problems?

Coexisting Medical or Surgical Problems: Has the patient suffered accidental trauma? Does the patient have acute appendicitis?

ETIOLOGIC OR PREDISPOSING FACTORS

Formulation of an optimal diagnostic and therapeutic plan must take into consideration all the possible etiologic and predisposing factors.

COMPLICATIONS OR ASSOCIATED PROBLEMS

Since every emergency problem can affect both the mother and the fetus, the possibilities for future complications in both mother and child must be considered when management plans are formulated.

SEVERITY OF PROBLEM

The assessment of severity determines the need for hospitalization. Patients with late-pregnancy bleeding, hypertensive disease, premature labor, and so forth should be hospitalized for evaluation and management.

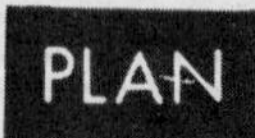

ADDITIONAL DIAGNOSTIC DATA

Laboratory Tests: Single laboratory values during pregnancy are often ambiguous. Consequently, laboratory tests are most helpful when serial determinations are available. A rising white blood cell count or an increasing shift to the left of the neutrophil count is always more meaningful than any single value.

Diagnostic Procedures:

X-ray: During the first half of pregnancy, direct pelvic radiation should be avoided unless essential for the mother's safety. During the second half of pregnancy, x-ray should also be limited. Whenever possible, the pelvis and lower abdomen are shielded from accidental exposure. X-ray pelvimetry may be indicated at the time of labor if there is a question of fetopelvic disproportion.

Ultrasound B-Scan: Sonography has recently become more widely available and is often a valuable diagnostic alternative to x-ray.

MANAGEMENT

During the latter half of pregnancy, all medical, surgical, and obstetric decisions must encompass the two lives involved: mother and fetus. Although specific therapy depends on the particular problem, a clear airway and an effective circulating blood volume are always essential.

Airway: Whenever there is any evidence of respiratory distress, an adequate airway and supplemental oxygen are essential in order to minimize the maternal and fetal risk of anoxia. The airway must be cleared of mucus and the patient positioned to avoid aspiration of vomitus.

Blood Volume: Whenever there is any evidence of hypovolemia, intravenous fluids are initiated immediately. The choice of fluid depends on the specific problem. Patients with active bleeding usually receive 5 per cent dextrose in lactated Ringer's solution.

PATIENT EDUCATION

Education for childbirth is an essential part of obstetric care. Emergency problems, however, may develop before the patient has completed her educational program and suddenly interfere with expectations for a natural, normal, uneventful labor and delivery. For optimal maternal and fetal well-being, the patient should understand the nature of the emergency problem and the reasons for the physician's diagnostic and therapeutic plans. This information should also become part of the patient's medical record.

If the immediate problem is not serious and does not require hospitalization, the patient should be instructed to return if symptoms progress or if any of the following occur or recur: vaginal bleeding, swelling of face or fingers, severe or continuous headache, severe dizziness, visual disturbances, abdominal pain, persistent vomiting, chills or fever, dysuria, or fluid leaking from the vagina.

4 DEFINED DATA BASE

In an emergency situation, it is rarely possible to obtain complete medical data. However, to provide comprehensive health care, additional data should be gathered at the earliest feasible opportunity. In order to identify *all* significant health problems — including those of medical, social, and psychologic origin — a defined data base is recorded. The data base includes the patient's chief complaint, present illness, and past history; a symptom review; a profile of how she spends her day and related social data; the physical examination; and laboratory tests.

A most important aspect of the problem-oriented record is the problem list, which is usually placed on the front of the chart. This master problem list codifies the patient's record and is a capsule summary of the patient's health status. The list contains the date of onset, active problems, inactive or resolved problems, and the date resolved.

Each problem is stated precisely at the level at which it is understood from the data at hand. For example, initially only an abnormal symptom may be known (postpartum hemorrhage or abdominal pain). This symptom is then recorded as the active problem. When additional data has indicated a physiologic mechanism or a definite diagnosis, the problem list is updated (for example, "postpartum hemorrhage → retained placental tissue".

The content of a defined data base, slightly modified from one prepared by the American College of Obstetricians and Gynecologists, is outlined in Table 4-1.

TABLE 4-1. The Content of a Defined Data Base

Identification

Name (last, first, maiden), address, age, phone number, religion, occupation, referring physician, primary physician, social history (married, separated, divorced, single, widowed, sexual partner)

Present Illness

Chief complaint — Onset, duration of symptoms, associated phenomena, phenomena that worsen, phenomena that relieve, modification by treatment

Health and Social History

Operations — Date, type, diagnosis, hospital

Hospitalizations — Date, type of illness

Pregnancies — Number, dates, full-term, premature, abortions, living children, infants' weights and sexes, maternal-fetal complications

Drug reactions and current medications

Immunizations — Polio, rubella, tetanus, small pox

Patient profile — Living situation (alone, with parents, with spouse, with friend, other; change in marital status), children (problems with drugs, school behavior, sex, recurrent illness), other family problems

Present means of support — Self, spouse, part-time work, pension, savings, welfare, other

Level of education

Level of satisfaction — With family, with occupation, with health care system

Family history — Number of siblings, health of parents and siblings

A list of current symptoms, past history, and indications of potential problems that may be included in the data base follows:

Gynecologic (Genital System)

Current — Menstrual abnormalities, dysmenorrhea, discharge, itching, dissatisfaction with sexual activity, dyspareunia, pelvic pain, protrusion, discharge from breasts, lumps or pain in breasts

Past — Menses (onset, interval, duration, last menstrual period), contraception, venereal disease, cytologic abnormalities, breasts (lactation)

Potential — Family history of cancer of uterus or breast or other cancer

Urinary

Current — Dysuria, urgency, incontinence, frequency, nocturia

Past — Renal disease, recurrent urinary infection, hematuria

Potential — Family history of polycystic disease

Endocrine

Current — Weight gain, weight loss, abnormal hair growth

Past — Thyroid disorder, diabetes mellitus

Potential — Exposure to radioactive material, family history of diabetes mellitus or hirsutism

Gastrointestinal

Current — Abdominal pain, melena, nausea, vomiting, diarrhea, changes in bowel habits

Past — Ulcer, gallbladder disease, jaundice or other liver diseases, diverticulosis, diverticulitis, colitis

Potential — Family history of cancer, rectal polyps

Hematopoietic

Current — Ecchymosis, abnormal bleeding, enlarged lymph nodes, B_{12} liver shots

Past — Blood transfusions, anemia, bleeding disorders

Potential — Family history of pernicious anemia, sickle cell disease, hemophilia

Cardiovascular

Current — Chest pain, dyspnea, edema (feet and ankles), varicose veins, leg ulcer

Past — Rheumatic fever or other heart disease, hypertension, phlebitis, embolic disease

Potential — Family history of hypertension or heart attack, limited physical activity, cigarette smoking, mental tension, high cholesterol

Mouth-Throat-Larynx

Current — Hoarseness, sore mouth or tongue, lump in neck

Past — Recurrent pharyngitis

Potential — Heavy smoking

Respiratory

Current — Chronic cough, hemoptysis, dyspnea

Past — Tuberculosis, heavy smoking, asthma

Potential — Smoking, family history of cystic fibrosis

Neurologic

Current — Headache, dizzy spells, drugs for seizures

Past — Seizures, paralysis, nervousness

Potential — Family history of Huntington's chorea

Psychiatric

Current — Anxiety, depression, difficulty in sleeping, weeping, suicidal thoughts, overuse of alcohol or other drugs

Past — Nervous breakdown, attempted suicide, psychiatric treatment

Potential — Drug abuse, family history of alcohol problem, suicide, or mental problems

Musculoskeletal

Current — Joint pain, stiff neck, backache

Past — Gout or other disease, injuries

Potential — Family history of dystrophy or arthritis

INITIAL PHYSICAL EXAMINATION

Information gained from physical examination of the following should be included in the defined data base: general appearance, body type, height, weight, blood pressure, eyes, ears, throat, skin, thyroid, lymph nodes, heart, lungs, breasts, abdomen, vulva, urethra, perineum, vagina (lesions, support, discharge), cervix (position, erosion, ulcers, lacerations), uterus (size, shape, position, mobility), adnexa (position, mass, tenderness), parametria, cul-de-sac, anorectal area, and extremities.*

INITIAL LABORATORY TESTS

A cervicovaginal cytologic test, a urinalysis (for protein and sugar), a hematocrit or hemoglobin test, and a serologic test for syphilis should be performed and their results recorded in the data base.†

---

*American College of Obstetricians and Gynecologists: Standards for Obstetric-Gynecologic Services, 1974.

†Ibid.

5 INFORMED CONSENT

Informed consent means that a patient agrees or consents to a specific diagnostic or therapeutic procedure after being informed of the benefits and risks of that specific procedure as well as possible diagnostic or therapeutic alternatives. It is becoming more and more generally accepted that before consenting to any procedure a patient is entitled to accurate and detailed information regarding

1. the projected operation, diagnostic procedure, or therapy;
2. recognized risks and possible complications and their effects; and
3. the available alternative methods of treatment.

Furthermore, this information must be described in lay terms so that the patient understands the nature of what is being proposed.

In the Cobbs versus Grant decision the California Supreme Court adopted the following four basic principles:

1. Patients are generally persons unlearned in the medical sciences.
2. An adult of sound mind has the right to determine whether to submit to lawful medical treatment.
3. The patient's consent to treatment, to be legally effective, must be an informed consent.
4. The patient, being unlearned in medical sciences, has dependence upon and trust in his or her physician for the information upon which he or she relies during the decision process. This raises an obligation for the physician that transcends the marketplace.

In California and many other states the courts have stated that it is the duty of a physician or surgeon to disclose to the patient all relevant information that will enable the patient to make an informed decision regarding the proposed operation or treatment.

There is no duty to discuss minor risks inherent in common procedures when such procedures very seldom result in serious ill effects. However, when a procedure inherently involves a known risk of death or serious bodily harm, it is the physician's or surgeon's duty to disclose to the patient the possibility of such outcome and to explain in lay terms the complications that might occur. The physician or surgeon must also disclose such additional information as a skilled practitioner of good standing would provide under the same or similar circumstances.

There is no duty to disclose risks when the patient requests that she not be so informed nor when the procedure is simple and the danger remote and commonly understood to be remote.

Also, a physician or surgeon has no duty of disclosure beyond that required of physicians or surgeons of good standing in the same or similar locality as long as the physician relies upon facts that would demonstrate to a reasonable person that the disclosure would so seriously upset the patient that the patient would not have been able to weigh rationally the risks of refusing to undergo the recommended treatment or operation.

Notwithstanding the patient's consent to a proposed treatment or operation, failure of the physician or surgeon to inform the patient as described before obtaining the consent is considered negligence and may render the physician or surgeon subject to liability for any injury resulting from the procedure if a reasonably prudent person in the patient's position would not have consented to the procedure if she had been adequately informed of all the significant perils.

Under emergency circumstances, a woman may not be able to weigh and evaluate the hoped-for benefits versus the possible hazards. The physician must evaluate the mental capacity of the patient, particularly her ability to understand sufficient information to give her consent. Under certain emergency situations when it is physically impractical or impossible for the patient to express her consent, the law implies that she has consented. Under other emergency situations the physician or surgeon may have to modify the extent of disclosure in accordance with the circumstances, keeping in mind the legal concept that the patient has the right of self-determination and that the courts may decide what is reasonable disclosure under a given set of circumstances. If the patient alleges that she was not given sufficient information for her to give her informed consent to a specific procedure, a court could require the patient to prove that a reasonable person would have refused treatment if the essential information had been provided. Under this rule, a patient is not going to make a convincing case in the face of strong medical necessity for the treatment given if she merely testifies that she would not have consented had she known certain facts.

Women in the reproductive age are *particularly* concerned with the risk of death or bodily harm, problems of recuperation, and future fertility. Under all but the most unusual circumstances these subjects should be discussed with the patient or her closest relative. If the patient on her own initiative informs the physician that she does not want to be informed of the details of an operation or its risks, the physician's duty to inform ceases as of that point. It is imperative, however, that the patient's decision be made freely and not as a result of any intimidation on the part of the physician.

Unless the patient specifically requests *not* to hear about any details of the proposed operation or its risks, and as long as the patient's condition permits the time required to discuss the proposed surgery, the following subjects should be discussed before the patient signs her name to the form authorizing surgery:

1. Infection: Any surgical procedure may be complicated by the development of a postoperative bacterial infection. In most instances, the natural defense mechanisms of the body heal the affected area without difficulty. Under certain circumstances, however, antibiotic medicines may be required, and at times, additional surgical procedures may be necessary.
2. Hemorrhage: Bleeding may occur with any surgical procedure. This is usually easily controlled. At times, however, blood transfusions may be required to replace excessive blood loss. Blood transfusions entail a certain risk of transfusion reactions, particularly affecting the liver or kidney. There is no way to completely predict the undesired reaction. There are also instances when excessive bleeding occurs after the original operation is completed, and additional surgery may be required to control delayed bleeding.
3. Drug reactions: Unexpected allergies or various adverse reactions may occur in response to specific medications. It is particularly important to discuss any past history of drug sensitivities or allergic reactions.
4. Anesthesia reactions: There may be unusual or expected responses to the gases, drugs, or methods used that can lead to difficulties with lung, heart, or nerve function.
5. Blood vessel inflammation and clotting: This is an uncommon complication of surgery but a possible one. A blood clot may form in the leg or pelvic vein and then move to the lung. Most of the time this complication can be treated with medication, but there is always the rare possibility of a fatal reaction.
6. Injury to other organs: Since other organs may be close to the area of surgery, unavoidable injuries, particularly to the intestinal tract, may occur.

7. Other concerns: The surgery's effect on future childbearing and sexual performance and the patient's psychologic feelings may also require discussion.

In summary, whenever the patient's condition permits, the physician should provide

1. a fair explanation of the management plan to be followed;
2. a description of the attendant discomforts and risks, including all major life-threatening risks and all common minor risks;
3. a description of the benefits to be expected;
4. an explanation of appropriate alternative treatment plans;
5. an offer to answer any questions concerning the proposed treatment plan.

Any physician who undertakes a patient's medical care unavoidably assumes certain legal risks. Physicians may be held liable for an injury to the patient for any one or more of many different reasons. The legal risk arising from lack of "informed consent" is only one of these reasons. No physician can eliminate all legal risks; at most, these risks can be minimized by the exercise of professional judgment and discretion.

For any proposed procedure, the individual physician knows the medical risks and is best able to judge the seriousness of the possible injuries. In addition, the physician must take into consideration the individual characteristics of the patient and the circumstances surrounding the need for treatment. With this knowledge, the physician must decide the appropriate amount of information that should be discussed with the patient or her family or both prior to the proposed procedure. Ultimately, however, the physician assumes the legal risk for the occurrence of any serious injury about which the patient was not forewarned.

EMERGENCY CONSENT PROCEDURE

The treatment of a patient under emergency conditions without a written consent is authorized by law under the doctrine of implied consent. This is based on the theory that if the patient were able or his personal representative were present, such consent would be given.

The following guidelines may help define the necessity for emergency consent:

1. The treatment should be immediately required and necessary to prevent deterioration or aggravation of the patient's condition. This may be a

Text continued on page 62

AUTHORIZATION FOR AND CONSENT TO SURGERY OR SPECIAL DIAGNOSTIC OR THERAPEUTIC PROCEDURES

1. I hereby authorize and direct the physicians and surgeons of ____________ Medical Center to perform the following operation(s) or special diagnostic and therapeutic procedure(s) upon me and to provide such additional services for me as he or they may deem reasonable and necessary, including, but not limited to, the administration and maintenance of the anesthesia and the performance of services involving pathology and radiology, and I consent thereto.

____

____

Dr. ____________ has explained to me that these surgical operation(s) and special diagnostic and therapeutic procedure(s) all may involve calculated risks of complications, injury, or even death, from both known and unknown causes and no warranty or guarantee has been made as to result or cure. I recognize that I have a right to be informed of the nature and purpose of the operation(s) or procedure(s), the risks of complications, and the alternative methods of treatment, if applicable. Further, I recognize that this form is not intended to be a substitute for the explanations of the nature and purpose of the operation(s) or procedure(s), the risks of complications, and the alternative methods of treatment, if applicable, which are to be provided by the physician mentioned above.

I have been told all I wish to know and consent to the performance of the above stated operation(s) or special diagnostic and therapeutic procedure(s) by Dr.(s) ____________ or his designee, and those under his immediate responsibility and supervision.

2. I hereby authorize the hospital pathologist to use his discretion in the disposal of any tissue or severed member removed in surgery, except ____________

____

Date: ____________ ____________________
Patient

Time: ____________ a.m. p.m ____________________
Witness (Signature of responsible family member or nurse)

If patient is a minor, or unable to sign, complete the following:

Patient is a minor, or is unable to sign because ____________________

____

Date: ____________ ____________________
Relationship

Time: ____________ a.m. p.m. ____________________
Witness

AUTHORIZATION FOR AND CONSENT TO SURGERY OR SPECIAL DIAGNOSTIC OR THERAPEUTIC PROCEDURES (TEACHING HOSPITALS)

1. I hereby authorize and direct the physicians and surgeons of __________ Hospital to perform the following operation or special diagnostic and therapeutic procedures upon me and to do any other diagnostic and therapeutic procedure that their judgment may dictate to be advisable for my well being:

____

____

____

Doctor __________ has explained to me that these surgical operations and special diagnostic and therapeutic procedures all may involve calculated risks of complications, injury or even death, from both known and unknown causes and no warranty or guarantee has been made as to result or cure. I recognize that I have a right to be informed of the nature and purpose of the operation or procedures, the risks of complications, and the alternative methods of treatment, if applicable. Further, I recognize that this form is not intended to be a substitute for the explanations of the nature and purpose of the operation or procedures, the risks of complications, and the alternative methods of treatment, if applicable, which are to be provided by the physician mentioned above. I understand and consent to the performance of the above stated operation or special diagnostic and therapeutic procedures by Doctor(s) __________,[1] or his designee,[2] and those under his immediate responsibility and supervision.

2. I hereby authorize and direct the physicians and surgeons of __________ Hospital to provide such additional services for me as he or they may deem reasonable and necessary, including, but not limited to, the administration and maintenance of the anesthesia and the performance of services involving pathology and radiology, and I consent thereto.

3. I hereby authorize the hospital pathologist to use his discretion in the disposal of any severed tissue or member removed in surgery, except __________

____

Witness __________ Signed __________

Date: __________ Time: __________ a.m. p.m. __________

(If the patient is a minor, or unable to sign, complete the following)

Patient is a minor, or unable to sign because __________

I hereby consent to the above for my __________

Witness __________ Signed __________

Date __________ __________

Relationship

Time: __________ a.m. p.m. __________

* * * * * * * * * *

1. If name of physician is added after patient signs under paragraph 3, the patient should at that time date and sign the following:

Date: __________ Signed: __________

2. It is understood and agreed by the hospital, physician and patient that the physician named in this form will perform the operation or special diagnostic and therapeutic procedures indicated unless unforeseen events render it necessary for such physician to designate that another physician perform such procedures. In this event, I expressly consent to the performance of the operation or special diagnostic and therapeutic procedures by the substitute physician(s).

AUTHORIZATION FOR AND CONSENT TO SURGERY OR SPECIAL DIAGNOSTIC OR THERAPEUTIC PROCEDURES (NONTEACHING HOSPITALS)

To ______________________
Name of Patient

Your admitting physician is ______________________, M.D.

Your surgeon is ______________________, M.D.

1. The hospital maintains personnel and facilities to assist your physicians and surgeons in their performance of various surgical operations and other special diagnostic and therapeutic procedures. These surgical operations and special diagnostic and therapeutic procedures all may involve calculated risks of complications, injury or even death, from both known and unknown causes and no warranty or guarantee has been made as to result or cure. Except in a case of emergency or exceptional circumstances, these operations and procedures are therefore not performed upon patients unless and until the patient has had an opportunity to discuss them with his physician. Each patient has the right to consent to or refuse any proposed operation or special procedure (based upon the description or explanation received).

2. Your physicians and surgeons have determined that the operations or special procedures listed below may be beneficial in the diagnosis or treatment of your condition. Upon your authorization and consent, such operations or special procedures will be performed for you by your physicians and surgeons and/or by other physicians and surgeons selected by them. The persons in attendance for the purpose of administering anesthesia or performing other specialized professional services, such as radiology, pathology and the like, are not the agents, servants or employees of the hospital or your physician or surgeon, but are independent contractors performing specialized services on your behalf and, as such, are your agents, servants or employees. Any tissue or member severed in any operation will be disposed of in the discretion of the pathologist, except ______________________

____

3. Your signature opposite the operations or special procedures listed below constitutes your acknowledgment (i) that you have read and agreed to the foregoing, (ii) that the operations or special procedures have been adequately explained to you by your attending physicians or surgeons and that you have all of the information that you desire, and (iii) that you authorize and consent to the performance of the operations or special procedures.

Operation or Procedure	Date	Time	
____________	______	______	______________
____________	______	______	Signature (Patient)
____________	______	______	______________
____________	______	______	Signature (Witness)

(If patient is a minor or unable to sign, complete the following):

Patient is a minor or is unable to sign, because ______________________

____

______________	______________
Father	Guardian
______________	______________
Mother	Other Person and Relationship

STERILIZATION PERMIT

Date ______ Hour ____________ .m.

I hereby authorize and direct Doctor ____________ and assistants of his choice to perform the following operation upon me at the above named hospital: ________________ __________ and to do any other procedure that his (their) judgment may dictate during the above operation. It has been explained to me that I may (or will probably) be sterile as a result of this operation but no such result has been warranted. I understand that the word "sterility" means that I may be unable to conceive or bear children and in giving my consent to this operation have in mind the possibility (probability) of such a result. I hereby absolve said doctor, his assistants and the hospital, from all responsibility for any condition of sterility which may result or fail to result from said operation.

Signed ____________________________

SIGNATURE WITNESSED:

By ____________________________

By ____________________________

RELEASE FROM RESPONSIBILITY FOR TREATMENT OF MISCARRIAGE OR PARTIAL ABORTION (OTHER THAN THERAPEUTIC)

Date __________ Hour ________.m.

I, the undersigned, a patient at the above named hospital, am advised by my doctor that I may be in a condition of abortion. I hereby declare that neither the physician nor any person employed by or connected with the said hospital has performed any act which may have contributed to the interruption of my pregnancy and do hereby absolve the said hospital and treating physician from any responsibility for my condition. My condition has been caused by the following facts occurring prior to the time of my admission to the hospital and treatment by my physician.

____

____

____

____
Patient

Signature witnessed:

By ______________________

By ______________________

This form to be completed in the case of patients who are or MAY BE in a condition of abortion. Patient should state facts of her case in her own handwriting whenever possible.

RELEASE FROM RESPONSIBILITY FOR ABORTION (MISCARRIAGE)

Date ________, 19____

Time ________ a.m. p.m.

This is to certify that I, ______________, a patient applying for admission to ____ __________ Medical Center, have been advised that I am in a condition of abortion (miscarriage).

I hereby declare that neither the attending physician nor any person employed by or connected with the said hospital has knowingly performed any act which may have contributed to the induction of the abortion (miscarriage).

Witness ________________ Signed ________________________
(Patient or nearest relative)

Witness ________________ ________________________
(Relationship)

Authorization must be signed by the patient or by the nearest relative when patient is physically or mentally incompetent.

matter of first aid or temporary medical care in lieu of surgery or actual surgical procedures.

2. The possibilities for obtaining necessary written consent must be weighed against the possibility that a delayed consent would jeopardize the health of the patient.
3. Medical consultation should be obtained in order to establish the existence of an emergency situation. (It must be remembered that the doctors are not consenting for the patient but are determining only that an emergency exists that requires treatment without further waiting to get a proper consent.)
4. The medical consultations should be carefully charted and should include a statement by each consultant such as follows: "The immediate treatment of the patient is necessary because..."

REFERENCES

Cobbs versus Grant, 104 Cal Rptr 505, 1972

Mills DH; Whither informed consent? JAMA *229*:305-310, 1974

Laforet EG: The fiction of informed consent. JAMA *235*:1579-1585, 1976

6 DRUG THERAPY DURING PREGNANCY AND LACTATION

GENERAL CONSIDERATIONS

Drugs with a high lipid solubility or a molecular weight of less than 1000 cross the placenta easily or diffuse into breast milk. Consequently, the fetus and newborn infant can be exposed to varying levels of maternal medications.

The most critical periods of fetal drug exposure are during the first trimester, when drugs may be responsible for congenital anomalies, and prior to delivery, when drugs may cause respiratory depression or fetal toxicity owing to the immaturity of fetal enzyme systems. Unless absolutely necessary, drugs of all types should be avoided during pregnancy.

Antibiotic Therapy: Bacterial infections during pregnancy are frequently life threatening, and antimicrobial drug therapy is essential. When one is selecting appropriate antibiotics one must take into consideration the potential toxicity for the pregnant patient, as well as the specific dangers to the fetus that may be created by transplacental passage. Of all the antibiotics, *ampicillin* tends to be the one most frequently prescribed during pregnancy as long as the mother has no history of penicillin allergy. Although ampicillin crosses the placenta, there has been no evidence of fetal toxicity. Ampicillin is usually preferred because of its broad spectrum of bactericidal activity against both penicillin-susceptible organisms and many common gram-negative pathogens.

A listing of various drugs and their potential fetal-neonatal risk follows.

Drug	Fetal-Neonatal Risk	Comment
Anti-infective agents		
Ampicillin	None known	
Carbenicillin	None known	
Cephalothin	None known	
Chloramphenicol	Cardiovascular collapse; "gray" cyanosis; death	Avoid during pregnancy
Chloroquine	Retinal damage	After high doses
Clindamycin	None known	Transplacental passage less than 10 per cent
Dicloxacillin	None known	Transplacental passage less than 10 per cent
Erythromycin	None known	Transplacental passage less than 10 per cent
Gentamycin	Potentially ototoxic and nephrotoxic	In severe infections the therapeutic balance (benefit versus risk) is favorable
Kanamycin	Potentially ototoxic and nephrotoxic	In severe infections the therapeutic balance (benefit versus risk) is favorable
Methicillin	None known	
Metronidazole	Unknown (Tumorigenic in rodents)	Contraindicated during first trimester and best avoided during pregnancy and lactation
Nalidixic acid	None known	Safe use during the first trimester has not been established
Nitrofurantoin	Hemolytic anemia	Avoid during third trimester and lactation
Oxacillin	None known	
Penicillin	None known	Drug of choice during pregnancy for therapy of sensitive organisms
Spectinomycin	Ototoxicity	Theoretical risk
Streptomycin	Ototoxicity	Only after long-term therapy
Sulfonamides	Congenital anomalies; kernicterus, particularly in premature infants; hemolysis in G6PD deficiency	Avoid during third trimester and lactation

Drug	Fetal-Neonatal Risk	Comment
Tetracyclines	Permanent staining of deciduous teeth; inhibition of bone growth	Avoid during pregnancy; may lead to maternal hepatic toxicity when given intravenously
Trimethoprim	Inhibition of folic acid metabolism	Avoid during pregnancy
Other Drugs		
Anesthetics, local	Bradycardia	
Barbiturates	Respiratory depression	
Chlordiazepoxide	Congenital anomalies; apnea, hypotonia	Data inconclusive
Coumarin anticoagulants	Congenital defects; hemorrhage; intrauterine death	Avoid during pregnancy unless benefits outweigh hazards
Cytotoxic drugs: Aminopterin Chlorambucil	Congenital anomalies; abortion	Avoid during pregnancy if possible
Diazepam	Congenital anomalies; hypotonia; hypothermia; respiratory depression; withdrawal symptoms	Data inconclusive
Diethylstilbestrol	Vaginal adenosis; ? vaginal adenocarcinoma	Avoid during pregnancy
Ergotamine	Vomiting; diarrhea; unstable blood pressure	Avoid during lactation
Furosemide	Fetal toxicity	For life-threatening situations only
Heparin	None known	Does not cross placenta
Heroin	Withdrawal symptoms	
Iodides	Thyroid enlargement	Avoid during pregnancy
Lithium carbonate	Electrolyte imbalance; congenital anomalies	
Narcotics	Respiratory depression	
Meprobamate	Congenital anomalies	Data inconclusive
Methadone	Withdrawal symptoms	
Phenytoin	Congenital anomalies	Potential maternal benefits usually necessitate therapy
	Hemorrhage	Prophylactic Vitamin K may be beneficial
Progestins	Congenital anomalies	Avoid during pregnancy

Drug	Fetal-Neonatal Risk	Comment
Propranolol	Beta adrenergic blockade	Avoid during pregnancy if possible
Reserpine	Nasal congestion; drowsiness	
Salicylates	Hemorrhage	Platelet dysfunction
Testosterone	Masculinization of female fetus	Avoid during pregnancy
Thiazide diuretics	Thrombocytopenia; jaundice	Can cross placenta; Secreted in breast milk
Warfarin	Congenital anomalies; hemorrhage; intra-uterine death	Avoid during pregnancy unless benefits outweigh hazards

REFERENCES

McCracken GH: Pharmacologic basis for antimicrobial therapy in newborn infants. Clin Perinatol *2*:139-161, 1975

Mead PB, Gump DW: Antibiotic therapy in obstetrics and gynecology. Clin Obstet Gynecol *19*:109-129, 1976

Oseid RJ: Breast feeding and infant health. Clin Obstet Gynecol *18*:149-173, 1975

Slone D, Siskind V, Heinonen OP, et al: Aspirin and congenital malformations. Lancet *1*:1373, 1976; Obstet Gynecol Surv *32*:16-18, 1977

Stirrat GM: Prescribing problems in the second half of pregnancy and during lactation. Obstet Gynecol Surv *31*:1-7, 1976

7 NORMAL LABORATORY VALUES

	Normal Female	Late Pregnancy
Complete Blood Count		
Hemoglobin (Hb)	12-16 gm/100 ml	10-14 gm/100 ml
Hematocrit (Hct) packed cell volume (PCV)	37-47 per cent	32-40 per cent
Red blood cells (RBC)	4.2-5.4 million/cu mm	3.6-4.8 million/cu mm
Red cell corpuscular values (red cell indices)		
Mean corpuscular volume (MCV) (Hct × 10/RBC)	82-92	82-92
Mean corpuscular hemoglobin (MCH) (Hb × 10/RBC)	27-31	27-31
Mean corpuscular hemoglobin concentration (MCHC) (Hb × 100)/(Hct)	32-36	32-36
White blood cells (WBC) (leukocytes)	5000-10,000	5000-12,500 (During and after labor may increase to 25,000)
Neutrophils, segmented	36-66 per cent	— or ↑
Neutrophils, band	5-11 per cent	— or ↑
Lymphocytes	24-44 per cent	— or ↓
Monocytes	4 per cent	—
Eosinophils	2-3 per cent	—
Basophils	0.5 per cent	—
Erythrocyte sedimentation rate (ESR)		
Westergren	0-22 mm/hr	30-70 mm/hr
Wintrobe	0-15 mm/hr	30-70 mm/hr
Reticulocyte count	0.5-1.5 per cent	—
Blood Coagulation Tests		
Platelet count	140,000-340,000	75,000-320,000
Bleeding time (Ivy)	< 4 min	—

	Normal Female	Late Pregnancy
Blood Coagulation Tests (Continued)		
Fibrin-split products	Minimal	Minimal
Prothrombin time	11-16 seconds (same as control)	—
Fibrinogen	200-400 mg/100 ml	300-600 mg/100 ml
Activated partial thromboplastin time	35-53 seconds	—
Thrombin time	12-18 seconds	—
Blood Chemistries		
Acetone	0.3-2.0 mg/100 ml	—
Ammonia	30-70 μg/100 ml	—
Amylase	60-180 Somogyi units/100 ml	— or ↑ (two fold)
	30-70 mg glucose/100 ml	50-200 mg glucose/100 ml
Bicarbonate (HCO_3^-)		
Venous	22-26 mEq/l	— or ↓
Arterial	20-24 mEq/l	— or ↓
Bilirubin		
Direct	0.1-0.4 mg/100 ml	— to slight ↑
Indirect	0.1-0.5	—
Total	0.2-0.9	— to slight ↑
Calcium	4.4-5.4 mEq/l	— to slight ↓
	8.5-10.5 mg/100 ml	— to slight ↓
Carbon dioxide		
Content (venous)	26-28 mEq/l	↓
Tension (pCO_2), arterial	32-42 mm Hg	↓
Tension (pCO_2), venous	39-52 mm Hg	↓
Ceruloplasmin	20-35 mg/100 ml	↑
Chloride	98-106 mEq/l	—
Cholesterol, total	120-330 mg/100 ml	↑ (two fold)
Creatine phosphokinase	0-12 Sigma units/ml	—
Creatinine	0.6-1.3 mg/100 ml	↓ 0.4-1.0 mg/100 ml
Glucose (fasting)	70-110 mg/100 ml	—
Haptoglobin	30-160 mg/100 ml	—
Iron	60-135 μg/100 ml	— or ↓
Iron-binding capacity	250-350 μg/100 ml	↑
Per cent saturation	20-55	
Lactic acid	6-16 mg/100 ml	—
Lactic dehydrogenase (LDH)	200-680 units/ml	Slight ↑
Magnesium	1.5-2.5 mEq/l	
	1.8-3.0 mg/100 ml	

	Normal Female	Late Pregnancy
Blood Chemistries (Continued)		
Osmolality	285-295 mOsm/l	275-285 mOsm/l
Oxygen tension (pO_2), arterial	80-100 mm Hg	—
pH		
Arterial	7.35-7.45	7.40-7.46
Venous	7.32-7.42	7.37-7.43
Phosphatase, alkaline	5-13 King-Armstrong units	7-41 King-Armstrong units
	20-100 International units/l	two to fourfold ↑
Phosphorus	2.0-4.5 mg/100 ml	—
Potassium	3.5-5.5 mEq/l	—
Protein-bound iodine (PBI)	3.6-8.8 mcg/100 ml	↑
Proteins, total	6.0-8.0 gm/100 ml	5.5-6.5 gm/100 ml
Albumin	3.5-5.5 gm/100 ml	2.5-3.5 gm/100 ml
Globulin	1.5-3.0 gm/100 ml	2.0-3.5 gm/100 ml
Sodium	136-145 mEq/l	—
T-3 resin sponge uptake	24-36 per cent	↓
T-4 (thyroxine by RIA)	5.0-11 mcg/100 ml	↑
Thyroxine binding globulin (TBG) (expressed as T_4 uptake)	10-26 mcg/100 ml	↑
Transaminase		
SGOT	5-40 units/ml	—
SGPT	5-35 units/ml	—
Triglycerides	10-150 mg/100 ml	↑
Urea nitrogen (BUN)	< 17 mg/100 ml	< 11/100 ml
Uric acid	3-7.5 mg/100 ml	3-5 mg/100 ml

— Same Range
↑ Increased
↓ Decreased
< Less than

REFERENCES

Sejeny SA, Eastham RD, Baker, SR: Platelet counts during normal pregnancy. J Clin Pathol *28*:812-813, 1975; Obstet Gynecol Surv *31*:368-369, 1976

Davidson I, Henry J: Clinical Diagnosis by Laboratory Methods. Philadelphia, W.B. Saunders Company, 1974

PART II

SPECIFIC PROBLEMS

8 ABDOMINAL PAIN

GENERAL CONSIDERATIONS

The three major sources of abdominal pain are:

Tension: Distention of a hollow viscus — intestine, ureter, uterus, fallopian tube — causes pain either by stretching of the muscular wall or by muscular contraction. Pain is also produced by traction on the mesentery and acute stretching of the capsules of solid organs such as the liver, spleen, kidney, and ovary. Since sensory impulses from several viscera overlap within the same segment of the spinal cord, visceral abdominal pain tends to be poorly localized.

Peritoneal Irritation: When inflammation from an adjacent viscus (appendicitis, salpingitis, or other inflammation) stimulates the sensitive parietal peritoneum, the pain tends to be well defined and localized.

Generalized peritonitis is caused by a diffuse spread of intestinal contents, blood, or pus throughout the peritoneal cavity. The peritoneal inflammation causes reflex spasm of the overlying muscles, resulting in rigidity and tenderness of the abdominal wall; peritoneal pain is aggravated by any movement that induces torsion, tension, or traction of the diseased peritoneum.

Ischemia of somatic, cardiac, or visceral muscle.

SUBJECTIVE DATA

CURRENT SYMPTOMS

Onset (Sudden versus Gradual): *Sudden* onset of abdominal pain suggests acute *perforation* of a hollow viscus; *rupture* of an intra-abdominal structure; intraperitoneal *hemorrhage* secondary to a ruptured ectopic pregnancy, ruptured ovarian cyst, or ruptured uterus;

intraperitoneal pus from a ruptured tuboovarian abscess; hemorrhage into an ovarian cyst or tumor; hemorrhage into a uterine tumor; or *torsion* of an ovarian tumor, pedunculated uterine tumor, paramesonephric cyst, or normal adnexa. The patient is frequently aware of the exact moment that she experienced the initial stabbing pain.

Gradual onset of pelvic pain suggests inflammation (salpingitis, appendicitis, diverticulitis); obstruction (ureteral or intestinal); or uterine contractions associated with abortion or labor. With a gradual onset, the pain may not reach its peak for several hours.

Location (Initial Site, Migration, Radiation): Generalized abdominal pain suggests flooding of the peritoneal cavity with an irritating fluid — blood, pus, or intestinal contents.

Epigastric pain is associated with structures innervated by the sixth to eighth thoracic nerves (T6–T8: stomach, duodenum, pancras, liver, and gallbladder). During the latter half of pregnancy, epigastric pain may be due to liver distention and can be a symptom of severe preeclampsia.

Periumbilical pain is associated with structures innervated by T9 and T10 (small intestine, appendix, upper ureters, and ovaries). The pain associated with appendicitis is initially located in the periumbilical area, since the appendicular nerves are derived from the same source as those that supply the small intestine. When the appendiceal inflammation extends to the parietal peritoneum, the pain "migrates" into the area overlying the appendix, usually the right lower quadrant. Such shifting of pain to a localized site, particularly when accompanied by local tenderness and muscle spasm, denotes inflammation of the parietal peritoneum.

Hypogastric or suprapubic pain has its origin in structures innervated by T11 and T12 (colon, bladder, lower ureters, and uterus).

Abdominal pain accompanied by shoulder pain suggests diaphragmatic irritation. Diffuse intraabdominal bleeding may cause diaphragmatic irritation, with pain referred to the corresponding part of the shoulder area on the same side of the body.

Pelvic pain always suggests reproductive tract disease. Afferent impulses from the cervix enter the sacral segments of the cord (S2, S3, S4). Uterine pain may be referred to the pubic and sacroiliac regions. Sensory stimuli from the ovaries and fallopian tubes are transmitted over sympathetic fibers that accompany the ovarian vessels and terminate at T10, T11, and T12.

Quality (Cramping versus Steady): *Cramping*, intermittent pain is the result of muscular contractions of a hollow viscus (stomach, intestine, bile duct, pancreatic duct, ureter, uterus, or fallopian tube). Cramping pain may also be caused by increased intraluminal pressure in a hollow viscus. Waves of pain interspersed with periods of complete relief or only a dull ache are typical of hollow viscus obstruction.

Steady pain without a periodic rhythm suggests a neoplastic or inflammatory process. One example is diffuse intraperitoneal irritation resulting from pus, blood, or a perforated viscus. Constant, progressive, or persistent pain may also be the result of swelling or overdistention of a solid viscus or intestinal obstruction after impairment of the blood supply.

Duration: The duration of pain, as well as the previous occurrence of similar episodes, helps establish the acute or chronic nature of the symptoms. If the patient states that she has had the same pain or similar pain for a prolonged period of time, the diagnosis of an acute surgical emergency is virtually excluded.

Metabolic diseases, such as porphyria, or nephrolithiasis may cause recurrent attacks of abdominal pain over long periods of time.

Ovulatory pain may be acute but of short duration and recurrent at periodic intervals.

Aggravating and Relieving Factors:

Body Movement: In cases of peritoneal inflammation, any movement that causes peritoneal tension or traction aggravates the patient's pain. Consequently, the patient with peritonitis prefers to lie in bed, as motionless as possible.

Patients with ureteral or uterine colic tend to be extremely restless and may even fling themselves about in an attempt to find relief from their spasmodic pain.

Pain of musculoskeletal origin tends to be aggravated by certain body movements and is often relieved by rest and the application of heat.

Foods: A burning pain associated with gastritis or peptic ulceration is aggravated by the ingestion of highly seasoned food and is usually relieved by milk or antacid medications.

Associated Symptoms:

Vaginal Bleeding: The combination of vaginal bleeding with abdominal pain usually indicates a pathologic process in the reproductive tract. Severe abdominal pain a few weeks after a missed menstrual period suggests ectopic pregnancy (p. 311). Acute abdominal pain associated with fever and chills during or shortly after menstruation suggests pelvic infection (p. 474).

Periodically recurrent uterine pain associated with most menstrual periods is usually dysmenorrhea (p. 293).

Lower abdominal pain periodically recurrent midway between the menstrual periods is frequently caused by ovulation (p. 459). Although the exact mechanism of ovulatory pain remains unknown, it may result from increased intrafollicular pressure prior to follicle rupture or the release or follicular fluid into the peritoneal cavity.

Anorexia, Nausea, Vomiting, and Constipation: Although gastrointestinal symptoms combined with abdominal pain suggest a pathologic process in the intestinal tract, these symptoms are frequently nonspecific, since they commonly occur during the first trimester of pregnancy. Severe persistent vomiting, however, is almost always the result of one or more of the following causes:

1. Severe irritation of the nerves of the peritoneum or mesentery. In cases of acute pancreatitis, for example, the celiac plexus is intimately associated with the inflamed organ. The reflex stimulus causes severe vomiting that persists until the stimulus is relieved. Torsion of the pedicle of an ovarian cyst can also cause sudden and severe stimulation of many sympathetic nerves with persistent vomiting.
2. Obstruction of an involuntary muscular tube (ureter, uterus, intestine, appendix). Although vomiting is frequent in cases of upper intestinal obstruction, this symptom may be absent in the case of a large bowel obstruction.
3. The action of absorbed toxins upon the medullary centers.

Syncope, Vascular Collapse, Shock: Abdominal pain accompanied by syncope, vascular collapse, or shock suggests intraperitoneal hemorrhage secondary to ectopic pregnancy or a ruptured ovarian cyst. Other possible causes for abdominal pain accompanied by syncope or shock are ruptured tuboovarian abscess, acute pancreatitis, mesenteric thrombosis, dissecting aneurysm, and myocardial infarction.

Urinary Symptoms: Abdominal pain accompanied by the urinary symptoms of frequency and dysuria suggest a pathologic process in the urinary tract, such as pyelonephritis or ureteral obstruction.

Fever and Chills: Associated symptoms of fever and chills are suggestive of an acute systemic infection, usually pelvic infection with bacteremia.

Sequence of Symptoms: The order of occurrence of symptoms may be helpful in the differential diagnosis of abdominal pain. In cases of appendicitis, for example, the typical sequence of symptoms is (1) epigastric or umbilical pain, (2) nausea or vomiting, (3) local iliac tenderness, (4) fever, and (5) leukocytosis.

PRIOR HISTORY

With a history of recent abortion, delivery, or surgery, the most common cause of abdominal pain is pelvic infection, particularly if the pain is accompanied by elevated temperature and leukocytosis.

A history of antecedent trauma suggests the possibility of a ruptured viscus (ruptured spleen or ruptured uterus).

Pain developing after the lifting of a heavy object suggests a musculoskeletal pathologic condition rather than a condition of gynecologic origin.

A prior diagnosis (diabetes, sickle cell disease, and so forth) may explain the current episode of pain.

OBJECTIVE DATA

PHYSICAL EXAMINATION

General examination includes observation of the temperature, pulse, blood pressure, respiration, general appearance, heart, and lungs. General examination of a patient may disclose the coexistence of vascular collapse and systemic infection or associated systemic disease.

Elevated temperature suggests infection. When the patient has a normal temperature, acute peritonitis may result from intraperitoneal bleeding (ruptured ectopic pregnancy) or possibly a perforated peptic ulcer.

The skin may be pallid in cases of acute blood loss or anemia. Yellow skin suggests biliary tract disease. In cases of acute blood loss and hypovolemia, the skin tends to be cold and clammy; diffuse perspiration is the result of the elevated level of circulatory epinephrine and norepinephrine.

The patient's activity is a significant feature of the general examination. A patient with general peritonitis prefers to lie quietly on her back, whereas a patient with an obstructed hollow viscus (ureteral stone, for example) is more likely to be rolling about in severe discomfort; the patient's movement may coincide with the periodic colic. A patient with appendicitis may pull up the right hip and knee in order to relax the psoas muscle, whereas the patient with pancreatitis may prefer to lie on her side with knees, hips, and back flexed.

Chest Examination: Since abdominal pain may be referred from intrathoracic lesions, such as pneumonia or empyema, the chest should be carefully examined to exclude the possibility of pulmonary disease.

Abdominal Examination:

Inspection of the abdomen should include observation of any distention, the contour, and any surgical scar. Abdominal pain accompanied by abdominal distention usually indicates intestinal obstruction. The presence of a surgical scar on the abdomen adds to the probability that an adhesion or band may be causing such an obstruction.

Palpation for tenderness, rebound tenderness, rigidity, and masses should be a part of the abdominal examination. Abdominal tenderness is a significant finding in cases of intraperitoneal disease. Rebound tenderness is an indication of peritoneal irritation.

Tenderness in the right upper quadrant suggests cholecystitis, hepatitis, pancreatitis, or gonococcal perihepatitis (Fitz-Hugh–Curtis syndrome). Renal pain or pleural pain may also be referred to the right upper quadrant. During pregnancy, the appendix may be displaced upward.

Tenderness in the lower abdomen suggests appendicitis, diverticulitis, or disease in the reproductive tract — uterus, tubes, or ovaries.

Abdominal rigidity usually indicates serious abdominal disease, particularly peritoneal irritation secondary to infection, chemical irritants, or blood. The degree of rigidity varies with the nature of the irritant and the suddenness of onset of the stimulus.

True rigidity secondary to intraabdominal disease must be distinguished from voluntary muscular contractions resulting from nervousness or anxiety. The examiner should gently lay one hand on the abdomen, palpating the surface with a light touch that cannot possibly hurt. This maneuver helps allay the patient's anxiety and gives the examiner an idea of the extent, intensity, and constancy of the rigidity. Voluntary muscular contractions tend to vary in intensity and often disappear when the patient is appropriately distracted.

Rigidity secondary to pleurisy or infection of the chest wall is usually limited to one side of the abdomen.

Masses palpable abdominally include tumors, abscesses, and pregnancy. Some patients are unaware of their menstrual periods and do not know when they are pregnant. Palpation of fetal movements makes the diagnosis of pregnancy evident.

Pelvic pathologic conditions to be considered in the evaluation of the distended abdomen include ovarian cysts, ovarian tumors, and leiomyomas of the uterus.

Percussion (Air, Fluid, Organ Size): Abdominal percussion yields information concerning gaseous or fluid distention, shifting dullness (free fluid), and the size of specific organs (liver, spleen, urinary bladder).

Auscultation (Bowel Sounds, Fetal Heart Sounds): Absent bowel sounds are a sign of paralytic ileus, usually secondary to peritonitis. Hyperactive bowel sounds are a sign of a mechanical intestinal obstruction or gastroenteritis.

The presence of fetal heart sounds confirms the diagnosis of pregnancy.

Pelvic Examination: Pelvic examination is essential in order to identify pelvic disease and evaluate the status of the reproductive organs (uterus, fallopian tubes, and ovaries). Unless a pregnant uterus has been palpated abdominally, pelvic examination is required to assess the possibility of intrauterine or extrauterine pregnancy. (See also p. 29.)

Rectal Examination: Rectal examination usually combined with vaginal examination, is particularly valuable for assessment of the cul-de-sac.

Bulging of the cul-de-sac may be caused by a pelvic abscess or profuse intraabdominal hemorrhage. (See p. 22.)

LABORATORY TESTS

Complete Blood Count with Differential Smear: Decreased hemoglobin values and decreased hematocrit suggest prior blood loss.

Elevated white blood count, particularly with a shift to the left, suggests systemic infection.

Urinalysis with Microscopic Examination: The presence of red cells or pus cells in the urine points to the urinary tract as the site of the pathologic process.

A metabolic imbalance may be suggested if the urine contains glucose or ketones.

Blood Type and Rh: Whenever intraperitoneal bleeding is suspected or blood transfusion may be indicated, blood should be sent to the blood bank for determination of type and for cross-matching.

ASSESSMENT

DIFFERENTIAL DIAGNOSIS

I. Reproductive Tract
   A. Uterus
      1. Abortion
      2. Adenomyosis
      3. Chorioamnionitis
      4. Dysmenorrhea
      5. Endometritis
      6. Hemangioma with intraperitoneal rupture
      7. Hematometra
      8. Labor
      9. Leiomyoma: degeneration, torsion
      10. Placental separation, premature
      11. Pyometra
      12. Round ligament: stretching or spasm
      13. Rupture
      14. Trauma

B. Fallopian Tube
   1. Ectopic pregnancy
   2. Pyosalpinx
   3. Salpingitis
   4. Torsion
   5. Tuboovarian abscess

C. Ovary
   1. Hemorrhage into an ovarian cyst or tumor
   2. Intraperitoneal hemorrhage from an ovarian cyst or tumor — usually corpus luteum or endometrioma
   3. Oophoritis
   4. Ovulation
   5. Rupture of an ovarian cyst
   6. Torsion of an ovarian cyst or tumor

D. Abdominal Pregnancy

E. Pelvic Thrombophlebitis

F. Endometriosis

II. Intestinal Tract
   1. Appendicitis
   2. Colitis
   3. Diverticulitis
   4. Enteritis: bacterial or regional
   5. Gastroenteritis
   6. Intestinal obstruction
   7. Intestinal perforation
      a. Burn associated with laparoscopic cauterization (see Post-operative Complications, p. 520)
   8. Mesenteric thrombosis
   9. Ruptured viscus
   10. Trauma
   11. Ulcer: gastric or duodenal; perforated, hemorrhaging

III. Biliary Tract; Pancreas; Spleen
   1. Biliary colic
   2. Cholecystitis
   3. Gallbladder perforation
   4. Hepatic adenoma with rupture
   5. Hepatic vein thrombosis

6. Hepatitis
7. Hepatomegaly
8. Pancreatitis
9. Pancreatic duct stone
10. Perihepatitis, gonococcal (Fitz-Hugh–Curtis syndrome)
11. Portal vein thrombosis
12. Splenic infarct
13. Splenic rupture
14. Trauma

IV. Urinary Tract
1. Cystitis
2. Pyelonephritis
3. Ureteral obstruction; renal calculus

V. Other Diagnoses to be Considered
1. Addisonian crisis
2. Aneurysm, aortic: rupture, dissecting
3. Cardiac failure with distention of liver capsule
4. Diabetic acidosis
5. Drug addiction; withdrawal symptoms
6. Epilepsy, abdominal
7. Herpes zoster
8. Hypercalcemia
9. Lead colic
10. Musculoskeletal pain
11. Myocardial infarction
12. Pericarditis
13. Pleural or pneumonic lesions
    a. Pneumonia
    b. Pulmonary embolus
    c. Empyema
14. Poisoning, acute
15. Porphyria, acute
16. Posterior nerve root pain from prolapsed intervertebral disc
17. Psychogenic causes
18. Tuberculous peritonitis
19. Sickle cell crisis
20. Retroperitoneal hemorrhage or effusion

SEVERITY OF DISEASE PROCESS

When patients with acute abdominal pain are initially seen the severity of the disease process is often difficult to evaluate. Reevaluation after one to four hours may be essential in order to assess the trend of the disease process.

Increasing pain, tenderness, guarding, or rigidity indicate that the condition is worsening. Extension of an area of tenderness associated with the development of rebound tenderness indicates a failure of localization of the underlying inflammatory condition. Increasing distention suggests an ongoing intestinal obstruction.

Frequently, serial determinations of the white blood count or hemoglobin can be helpful in the evaluation of infection or occult blood loss.

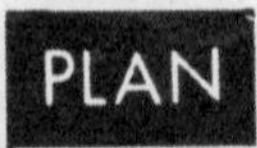

ADDITIONAL DIAGNOSTIC DATA

Many cases of acute abdominal pain are a diagnostic challenge, particularly when the symptoms do not fit the typical textbook picture. The following tests may provide valuable diagnostic information, depending on the presumptive diagnosis.

Cervical culture is indicated whenever pelvic infection is suspected. A Gram stain of the cervical secretion may also be helpful.

Culdocentesis can be diagnostic when intraperitoneal bleeding is suspected.

Liver Function Tests: Bilirubin, SGOT, and SGPT are elevated in cases of hepatic disease. Alkaline phosphatase is increased in cases of complete biliary obstruction but also is elevated during normal pregnancy.

Amylase is elevated within 24 to 48 hours in cases of acute pancreatitis. Other possible causes of hyperamylasemia include perforated peptic ulcer, and biliary, intestinal, salivary gland, or fallopian tube disease.

Erythrocyte sedimentation rate (ESR) is elevated with pelvic inflammatory disease and after the third month of pregnancy. Normal values would be expected in cases of early appendicitis or unruptured ectopic pregnancy.

Glucose elevation is usually indicative of diabetes mellitus. Glucose may also be elevated in cases of pancreatitis.

Blood Urea Nitrogen, Creatinine, Uric Acid: These tests evaluate renal function and tend to be elevated with chronic renal disease. Uric acid may be differentially elevated in cases of preeclampsia.

Blood electrolyte determinations are particularly important in the evaluation of fluid loss associated with vomiting or diarrhea.

Coagulation Studies: Whenever a coagulation defect is suspected, a platelet count, prothrombin time, partial thromboplastin time, fibrinogen, and fibrin-split products should be determined.

X-rays: Abdominal x-rays, including an upright film, supine film, and lateral decubitus film, may reveal (1) free air under the diaphragm, which is suggestive of intestinal perforation or uterine perforation; (2) free fluid, suggestive of a ruptured viscus, ruptured cyst, or intraperitoneal bleeding; (3) air in an abscess cavity; (4) calcifications (appendicoliths, renal calculi, or gallstones); (5) evidence of intestinal obstruction; or (6) an intrauterine device.

A chest film may be helpful when there is any question of pulmonary disease. The chest film may also reveal free air under the diaphragm.

Ultrasound B-scan is preferable to x-ray when the patient is pregnant. The sonogram may be particularly helpful in the diagnosis of an early intrauterine pregnancy, the diagnosis of molar pregnancy, or the assessment of an equivocal pelvic mass.

Electrocardiogram is performed when cardiac disease is suspected.

Laparoscopy often clarifies the existence of tubal or ovarian disease.

Other diagnostic procedures or tests that may be indicated under special circumstances include

1. Cholecystogram
2. Intravenous pyelogram
3. Sigmoidoscopy
4. Esophagoscopy, gastroscopy
5. Barium enema or barium meal
6. Angiography
7. Abdominal paracentesis

8. Blood gases
9. Radioisotope scans: liver, lungs
10. Urinalysis for porphyrins
11. Sickle cell preparation

MANAGEMENT

Conditions requiring immediate abdominal surgery whether or not the patient is pregnant include

1. Appendicitis, acute
2. Bladder rupture
3. Cholecystitis, acute, with perforation
4. Ectopic pregnancy
5. Gastrointestinal hemorrhage, massive and unresolved
6. Intestinal obstruction, mechanical
7. Intraabdominal abscesses, including pancreatic abscess
8. Mesenteric vascular occlusion
9. Ovarian cyst or tumor: hemorrhage or torsion
10. Perforated hollow viscus: stomach, duodenum, intestine, or colon
11. Splenic rupture
12. Strangulated hernia: internal or external
13. Trauma with visceral injury or hemorrhage
14. Tuboovarian abscess, ruptured
15. Vascular emergencies: ruptured abdominal aneurysm
16. Volvulus or intussusception

Hemorrhage, perforation or rupture of a viscus, and torsion always require surgical repair.

Conditions *not* requiring immediate surgery include

1. Abdominal abscess, localized
2. Cholecystitis, acute
3. Diverticular disease of the colon
4. Gastrointestinal hemorrhage: responsive to blood replacement and giving evidence of cessation
5. Ovarian follicle, ruptured
6. Pancreatic pseudocyst
7. Pancreatitis
8. Retroperitoneal hemorrhage, localized
9. Salpingitis

REFERENCES

Barber HRK, Graber EA: Surgical Disease in Pregnancy. Philadelphia, W.B. Saunders Company, 1974

Botsford TW, Wilson RE: The Acute Abdomen. 2nd edition. Philadelphia, W.B. Saunders Company, 1977

Cope Z: The Early Diagnosis of the Acute Abdomen. 14th ed. London, Oxford University Press, 1972

Hochberg CJ: Tubal amylase. Obstet Gynecol *43*:129-131, 1974

9 ABORTION

DEFINITIONS

Abortion—the term applied to all pregnancies that terminate before the period of fetal viability, that is, that terminate before the fetal weight is 500 grams. In the absence of known weight, an estimated length of gestation of less than 20 completed weeks (139 days), calculated from the first day of the last normal menstrual period, may be used.

Complete abortion—the expulsion of all the products of conception before the twentieth completed week of gestation.

Habitual abortion—the occurrence of three or more consecutive spontaneous abortions.

Incomplete abortion—the expulsion of some, but not all, of the products of conception before the twentieth completed week of gestation (Fig. 9-1).

Induced abortion—the deliberate interruption of pregnancy by any means before the twentieth completed week of gestation. It may be therapeutic or nontherapeutic.

Inevitable abortion—the state in which bleeding of intrauterine origin occurs with continuous and progressive dilatation of the cervix but without expulsion of the products of conception before the twentieth completed week of gestation (Fig. 9-1).

Infected abortion—an abortion associated with infection of the genital organs.

Missed abortion—an abortion in which the embryo or fetus dies *in utero* before the twentieth completed week of gestation but the products of conception are retained *in utero* for eight weeks or more (Fig. 9-1).

Septic abortion—an infected abortion in which there is dissemination of microorganisms and their products into the maternal systemic circulation.

Spontaneous abortion—the expulsion of the products of conception without deliberate interference before the twentieth completed week of gestation.

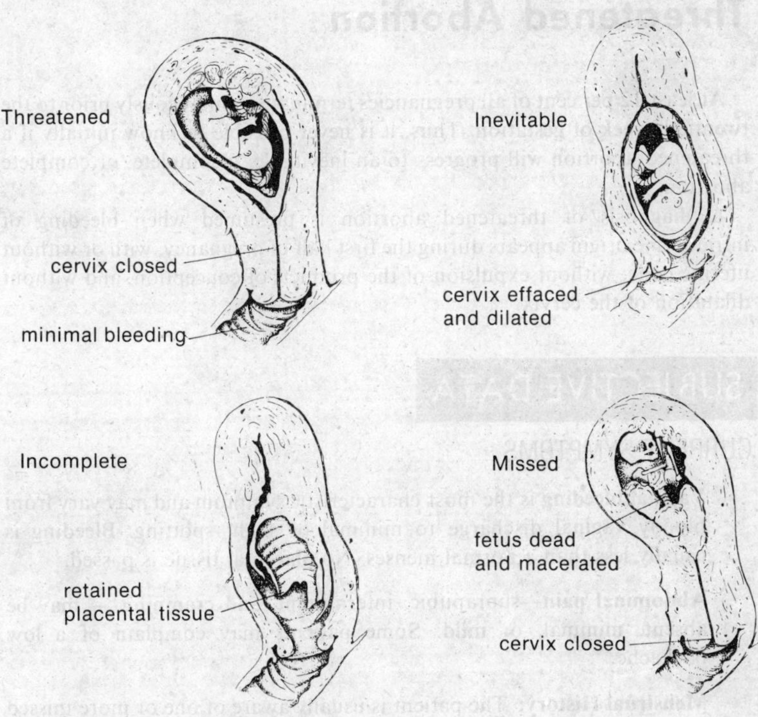

Figure 9-1. Types of abortion.

Therapeutic abortion—the interruption of pregnancy before the twentieth completed week of gestation for legally acceptable, medically approved indications.

Threatened abortion—a state in which bleeding of intrauterine origin occurs before the twentieth completed week of gestation, with or without uterine colic, without expulsion of the products of conception, and without dilatation of the cervix (Fig. 9-1).

Threatened Abortion

At least 12 per cent of all pregnancies terminate spontaneously prior to the twentieth week of gestation. Thus, it is never possible to know initially if a threatened abortion will progress to an inevitable, incomplete, or complete abortion.

A diagnosis of threatened abortion is presumed when bleeding of intrauterine origin appears during the first half of pregnancy, with or without uterine colic, without expulsion of the products of conception, and without dilatation of the cervix.

SUBJECTIVE DATA

CURRENT SYMPTOMS

Vaginal bleeding is the most characteristic symptom and may vary from bloody vaginal discharge to minimal or slight spotting. Bleeding is usually less than a normal menses. No placental tissue is passed.

Abdominal pain—suprapubic, intermittent, and cramping — may be absent, minimal, or mild. Some patients may complain of a low backache.

Menstrual History: The patient is usually aware of one or more missed menstrual periods.

Pregnancy Symptoms: As long as the pregnancy is viable there is usually no change in subjective pregnancy symptoms: breast tenderness, morning nausea, and so forth.

OBJECTIVE DATA

PHYSICAL EXAMINATION

General examination findings are normal.

Abdominal examination findings are normal (soft, nontender).

Pelvic Examination: On speculum examination there is usually only a minimal amount of blood or brownish discharge in the vagina. The cervical os is closed.

On bimanual examination, the uterus is enlarged, softened, and nontender. Uterine size is consistent with the menstrual history. The cervix is closed, uneffaced, and of normal pregnancy consistency.

LABORATORY TESTS

Complete Blood Count with Smear: Normal values would be expected.

Urinalysis: In cases of threatened abortion urinalysis is normal. If red or white cells were found, the possibility of a urinary tract problem must be suspected, since cystitis or ureteral obstruction could produce symptoms that mimic those of threatened abortion.

ASSESSMENT

DIFFERENTIAL DIAGNOSIS

The differential diagnosis of threatened abortion includes implantation bleeding, inevitable or incomplete abortion, missed abortion, ectopic pregnancy, molar pregnancy, cervical lesions, and vaginal trauma. (See Vaginal Bleeding, p. 686.)

Implantation bleeding (Hartman's sign) may appear about the time of the expected menses. Usually the amount is no more than that of the first day of a normal cycle. There is no associated pain or backache.

Inevitable or incomplete abortion is characterized by more profuse bleeding and cervical effacement and dilatation.

Missed Abortion: The uterus is smaller than expected for the duration of amenorrhea. A pregnancy test for chorionic gonadotropin is usually negative.

Ectopic pregnancy must be considered whenever a patient complains of unilateral pelvic pain during early pregnancy. Findings of unilateral tenderness and a corpus smaller than expected for the duration of amenorrhea are additional suspicious signs. The symptoms and signs of an ectopic pregnancy can be very similar to those of a threatened abortion complicated by a bleeding corpus luteum.

Molar Pregnancy: The uterus may be larger than expected for the gestational age. Grapelike vesicles may be observed in the vagina.

Cervical Lesions or Vaginal Trauma: Polyps presenting at the external cervical os, as well as decidual reactions of the cervix, may bleed in early gestation. Pain is usually absent. Speculum examination of the cervix and vagina would establish the diagnosis.

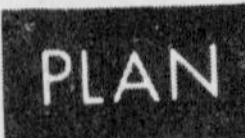

ADDITIONAL DIAGNOSTIC DATA

Pregnancy Test for Chorionic Gonadotropin: In the case of a viable intrauterine pregnancy, the pregnancy test is positive.

Ultrasound B-Scan: When the diagnosis of a viable intrauterine pregnancy is questionable, the presence of a normal gestational sac on a sonogram is reassuring. With a real time scan, fetal activity and the fetal heart beat may be visualized.

MANAGEMENT

Bed rest and restricted activity at home are usually recommended. Hospitalization is rarely required. The patient is advised to abstain from coitus in order to minimize the possibility of prostaglandin stimulation. If an intrauterine device is present, it should be removed.

Mild sedation may be prescribed. Hormonal therapy with estrogen or progesterone is *not* recommended.

Cervical circlage may be indicated during the second trimester for a patient with cervical incompetence. (See Cervical Incompetence, p. 194.)

PATIENT EDUCATION

It is never possible to know whether symptoms of threatened abortion represent the first stage of an inevitable spontaneous abortion, placental bleeding, or clinically insignificant bleeding from the implantation site or elsewhere in the uterus. When spontaneous abortions are caused by chromosomal or developmental abnormalities incompatible with fetal life, no treatment could possibly be effective and abortion is inevitable. In general, approximately 50 per cent of women with symptoms of threatened abortion lose the pregnancy, a small percentage have a premature delivery, and the others continue to term delivery. Follow-up care is essential in order to evaluate persistent symptoms, signs of fetal life, and uterine growth.

Inevitable Abortion

Inevitable abortion is the state in which bleeding of intrauterine origin occurs with continuous and progressive dilatation of the cervix, without expulsion of the products of conception before the twentieth completed week of gestation.

SUBJECTIVE DATA

CURRENT SYMPTOMS

Abdominal Pain: Intermittent, progressive suprapubic cramps are the result of the uterine contractions that produce cervical effacement and dilatation.

Vaginal Bleeding: The amount of bleeding tends to be very variable. Some patients bleed profusely, whereas others may have minimal symptoms.

Menstrual History: Although most abortions occur prior to the twelfth week after the last menstrual period, late abortions may occur during the second trimester.

Leakage of Amniotic Fluid: Abortion is inevitable when the amniotic sac ruptures. (Rarely, fluid that has collected between the amnion and chorion escapes and the pregnancy continues without serious consequence).

PRIOR HISTORY

Patients who have had a previous abortion frequently recognize the earliest symptoms of a repeat abortion.

OBJECTIVE DATA

PHYSICAL EXAMINATION

General Examination: Temperature, pulse, blood pressure, and respiration are usually normal.

Abdominal Examination: The abdomen is soft and nontender. The uterus may be palpable abdominally, depending on the gestational age.

Pelvic Examination: On speculum examination the cervix is often effaced and dilated. The amniotic sac may be seen bulging through the cervix or it may be ruptured, with amniotic fluid present in the vagina.

Bimanual examination reveals an enlarged and softened uterus; the size is more or less consistent with the duration of amenorrhea. The adnexa are normal.

LABORATORY TESTS

Complete Blood Count and Blood Smear: Hemoglobin and hematocrit reflect preexisting anemia and blood loss. White blood count and differential count may identify a systemic infection.

Urinalysis: The results of urinalysis are normal.

ASSESSMENT

DIFFERENTIAL DIAGNOSIS

See Incomplete Abortion, and Threatened Abortion, p. 87 and 93.

ETIOLOGIC FACTORS

See Incomplete Abortion, p. 93.

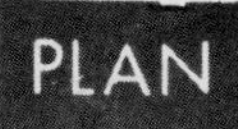

MANAGEMENT AND PATIENT EDUCATION

The patient should be hospitalized. Since there is no possibility of fetal survival in inevitable abortion, oxytocin is administered intravenously (20 units per 1000 ml of lactated Ringer's solution) to promote delivery of the fetus. Analgesics may be required to relieve pain and apprehension.

After the fetus has passed, curettage may be necessary if there is any possibility of retained placental tissue.

The Rh-negative, unsensitized patient should be given Rh immune globulin prophylaxis.

See Incomplete Abortion.

Incomplete Abortion

Even when the fetus and placenta appear to be expelled as an intact conceptus, some placental tissue frequently tears loose and remains adherent to the uterine wall.

SUBJECTIVE DATA

Abdominal Pain: Suprapubic, cramping pain is the result of uterine contractions attempting to expel intrauterine contents. Initially, the pain tends to be slight and intermittent, but it gradually becomes more severe.

Vaginal Bleeding: This is the most characteristic symptom of incomplete abortion. The amount of blood lost tends to be greater than the usual menstrual flow; it may be profuse and even extensive enough to cause hypovolemic shock.

As long as placental tissue remains partially attached to the uterine wall, myometrial contraction is impaired; the blood vessels in the denuded segment of the placental site bleed profusely. The patient may pass large blood clots or recognizable fetal or placental tissue.

Menstrual Symptoms: Usually the patient has missed two menstrual periods, since incomplete abortions tend to occur approximately ten weeks after the onset of the last menstrual period.

Pregnancy Symptoms: Many patients are aware of the disappearance of subjective pregnancy symptoms. This may signify intrauterine fetal death preceding a spontaneous abortion.

OBJECTIVE DATA

PHYSICAL EXAMINATION

General Examination: Temperature is normal unless there is an associated infection. Pulse, blood pressure, and respiration are normal unless the abortion is infected or hypovolemia has resulted from excessive blood loss.

Abdominal Examination: The abdomen is usually soft and nontender.

Pelvic Examination: On speculum examination, the vagina frequently contains numerous blood clots and the cervix appears dilated and effaced. Placental tissue may be visible in the cervical os or vagina.

On vaginal examination, the cervix is soft, dilated, and effaced. Placental tissue or blood clots or both may be palpable. The uterus is enlarged and softened. Adnexal areas are normal.

The diagnosis is established by the visualization of placental or fetal tissue.

LABORATORY TESTS

Complete Blood Count with Blood Smear: The white blood count is usually within normal limits unless there is an associated infection. The blood smear, hemoglobin, and hematocrit values are indicative of prior blood loss or preexisting anemia.

Urinalysis is normal.

Blood Type and Rh: Blood should be sent to the blood bank for type and Rh determinations. Whenever blood replacement is anticipated, cross-matched blood is ordered from the blood bank.

ASSESSMENT

DIFFERENTIAL DIAGNOSIS

The differential diagnosis of incomplete abortion includes threatened abortion, inevitable abortion, complete abortion, molar pregnancy, ectopic pregnancy, and torsion of an ovarian cyst.

Threatened Abortion: The cervix is closed and bleeding is minimal.

Inevitable Abortion: Once the cervix has dilated or the amniotic sac ruptures, abortion is inevitable.

Complete Abortion: Expulsion of the fetus and the intact placenta is considered a complete abortion. Bleeding is usually minimal and curettage is not required. Ergonovine or methylergonovine maleate — 0.2 mg orally three times daily for three days — may help stimulate uterine contractions.

Molar Pregnancy: The possibility of a molar pregnancy must be considered if the patient notes the passage of grapelike vesicles or if such vesicles are seen in the vagina.

Ectopic Pregnancy: When placental tissue has not been visualized, and pain and tenderness are lateral to the uterus rather than midline, the possibility of ectopic gestation must be considered.

Torsion of an Ovarian Cyst: On pelvic examination a tender adnexal mass should be palpable.

ETIOLOGIC FACTORS

Fetal death nearly always precedes spontaneous abortions occurring during the early months of pregnancy. Chromosomal abnormalities have been identified in 28 to 60 per cent of spontaneously aborted fetuses.

Radiation, virus infections (rubella and cytomegalovirus), and cytotoxic drugs have an embryotoxic potential. Exerting their effect at a particular time and in a particular concentration, they may produce abortion either by direct action on the embryo or by alteration of its chromosomal constitution.

Placental separation, particularly abnormally low implantation of the placenta, may be responsible for abortion at any stage of gestation.

Cervical and uterine abnormalities — cervical incompetence, submucous leiomyomas, and uterine developmental anomalies — may be responsible for abortion during the second trimester.

POTENTIAL COMPLICATIONS

These include septic abortion (see Septic Abortion, p. 106), shock, either hypovolemic or septic (see Shock, p. 612), and anemia.

SEVERITY OF DISEASE PROCESS

The severity of anemia or hypovolemia or both depends on the duration and quantity of bleeding. Profuse bleeding tends to persist as long as the uterine cavity contains adherent placental tissue. Patients with preexisting anemia are most susceptible to hypovolemic shock.

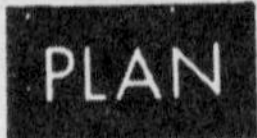

MANAGEMENT

Once any part of the products of conception has been expelled or bleeding has become excessive, prompt evacuation of the uterus is indicated in order to minimize blood loss and the risk of pelvic infection.

Hospitalization is not necessarily required; vacuum curettage can be carried out in the emergency room as an outpatient procedure. Hospitalization may be preferred for an anxious, frightened patient who requires general anesthesia for curettage. Hospitalization is also indicated for any patient with profuse blood loss, hypovolemia, severe anemia, actual or suspected intrauterine infection, an unusually large uterus, or associated medical problems.

Prior to curettage, the patient is asked to empty her bladder and intravenous fluids are initiated — usually 5 per cent dextrose in lactated Ringer's solution containing 20 units of oxytocin per 1000 ml. The oxytocin helps reduce the rate of bleeding by stimulating uterine contractions while the curettage is being performed.

Systemic analgesics [alphaprodine (Nisentil) or meperidine hydrochloride (Demerol)] or systemic sedatives [promethazine hydrochloride (Phenergan) or diazepam (Valium)] or both may be administered to reduce the patient's discomfort.

Uterine size, shape, and position are determined by bimanual examination. A sterile speculum is inserted into the vagina and the cervix visualized. The upper vagina and cervix are cleansed with a mild antiseptic solution such as povidone-iodine. The anterior lip of the cervix is grasped with a tenaculum. Any placental tissue present in the lower uterine segment or cervical canal is removed with an ovum or sponge forceps. A paracervical block using 1 per cent lidocaine may reduce the patient's discomfort.

Since the cervix is already dilated by the prior passage of fetal or placental tissue, an 8 or 10 mm suction cannula can usually be inserted easily through the cervical canal. The cannula is then attached to aspiration equipment with vacuum tubing (Fig. 9-2). Suction is built up to 70 cm Hg; the cannula is rotated gently until blood and tissue flow cease. All tissue is sent to the laboratory for pathologic examination.

If residual placental tissue is suspected after the uterine aspiration, the uterine cavity is explored with an ovum forceps or curette or both.

After the procedure has been completed, the patient may be given an intramuscular injection of 0.2 mg. of methylergonovine or ergonovine to stimulate uterine contractions and minimize any further bleeding.

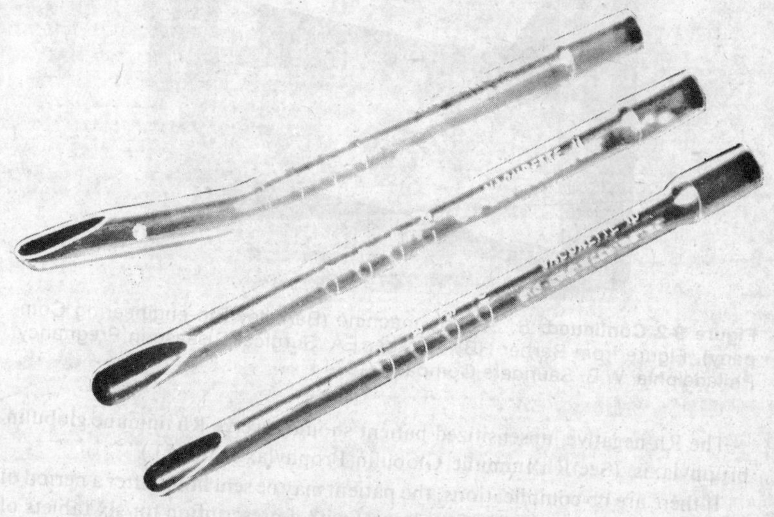

Figure 9-2. *A*, Vacurettes.

Illustration continued on the following page

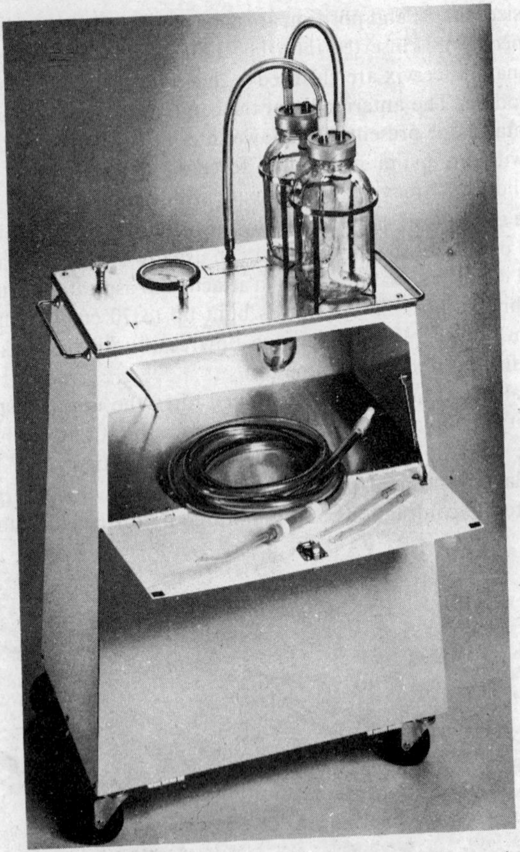

Figure 9-2 Continued. *B*, Suction machine (Berkeley Bio-engineering Company). Figure from Barber HBK, Graber EA: Surgical Disease in Pregnancy. Philadelphia, W.B. Saunders Company, 1974.)

The Rh-negative, unsensitized patient should receive Rh immune globulin prophylaxis. (See Rh Immune Globulin Prophylaxis, p. 853.)

If there are no complications, the patient may be sent home after a period of observation (usually two to four hours) with a prescription for six tablets of ergonovine or methylergonovine to be taken orally — one tablet three times daily for two days. In addition, the patient may be given a prescription for analgesic medication — acetaminophen 325 mg with codeine 30 mg, or pentazocine 50 mg. Every patient should be encouraged to take supplemental iron medication in order to restore hemoglobin concentration.

If bleeding has been profuse, blood transfusion may be required. The decision depends on the patient's clinical condition, initial hematocrit, and known blood loss.

PATIENT EDUCATION

The patient should be advised that she may have intermittent menstrual-like flow and cramps during the following week. Although she may resume her usual activities as soon as she feels well, intercourse and douching should be deferred for two weeks. The next menstrual period usually occurs within four to five weeks.

The patient should also be advised that she should seek further emergency care if bleeding becomes profuse, if severe pelvic pain develops, or if her temperature rises above 100.4° F (38° C).

A single spontaneous abortion is usually ascribed to chance. Unless specific reproductive problems are identified, the patient may be reassured that 10 to 15 per cent of all pregnancies terminate in spontaneous abortion and that conception is likely to reoccur unless she uses contraceptive precaution. For patients having their second or third abortion, follow up gynecologic evaluation is recommended.

Arrangements should be made for a follow-up visit in two weeks.

Induced Abortion: Complications

GENERAL CONSIDERATIONS

Prior to the period of fetal viability, some women request that pregnancy be terminated. In most instances, abortion is induced in a healthy woman because pregnancy is unwanted or a fetal abnormality is diagnosed. In some instances, pregnancy is terminated because of a maternal medical problem that could be exacerbated by pregnancy per se or by maternal responsibility.

During the first trimester, suction curettage is the most commonly used technique for pregnancy termination. After 16 weeks' gestation, abortion may be induced by the intraamniotic injection of hypertonic, saline, prostaglandin $F_2\alpha$, or urea.

Complications of an induced abortion may become apparent immediately or may develop a few hours or days after the patient has returned to her home.

SUBJECTIVE DATA

Abdominal pain may be caused by intrauterine infection, intraperitoneal bleeding, or intestinal injury.

Vaginal bleeding is usually due to retained placental fragments that interfere with normal uterine contractility. Other causes of bleeding include trauma or a coagulation disorder.

Fever may indicate uterine infection and possibly septicemia.

Convulsions or coma may result from water intoxication or severe hypernatremia. This has occurred with the use of intraamniotic hypertonic saline accompanied by the intravenous administration of oxytocin infusion. Thirst and headache may be symptoms of mild hypernatremia.

Nausea, vomiting, diarrhea, or bronchospasm may be associated with the administration of prostaglandins. Nausea, vomiting, and mental confusion are also early symptoms of water intoxication.

Essential diagnostic information includes the date of the last menstrual period, the gestational age of the fetus, and the date and method of the abortion.

OBJECTIVE DATA

PHYSICAL EXAMINATION

General Examination: Shock, hypotension, and tachycardia may signify profuse hemorrhage, either external or concealed. Shock may also result from sepsis. (See Shock, p. 612.)

Abdominal Examination: Tenderness of the abdomen, particularly rebound tenderness, suggests peritoneal irritation due to infection or intraabdominal bleeding.

Pelvic Examination: Speculum examination may disclose vaginal or cervical trauma, as well as the quantity and extent of active bleeding.

Bimanual examination determines the uterine size. When a mass is palpable adjacent to the uterus the possibility of uterine perforation with a broad ligament hematoma must be considered. (The uterine perforation may or may not have been recognized during the abortion procedure). If the uterine size is compatible with that present at the calculated gestational age or larger, it is possible that the abortion has not been completed and that products of conception still remain in the uterus.

LABORATORY TESTS

Complete Blood Count and Blood Smear: Hemoglobin and hematocrit values are indicators of blood loss. Serial determinations are particularly helpful in the evaluation of continued concealed bleeding. Leukocytosis, with increased neutrophils and band forms, suggests intrauterine infection.

Urinalysis: The presence of blood or red cells in the urine suggests the possibility of urinary tract trauma.

Blood Type and Rh: Blood should be sent to the blood bank to be typed and cross-matched for transfusion when indicated.

ASSESSMENT

Complications of suction curettage include

1. Hemorrhage due to
   a. Incomplete evacuation of the products of conception and resulting uterine atony
   b. Incomplete involution of the uterus or placental site
   c. Uterine lacerations or perforations
2. Infection — endometritis, parametritis, peritonitis, pelvic abscess
3. Uterine perforation. Most injuries are caused by cervical dilators and usually involve the isthmus. Occasionally, fundal injuries may occur.

Although many perforations are asymptomatic, the possibility of intra-abdominal hemorrhage, laceration of the uterine artery with broad ligament hematoma, or damage to the omentum or small bowel must be considered. (See Uterine Perforation, p. 670.)

4. Cervical laceration

Complications of intraamniotic hypertonic saline administration include

1. Hemorrhage due to retained placental tissue, trauma, uterine atony, or coagulation defects
2. Infection — endometritis, parametritis
3. Cervical rupture, which although rare may occur if the cervix does not dilate properly
4. Mild hypernatremia, which may develop in approximately 1 of 200 patients. Signs and symptoms include thirst, headache, and cardiorespiratory abnormalities (hypotension and bradycardia). Sudden hypernatremia, resulting from either intravascular injection or rapid absorption of hypertonic saline, may cause cardiovascular collapse. Severe hypernatremia characterized by the development of convulsive seizures or coma is a life-threatening crisis that occurs rarely.
5. Water intoxication associated with intraamniotic saline does not seem to be directly related to the saline instillation but rather to the use of high doses of oxytocin in association with a substantial intake of electrolyte free fluids, since oxytocin has a dose-related antidiuretic effect. (Burnett, 1974). Clinical symptoms in addition to oliguria include headache, confusion, and changes in the state of consciousness progressing to coma and seizures.
6. Coagulation defects. Disseminated intravascular coagulation is a rare complication apparently caused by tissue thromboplastin released into the maternal circulation either from the placenta or from the amniotic fluid. In a review of over 4000 saline-induced abortions, Cohen and Ballard (1974) found only ten cases of serious coagulopathy.

Complications of intraamniotic prostaglandin $F_2\alpha$ include nausea, vomiting, diarrhea, and rarely, bronchospasm. Although cervical rupture has occurred following intraamniotic prostaglandin, this complication would be expected mostly when laminaria tents have not facilitated cervical dilatation and oxytocin infusion has induced excessive uterine contractions.

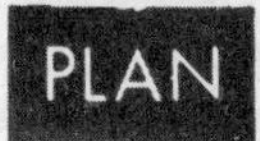

ADDITIONAL DIAGNOSTIC DATA

Abdominal x-ray may reveal free air, suggesting uterine or intestinal perforation.

Coagulation Studies: Platelet count, fibrinogen, fibrin-split products, prothrombin time, and partial thromboplastin time — may be helpful when bleeding is unexplained and disseminated intravascular coagulation is suspected (See Coagulation Disorders, p. 210.)

Serum sodium greater than 160 mEq/l indicates hypernatremia.

MANAGEMENT

When serious complications are suspected the patient should be hospitalized for observation. Intravenous fluids are initiated and blood is administered for severe anemia or hypovolemia.

Patients who continue to bleed a number of days after an induced abortion usually have retained placental tissue in the uterus. Uterine curettage and oxytocic medication are indicated. Management is essentially similar to the management of incomplete abortion.

When there is any evidence of an infection, antibiotic therapy is initiated. (See Septic Abortion, p. 106.)

Uterine Perforation: Treatment of *uterine perforation* depends on the total blood loss, both external and internal; the size and location of the injury; and the likelihood of trauma to other viscera. A simple perforation by sound or dilator can usually be managed by careful observation in the hospital. Whenever there is evidence of continued internal bleeding or damage to the bowel or omentum, exploratory laparotomy is essential in order to carry out appropriate repairs. Hysterectomy may be necessary if there is extensive damage to the lower uterine segment. When the uterus is removed, the vaginal vault is usually left open to allow drainage from the contaminated peritoneal cavity.

Laparoscopy may aid in the evaluation of intraabdominal injury. With the use of this technique, laparotomy can be avoided if unnecessary or performed more promptly if indicated. In some cases the abortion can be completed under laparoscopic visualization.

(See Uterine Perforation, p. 670.)

Cervical lacerations frequently can be repaired vaginally. Laparotomy is necessary if the tear has extended above vaginally visible areas.

Hypernatremia is treated by the intravenous administration of 5 per cent dextrose solution to accelerate urinary excretion of the excess sodium load.

Water intoxication is treated by the immediate discontinuance of oxytocin. Because of the short half-life of oxytocin, urine flow, in the absence of renal damage, can be expected to resume within about 30 minutes. In severe cases, with seizures, coma, and documented hyponatremia, 500 ml of hypertonic (5 per cent) sodium chloride solution may hasten recovery.

Coagulation disorders are usually managed with intravenous fluids and blood replacement. In general, the bleeding diathesis ceases, and coagulation factors rapidly return toward normal, as soon as the abortion is completed. The need for fresh-frozen plasma and platelet packs would depend on the clinical condition. (See Coagulation Disorders, p. 210.)

Missed Abortion

Missed abortion is defined as the prolonged retention of the products of conception after the death of the fetus.

SUBJECTIVE DATA

Vaginal spotting or staining may be persistent and precipitate an emergency visit.

Menstrual Symptoms: Usually, the patient is aware of an interval of amenorrhea and reports that her last normal menstrual period occurred three to five months previously.

Pregnancy Symptoms: Although early pregnancy has been normal with amenorrhea, morning nausea, breast changes, and abdominal enlargement, these symptoms often cease after fetal death.

Other Symptoms: Rarely, skin ecchymoses, epistaxis, or bleeding gums may be the patient's only symptom, representing an associated coagulation defect.

OBJECTIVE DATA

PHYSICAL EXAMINATION

General examination findings are usually completely normal. Rarely, skin ecchymoses may be observed, suggesting the possibility of an associated coagulation disorder.

Abdominal Examination: The uterus may or may not be palpable on abdominal examination. When palpable, uterine size is smaller than expected considering the dates of the last normal menstrual period.

Fetal heart tones are not audible.

Pelvic Examination: The cervical os is closed. Although the uterus usually feels enlarged and softened, the size is smaller than expected for the presumed length of gestation.

LABORATORY TESTS

Complete Blood Count and Blood Smear: Decreased platelets may be the first clue to an associated coagulation disorder.

Urinalysis is normal.

ASSESSMENT

DIFFERENTIAL DIAGNOSIS

The differential diagnosis includes threatened abortion and delayed ovulation.

Although a missed abortion should be suspected when the uterine size is smaller than expected for the duration of amenorrhea, the possibility of delayed ovulation coupled with a viable intrauterine pregnancy must always be considered. After discontinuation of the use of oral contraceptive medications, for example, ovulation is frequently delayed two or more months after the last withdrawal bleeding. Under these circumstances, a patient may believe herself to be five months pregnant, when, in reality, she is only two months pregnant. A pregnancy test for chorionic gonadotropin or ultrasound B-scan or both may be helpful in diagnosis.

COMPLICATIONS

Those to be anticipated include coagulation defects that may be associated with a retained dead fetus.

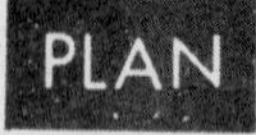

ADDITIONAL DIAGNOSTIC DATA

Pregnancy Test for Chorionic Gonadotropin: This is usually negative.

Ultrasound B-scan may demonstrate the absence of a normal gestational sac with irregular fragmented echoes within the uterus consistent with fetal demise (Fig. 9-3).

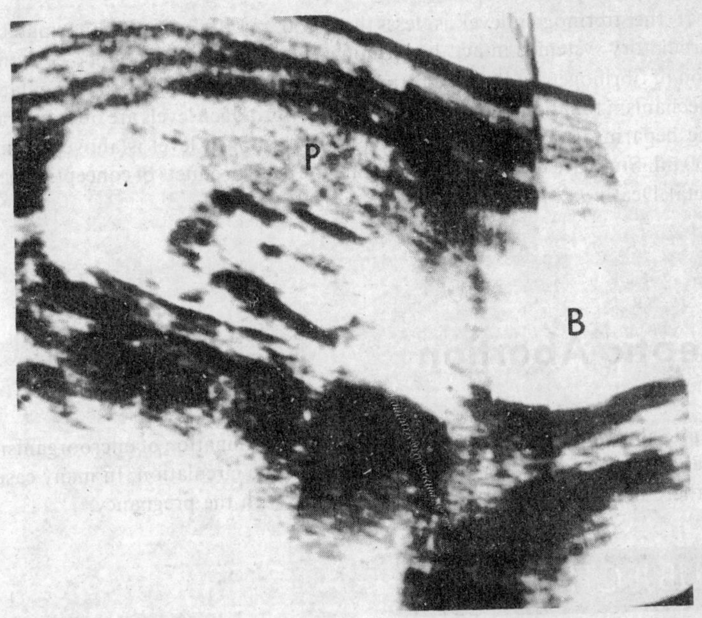

Figure 9-3. Ultrasound B-scan of the uterus of a patient 22 weeks pregnant. The uterine size is consistent with a pregnancy of only 12 weeks' gestation. The compact central echoes, which are disproportionate to uterine size, indicate the fetal residua of a missed abortion. (From Sanders BC, Conrad MR: Sonography in obstetrics. Radiol Clin North Am *13*:435-455, 1975.)

Coagulation tests—fibrinogen, fibrin-split products, and platelet count — assess the possibility of a coagulation disorder.

MANAGEMENT AND PATIENT EDUCATION

As long as the fibrinogen level is above 150 mg/100 ml and fetal death is certain, the uterus should be emptied. The cervix may be dilated with laminaria tents. The uterus less than 14 to 16 weeks' size can be emptied by suction curettage. If the uterus is larger, intraamniotic prostaglandin injection may be followed after six hours with intravenous oxytocin (50 to 100 units per 1000 ml of 5 per cent dextrose in lactated Ringer's solution). The Rh-negative patient should receive Rh immune globulin prophylaxis.

If the fibrinogen level is less than 150 mg/100 ml and the maternal circulatory system is intact, heparin may block further pathologic consumption of fibrinogen and other clotting factors and thereby allow the coagulation mechanism to repair spontaneously. Serial fibrinogen levels are obtained, and the heparin discontinued as soon as the fibrinogen level is above 200 mg/100 ml. Steps are then taken to evacuate the dead products of conception. (See Fetal Death *in Utero*, p. 344.)

Septic Abortion

Septic abortion is an infected abortion, with dissemination of microorganisms and their products into the maternal systemic circulation. In many cases, there has been some external interference with the pregnancy.

SUBJECTIVE DATA

CURRENT SYMPTOMS

Abdominal pain associated with a septic abortion is usually suprapubic, severe, and constant. In cases of parametritis and peritonitis more diffuse abdominal pain is evident.

Vaginal Bleeding: The amount of bleeding is variable. Some patients bleed minimally, whereas others have profuse hemorrhage.

Menstrual Symptoms: Most patients with a septic abortion are aware of their pregnancy and report that their last normal menstrual period had occurred two or more months prior to the onset of current symptoms.

Chills and fever are characteristic symptoms of serious infection. The patient often feels weak and is extremely ill.

PRIOR HISTORY

Septic abortion may follow an induced abortion or may be associated with an intrauterine device.

OBJECTIVE DATA

PHYSICAL EXAMINATION

General Examination: The patient is usually febrile, with a temperature above 102° F. Normal or subnormal temperature associated with hypotension and tachycardia suggests endotoxic shock. Hypotension and tachycardia can also be caused by intraperitoneal bleeding secondary to uterine perforation or laceration or both.

Abdominal Examination: Suprapubic tenderness is a characteristic finding. Generalized abdominal tenderness with rebound tenderness, guarding, rigidity, or distention indicates peritoneal involvement.

Pelvic Examination: On speculum examination, products of conception or a bloody, purulent discharge may be seen in the vagina. The cervix may be dilated, with a foul-smelling discharge exuding from the external os.

On bimanual examination, the uterus is usually enlarged and tender. Cervical motion is very painful. Often the internal os is dilated and admits one finger. Broad ligament tenderness is evidence of parametritis and pelvic cellulitis.

LABORATORY TESTS

Complete Blood Count with Blood Smear: The white cell count almost invariably is elevated, with increased neutrophils and bands on the differential smear. The peripheral smear should also be screened for any evidence of hemolysis.

Urinalysis is normal unless there is associated hemolysis or urinary tract infection.

Blood Type and Rh: Blood should be cross-matched for transfusion if necessary.

ASSESSMENT

DIFFERENTIAL DIAGNOSIS

This includes the very rare cases of cervical pregnancy or other ectopic pregnancies that may present as a septic abortion.

ETIOLOGIC FACTORS

Uterine Instrumentation: Many cases of septic abortion are associated with nonsterile attempts to terminate the pregnancy.

Intrauterine devices have been associated with septic abortions.

Bacteria: An abortion may become infected by exogenous or endogenous organisms. In the presence of necrotic tissue, normally nonvirulent anaerobic organisms endogenous to the genital tract may become pathogenic.

POTENTIAL COMPLICATIONS

These include peritonitis (localized or generalized), bacteremia, septicemia, pelvic abscess, intravascular hemolysis, shock (septic or hemorrhagic), pelvic thrombophlebitis, disseminated intravascular coagulation, and renal failure.

SEVERITY OF DISEASE PROCESS

Temperature spiking to 104°, shaking chills, and a leukocytosis greater than 20,000 are manifestations of a severe, fulminating infection. These patients appear severely ill, invariably have an associated bacteremia or peritonitis, and may be on the verge of septic shock.

Abortion complicated by clostridial sepsis and intense hemolysis is a highly lethal disease. Immediate diagnosis must be attempted by Gram-stain cervical smear, abdominal x-ray for intrauterine gas, and evaluation of the serum for hemolysis.

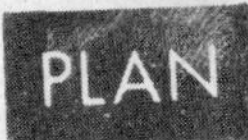

ADDITIONAL DIAGNOSTIC DATA

Gram Stain and Bacteriologic Culture: A specimen should be taken from the cervical os and any purulent placental tissue for Gram stain and culture. The Gram stain provides a presumptive bacteriologic diagnosis and is particularly helpful when clostridia are suspected. A list of Gram-stain characteristics of common organisms follows:

Gram-negative intracellular diplococci — Neisseria
Gram-positive cocci — streptococci
Gram-positive rods — clostridia (Fig. 9-4)

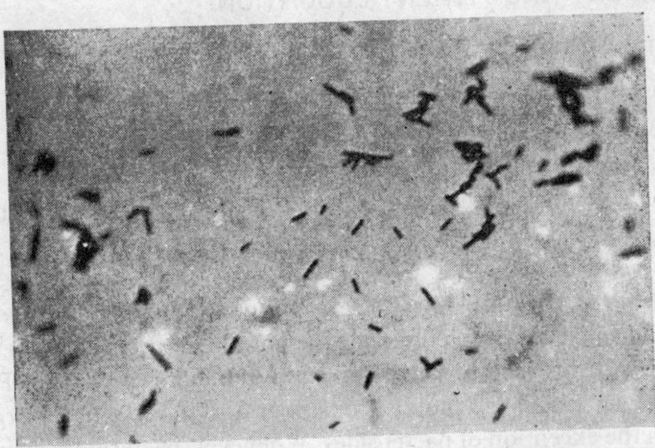

Figure 9-4. Clostridial gas gangrene. (From Frobisher M Jr, Sommermeyer L, Goodale RH: Microbiology and Pathology for Nurses. 5th edition. Philadelphia. W.B. Saunders Company, 1960.)

Gram-negative rods — Bacteroides, enteric bacilli

Blood should be drawn for aerobic and anaerobic cultures.

Coagulation tests—fibrinogen, fibrin-split products, prothrombin time, partial thromboplastin time, and platelet count — should be performed. Gross disruption of the coagulation mechanism is an uncommon but serious complication of septic abortion.

Abdominal X-ray (Three Way): Abdominal x-rays may reveal free air, suggesting uterine or intestinal perforations; the presence of a foreign body in the uterus or peritoneal cavity; or intrauterine gas, suggesting clostridia.

Other Blood Tests: Additional blood tests that may be helpful include blood urea nitrogen and creatinine to evaluate the renal status and electrolyte determinations to assess electrolyte balance. If hemolysis is suspected, a serum hemoglobin may be helpful.

Urine Output: Urine output should always be closely monitored. Oliguria combined with hypotension may be the result of blood loss, clostridial sepsis, or endotoxic shock.

MANAGEMENT AND PATIENT EDUCATION

General Therapeutic Principles:

1. Infection must be controlled with appropriate antibiotics.
2. Effective intravascular volume must be maintained in order to provide adequate tissue perfusion.
3. The uterus must be evacuated at the earliest possible time.

Specific Measures: The patient should be hospitalized.

Antibiotic therapy is initiated intravenously even before specific organisms have been cultured. The antibiotics are chosen on the basis of organisms seen on the Gram stain of the cervical smear. Penicillin and gentamicin in combination cover all the most likely organisms, with the exception of bacteroides. Whenever, bacteroides is suspected, clindamycin, chloramphenicol, or carbenicillin should be selected.

Initial intravenous dosages are

Penicillin: 3 to 5 million units every four hours
Gentamicin: 60 to 80 mg every eight hours
Clindamycin: 450 to 600 mg every six hours
Carbenicillin: 5 grams every four hours.

As soon as the specific responsible bacteria have been identified on culture and antibiotic sensitivities have been established, unnecessary antibiotics are discontinued.

Intravenous Fluids with Oxytocin: Twenty to 40 units of oxytocin diluted in 1000 ml of 5 per cent dextrose in lactated Ringer's solution aid in the expulsion of infected intrauterine contents. In addition, oxytocin stimulates uterine contraction, to diminish uterine bleeding.

Blood transfusions are administered as indicated, depending on the degree of anemia and blood loss.

Curettage: The uterus should be evacuated promptly. Large pieces of necrotic tissue may be removed with a ring forceps. Suction curettage is usually the most efficient method.

Rh immune globulin is administered to the Rh-negative, unsensitized patient.

Exploratory laparotomy is necessary if there is any evidence of active intraperitoneal bleeding or intestinal injury following a traumatic uterine perforation, or if an intraperitoneal foreign body is seen on X-ray.

Hysterectomy is usually advised when clostridial sepsis is accompanied by overt hemolysis; the uterus has been traumatized grossly, clostridial gas formation with necrosis being present, or the patient fails to improve within 48 to 72 hours despite curettage and vigorous medical therapy.

REFERENCES

Beric B, Kupresanin M, Kapor-Stanulovic N: Accidents and sequelae of medical abortions. Am J Obstet Gynecol *116*:813-821, 1973

Boue J, Boue A, Lazar P: Retrospective and prospective epidemiological studies of 1500 karyotyped spontaneous human abortions. Teratology *12*:11-26, 1975; Obstet Gynecol Surv *31*:617-620, 1976

Brenner WE: Second trimester interruption of pregnancy. In Taymor ML, Green TH: Progress in Gynecology. Vol 6. New York, Grune & Stratton, 1975, pp. 421-444

Burman RT, Atienza MF, King TM, et al: Intra-amniotic urea and prostaglandin $F_2\alpha$ for midtrimester abortion: a modified regimen. Am J Obstet Gynecol *126*:328-333, 1976

Burnett LS, Wentz AC, King TM: Techniques of pregnancy termination. Obstet Gynecol Surv *29*:6-42, 1974

Chow AW, Marshall JR, Guze LB: Anaerobic infections of the female genital tract. Obstet Gynecol Surv *30*:477-494, 1975

Cohen E, Ballard CA: Consumptive coagulopathy associated with intra-amniotic saline instillation and the effect of intravenous oxytocin. Obstet Gynecol *43*:300-303, 1974

Eaton CJ, Peterson EP: Diagnosis and acute management of patients with advanced clostridial sepsis complicating abortion. Am J Obstet Gynecol *109*:1162-1166, 1971

Jouppila P, Koivisto M: The prognosis in pregnancy after threatened abortion. Ann Chir Gynaecol Fenn *63*:439-444, 1974; Obstet Gynecol Surv *30*:506-507, 1975

McDonald TW, Aaro LA: Medical complications of induced abortions. South Med J *67*:560-566, 1974; Obstet Gynecol Surv *30*:30-33, 1975

Nathanson BN: Ambulatory abortion: experience with 26,000 cases. N Engl J Med *286*:403-407, 1972

Pritchard JA, Whalley PJ: Abortion complicated by *Clostridium perfringers* infection. Am J Obstet Gynecol *111*:484-492, 1971

10 ACCIDENTAL TRAUMA DURING PREGNANCY

GENERAL CONSIDERATIONS

Minor accidental injuries are common occurrences during pregnancy. Fainting spells, hyperventilation, and easy fatigability set the stage for accidents during early pregnancy; the protuberant abdomen and loosening of the pelvic joints are responsible for unsteadiness during the later stages of gestation.

The developing infant is well protected within the confines of the uterine cavity. Amniotic fluid acts as an excellent shock absorber, and it is extremely rare for a fetus to experience physical trauma as a result of anything but direct penetrating wounds or extensive blunt trauma.

Serious accidental injuries (automobile accidents, stabbings, and gunshot wounds) are no more likely to occur during pregnancy than during the nonpregnant state. If an accident does occur, however, increased vascularity surrounding the gravid uterus renders a patient more vulnerable to hemorrhage.

SUBJECTIVE DATA

Abdominal pain may be caused by any serious injury during pregnancy. The likelihood of uterine injury depends on the gestational age as well as on the extent of the trauma. Whenever a pregnant patient complains of diffuse intra-abdominal pain following a traumatic injury, intraperitoneal hemorrhage must be suspected. If pain is confined to the uterus and associated with an increased uterine tone, the possibility of premature placental separation must be considered.

Vaginal bleeding may be the earliest symptom of placental separation preceding abortion or premature labor. Vaginal bleeding may also be associated with a traumatic injury to any portion of the genital tract.

Other Symptoms:

Loss of consciousness is an indication of the severity of the trauma and may be a symptom of occult bleeding.

Absence of Fetal Movements: Women become aware of fetal movements between the sixteenth and twentieth weeks of gestation. Sudden cessation of previously active fetal movements is an ominous sign portending fetal demise. Occasionally, excessive fetal activity may be noted.

Electronic monitoring of the fetal heart rate provides the most accurate estimate of fetal well-being.

OBJECTIVE DATA

PHYSICAL EXAMINATION

General Examination: Pulse, blood pressure, and respiration are indicators of the patient's general condition. Tachycardia and hypotension may be early signs of intraperitoneal bleeding, ruptured viscus, or premature placental separation.

Fractured bones, actively bleeding lacerations, contusions, and hematomas are evidence of extensive traumatic injury.

Abdominal Examination: Contusions or hematomas of the abdominal wall are an indication of the severity of the injury. Diffuse abdominal tenderness with rebound tenderness suggests intraperitoneal hemorrhage.

Uterine tenderness, particularly if associated with increased uterine tone, suggests premature placental separation. (See Placenta, Premature Separation, p. 502.) Palpable uterine contractions suggest premature labor.

Auscultation of the fetal heart provides an initial assessment of fetal life. If the pregnancy is close to viability and fetal heart tones are absent, either uterine rupture or premature placental separation must be suspected.

LABORATORY TESTS

Complete Blood Count with Blood Smear: Hemoglobin and hematocrit determinations provide an estimate of blood loss. Serially decreasing values suggest occult bleeding.

Urinalysis: Hematuria suggests an associated injury to the urinary tract.

Blood Type and Rh: Blood should be sent to the blood bank to be cross-matched in order that transfusions can be administered if necessary.

ASSESSMENT

DIFFERENTIAL DIAGNOSIS

Fetal Injury or Death: Severe trauma may cause fetal injury or death. The most commonly reported fetal injury apparent at birth is skull fracture. Other, rarer, injuries include fractures of the tibia, clavicle, and femur.

The leading single cause of fetal death is maternal death. When the mother survives a serious accident placental separation is the most frequent cause of fetal death. Other causes of fetal death are maternal shock, with uterine artery constriction and reduced blood flow through the intervillous space; uterine rupture; and fetal head injury.

If the mother is in an automobile accident but restrained by a lap belt, fetal head injury may occur without pelvic fracture, apparently owing to compression of the fetal skull between the lap belt and the maternal spine.

Premature separation of the placenta may result from abrupt vehicular deceleration in late pregnancy. Clinical symptoms depend on the extent of the placental surface involved. If decidual bleeding is limited, only a small hematoma may form, with or without external bleeding. Larger areas of placental separation threaten fetal survival. The fetus usually dies when more than 50 per cent of the placenta has separated.

Premature placental separation should always be suspected when vaginal bleeding follows trauma. If placental separation has proceeded to the point of producing uterine tetany and fetal death, shock is usually profound; the degree of hypotension cannot be explained by the observed external bleeding. (See Placenta, Premature Separation, p. 502.)

Pelvic Fracture: Fracture of the pelvic ring during pregnancy produces not only pain and pelvic deformity but also increased risks for fetal injury and retroperitoneal hemorrhage. Retroperitoneal hemorrhage around the fracture site may be exceptionally severe because of the increased vascularity of the pelvic region during pregnancy.

Uterine Trauma and Other Injuries: Although rare, the gravid uterus can be ruptured during an automobile collision whether or not the victim wears a lap belt. With any serious injury there is always a possibility of parametrial hemorrhage. When a serious accident occurs, multiple intra-abdominal injuries may be expected. Splenic or hepatic rupture can cause profuse intraabdominal hemorrhage. Rupture of an epigastric vessel may simulate an acute abdomen or concealed placental abruption. The signs and symptoms are evidence of hidden blood loss, abdominal pain, and uterine irritability. Treatment includes blood transfusion and surgical repair.

Premature Labor or Abortion: A casual relationship between trauma and any given post-trauma abortion is difficult to establish because an abortion that occurs within a few days of the accident may have already been in progress at the time the injury occurred.

SEVERITY OF INJURY IN AUTOMOBILE ACCIDENTS

The extent of injury following automotive trauma varies considerably with the physical damage to the vehicle, the seating position of the victim, the type of collision, the weight and size of the vehicle, and the use of occupant restraints. In general, the severity of maternal and fetal injury parallels the severity of vehicular damage. Unless there is severe damage to the automobile, the likelihood of major or life-threatening injury to the pregnant occupant is minimal.

However, an *unrestrained* individual may be buffeted about the interior of the vehicle during secondary and tertiary impacts. *Ejection* increases the number and severity of the injuries; multiple fractures are frequent. Belted pregnant women are nearly immune to pelvic fracture.

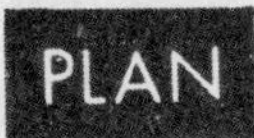

ADDITIONAL DIAGNOSTIC DATA

Abdominal X-rays: If pelvic fracture, uterine rupture, or intra-abdominal trauma is suspected, pelvic and abdominal x-ray films are indicated. During early pregnancy the risk of fetal radiation must always be carefully weighed against the need for accurate maternal evaluation.

Other X-rays: X-rays should be taken of any suspected bone fractures.

Fetal Heart-Rate Monitoring: During the immediate post-trauma period the fetal status may be assessed with electronic monitoring of the fetal heart rate and uterine contractions. Patients past 28 weeks of pregnancy should be carefully observed for any evidence of utero-placental insufficiency. Fetal monitoring reveals the frequency of spontaneous uterine contractions, the base-line fetal heart rate, and any alterations in heart rate in response to uterine contractions or spontaneous fetal movements.

Oxytocin Challenge Test: If the patient is not having spontaneous uterine contractions, an oxytocin challenge test may be used to assess the possibility of uteroplacental insufficiency. Usually this test should be performed only after the mother has been hospitalized and her general condition has well stabilized.

Amniocentesis may be indicated to evaluate the possibility of intra-amniotic bleeding as well as to obtain evidence of fetal maturity.

Culdocentesis is a relatively simple procedure for the diagnosis of intra-peritoneal bleeding.

Central Venous Pressure: When maternal hypotension and profuse bleeding are present, volume replacement should be monitored by continuous central venous pressure determinations.

MANAGEMENT

Immediate therapeutic priorities are the same whether or not the victim is pregnant: (1) adequate airway with oxygen, (2) adequate circulatory volume, (3) control of bleeding, and (4) fracture immobilization. Blood transfusions are administered as indicated for acute hemorrhage.

During late pregnancy, vena caval compression tends to occur if the patient lies supine. Since elevated venous pressure in the lower half of the body may produce increased hemorrhage in injured areas, the pregnant trauma victim should be instructed to lie on her side.

Vasoconstrictor drugs rarely are advisable for pregnant accident victims because of the extreme sensitivity of the uterine arteries to these drugs. Uterine blood flow can be so compromised by the combination of drug-induced uterine vasospasm and hypotension that the fetus may die.

Since gastric rupture is always possible in trauma victims, a nasogastric tube should be placed in every pregnant trauma victim prior to laparotomy.

Pregnancy imposes a great urgency to correct hypotension quickly. When intraperitoneal bleeding is suspected, the earlier the laparotomy and control of bleeding are achieved, the better the prognosis for both mother and fetus.

Regardless of fetal status, exploratory laparotomy is indicated after a knife wound, gunshot wound, or other penetrating injury, that is, whenever a ruptured uterus or viscus is suspected. Surgery may be required for the management of an expanding retroperitoneal hematoma associated with a pelvic fracture. Decisions concerning cesarean section at the time of laparotomy depend on the length of gestation, fetal status, and maternal status.

If the fetus is immature and there is no evidence of fetal danger, premature labor may be suppressed. (See Labor, Premature, p. 413.)

If the fetus is alive and near term, signs of placental separation may warrant immediate delivery. (See Placenta, Premature Separation, p. 502.)

In the case of a pelvic fracture, cesarean section may be recommended if the fetus is mature and vaginal delivery could disrupt the orthopedic fixation and immobilization.

REFERENCES

Crosby WM: Trauma during pregnancy: maternal and fetal injury. Obstet Gynecol Surv *29*:683-699, 1974

Mussalli NG: Uterine, fetal and placental injuries due to a motor car accident. J Obstet Gynaecol Brit Commw *79*:379-380, 1972

11 ADENOMYOSIS

DEFINITION

Adenomyosis—a benign disorder of the uterus characterized by the presence of ectopic foci of endometrial glands and stroma in the myometrium. This condition may explain the progressive secondary dysmenorrhea seen in women who have heavy menstrual bleeding associated with generalized pelvic discomfort during their late thirties and forties.

SUBJECTIVE DATA

Vaginal Bleeding: Menorrhagia (excessive or prolonged menstrual bleeding) is the most frequent symptom. Intermenstrual bleeding, irregular bleeding, and premenstrual staining are other possible symptoms. Although the precise cause of the abnormal uterine bleeding is not known, ovarian dysfunction, endometrial hyperplasia, increased uterine vascularity, and interference with myometrial contractility are possible explanations.

Pelvic Pain and Secondary Dysmenorrhea: These symptoms may be due to the painful uterine contractions induced by menstrual swelling of endometrial islands.

OBJECTIVE DATA

Pelvic Examination: The uterus may be moderately or diffusely enlarged and occasionally tender. Adnexa are normal. Associated leiomyomas may cause significant uterine enlargement.

ASSESSMENT

Differential diagnosis includes endometrial hyperplasia, endometrial malignancy, and other causes of endometrial bleeding. (See Vaginal Bleeding, p. 686.)

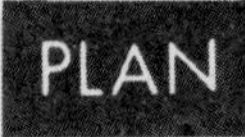

MANAGEMENT

Minor symptoms require only palliative treatment. Persistent symptoms may eventually require hysterectomy for definitive therapy.

PATIENT EDUCATION

Adenomyosis is a benign condition that is not life-threatening.

REFERENCE

Molitor JJ: Adenomyosis: A clinical and pathologic appraisal. Am J Obstet Gynecol *110*:275-284, 1971

12 ADNEXAL TORSION

GENERAL CONSIDERATIONS

Although rare, torsion (twisting) of a fallopian tube or of both a tube and an ovary (Fig. 12-1) may occur at any age — prior to puberty, during the postovulatory phase of the menstrual cycle, during pregnancy, or after the menopause. The more severe the torsion, the more likely is the development of tissue necrosis. Consequently, the clinical picture is determined by the extent of interference with the adnexal blood supply. Early abdominal surgery may permit preservation of adnexa that might otherwise become gangrenous.

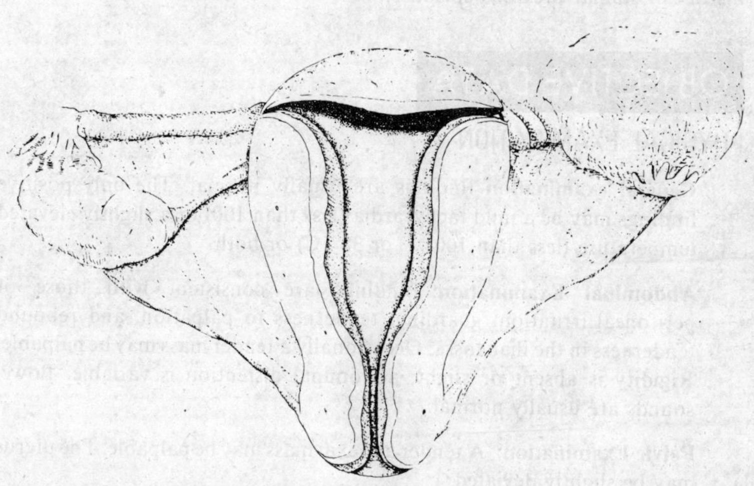

Figure 12-1. Adnexal torsion.

SUBJECTIVE DATA

CURRENT SYMPTOMS

Abdominal pain may develop suddenly or gradually. Usually sharp, paroxysmal, and intermittent, the pain tends to be unilateral and localized to the area of the involved adnexa but may radiate to the thigh or flank. The pain gradually increases in intensity as the vascular occlusion produced by torsion becomes more complete and the ischemia more extensive.

Associated Symptoms: Nausea and vomiting are variable symptoms. Some patients complain of a sense of fullness in the lower abdomen.

PRIOR HISTORY

Some patients give a history of unusual physical activity; others give a history of similar previous episodes.

OBJECTIVE DATA

PHYSICAL EXAMINATION

General examination findings are usually normal. The only positive findings may be a mild tachycardia (less than 100) or a slightly elevated temperature (less than 100° F or 38° C) or both.

Abdominal Examination: Findings are consistent with those of peritoneal irritation: guarding, tenderness to palpation, and rebound tenderness in the iliac fossa. Occasionally a tender mass may be palpable. Rigidity is absent or slight; abdominal distention is variable. Bowel sounds are usually normal.

Pelvic Examination: A tender adnexal mass may be palpable. The uterus may be slightly deviated.

Rectal Examination: In the prepuberal child, a small tender mass may be felt at the brim of the pelvis or in the lower abdomen.

LABORATORY TESTS

The white blood count is either normal or slightly elevated. Urinalysis is normal.

ASSESSMENT

DIFFERENTIAL DIAGNOSIS

Other diagnostic possibilities include appendicitis, diverticulitis, salpingitis, ectopic pregnancy, ureteral colic, ruptured follicle cyst, and twisted ovarian cyst.

Appendicitis is the preoperative diagnosis in many patients, since adnexal disease may be unrecognized until the time of surgery.

PREDISPOSING FACTORS

These include hydrosalpinx, tubal neoplasm, ovarian cysts or tumors, and paraovarian cysts. Adnexal torsion may also occur in the posthysterectomy female whose preserved adnexa were permitted to dangle loosely from the infundibulopelvic ligament.

Some patients have a history of a sudden body movement or trauma that may be a precipitating factor.

PLAN

ADDITIONAL DIAGNOSTIC DATA

Culdocentesis may help to rule out ectopic pregnancy or pelvic infection. In the case of adnexal torsion there is usually no peritoneal fluid or a minimal amount of serosanguinous fluid.

MANAGEMENT AND PATIENT EDUCATION

Although the diagnosis may be difficult to establish preoperatively, evidence of an acute surgical abdomen warrants exploratory laparotomy. If the ovary and tube are obviously strangulated and infarcted, they should be removed without untwisting the pedicle in order to avoid the possible release of thrombotic emboli. If no thrombi are evident, the adnexa are healthy and viable, and the twist is incomplete, the tube and ovary can be preserved.

Prior to surgery, the patient should be advised that removal of the tube and ovary may be necessary.

REFERENCES

Huffman JW: Gynecology of Childhood and Adolescence. Philadelphia, W.B. Saunders Company, 1968, pp. 327-328

James DF, Barber HRK, Graber EA: Torsion of normal uterine adnexa in children. Obstet Gynecol *35*:226-230, 1970

Lomano JM, Trelford JD, Ullery JC: Torsion of the uterine adnexa causing an acute abdomen. Obstet Gynecol *35*:221-225, 1970

Powell JL, Foley GP, Llorens AS: Torsion of the fallopian tube in postmenopausal women. Am J Obstet Gynecol *113*:115-118, 1972

Provost RW: Torsion of the normal fallopian tube. Obstet Gynecol *39*:80-82, 1972

13 ANAPHYLAXIS

DEFINITION

Anaphylaxis—an acute, life-threatening allergic reaction in which hypotension, bronchospasm, urticaria, diffuse erythema, pruritus, laryngeal edema, cardiac arrhythmias, and hyperperistalsis occur either in combination or as isolated manifestations. The mechanism of the reaction involves the interaction of antigen and antibody in a suitably immunized individual, with the release of pharmacologically active mediators causing the clinical manifestations.

GENERAL CONSIDERATIONS

Drugs that are most likely to be associated with an anaphylactic reaction or an acute systemic reaction include penicillin, radiographic contrast media, sodium sulfobromophthalein (Bromsulphalein), iron dextran injection, nitrofurantoin, and local anesthetics. Other antigens associated with anaphylaxis include foreign antisera, allergen extracts, hormones, and venoms from various insects, especially bees and wasps. Typically, the reaction develops rapidly, reaching a maximum within 5 to 30 minutes.

SUBJECTIVE DATA

The symptom complex may involve the respiratory tract, cardiovascular system, skin, eyes, and gastrointestinal tract, either singly or in combination.

Respiratory symptoms are the most common clinical manifestations of anaphylaxis and include dyspnea, wheezing, and cough . Symptoms are due to bronchospasm or laryngeal edema. Nasal congestion and itching are due to rhinitis.

Cardiovascular Symptoms: Syncope or a feeling of faintness may be due to hypotension. Uneasiness, anxiety, and restlessness are other symptoms that may develop suddenly and presage an acute anaphylactic reaction.

Cutaneous symptoms, also common, include erythema, itching, skin wheals, swelling of an extremity, and perioral or periorbital edema. Cyanosis or pallor or both may be caused by the severe anoxia associated with anaphylactic shock.

Ocular symptoms include itching and lacrimation.

Gastrointestinal symptoms include abdominal cramps, nausea, vomiting, and diarrhea.

OBJECTIVE DATA

PHYSICAL EXAMINATION

General Examination: Tachycardia, hypotension, and tachypnea are signs of anaphylactic shock. A severe anaphylactic reaction can cause cardiac arrest. Cyanosis may be due to laryngeal edema or bronchospasm. Urticaria or angioedema or both may be present.

Pulmonary Examination: Wheezing, rales, respiratory distress, and tachypnea are caused by laryngeal edema or bronchospasm.

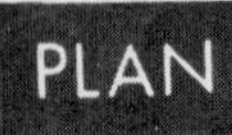

MANAGEMENT

Epinephrine is the initial treatment of choice and is generally the most effective therapy. A dose of 0.3 to 1.0 mg is administered subcutaneously or intramuscularly (0.3 to 1.0 ml of 1:1000 epinephrine). If shock is profound, 1.0 ml of a 1:10,000 solution of epinephrine is administered intravenously (0.1 ml of 1:1000 solution mixed with 10 ml of normal saline). Prompt therapy is essential. Tourniquets may be applied proximal to the injection site, or epinephrine may be injected locally at the injection site to slow the absorption of the antigen.

Adequate ventilation, oxygenation, and artificial respiration if necessary are included in essential supportive therapy. Intubation or tracheotomy must be considered if the patient shows any evidence of airway obstruction.

Intravenous fluids with 1000 ml of 5 per cent dextrose in water are initiated immediately.

Antihistamines are competitive inhibitors of histamine at the target cell. Because histamine has been implicated as a mediator of anaphylaxis, an antihistamine is prescribed intravenously or intramuscularly. Diphenhydramine hydrochloride (Benadryl), 50 mg, or an equivalent drug is recommended.

Aminophylline is a potent bronchodilator and is particularly helpful if bronchospasm has not responded to epinephrine. A dose of 250 to 500 mg is administered slowly intravenously. Persistent bronchospasm requires therapy similar to that for status asthmaticus. Monitoring of blood gases is necessary for the evaluation of pulmonary function. Intubation and assisted ventilation may be required in severe cases progressing to respiratory failure.

Vasopressor agents may be indicated for severe hypotension. If 15 to 100 mg of metaraminol bitartrate are diluted in 500 ml of 5 per cent dextrose solution, the rate of infusion is adjusted to the blood pressure response. During pregnancy, however, the risk of impaired uterine blood flow must be considered.

Corticosteroids may also provide a beneficial effect, particularly in severe cases. Dexamethasone, 4 to 20 mg intravenously, or methylprednisolone, 20 to 100 mg intravenously, may be given at four-hour intervals for 24 to 48 hours, depending on the duration of the reaction.

An outline of suggested therapy for anaphylaxis is provided in Table 13-1.

REFERENCE

Kelly JF, Patterson R: Anaphylaxis. JAMA *227*:1431-1436, 1974

TABLE 13-1. Outline of Suggested Therapy for Anaphylaxis*

Reaction	Immediate Treatment	Supportive Treatment	
		Mild	*Severe*
Conjunctivitis Rhinitis Urticaria Pruritus Erythema	Epinephrine hydrochloride,† 0.3 ml of 1:1000 IM‡ Diphenhydramine hydrochloride, 50 mg orally	Diphenhydramine hydrochloride, every six hr	—
Laryngeal edema	Epinephrine hydrochloride, 0.3 ml of 1:1000 IM Diphenhydramine hydrochloride, 50 mg IV§	Diphenhydramine hydrochloride, 50 mg every six hr Ephedrine sulfate, 25 mg every six hr	Oxygen Monitor blood gases Tracheostomy Diphenhydramine hydrochloride 50 mg every six hr Ephedrine sulfate, 25 mg every six hr Hydrocortisone
Bronchospasm	Epinephrine hydrochloride, 0.3 ml of 1:1000 IM‡ Diphenhydramine hydrochloride, 50 mg IV§ (one dose only)	Epinephrine hydrochloride, 0.3 ml of 1:1000 IM Aminophylline, 250 mg IV over ten min	Oxygen Monitor blood gases Aminophylline, 500 mg IV§ every six hr Intravenous fluids Hydrocortisone Observe for respiratory failure

TABLE 13-1. Outline of Suggested Therapy for Anaphylaxis* (Continued)

Reaction	Immediate Treatment	Supportive Treatment: Mild	Supportive Treatment: Severe
Hypotension	Epinephrine hydrochloride, 0.3 ml of 1:1000 IM‡ Diphenhydramine hydrochloride, 50 mg IV§	Metaraminol bitartrate, 100 mg in 1000 ml of 5 per cent dextrose in water	Oxygen Metaraminol bitartrate or norepinephrine IV Monitor urine output Monitor ECG Monitor blood volume Intravenous fluids Isoproterenol hydrochloride in normovolemic low cardiac output hypotension
Arrhythmia			Treat primary manifestations with oxygen, vasopressors Treat arrhythmia with antiarrhythmic agents

* From Kelly JF, Patterson R: Anaphylaxis. JAMA *227*:1431-1436, 1974.
† Initial drug to be used: See text regarding route of administration.
‡ IM indicates intramuscularly.
§ IV indicates intravenously.

14 ANEMIA DURING PREGNANCY

GENERAL CONSIDERATIONS

Anemia is a condition in which either the number of circulating red blood cells or their hemoglobin concentration is decreased. As a result, there is decreased transport of oxygen from the lung to the peripheral tissues. During pregnancy, anemia is common and is usually due to iron deficiency, secondary either to previous blood loss or to inadequate iron intake.

Although anemia, per se, rarely creates an acute emergency crisis during pregnancy, virtually every emergency problem can be aggravated by pre-existing anemia.

By the thirty-sixth week of pregnancy, maternal blood volume increases an average of 40 to 50 per cent over that of the nonpregnant state. Despite augmented erythropoiesis and an increased red cell volume, more plasma is added to the maternal circulation. Consequently, the hemoglobin concentration as well as the hematocrit decreases during pregnancy.

SUBJECTIVE DATA

CURRENT SYMPTOMS

Fatigue and general weakness may be the only symptoms of decreased oxygen-carrying capacity. Many patients are asymptomatic even with a moderate degree of anemia.

Palpitations or dyspnea at rest or both are rarely noted unless the hemoglobin is 5 gm or less. Even more rarely, bone, joint, or abdominal pains may be caused by thrombotic crises associated with sickle cell anemia or hemoglobin SC disease.

PRIOR HISTORY

A prior history of refractory anemia, frequent infections, or cholelithiasis, or a family history of anemia suggest the possibility of a genetic hemoglobinopathy.

OBJECTIVE DATA

PHYSICAL EXAMINATION

General Examination: Tachycardia, tachypnea, and a widened pulse pressure are compensatory mechanisms to increase blood flow and the delivery of oxygen to the major organs. The skin and conjunctiva appear pale. Jaundice may be observed with a hemolytic anemia.

Other physical findings associated with severe anemias include cardiomegaly, a "hemic" murmur, hepatomegaly, and splenomegaly.

LABORATORY TESTS

Complete Blood Count and Blood Smear: For practical purposes, anemia during pregnancy may be defined as a hemoglobin of less than 10 or 11 grams/100 ml and a hematocrit of less than 30 to 33 per cent (McFee, 1973) see Normal Laboratory Values, p. 67.

The peripheral blood smear provides an evaluation of red cell morphology, the differential white cell count, and an estimate of platelet adequacy.

Definitions of common terms are the following:

Anisocytosis—variability in size of red cells.
Poikilocytosis—variability in shape of red cells.
Hypochromia—decreased hemoglobin content of red cells.

Hypochromia and microcytosis are characteristic of iron deficiency anemia as well as of the anemia of infection.

Basophilic or polychromatophilic macrocytes are an indication of increased erythropoiesis, which may be associated with hemorrhage or hemolysis.

Oval macrocytes, with an increased number of lobules in the polymorphonuclear leukocytes, are seen with megaloblastic anemia.

Target cells are seen in hemoglobinopathies (thalassemia and so forth).

Hypersegmentation of neutrophil nuclei may be seen in the early stages of folic acid deficiency and may predict megaloblastic anemia. More than 3 per cent of polymorphonuclear leukocytes with five or more nuclear segments is indicative of folate insufficiency.

Fragmented red cells, schistocytes, burr cells, helmet cells, and other bizarre forms, as well as decreased platelets, are seen in microangiopathic hemolytic anemia.

Anisocytosis and persistent reticulocytosis, with or without nucleated red cells, are associated with hemolytic disorders.

ASSESSMENT

DIFFERENTIAL DIAGNOSIS

Microcytic Hypochromic Anemia (MCV<80; MCHC<30): Red cell production is normal, but hemoglobin synthesis is impaired. Iron deficiency interferes with heme synthesis. Thalassemia impairs globin synthesis. The cells are small, with decreased hemoglobin concentration. *Serum iron* values help distinguish the two disorders: serum iron is decreased with iron deficiency and normal (or increased) with thalassemia.

Macrocytic megaloblastic anemia is caused by any disorder that interferes with cellular DNA synthesis but allows normal hemoglobinization (for example, folate deficiency).

Normocytic normochromic anemia is associated with excessive blood loss or impaired bone marrow activity.

ETIOLOGIC FACTORS

Blood Loss (Acute or Chronic, Internal or External, Overt or Occult): Overt blood loss (from vaginal bleeding, epistaxis, and so forth) is an obvious explanation for anemia. Occult blood loss may be due to gastrointestinal bleeding. Whenever occult blood loss is suspected, the stool should be examined through a guaiac or similar test.

Nutritional Deficiencies:

Iron deficiency anemia is a consequence of dietary iron deficiency or depleted iron reserves from prior pregnancies, menstrual loss, or occult bleeding. Normally, the total body iron is 3500 to 4000 mg. Approximately 70 per cent is contained in the circulating hemoglobin; 25 per cent is stored as ferritin in the bone marrow, spleen, and liver; and the remainder is in myoglobin and oxidative enzymes.

Iron is absorbed in its ferrous state from the upper small intestine. The amount absorbed depends on the amount ingested and on the body needs. Usual absorption is in the range of 5 to 15 per cent.

During a normal pregnancy approximately 1000 mg of iron are required by the fetus and placenta and for increased maternal red cell volume. At delivery, a minimum of 300 to 350 mg of iron are lost with the fetus and placenta. In addition, the average amount of blood lost at delivery contains 150 mg of iron (100 ml of blood contains 50 mg of iron). Consequently, the minimal net cost of pregnancy is approximately 500 mg of iron. Additional iron is lost if bleeding is more than average. Women with depleted iron stores are unable to meet the iron needs of pregnancy and consequently iron deficiency anemia results. (With twins, the fetal iron requirements are even greater; iron deficiency is common.)

Folate Deficiency: Megaloblastic anemia of pregnancy results from dietary folic acid deficiency or a defect in the normal conversion of folic acid into folinic acid. This is rarely seen in the United States.

The diagnosis is suggested by the presence of a macrocytic anemia on peripheral smear and verified by the identification of abnormal megaloblasts on bone marrow examination. Other laboratory findings are neutrophil hypersegmentation. Serum iron values are elevated unless there is a coexisting iron deficiency. In late pregnancy hemoglobin levels may drop as low as 3 to 5 gm/100 ml.

Hemoglobinopathies: Inherited genetic defects in the synthesis of the globin moiety of hemoglobin. Various types of hemoglobin can be identified by electrophoresis.

Thalassemia: Red cells are microcytic and hypochromic with diminished survival time. The bone marrow tends to be hyperactive in an effort to combat the anemia.

Sickle Cell Disease: Individuals homozygous for hemoglobin S have sickle cell disease (Hb S/S). With decreased oxygen tension, sickling deformity of the red cells occurs. This increases blood viscosity, leading to stasis, agglutination, thrombosis, tissue hypoxia, perivascular hemorrhage, and even necrosis. Chronic hemolysis results in severe anemia.

Laboratory findings include a hemoglobin value of 5 to 9 gm/100 ml associated with bizarre red blood cell shapes — many in the sickled form — reticulocytosis (usually 10 to 20 per cent), and variable hyperbilirubinemia.

Sickle Cell – Hemoglobin C Disease: Patients who inherit both hemoglobin C and hemoglobin S may remain asymptomatic until the stress of pregnancy.

Bone Marrow Depression:

Chronic Infection: The anemia of infection is usually normocytic and normochromic, although it may be microcytic and hypochromic. Serum iron levels and iron-binding capacity tend to be reduced, marrow iron is present and occasionally increased, and toxic granulopoiesis may be found in the marrow.

Aplastic Anemia: Pancytopenia (anemia, granulocytopenia, and thrombocytopenia) may be caused by various drugs and chemicals that depress bone marrow.

Hemolysis:

Congenital Hemolytic Anemia: Hereditary spherocytosis is characterized by the presence of spherocytes, small hyperchromic cells with increased osmotic fragility.

Nonspherocytic congenital hemolytic anemia may be caused by an inherited deficiency of glucose 6-phosphate dehydrogenase. The disease is seen in severe form in about 2 per cent of black women and in a milder form in about 10 to 15 per cent. This disorder is inherited as an X-linked trait. Hemolytic episodes are precipitated by infections and various oxidative drugs (aspirin, phenacetin, sulfonamides, nitrofurantoin, primaquine, probenecid, and so forth).

Coombs' positive acquired hemolytic anemia may be idiopathic or associated with diseases such as leukemia, lymphoma, and lupus erythematosus. The shortened life of the red cell is the result of an autoimmune hemolysin. The direct Coombs test is positive.

Other Causes of Intravascular Hemolysis:

1. Isoantibodies — blood transfusion reactions.
2. Chemical agents, drugs, and poisons — toluene, benzene, phenacetin, copper, castor beans, snake and spider venoms.
3. Infectious agents — clostridial sepsis, malaria.
4. Intravascular fragmentation — microangiopathic hemolytic anemia (disseminated intravascular coagulation, hemolytic uremic syndrome,* thrombotic thrombocytopenic purpura).
5. Severe thermal burns.
6. Intravascular hypotonic solution — hypotonic saline, water.
7. Ovarian tumor.

COMPLICATIONS

Complications of sickle cell anemia and sickle cell–hemoglobin C disease include thrombotic crises, urinary tract infection, congestive heart failure, hemolytic crises (pain, fever, jaundice, hemoglobinuria), retinopathy, and hypertension. There is a high incidence of abortion, low birth-weight infants, and perinatal deaths.

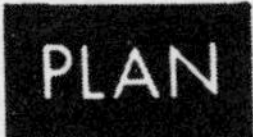

ADDITIONAL DIAGNOSTIC DATA

Iron, Total Serum: Normal value is 60 to 135 mcg/100 ml. Total serum iron is decreased in iron-deficiency anemia, anemias of infection, and chronic diseases. Increased serum iron occurs with increased destruction of red cells (hemolytic anemias).

Total Iron-Binding Capacity (TIBC): Normal value is 250 to 350 mcg/100ml (elevated approximately 15 per cent in pregnancy). Total iron-binding capacity is decreased in thalassemia major, anemias of

*Hemolytic uremic syndrome may occur two weeks to six months after delivery.

infection, and chronic diseases. It is increased in iron deficiency anemia and with acute and chronic blood loss.

Transferrin Saturation [Ratio of Serum Iron to Iron-binding Capacity (Fe/TIBC)]:

Normal value is 20 to 40 per cent. Values less than 15 per cent indicate iron deficiency anemia. Values in the 30 per cent range accompanied by total iron-binding capacity in the vicinity of 350 mcg/100 ml suggest the possibility of β-thalassemia minor. The diagnosis is established by hemoglobin electrophoresis.

Sickle Cell Test: Exposure of blood to a reducing agent produces a characteristic change associated with hemoglobin S.

Hemoglobin electrophoresis can identify the different forms of hemoglobin. Those that are clinically most important are hemoglobin S,C,F (fetal), and A (adult).

Reticulocyte Count: Normal value is 0.5 to 1.5 per cent erythrocytes.

Increased values are found with increased red cell destruction owing to hemolysis (in sickle cell disease the reticulocyte count may be increased up to 30 per cent). An increased reticulocyte count is also a useful index of a therapeutic response to iron in iron deficiency anemia and of specific therapy in megaloblastic anemias.

Bone Marrow Examination: The lack of stainable iron in an otherwise normal bone marrow is the most reliable measure of iron deficiency. In cases of megaloblastic anemia, abnormal megaloblasts are seen.

Serum hemoglobin is slightly increased in sickle cell–thalassemia and hemoglobin C disease and moderately increased in sickle cell–hemoglobin C disease, sickle cell anemia, thalassemia major, and acquired hemolytic anemia. Serum hemoglobin is markedly increased with any rapid intravascular hemolysis.

Coombs' "Direct" Antiglobulin Test: This test serves to demonstrate the presence of "incomplete" antibodies, those that are attached at some points on the surface of the red cell but require a completing substance, such as antihuman globulin, to cause agglutination. A positive result is seen with erythroblastosis fetalis and autoimmune hemolytic anemia. The test is negative in hemolytic anemias due to intrinsic defects in red cells (for example, enzyme deficiencies or hemoglobinopathies).

An indirect Coombs test permits detection of circulating antibodies in the patient's serum. Positive results may indicate isoimmunization (Rh-sensitized mother) or "nonspecific" autoantibody in acquired hemolytic anemia.

MANAGEMENT AND PATIENT EDUCATION

Iron Deficiency Anemia:

Oral iron therapy is preferred, usually 325 mg tablets of ferrous sulfate three times daily. Each tablet provides 65 mg of elemental iron. A reticulocyte response should be seen within one week, and the hematocrit and hemoglobin should begin to rise shortly thereafter.

The importance of continued therapy must be stressed, since bone marrow iron stores must be replenished.

Parenteral iron therapy may be indicated when a patient cannot tolerate oral iron. Approximately 250 mg of iron dextran (Imferon) is needed for each 1.0 gm/100 ml deficit in hemoglobin concentration. Iron dextran may be administered either intramuscularly or intravenously. For intravenous administration a small-gauge needle limits the speed of injection. The most serious adverse effect is an anaphylactic reaction.

For intravenous use the total dose is calculated on the basis of the patient's weight and observed hemoglobin. The total cumulative amount required to restore hemoglobin and replenish iron stores may be approximated from this formula:

$$0.3 \times \text{body weight (lbs)} \times \left(100 - \frac{\text{Hb (gm/100 ml} \times 100)}{14.8}\right) =$$

Mg total iron to be injected.

One ml of iron dextran contains 50 mg of iron.

Megaloblastic Anemia — Folate Deficiency: Folic acid, 1 mg orally once a day, usually produces a striking reticulocytosis within four or five days. *Iron* supplementation should be provided since rapid hemoglobin synthesis requires additional iron.

Anemia of Infection: The underlying infection must be treated with appropriate antibiotics. The most common site of chronic infection during pregnancy is the urinary tract. Iron supplementation may also be required.

Sickle Cell Anemia: During pregnancy there is no need to raise the patient's hemoglobin level above her usual nonpregnant value (often in the range of 7 gm/100 ml). During labor and delivery transfusion of packed red cells may be necessary.

Supplementary folic acid, 1 mg per day, is recommended. Iron supplementation, however, is usually not required.

Oxygen therapy should be initiated during times of increased oxygen need.

Hemolytic Anemia: Whenever possible the hemolytic agent (incompatible blood, chemical or bacterial toxin) must be eliminated. Aquired hemolytic anemias may respond to corticosteroid therapy or splenectomy.

REFERENCES

Carr MC: Serum iron/TIBC in the diagnosis of iron deficiency anemia during pregnancy. Obstet Gynecol *38*:602-608, 1971

Dawson MA, Talbert W, Yarbro JW: Hemolytic anemia associated with an ovarian tumor. Am J Med *50*:552-556, 1971

McFee JG: Anemia in pregnancy — a reappraisal. Obstet Gynecol Surv *28*:769-793, 1973

Stohlman F: Drug-related haematological problems during pregnancy. Clin Haematol *2*:525-542, 1973

Wallerstein RO: Iron metabolism and iron deficiency during pregnancy. Clin Haematol *2*:453-460, 1973

15 ANESTHETIC EMERGENCIES

Anesthetic emergencies may develop any time a patient receives general, conduction, or local anesthesia. Complications to be anticipated include respiratory depression and cardiac arrest (See Cardiopulmonary Resuscitation, p. 832, pulmonary aspiration of gastric contents (see p. 577), hypotension, total spinal block, and local anesthetic toxicity.

Immediate resuscitation is imperative! The airway must be *patent.* Mucus blood, and vomitus must be aspirated. Oxygen is administered by artificial respiration if respiration is depressed.

Circulation must be supported with intravenous fluids and possibly blood or vasopressor medications. Cardiac arrest demands immediate cardiac resuscitation.

Hypotension Following Conduction Anesthesia: During labor, cardiovascular changes, particularly the supine hypotensive syndrome (vena cava compression), may increase the susceptibility to severe hypotension and sudden cardiovascular collapse following conduction anesthesia (epidural or spinal block). In order to prevent fetal distress and to assure maternal consciousness and preservation of upper airway reflexes, hypotension must be treated immediately:

Oxygen is administered by face mask.

Left Uterine Displacement: The patient is positioned on her left side in order to displace the uterus and avoid vena cava compression.

Intravenous Fluids: 1000 ml of 5 per cent dextrose in lactated Ringer's solution is infused rapidly.

Vasopressor Medications: If the preceding measures are not effective, 10 to 15 mg of ephedrine may be administered intravenously.

Total Spinal or Epidural Block: The obstetric patient is particularly susceptible to high levels of subarachnoid or epidural block because of increased cerebrospinal fluid pressure during uterine contractions and voluntary expulsive efforts. Total spinal block produces unconsciousness, respiratory rrest, and cardiovascular collapse, resulting from generalized vasodilation compounded by blockage of sympathetic cardioaccelerator fibers. All muscles are paralyzed except those of the face and neck innervated by cranial nerves.

Treatment includes oxygenation, left uterine displacement, rapid intravenous hydration, and 10 to 15 mg of ephedrine. *Oxygen* must be administered immediately with positive pressure ventilation. If the patient is unconscious, intubation can be accomplished easily and directly. If there is resistance to intubation, a small intravenous dose of thiopental (Pentothal) followed by succinylcholine chloride may be required to facilitate the intubation. Ventilation is then maintained with oxygen alone until the patient regains consciousness. These patients should not be seated or placed in reverse Trendelenburg's position, since these positions, when combined with sympathetic block and aortocaval compression, result in additional pooling of blood and cardiovascular collapse. The patient should remain supine, with left uterine displacement; the head should be slightly elevated with a small pillow to accentuate the thoracic kyphosis (Gutsche, 1976).

Local Anesthetic Toxicity: Elevated toxic blood levels of local anesthetic drugs are caused by accidental intravascular injection, extremely rapid absorption through a vascular area, or overdosage. Since lidocaine, mepivacaine, and bupivacaine are slowly metabolized, repeated injection of these drugs may result in a toxic accumulation in both maternal and fetal blood. The toxic blood level can persist even after the block has dissipated. Chloroprocaine hydrochloride is metabolized more rapidly to nontoxic substances in both fetal and maternal blood.

Immediate toxic reactions are usually caused by accidental injection into a blood vessel or by extremely rapid absorption through a highly vascular area. Acute circulatory or respiratory collapse can occur within one or two minutes.

Allergic or anaphylactic reactions are rare. (See Anaphylaxis, p. 125.)

Delayed toxic reactions result from the slow build-up of a toxic blood level. Commencing 5 to 30 minutes after injection, somnolence may progress to coma. In certain patients, the sleepy stage may be replaced by marked euphoria, excitement, and elation. Very often the patient senses that something is wrong. There may be a progressive decrease in rate and quality of the pulse; development of facial pallor; cold, clammy skin; or twitching of the face, hands. and feet, with hypotension, syncope, and convulsions.

Mental changes require no specific treatment. Hypotension with a slow weak pulse, cold clammy skin, and intermittent apnea and dyspnea is treated with intravenous fluids, oxygen, and possibly vasopressors. (See Shock, p. 612.)

Convulsions must be controlled as rapidly as possible with intravenous rapid-acting barbiturates or diazepam.

Fetal bradycardia and depression may occur when a paracervical block is administered during the first stage of labor. Although the bradycardia is usually transitory, fetal acidosis and depression have occurred (Shnider, 1970). Paracervical block should be avoided when there is any evidence of preexisting fetal distress, prematurity, or placental insufficiency. An overdose of regional blocking agents may intoxicate the fetus, causing apnea and vascular collapse from medullary depression.

Management of local anesthetic toxicity includes

1. Discontinuation of *local anesthetic injection* at the first sign of toxicity
2. Immediate administration of *oxygen*
3. Maintenance of a clear *airway*. To minimize the risk of pulmonary aspiration, the patient is turned on her side in the head-down position. Mucus and regurgitated material are removed by suction. If apnea occurs, intubation and positive pressure ventilation are usually required.
4. Administration of *intravenous fluids*
5. Control of *convulsions* with anticonvulsant medication. Usually 5 to 10 mg of diazepam are administered intravenously. Thiopental may be preferred, particularly if an anesthetist is present. Other anticonvulsant medications that may be useful include pentobarbital or secobarbital, 50 to 100 mg.

6. Treatment of *hypotension* with oxygen, rapid hydration, and intravenous ephedrine. Left uterine displacement is always indicated in late pregnancy.
7. Artificial ventilation and cardiac massage *in cases of cardiac arrest.* (See Adult Cardiopulmonary Resuscitation, p. 832.)
8. Giving the mother oxygen and turning her to the left lateral position if fetal bradycardia develops. The natural metabolism of the local anesthetic agent appears to be preferable to accelerated delivery of a fetus with myocardial depression.

REFERENCES

Finster M: Toxicity of local anesthetics in the fetus and the newborn. Bull NY Acad Med *52*:222-225, 1976; Obstet Gynecol Surv *31*:724-725, 1976.

Gutsche BB: Anesthetic emergencies in obstetrics. Clin Obstet Gynecol *19*:519-531, 1976.

Shnider SM, Asling JH, Holl JW, Margolis AJ: Paracervical block anesthesia in obstetrics. Am J Obstet Gynecol *107*:619-625, 1970

16 APPENDICITIS DURING PREGNANCY

GENERAL CONSIDERATIONS

Although appendicitis is one of the most serious abdominal surgical disorders complicating pregnancy, the incidence of appendicitis is not altered by pregnancy, ranging from 1 in 1,000 to 1 in 3,000 pregnant patients. Maternal risk is increased, however, since the symptoms and signs of appendicitis tend to be masked by pregnancy. Furthermore, if the appendix should perforate during late pregnancy, the enlarged uterus could make it difficult for the omentum to wall off the intraperitoneal infection.

SUBJECTIVE DATA

CURRENT SYMPTOMS

Abdominal Pain: The initial pain of appendicitis, visceral in origin, is usually experienced in the epigastrium or the periumbilical area. The onset is gradual and often colicky, since the primary lesion may be a fecalith or band obstructing the appendix. With increasing inflammation of the appendiceal serosa and subsequent involvement of the overlying parietal peritoneum, the pain localizes within 6 to 12 hours in the area overlying the appendix. As pregnancy progresses the appendix is displaced upward by the enlarging uterus. For this reason the pain of appendicitis is not confined to the right lower quadrant but is located at the site where the appendix is located for that stage of pregnancy.

Anorexia, nausea, or vomiting generally occurs a few hours after the initial pain. The degree of nausea or vomiting depends on two factors: first, the amount of distention of the inflamed appendix and, second, the reflex susceptibility of the patient.

During the first trimester, nausea and vomiting are common pregnancy symptoms that may be difficult to interpret. After the fourth month, however, the sudden occurrence of nausea or vomiting must always be considered to have potential pathologic significance.

The severity and frequency of vomiting at the onset of an appendicitis attack may be a manifestation of the degree of appendiceal distention and, consequently, of the immediate risk of perforation.

PRIOR HISTORY

A history of repeated attacks of right lower quadrant pain prior to pregnancy appears to be correlated with acute appendicitis during pregnancy.

OBJECTIVE DATA

PHYSICAL EXAMINATION

General Examination: The temperature may be normal or slightly elevated, to 101°F (38°C).

Abdominal Examination: Tenderness is usually localized to the area immediately overlying the appendix. Rebound tenderness is a sign of peritoneal irritation.

After the fourth month of pregnancy, the appendix is displaced upwards; consequently, the point of maximal tenderness is higher than McBurney's point. By the sixth month, the ileum and the base of the appendix are situated at the level of the iliac crest, lying adjacent to the anterior iliac spine (unless previously fixed by adhesions). In the third trimester, pain and tenderness may rise as high as the right costal margin (Fig. 16-1).

Abdominal distention is usually moderate.

Muscle spasm, guarding, and rigidity may be expected in approximately 50 per cent of patients.

Movement of the uterus from the left to the right side often causes pain in the appendiceal area.

To distinguish pain of uterine origin from extrauterine disease, Alders (1951) suggested the following maneuver: While the physician maintains the examining fingers at the point of maximal tenderness, the patient is asked to turn onto her left side. The pain produced by the pressure of the

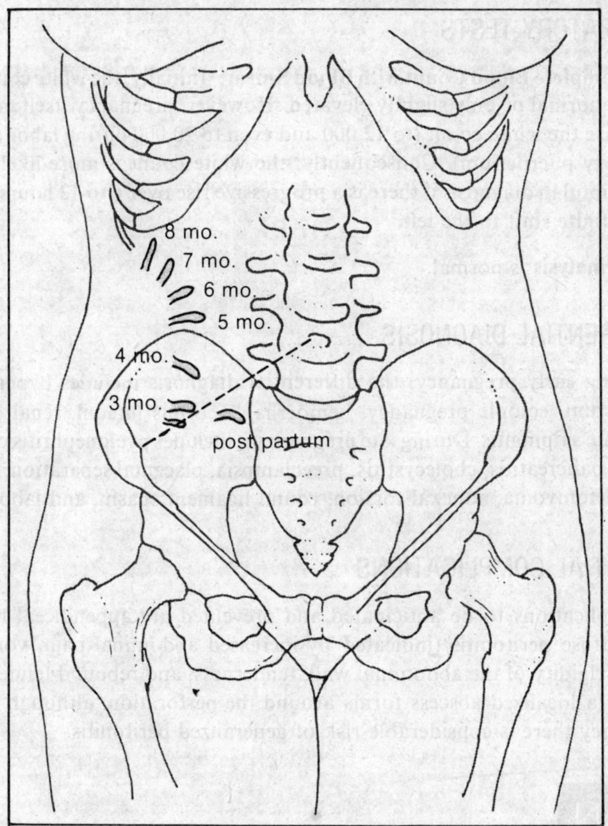

Figure 16-1. During pregnancy, the enlarging uterus displaces the vermiform appendix upward.

fingers becomes less or disappears entirely if the lesion is uterine, since the uterus has fallen away from the examining fingers: The tender area has shifted. If the lesion is extrauterine, however, the pain sensation remains unaltered: The tenderness is fixed (Alder's sign).

Rectal Examination: Rectal tenderness confined to the right side is a finding in approximately 80 per cent of patients (Cunningham, 1975).

LABORATORY TESTS

Complete Blood Count with Blood Smear: Initially, the white count may be normal or only slightly elevated. However, pregnancy itself may also raise the white count (to 12,000 and even to 20,000 during labor and the early puerperium). Consequently, the white count is more likely to be helpful in diagnosis if there is a progressive rise over 6 to 12 hours, with a definite shift to the left.

Urinalysis is normal.

DIFFERENTIAL DIAGNOSIS

During early pregnancy, the differential diagnosis includes hyperemesis gravidarum, ectopic pregnancy, hemorrhagic corpus luteum, renal calculi, and acute salpingitis. During late pregnancy it includes pyelonephritis or renal calculi, pancreatitis, cholecystitis, preeclampsia, placental separation, degenerated leiomyoma, adnexal torsion, round ligament spasm, and labor.

POTENTIAL COMPLICATIONS

Complications to be anticipated and prevented are appendiceal rupture with diffuse peritonitis (indicated by increased abdominal pain, vomiting, intense rigidity of the abdominal wall, tenderness, and rebound tenderness). Usually a localized abscess forms around the perforation, although during pregnancy there is considerable risk of generalized peritonitis.

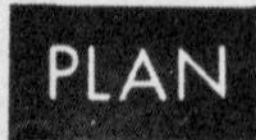

ADDITIONAL DIAGNOSTIC DATA

Abdominal x-rays may be helpful in the differential diagnosis of ambiguous problems, even though there are no characteristic x-ray findings in appendicitis. The potential benefits of radiologic information must always be weighed against the risks of radiation.

Exploratory Laparotomy: When the clinical picture suggests appendicitis (initial epigastric or periumbilical pain, followed by nausea or vomiting, with localization into the area overlying the appendix; low-grade fever; and leukocytosis), *exploratory laparotomy* may be the only way to make an accurate diagnosis.

MANAGEMENT AND PATIENT EDUCATION

The patient should always be hospitalized whenever appendicitis is suspected, since the risk is even greater to a pregnant woman than it is to a nonpregnant person.

Intravenous fluids are initiated for hydration. In anticipation of surgery, the patient is not permitted to take food or liquids orally.

As soon as the diagnosis is established, *exploratory laparotomy* is mandatory. The fact that maternal mortality has been associated with missed diagnoses justifies exploration in all suspicious cases. Appendectomy is virtually always the procedure of choice. With evidence of appendiceal rupture, antibiotics are administered intravenously (often penicillin, gentamicin, and clindamycin). At the time of surgery, cesarean section is recommended only for obstetric indications.

REFERENCES

Alders N: A sign for differentiating uterine from extrauterine complications of pregnancy and puerperium. Br Med J *2*:1194-1195, 1951

Babaknia A, Parsa H, Woodruff JD: Appendicitis during pregnancy. Obstet Gynecol *50*:40-44, 1977

Cunningham FG, McCubbin JH: Appendicitis complicating pregnancy. Obstet Gynecol *45*:415-420, 1975

Mohammed JA, Oxorn H: Appendicitis in pregnancy. Can Med Assoc J *112*:1187-1188, 1975; Obstet Gynecol Surv *31*:199-201, 1976

17 ASTHMA DURING PREGNANCY

GENERAL CONSIDERATIONS

Asthma can be defined as paroxysmal dyspnea accompanied by the adventitious sounds caused by a spasm of the bronchial tubes or swelling of bronchial mucosa. Characterized by reversible bronchoconstriction, asthmatic attacks may be triggered by allergens, respiratory infections, environmental pollutants, or psychogenic factors. Airway obstruction results from bronchial spasm, mucosal edema, and the reactive increase in bronchial secretions.

SUBJECTIVE DATA

Paroxysmal dyspnea is the most characteristic symptom. Usually an asthmatic attack begins with a sensation of chest tightness followed by coughing and wheezing. Fever suggests respiratory infection. The patient is usually aware of her diagnosis, having experienced multiple previous attacks.

OBJECTIVE DATA

Chest examination reveals diffuse inspiratory and expiratory wheezes and rhonchus. Expiration is prolonged. In status asthmaticus breathing is intensely labored and wheezing may be audible without a stethoscope.

ASSESSMENT

DIFFERENTIAL DIAGNOSIS

This includes bronchitis, foreign body in airway, and pulmonary embolism with bronchospasm. (See Dyspnea during Pregnancy, p. 298.)

PRECIPITATING AND AGGRAVATING FACTORS

These include allergens, respiratory infections, environmental pollutants, and psychogenic factors.

POTENTIAL COMPLICATIONS

Complications to be anticipated include mediastinal emphysema and fetal mortality due to severe hypoxemia.

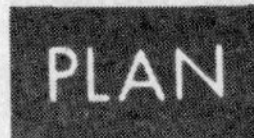

ADDITIONAL DIAGNOSTIC DATA

Arterial blood gases are evaluated to determine the severity of the disease process. They also serve as a guide to therapeutic response. Reduced arterial pO_2 is an indication of disturbed ventilation-perfusion relationships. In status asthmaticus the arterial pO_2 may be decreased considerably. In moderate asthma, the pCO_2 is often low, indicating hyperventilation. Elevation of pCO_2 is a grave sign, indicating that the patient's ventilation is virtually the maximum possible and that increased airway resistance or reduction in drive to breathe could be rapidly fatal.

The objective of therapy is an arterial pO_2 of 70 mm Hg or greater.

Chest x-ray may be helpful when pneumonitis or other complications are suspected.

MANAGEMENT

Acute asthmatic attacks are usually relieved by one or more of the following measures:

1. Epinephrine (1:1000) solution—0.2 to 0.5 ml subcutaneously.
2. Isoproterenol (1:100) solution—three to seven deep inhalations.
3. Oxygen by mask or nasal catheter.
4. Intermittent positive pressure breathing therapy to deliver the bronchodilator isoproterenol.
5. Hydration—1000 ml 5 per cent dextrose in water.
6. Aminophylline—250 to 500 mg (6 mg/kg) added to 100 ml of 5 per cent dextrose in water and infused over 20 to 30 minutes—if bronchospasm has not responded to previous measures.
7. Hydrocortisone—250 to 1000 mg slowly intravenously or diluted into 200 ml of 5 per cent dextrose infusion.
8. Phenobarbital—60 mg intramuscularly—only if sedation appears necessary. Facilities for artificial ventilation should be available.

Iodides are avoided during pregnancy, since their value is questionable and chronic use may be injurious to the fetus.

Antibiotics are prescribed if there is any evidence of infection. After the acute attack has been relieved, the patient may be sent home with a prescription for one of the following bronchodilators:

1. Isoproterenol for inhalation;
2. Ephedrine—25 mg orally three to four times a day; or
3. Metaproterenol—oral tablets or metered dose inhaler.

PATIENT EDUCATION

The influence of pregnancy on asthma tends to be variable; some patients note improvement, whereas others remain stable or have more frequent attacks. The effect of asthma on pregnancy appears to depend primarily on the severity of the condition. Unless the asthma is very severe, maternal morbidity and mortality rates are rarely increased. Perinatal morbidity and mortality may be increased, however, particularly among infants born to severely affected mothers (Bahna, 1972). Opinions differ on the relationship between maternal asthma and premature delivery or fetal growth retardation.

Pregnant asthmatic patients should receive psychogenic support and avoid allergenic drugs or environmental factors known to precipitate asthmatic attacks. (Common allergens include grass pollen, various foods, animal dander, household dust, feathers, and drugs, particularly aspirin.) The patient should also be advised to seek immediate medical attention at the earliest sign of upper respiratory tract infection.

REFERENCES

Bahna SL, Bjerkedal T: The course and outcome of pregnancy in women with bronchial asthma. Acta Allergol *27*:397-406, 1972

Gordon M, Niswander KR, Berendes H et al: Fetal morbidity following potentially anoxigenic obstetric conditions. VII. Bronchial asthma. Am J Obstet Gynecol *106*:421-429, 1970

Senior RM, Lefrak SS, Korenblat PE: Status asthmaticus. JAMA *231*:1277-1279, 1975

Wilson AF: Drug treatment of acute asthma. JAMA *237*:1141-1143, 1977

18 BARTHOLIN'S ABSCESS

Bartholin's abscess is an infected Bartholin duct cyst caused by gonococcal infection, coliform bacilli, or other organisms.

SUBJECTIVE DATA

Perineal pain may be so severe that the patient is unable to sit or walk comfortably. An acute, painful swelling is noted in the lower lateral margin of the vaginal orifice. Vulvar irritation is often associated.

OBJECTIVE DATA

Vulvar Examination: There is a discrete, spherical, soft, exquisitely tender fluctuant mass located lateral to and near the posterior fourchette, surrounded by red and markedly tender tissue. The labia majora are often edematous.

ASSESSMENT

DIFFERENTIAL DIAGNOSIS

This includes perirectal abscess.

PLAN

ADDITIONAL DIAGNOSTIC DATA

Cervical and urethral cultures should be sent to the bacteriologic laboratory.

MANAGEMENT

Incision and drainage is usually advisable to relieve the acute discomfort. After cleansing the area, an incision is made in the mucosa of the vestibule just distal to the hymeneal ring. Often there is marked pain relief with the escape of the pus. A small Penrose drain or catheter is inserted into the abscess cavity to promote continued drainage. Alternatively, the abscess cavity may be packed with iodoform gauze for 24 hours.

Analgesic medications are prescribed for pain. Hot sitz baths are conducive to healing.

The purulent material should be sent to the bacteriology laboratory for culture and Gram stain.

Appropriate antibiotic therapy is prescribed.

PATIENT EDUCATION

The patient should be advised that recurrences are possible. Consequently, marsupialization or excision of a persistent cyst should be considered after the infection has fully subsided.

19 BREAST ENGORGEMENT, POSTPARTUM

Postpartum breast engorgement is a temporary inflammatory condition that represents an exaggeration of the venous and lymphatic breast engorgement preceding lactation.

SUBJECTIVE DATA

Breast pain may become severe on or about the third or fourth postpartum day.

OBJECTIVE DATA

General Examination: Temperature is usually normal or slightly elevated.

Breast Examination: Breasts are swollen, firm, and tender. There is no evidence of infection.

PLAN

MANAGEMENT

The patient is provided with a firm binder for breast support. Ice compresses and analgesic medication usually relieve the severe discomfort.

If the patient wishes to nurse her baby, breast pumping or manual expression may be helpful. Oxytocin may encourage milk letdown and aid certain patients with engorged breasts.

PATIENT EDUCATION

Breast engorgement is usually a self-limited process that regresses within 24 to 48 hours. Symptomatic medication tides the patient over the period of acute discomfort.

20 BREAST INFECTION

DEFINITIONS

Acute mastitis—an acute inflammation of the breast, usually associated with a cracked or fissured nipple, occurring during the period of lactation.

Breast abscess—a late and usually suppurative sequel to acute mastitis.

Subareolar abscess and fistula formation—a chronic recurring infection unrelated to pregnancy that may occur in young women.

SUBJECTIVE DATA

Breast pain usually devélops during the period of lactation, one or more weeks after delivery.

Fever and chills are frequently associated with breast infections.

OBJECTIVE DATA

General Examination: Temperature is usually elevated above 100.4° F (38° C).

Breast Examination: A localized, tender, indurated, and erythematous area is characteristic of mastitis. Often a nipple fissure is observed. Palpable fluctuation is characteristic of a breast abscess. Painful axillary lymphadenopathy may be an associated finding.

ASSESSMENT

ETIOLOGIC FACTORS

Coagulase-positive staphylococci are the most common pathogenic organisms. The next most common organisms are the alpha-hemolytic streptococci.

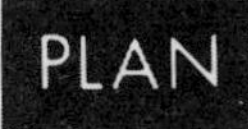

ADDITIONAL DIAGNOSTIC DATA

Gram Stain and Culture: Breast milk is sent to the bacteriology laboratory for culture and sensitivity studies.

MANAGEMENT AND PATIENT EDUCATION

Antibiotic Therapy: The initial choice is usually a penicillinase-resistant penicillin or a cephalosporin for ten days. Culture and sensitivity reports may indicate the need for alternative therapy.

Lactation is usually discontinued, although Marshall (1975) has recommended continuing lactation during antibiotic therapy of sporadic mastitis.

Adjunctive therapy includes heat applied locally to the breast, breast support, and analgesics for pain.

Surgical Drainage: A fluctuant breast abscess requires surgical drainage, usually under general anesthesia. The incision is made radially, extending from the areolar margin to the periphery of the gland.

REFERENCE

Marshall BR, Hepper JK, Zirbel CC: Sporadic puerperal mastitis. JAMA *233*:1377-1379, 1975; Obstet Gynecol Surv *31*:663-665, 1976

21 BREAST MASSES

Breast masses may be caused by infection, benign cysts, benign tumors, or malignant tumors.

SUBJECTIVE DATA

The length of time the mass has been noted, any change in size with menses, and pain or tenderness are important diagnostic considerations.

OBJECTIVE DATA

Breast Examination: On *inspection*, skin retraction, local edema, erythema, surface lesions, or distortions are noted. Skin retraction or nipple retraction of recent onset may be a sign of breast malignancy. Erythema is associated more frequently with a breast infection, although it may be seen with an inflammatory carcinoma.

On *palpation*, the size, shape, firmness, tenderness, and fixation of the mass are identified. Cystic masses are frequently benign; hard, irregular fixed masses are likely to be malignant.

ASSESSMENT

DIFFERENTIAL DIAGNOSIS

Carcinoma: The mass is frequently hard and indurated, with decreased mobility, ill-defined borders, and fixation to surrounding tissues and skin. Retraction of the skin over the palpable lesion, evidence of inflammation, and edema are additional suspicious signs of malignancy. Initially carcinoma is usually a painless tumor.

Cystic breast disease (chronic cystic mastitis) is the most frequent cause of mammary cysts. Although frequently asymptomatic, the cysts may be tender and increase in size during the premenstrual days of the cycle, with improvement following menstruation. The cysts tend to be firm, mobile, well-defined, frequently bilateral, and multifocal.

Fat necrosis usually results from breast trauma. A small, firm tumor may be palpable just below the skin in the most superficial breast tissue. Ecchymosis and erythema of the overlying skin are frequently associated findings.

Fibroadenomas are the most common benign breast tumors. Although usually solitary, they may be multiple and bilateral. Characteristically, they are well circumscribed and movable.

Galactoceles are cysts with a thick, creamy secretion, rounded structures with sharply defined borders, and good mobility within the breast tissue.

Mammary Duct Ectasia: Dilatation of the mammary ducts in the area of the nipple and areola may occur in perimenopausal and menopausal women. The cystic tumors tend to be 1 to 3 cm in diameter. Symptoms associated with ductal ectasia include nipple retraction and nipple discharge. Initially painless, ductal ectasia may become painful with time.

Mastitis is most likely to occur during puerperal lactation and is characterized by a localized tender, indurated area of the breast.

Sclerosing adenosis is a benign condition. The mass can be firm, poorly defined, and fixed.

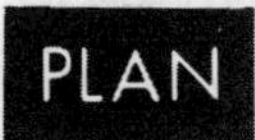

ADDITIONAL DIAGNOSTIC DATA

Mammography may be helpful in the evaluation of suspicious breast lesions.

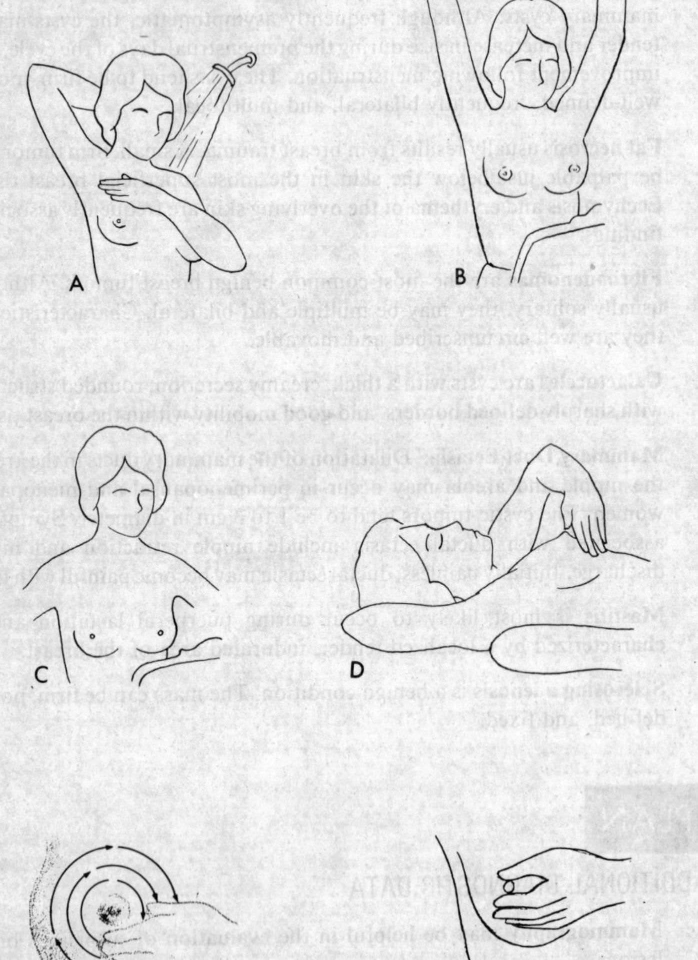

Figure 21-1. The steps of breast self-examination.

MANAGEMENT AND PATIENT EDUCATION

Aspiration: Cystic lesions may be aspirated with a syringe and needle. The fluid is sent to the cytologic laboratory for evaluation. As long as there are no malignant cells and the lump disappears, the patient may be reassured that carcinoma is unlikely. She should be instructed, however, to examine her breasts at home monthly in order to report any additional masses (Fig. 21-1).

Biopsy: If the mass persists despite fluid aspiration, or if no fluid is obtained, excisional biopsy should be scheduled so that a microscopic tissue diagnosis can be made in order to be certain that there is no evidence of carcinoma.

22 BREECH PRESENTATION

GENERAL CONSIDERATIONS

Breech presentation occurs in approximately 3 or 4 per cent of deliveries near term and is more frequent prior to the thirty-second gestational week. Breech presentation is also more likely if the uterine cavity is distorted by placenta previa, lower segment leiomyoma, hydramnios, or multiple pregnancy.

Fetal position is designated by the location of the fetal sacrum in relation to the maternal pelvis. The varying relations between the lower extremities and buttocks of the fetus are designated as complete breech, frank breech, or incomplete breech presentations.

DEFINITIONS

Complete breech presentation—the buttocks descend first. The legs are flexed on the fetal abdomen, and the feet are alongside the fetal buttocks.

Frank breech presentation—the legs lie extended alongside the fetal body so that the buttocks descend first.

Incomplete breech presentation—a breech presentation with one or both feet or knees prolapsed into the vagina.

Double footling presentation—both feet have prolapsed into the vagina.

Single footling presentation—one foot has prolapsed into the vagina.

Sacrum right anterior (SRA)—a position of the fetus in which the sacrum is located in the right anterior quadrant of the maternal pelvis.

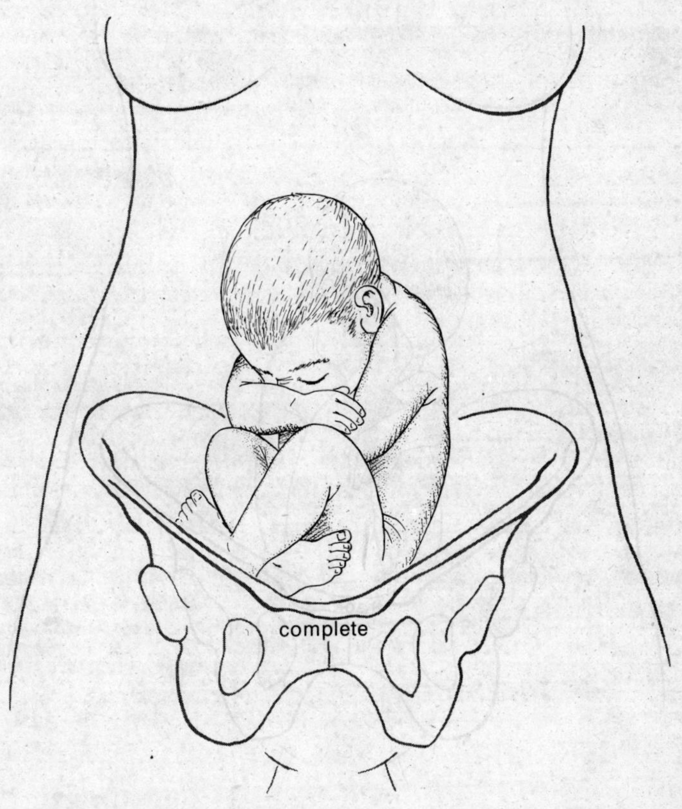

Figure 22-1. Types of breech presentation.

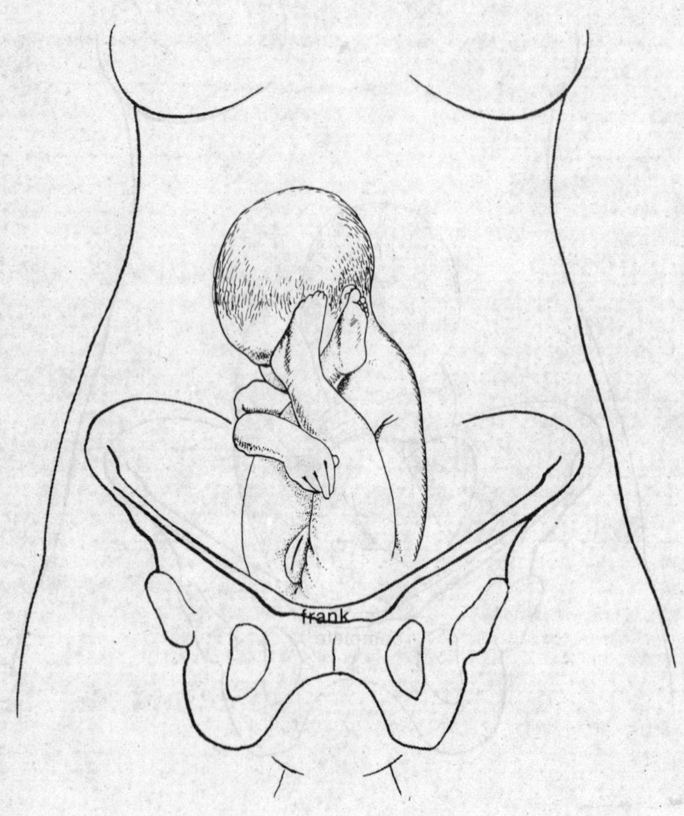

Figure 22-1 Continued.

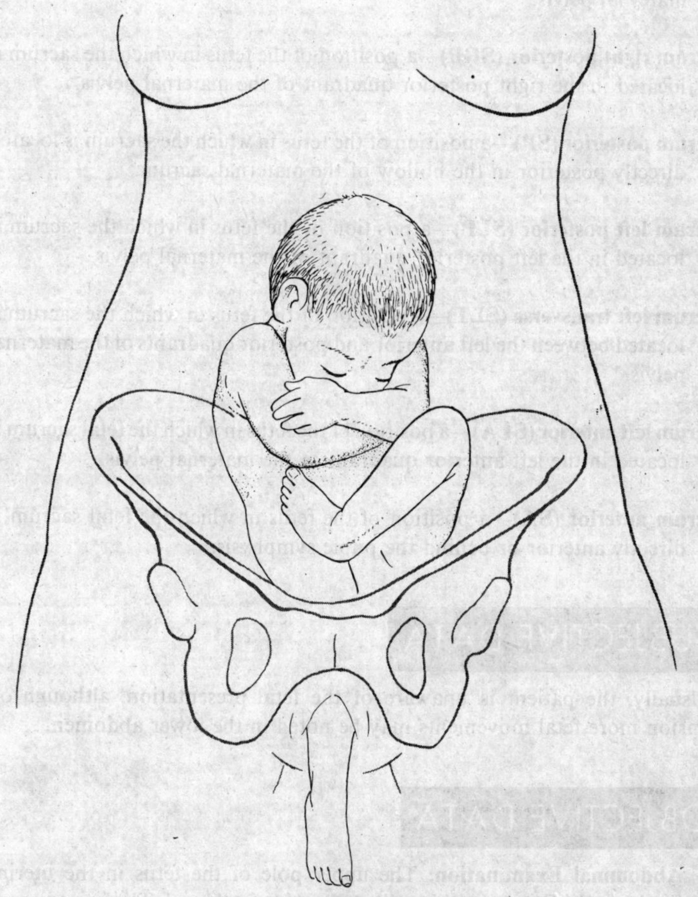

Figure 22-1 Continued.

Sacrum right transverse (SRT)—a position of the fetus in which the sacrum is located between the right anterior and posterior quadrants of the maternal pelvis.

Sacrum right posterior (SRP)—a position of the fetus in which the sacrum is located in the right posterior quadrant of the maternal pelvis.

Sacrum posterior (SP)—a position of the fetus in which the sacrum is located directly posterior in the hollow of the maternal sacrum.

Sacrum left posterior (SLP)—a position of the fetus in which the sacrum is located in the left posterior quadrant of the maternal pelvis.

Sacrum left transverse (SLT)—a position of the fetus in which the sacrum is located between the left anterior and posterior quadrants of the maternal pelvis.

Sacrum left anterior (SLA)—a position of the fetus in which the fetal sacrum is located in the left anterior quadrant of the maternal pelvis.

Sacrum anterior (SA)—a position of the fetus in which the fetal sacrum is directly anterior or behind the pubic symphysis.

SUBJECTIVE DATA

Usually, the patient is unaware of the fetal presentation, although on occasion more fetal movements may be noted in the lower abdomen.

OBJECTIVE DATA

Abdominal Examination: The upper pole of the fetus in the uterine fundus is the firm, round, readily ballotable fetal head. The heart sounds are usually heard above the umbilicus. The lower fetal pole is often indistinct, especially if engagement has occurred.

Vaginal Examination: The feet or sacrum may be palpable. The breech is felt as a soft, smooth, irregularly rounded surface with a dimpled depression (anus). In a complete breech presentation, the feet may be felt alongside the buttocks. In a footling presentation, one or both feet are easily palpable.

ASSESSMENT

POTENTIAL COMPLICATIONS

Complications that should be anticipated in cases of breech presentation include perinatal morbidity and mortality from difficult delivery; low birth weight from prematurity, growth retardation, or both; prolapsed cord; placenta previa and placental abruption; fetal anomalies; uterine anomalies and tumors; and multiple fetuses.

PLAN

ADDITIONAL DIAGNOSTIC DATA

X-ray or ultrasound B-scan can be helpful when fetal presentation is doubtful. Either test may also identify a fetal anomaly. Anencephalus—a malformation characterized by complete or partial absence of the brain and overlying skull—may feel like a breech presentation on vaginal examination.

X-ray pelvimetry provides an assessment of pelvic size, pelvic architecture, type of breech presentation (footling or frank), and hyperextension of the fetal head.

MANAGEMENT AND PATIENT EDUCATION

Breech presentation is associated with a three- to fourfold greater risk for the baby than vertex presentation. Delivery trauma and anoxia due to cord compression or cord prolapse are two factors that account for the increased perinatal morbidity and mortality. Cord prolapse, for example, is approximately 20 times greater with a complete or a footling breech than with a term vertex presentation.

The increased perinatal loss associated with breech presentation also results from factors that play a role in the causation of the breech presentation, such as prematurity and placenta previa.

External cephalic version is advocated by some obstetricians when a breech presentation is diagnosed in the third trimester. However, this maneuver is not without intrinsic risk: cord or placental accident, antepartum hemorrhage, premature labor, premature rupture of the membranes, and fetal death are possible hazards.

Vaginal versus Abdominal Delivery: When the patient with a breech presentation presents in active labor or with ruptured membranes prior to the onset of labor, opinions differ over optimal obstetric management.

Vaginal Delivery: There are three types of vaginal breech deliveries:

Spontaneous Breech Birth: The entire infant is expelled by natural forces of labor (uterine contractions supplemented by voluntary bearing-down efforts) without any traction or manipulation except for support of the infant (Fig. 22-2).

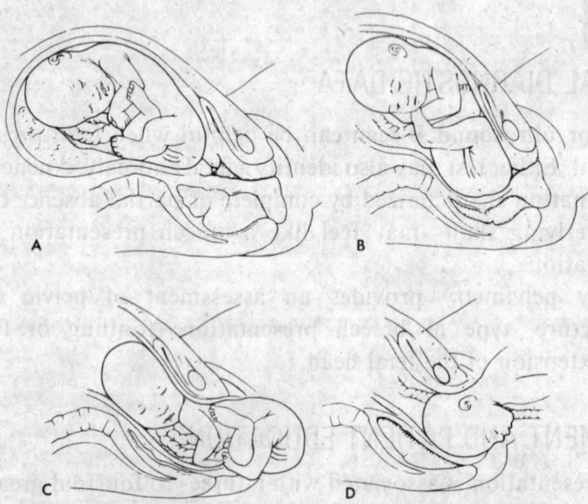

Figure 22-2. Spontaneous breech delivery. *A*, Engagement of the fetus. *B*, Descent in an oblique diameter with concurrent internal rotation and lateral flexion. *C*, The hips deliver in an anteroposterior position, and the shoulders engage in the oblique. *D*, The shoulder rotated and delivered in an anteroposterior position while the flexed head entered the pelvis in an oblique position and then rotated so that the nape of the neck stemmed under the symphysis. The head now delivers by flexion, the chin first and the occiput last. (Modified from Huffman JW: Gynecology and Obstetrics. Philadelphia, W.B. Saunders Company, 1962.)

Partial Breech Extraction: The baby is delivered spontaneously as far as the umbilicus; the remainder of the body is extracted by the obstetrician (Fig. 22-3).

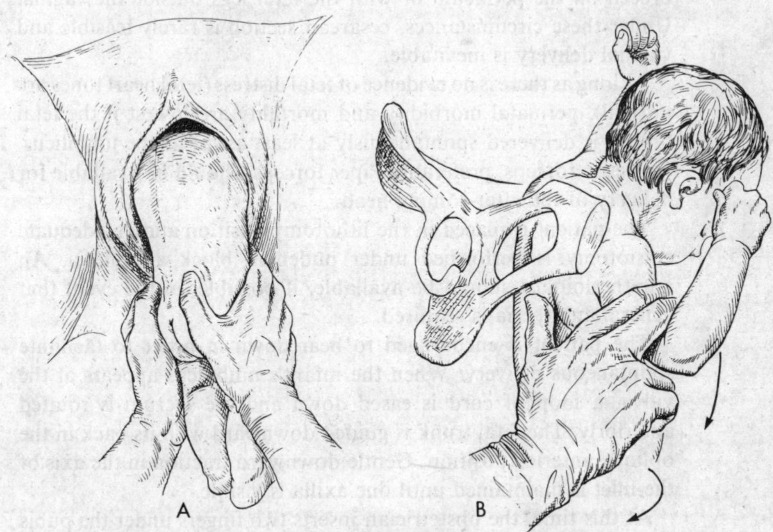

Figure 22-3. *A*, Delivery from the umbilicus to the shoulders in partial breech extraction. The breech is grasped with the thumbs over the back of the sacrum, and the index fingers rest on the anterior superior iliac spines. Gentle, even traction is made downward in the direction of the axis of the inlet, until the anterior shoulder blade comes well under the pubis. *B*, Bringing down the anterior arm. The arms are delivered as they lie. Two fingers are slipped upward under the pubis over the fetal back and down to its elbow flexure. By flexing the fingers and twisting the wrist, the physician sweeps the arm of the fetus down over its chest and out. (Modified from Greenhill JP, Friedman EA: Biological Principles and Modern Practice of Obstetrics. Philadelphia, W.B. Saunders Company, 1974.)

Total Breech Extraction: The entire body of the infant is extracted.

Successful vaginal delivery can usually be anticipated when the baby is in a frank breech presentation, the breech is engaged, the child is estimated to weigh between 2500 and 3500 grams, the pelvis is known to be roomy (either by x-ray pelvimetry or previous delivery of a full-term infant), the pregnancy is uncomplicated, and labor progresses spontaneously and normally.

Occasionally the patient arrives in extremely active labor with the breech on the perineum or with the fetal legs outside the vagina. Under these circumstances, cesarean section is rarely feasible and vaginal delivery is inevitable.

As long as there is no evidence of fetal distress (fetal heart tones are normal), perinatal morbidity and mortality are lowest if the fetal breech is delivered spontaneously at least as far as the umbilicus. Obstetric forceps, preferably Piper forceps, should be available for delivery of the after-coming head.

The patient is placed in the lithotomy position and an adequate episiotomy is performed under pudendal block anesthesia. An anesthesiologist should be available, if possible, in the event that general anesthesia is required.

The patient is encouraged to bear down in order to facilitate spontaneous delivery. When the infant's umbilicus appears at the vulva, a loop of cord is eased down and the sacrum is rotated anteriorly. The fetal trunk is guided downward with its back in the oblique anterior position. Gentle downward traction in the axis of the inlet is maintained until one axilla is visible.

At this time, the obstetrician inserts two fingers under the pubis over the fetal back down to the elbow flexure in order to deliver the fetal arm by gently sweeping it across the chest. Once this is accomplished, the other arm emerges spontaneously or is similarly delivered.

The infant's back is then rotated anteriorly so that the occiput is anterior and the chin posterior. With the fetal body straddling the obstetrician's forearm, two fingers are introduced into the infant's mouth and applied over the maxilla to facilitate flexion of the head. Gentle fundal pressure aids in the descent of the fetal head into the pelvic cavity. The body of the child is gently elevated and the mouth, nose, and brow spontaneously emerge over the perineum.

If the head is not delivered easily with flexion and gentle fundal pressure, obstetric forceps should be applied. Indeed, many obstetricians feel that delivery of the after-coming head is generally accomplished with the greatest degree of safety by use of Piper forceps. Piper forceps are especially useful because the backward curve of the shank facilitates application to the head from beneath the baby's body. Gentle traction and flexion with the forceps combined with gradual elevation of the fetal body complete the delivery (Fig. 22-4).

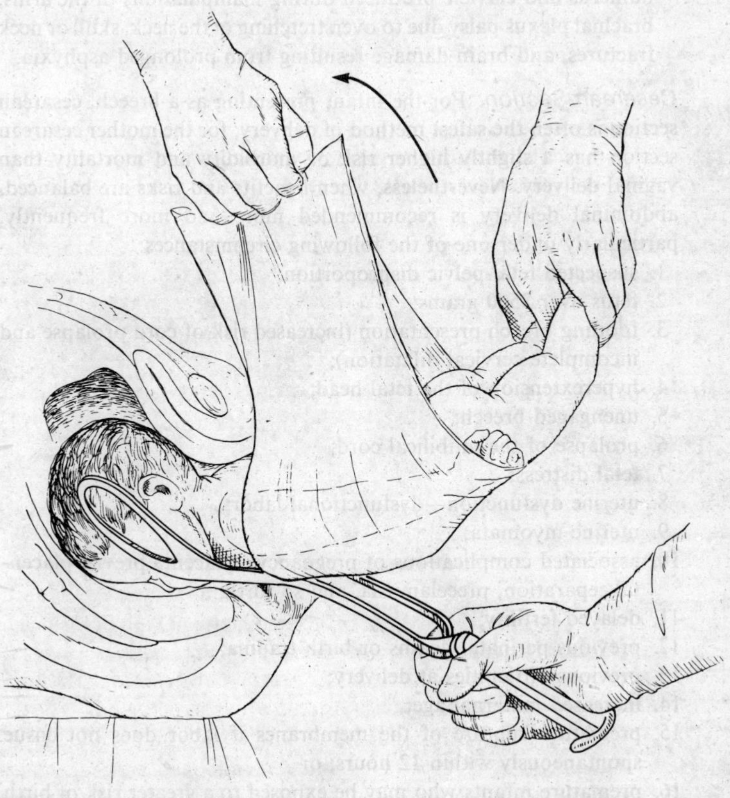

Figure 22-4. Piper forceps aid in the delivery of the head. Note the towel used to lift slightly the child's body and arms.

Since birth trauma is a significant risk in vaginal breech delivery, errors to be guarded against include

1. exaggerated haste;
2. failure to maintain the head in an attitude of flexion;
3. overextension of the fetal cervical spine; and
4. excessive fundal pressure.

Serious complications to be avoided include fractures of the humerus and clavicle produced during manipulations of the arms, brachial plexus palsy due to overstretching of the neck, skull or neck fractures, and brain damage resulting from prolonged asphyxia.

Cesarean Section: For the infant presenting as a breech, cesarean section is often the safest method of delivery; for the mother cesarean section has a slightly higher risk of morbidity and mortality than vaginal delivery. Nevertheless, when benefits and risks are balanced, abdominal delivery is recommended more and more frequently, particularly under one of the following circumstances:

1. suspected fetal-pelvic disproportion;
2. fetus over 3500 grams;
3. footling breech presentation (increased risk of cord prolapse and incomplete cervical dilatation);
4. hyperextension of the fetal head;
5. unengaged breech;
6. prolapse of the umbilical cord;
7. fetal distress;
8. uterine dysfunction—dysfunctional labor;
9. uterine myomata;
10. associated complications of pregnancy—placenta previa, placental separation, preeclampsia, and so forth;
11. delayed fertility;
12. previous perinatal deaths or birth trauma;
13. previous difficulties at delivery;
14. increased maternal age;
15. premature rupture of the membranes if labor does not ensue spontaneously within 12 hours; or
16. premature infants who may be exposed to a greater risk of birth trauma during vaginal delivery.

REFERENCES

Bradley-Watson PJ: The decreasing value of external cephalic version in modern obstetric practice. Am J Obstet Gynecol *123*:237-240, 1975

Brenner WE, Bruce RD, Hendricks CH: The characteristics and perils of breech presentation. Am J Obstet Gynecol *118*:700-712, 1974; Obstet Gynecol Surv *29*:707-710, 1974

Caterini H, Langer A, Sama JC, et al: Fetal risk in hyperextension of the fetal head in breech presentation. Am J Obstet Gynecol *123*:632-636, 1975; Obstet Gynecol Surv *31*:488-490, 1976

Marcus RG, Drewe-Brown H, Krawitz S, et al: Fetomaternal haemorrhage after external cephalic version. Br J Obstet Gynaecol *82*:578-580, 1975

Milner RDG: Neonatal mortality of breech deliveries with and without forceps to the aftercoming head. Br J Obstet Gynaecol *82*:783-785, 1975; Obstet Gynecol Surv *31*:289-290, 1976

Rovinsky JJ, Miller JA, Kaplan S: Management of breech presentation at term. Am J Obstet Gynecol *115*:497-513, 1973

23 BURNS IN PREGNANCY

Emergency management of the burned pregnant patient is essentially the same as the emergency management of any burned patient. The severity of injury depends on the percentage of body surface affected, the depth of the injury, the anatomical location, and the etiologic factors (hot liquids, fire, electricity, chemicals, radiation, or sun). Perineal burns, being located in an area where sepsis is difficult to prevent, compound the patient's problem.

Minor burns involve less than 2 per cent of the body surface. They are treated by local cleansing and then dressed with petrolatum gauze.

More extensive burns require hospital care. Initial treatment consists in cutting off clothing and estimating the extent of the burned area. First-aid treatment for thermal burns is the application of cold. Chemical burns should be irrigated copiously.

Critical burns include those complicated by respiratory tract injury; partial thickness burns of more than 30 per cent of the body surface; full thickness burns of more than 10 per cent of the body surface including burns of the face, hands, feet or genitalia; burns complicated by fractures or major soft tissue injury; and burns associated with electrical injury.

Since the most significant systemic effect of thermal injury is *shock*—due to the escape of fluid and protein from the vascular tree into the interstitial space—circulatory and renal integrity must be restored and maintained. Intravenous fluid therapy with lactated Ringer's solution is initiated immediately in order to avoid even transitory hypovolemia, which may have a deleterious effect on the mother or fetus. Both mother and fetus must be carefully monitored (see Shock, p. 612.)

If products of combustion have been inhaled, repeated examinations of the chest and arterial blood gases are advisable. Treatment of inhalation injury includes endotracheal intubation, humidified air, and positive pressure ventilation. Morphine (3 to 4 mg intravenously) may be administered for sedation and analgesia.

After airway evaluation and the initiation of fluid therapy, the burn wound is cleansed with soap and water. Acceptable methods of local wound care include occlusive dressings, exposure, initial excision, and topical antibacterial agents. Tetanus immunization and prophylactic antibiotics are given to prevent sepsis.

When second- and third-degree burns involve over 30 per cent of the body surface, premature labor is a hazard (Stage, 1973). In the case of a patient with a life-threatening burn, cesarean section must be considered in order to save a viable infant. When possible, the patient is transferred to a center with a neonatal intensive care unit *prior* to delivery. *For a fetus in danger, the uterus is the best transport vehicle.* Surgical, obstetric, and pediatric consultations are advisable.

REFERENCES

Artz C, Moncrief JA and Pruitt BA: Burns: A Team Approach. Philadelphia, W.B. Saunders Company, 1978

Stage AH: Severe burns in the pregnant patient. Obstet Gynecol *42*:259-262, 1973

24 CARDIAC FAILURE DURING PREGNANCY

GENERAL CONSIDERATIONS

Cardiovascular changes during pregnancy—increased cardiac output, blood volume, and oxygen consumption—may contribute to cardiac failure when a pregnant patient has heart disease. Formerly, rheumatic heart disease, particularly mitral stenosis, accounted for the majority of cases of heart disease during pregnancy. In recent years, cardiac complications of rheumatic fever have become less frequent, whereas more women with congenital heart disease are likely to become pregnant.

Cardiac output at rest, measured in the lateral recumbent position, increases appreciably during the first trimester and then increases only slightly more during the second and third trimesters. By 20 to 24 weeks' gestation, resting cardiac output is at or near its peak: 30 to 40 per cent above nonpregnant values (Ueland, 1975).

During late pregnancy, cardiac output is appreciably higher in the lateral recumbent position than in the supine position, since the enlarged uterus impedes venous return in the supine position.

Heart rate rises slowly and progressively throughout pregnancy, reaching a peak of about 15 beats per minute above nonpregnant levels at term. With physical activity, cardiac output tends to be increased more in the pregnant patient than in the nonpregnant patient.

During the first stage of labor, maternal cardiac output increases moderately; during the second stage of labor, vigorous expulsive efforts are associated with an appreciably greater cardiac output.

Blood volume increases markedly during pregnancy. Although the rise begins during the first trimester, maternal blood volume expands most rapidly during the second trimester, subsequently rising at a much slower rate during the third trimester. The increase in blood volume during normal pregnancy varies greatly (20 to 100 per cent above pregravid values) and is influenced by maternal weight, weight of the products of conception, and maternal nutrition.

Since total body water increases throughout pregnancy, edema is a common accompaniment of normal pregnancy (Robertson, 1971). Normal gestational edema must not be confused with the fluid accumulation secondary to renal or cardiac disease.

Oxygen consumption begins to increase during the second month of pregnancy and reaches a value 10 to 20 per cent above normal at term. The rise is due primarily to fetal metabolic demands superimposed on the increased needs of the maternal tissues, particularly the uterus and breasts.

Although the peak physiologic cardiovascular changes of pregnancy are reached by the thirty-second week of pregnancy, cardiac failure may develop at any time during pregnancy, labor, or the puerperium—whenever the cardiac load exceeds the functional capacity of the heart. With failure, there is diminished cardiac output, prolonged circulation time, gradual increase in intra- and extravascular fluid volume, and functional changes in various organs. Retained salt and water owing to altered renal function produce hypervolemia, aggravating the congestive state. Pulmonary edema results from pulmonary congestion and increased pulmonary capillary pressure.

SUBJECTIVE DATA

CURRENT SYMPTOMS

Dyspnea and cough may be the earliest symptoms of congestive heart failure. Other symptoms include orthopnea, hemoptysis, fatigue, palpitation, anxiety, limited physical activity, fluid retention, and weight gain.

PRIOR HISTORY

A history of congenital or rheumatic heart disease would be expected.

OBJECTIVE DATA

General Examination: The heart rate increases to 110 per minute or more. Excessive weight gain, edema, cyanosis, and engorged jugular veins are frequently noted.

Cardiac Examination: Cardiac murmurs (diastolic, presystolic, or continuous), arrhythmias, and cardiac enlargement are indicative of heart disease.

In cases of cardiac failure, a third heart sound is heard early in diastole. The fixed sequence of two normal heart sounds and a third abnormal sound, in conjunction with an increased heart rate, is responsible for the characteristic cadence of a gallop rhythm (S 3 gallop). As a result of increased pulmonary arterial pressure, the pulmonary second sound—the heart sound attributed to pulmonary valve closure—increases in intensity.

Pulmonary Examination: Bilateral basal rales are a sign of alveolar edema and fluid in the terminal bronchioles.

Abdominal Examination: The liver may be enlarged and tender. Ascites may be present.

ASSESSMENT

FUNCTIONAL CLASSIFICATION

Class I: This includes the patients with cardiac disease but without resulting limitation of physical activity. Ordinary physical activity does not cause undue fatigue, palpitation, dyspnea, or anginal pain.

Class II: Patients with cardiac disease resulting in a slight limitation of physical activity compose Class II. Although comfortable at rest, these patients experience fatigue, palpitation, dyspnea, or anginal pain with ordinary physical activity.

Class III: Patients with cardiac disease resulting in marked limitation of physical activity are included in Class III. Comfortable at rest, these patients experience fatigue, palpitation, dyspnea, or anginal pain with less than ordinary activity.

Class IV: These patients have cardiac disease that results in inability to carry on any physical activity without discomfort. Symptoms of cardiac insufficiency or of the anginal syndrome may be present even at rest. Discomfort is increased by any physical activity.

THERAPEUTIC CLASSIFICATION

Class A: Patients with cardiac disease whose physical activity need not be restricted compose this class. This is seldom the case in pregnancy because of the added burdens involved.

Class B: In this category are patients with cardiac disease whose ordinary physical activity need not be restricted but who should be advised against severe or competitive physical efforts.

Class C: Patients with cardiac disease whose ordinary physical activity should be restricted moderately and whose more strenuous effort should be discontinued are included in this group.

Class D is made up of patients with cardiac disease whose ordinary physical activity should be restricted markedly.

Class E comprises patients with cardiac disease who should be at complete rest or confined to bed or chair.

PREDISPOSING FACTORS

These include physiologic cardiovascular changes during pregnancy, physical activity, infections, anemia, thyrotoxicosis, obesity, and hypertension.

POTENTIAL COMPLICATIONS

Complications of heart disease that should be anticipated include congestive failure, pulmonary edema, atrial arrhythmias, and pulmonary embolism. Extremely rare complications of heart disease during pregnancy include aortic rupture and bacterial endocarditis.

Hypotensive episodes may be fatal in patients with cardiac shunts if flow is reversed from the right to the left side of the heart, thereby bypassing the lungs.

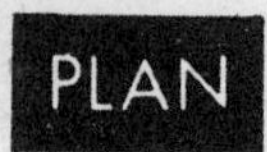

ADDITIONAL DIAGNOSTIC DATA

Chest x-ray may be helpful in the assessment of cardiac enlargement, pulmonary edema, and pleural effusion.

Electrocardiograms aid in the determination of cardiac rate and rhythm and in the estimation of specific chamber enlargement.

Serum electrolytes, particularly potassium, are a guide to fluid and electrolyte therapy.

MANAGEMENT AND PATIENT EDUCATION

Pregnant Cardiac Patients with Intercurrent Problems

During pregnancy all cardiac patients must be observed carefully in order to reduce, prevent, or eliminate any contributory cardiac burden.

Infections increase cardiac output and should be treated in the hospital. Upper respiratory tract infections may progress to bronchitis and pneumonia—important contributory causes of severe heart failure during pregnancy.

Overactivity: Physical exertion may also lead to heart failure. Patients with a limited cardiac reserve should compensate for the burden of pregnancy by resting more than usual and by avoiding undue physical and emotional stresses.

Arrhythmias: In the presence of structural heart damage, atrial tachycardia, fibrillation, or flutter may precipitate failure. Consequently, these disorders should be treated promptly.

Anemia: Cardiovascular complications may occur in patients with sickle cell anemia and sickle cell–hemoglobin C disease. Decompensation may also occur when anemia aggravates other types of heart disease.

Hypervolemia may lead to pulmonary edema. Infusions and transfusions should be avoided unless essential, in which case the rate of infusion must be very carefully observed. Sodium intake should be limited.

Obesity: With increased bodily bulk, the cardiac burden becomes greater. Dietary intake should be restricted to meet maternal and fetal nutritional needs without causing excess fat deposition. Sodium intake should be limited to approximately 2000 mg daily.

Cardiac Failure during Pregnancy

The patient in cardiac failure should be hospitalized and placed at *complete bed rest* in order to decrease cardiac work demands.

Oxygenation: Oxygen is administered by nasal catheter, mask, or intermittent positive pressure as necessary.

Sedation: Morphine (10 to 15 mg) helps allay anxiety and agitation. Both physical and mental rest are extremely important aspects of successful therapy.

Reduction in Blood Volume:

Diuresis: Furosemide (Lasix) (40 mg intravenously) usually produces a rapid diuresis, beginning within 5 to 15 minutes and reaching a maximum within one to two hours. Subsequent doses may be given orally or parenterally as necessary. (Because animal reproductive studies have shown that furosemide may cause fetal abnormalities, the drug is contraindicated in women of childbearing potential except in life-threatening situations.)

Rotating tourniquets on the extremities (releasing one at a time for five minutes every half hour) decreases venous return to the right heart.

Digitalization: Digitalis (digoxin or deslanoside) is particularly useful in the treatment of heart failure associated with supraventricular arrhythmias with rapid ventricular response, since digitalis slows the ventricular rate. As long as the patient has not received digitalis during the preceding two weeks, rapid intravenous digitalization may be indicated. An initial dose of 0.5 mg digoxin is followed by 0.25 mg every two to four hours; the average digitalizing dose of digoxin is 0.75 to 1.0 mg intravenously or 1.25 to 1.5 mg orally (Smith, 1973). The onset of action is 15 to 30 minutes following intravenous administration. The usual daily oral maintenance dose is 0.25 to 0.5 mg.

Factors influencing individual sensitivity to digitalis include potassium, magnesium, and calcium levels; myocardial hypoxia or necrosis; thyroid function; renal function; and the type and severity of the underlying heart disease. With hypokalemia, there is an increased tendency toward digitalis intoxication. Intravenous administration of a bolus of a digitalis preparation to a patient who has recently taken digitalis may precipitate ventricular tachycardia or fibrillation. Clinical manifestations and the electrocardiogram are the key guides to dosage.

Additional Measures: Fluid and sodium intake are restricted. Potassium supplementation may be required. After heart failure has been treated, the patient should remain under close observation, preferably in the hospital, until after delivery.

Management of Labor and Delivery

Hospitalization prior to delivery is usually recommended. Labor is not ordinarily induced prematurely, since premature induction may result in a prolonged, difficult labor that would impose an unnecessary burden on the patient. Consequently, the onset of spontaneous labor is awaited and normal vaginal delivery is anticipated, unless obstetric complications require cesarean section.

During labor, adequate pain relief is essential; pain evokes tachycardia and increased cardiac output. The patient is kept on her side, since cardiac output tends to be more stable in the lateral position. Careful monitoring for pulse rate, blood pressure, respiratory rate, temperature, and urinary output is necessary. In addition, an electrocardiogram, evaluation of central venous pressure and arterial blood gases may be indicated.

Continuous epidural anesthesia provides maximal pain relief during labor and delivery. In addition, epidural anesthesia tends to eliminate the bearing-down reflex in the second stage. If transient hypotension is life threatening, however, this form of anesthesia may be contraindicated. Consultation with an anesthesiologist aware of the patient's cardiovascular and pulmonary pathophysiologic condition is recommended.

The cardiac patient is given oxygen by nasal catheter or face mask throughout labor, and the fetus is delivered as soon as feasible after full cervical dilatation, in order to shorten the time of bearing down during the second stage.

In the absence of fever, a pulse rate of 110 per minute or higher suggests impending cardiac failure. Dyspnea, tachypnea, and moist basal rales are additional signs of cardiac failure.

Treatment includes oxygen, a potent diuretic, rotating tourniquets, and a digitalis preparation. Intravenous digoxin may be indicated if the patient has not received digitalis during the preceding two weeks.

After delivery, during the third stage of labor, blood loss should be minimized. Intravenous therapy is limited, since intravascular expansion can aggravate the cardiac burden. When oxytocin is required for the control of uterine atony, it should be administered intramuscularly. (A sudden intravenous bolus of undiluted oxytocin can precipitate immediate hypotension and tachycardia.) Ergonovine maleate must be used cautiously because of its tendency to produce transient hypertension. If hemorrhage occurs and transfusion is considered essential, packed red cells rather than whole blood are preferable.

Prophylaxis of bacterial endocarditis in patients with a predisposing cardiovascular deformity is directed at preventing bacteremia and eradicating microorganisms after intravascular invasion. Opinions differ over the optimal regimen and even the necessity for prophylaxis after uncomplicated vaginal delivery, since the likelihood of bacteremia is minimal (Everett, 1977).

Although there is no proof that antibiotic agents are effective in preventing bacterial endocarditis in persons undergoing traumatic procedures associated with transient bacteremia, experimental animal data suggest that prophylactic antibiotics offer a reasonable approach to the potential problem. Following genitourinary tract surgery or instrumentation, enterococci are the organisms most frequently responsible for endocarditis. Thus, antibiotic prophylaxis to prevent endocarditis should be directed primarily against enterococci. The Committee on Prevention of Rheumatic Fever and Bacterial Endocarditis of the American Heart Association suggests the following regimen for adults: aqueous crystalline penicillin G (2,000,000 units intramuscularly or intravenously) or ampicillin (1.0 gm intramuscularly or intravenously) *plus* gentamicin (1.5 mg/kg, not to exceed 80 mg, intramuscularly or intravenously) or streptomycin (1.0 gm intramuscularly). The initial dose is given 30 minutes to one hour prior to the procedure. If gentamicin is used, both drugs are repeated 8 and 16 hours later. If streptomycin is used, both drugs are repeated 12 and 24 hours later. For adults allergic to penicillin, the Committee suggests vancomycin (1.0 gm intravenously given over 30 minutes to an hour) *plus* streptomycin (1.0 gm intramuscularly). A single dose of these antibiotics begun 30 minutes to an hour prior to the procedure is probably sufficient, though the same dose may be repeated in 12 hours (Kaplan, 1977).

REFERENCES

Everett ED, Hirschmann JV: Transient bacteremia and endocarditis prophylaxis. A review. Medicine *56*:61-77, 1977

Kaplan EL, Anthony BF, Bisno A, et al: Prevention of bacterial endocarditis. Circulation *56*:139A-143A, 1977

Robertson EG: The natural history of oedema during pregnancy. J Obstet Gynaecol Br Commonw *78*:520-529, 1971

Smith TW: Digitalis glycosides. N Engl J Med *288*:719-722, 942-946, 1973

Ueland K: Pregnancy and cardiovascular disase. Med Clin North Am *61*:17-41, 1977

Ueland K, Metcalfe J: Heart disease in pregnancy. clin Perinatol *1*:349-367, 1974

Ueland K, Metcalfe J: Circulatory changes in pregnancy. Clin Obstet Gynecol *18*:41-50, 1975

25 CEREBROVASCULAR ACCIDENT DURING PREGNANCY

GENERAL CONSIDERATIONS

Cerebrovascular accidents—subarachnoid hemorrhage or cerebral vascular occlusion—are unusual but formidable complications of pregnancy. Maternal mortality ranges from 30 to 45 per cent.

The source of subarachnoid hemorrhage is usually an arteriovenous anomaly or an aneurysm. The former may bleed at any time during pregnancy, while an aneurysm is more likely to bleed during the second half of pregnancy. In general, the relationship between pregnancy and intracranial bleeding is probably fortuitous, although hypertension may provoke rupture of a preexisting vascular anomaly. Labor does not appear to increase the likelihood of a vascular accident.

Occlusive cerebral disease—either arterial or venous—is even rarer than hemorrhage.

SUBJECTIVE DATA

Recurrent severe headache or neck pain or both tend to be the most characteristic presenting symptoms. The pain associated with intracerebral hemorrhage usually develops suddenly, is often localized at first, and has been described as a bursting, bubbling, or cracking sensation or as a constricting pain in the back of the neck.

Coma is a serious prognostic symptom that may portend maternal mortality.

Convulsive seizures with headaches and some degree of paralysis suggest venous or arterial thrombosis. Visual aberrations, aphasia, and psychiatric symptoms may indicate a local cerebral lesion.

OBJECTIVE DATA

General and Neurologic Examination: Blood pressure is elevated in approximately 25 per cent of patients. Papilledema indicates increased intracranial pressure, often associated with cerebral vascular occlusion. Neurologic findings include neck rigidity, pupillary inequality, and motor or sensory impairment. The distribution of neurologic deficits helps to locate the involved blood vessels.

TABLE 25-1. Comparison of Signs and Symptoms in Eclampsia and Subarachnoid Hemorrhage*

	Eclampsia	Subarachnoid Hemorrhage
Headache	60 % (Frontal—throbbing)	80% (Severe sudden—frontal or suboccipital)
Coma	100%	45%
Convulsions	90% (Generalized)	15% (May be focal)
Nausea and vomiting	20% (Usually associated with epigastric pain)	60% (Not usually associated with epigastric pain)
Hypertension	Severe	Present in 40%, but usually moderate
Focal lateralizing neurologic signs	Rare	15%
C.S.F.	Clear—normal pressure	Bloody—usually increased pressure
Albuminuria	99%	50%—mild
Arteriogram	Normal	Aneurysm, 51% Arteriovenous malformation, 6%

*From Barber HRK, Graber EA: Surgical Disease in Pregnancy. Philadelphia, W.B. Saunders Company, 1974, p. 211.

ASSESSMENT

DIFFERENTIAL DIAGNOSIS

This includes eclampsia (see Table 25-1), epilepsy, intracranial infection, and psychosis.

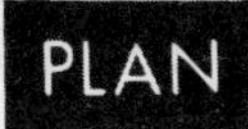

ADDITIONAL DIAGNOSTIC DATA

Lumbar puncture is indicated when subarachnoid hemorrhage is suspected. Heavily blood-stained fluid confirms the diagnosis.

Cerebral angiography or computed tomography may identify the bleeding site or a suspected occlusion.

MANAGEMENT AND PATIENT EDUCATION

Hospitalization and neurosurgical consultation are mandatory. The primary concern is appropriate treatment of the cerebral lesion. In general, neurosurgical management is carried out in the same manner as it would have been if the patient were not pregnant.

Obstetric management is based on the concept of vaginal delivery whenever possible, since cesarean section does not appear to afford any protection against subsequent intracranial hemorrhage (Hunt, 1974). Epidural anesthesia and forceps delivery may obviate preventable cardiovascular stresses (Robinson, 1972).

REFERENCES

Amias AG: Cerebral vascular disease in pregnancy. 1. Hemorrhage. J Obstet Gynaecol Br Commonw *77*:100-120, 1970

Amias AG: Cerebral vascular disease in pregnancy. 2. Occlusion. J. Obstet Gynaecol Br Commonw *77*:312-325, 1970

Carmel PW: Neurologic surgery in pregnancy. *In* Barber HRK, Graber EA: Surgical Disease in Pregnancy. Philadelphia, W.B. Saunders Company, 1974

Dalessio DJ: Neurologic complications. *In* Burrow GN, Ferris TF: Medical Complications during Pregnancy. Philadelphia, W.B. Saunders Company, 1975

Hunt HB, Schifrin BS, Suzuki K: Ruptured berry aneurysms and pregnancy. Obstet Gynecol *43*:827-837, 1974

Robinson JL, Hall CJ, Sedzimir CB: Subarachnoid hemorrhage in pregnancy. J Neurosurg *36*:27-33, 1972

26 CERVICAL LESIONS

Cervical lesions responsible for emergency symptoms may be benign or malignant. Benign cervical pathologic disorders include polyps and inflammatory lesions; malignancies are usually carcinomas.

SUBJECTIVE DATA

Leukorrhea: Increased mucus or mucopurulent vaginal discharge is frequently associated with cervical disease.

Bleeding is usually painless and unrelated to menses but associated with cervical contact (for example, in douching, intercourse). The most likely causes of cervical bleeding are inflammatory lesions, polyps, and malignancy.

OBJECTIVE DATA

Cervical Examination: The cervix may be hypertrophied with single or multiple lacerations. Mucopurulent discharge, reddened areas, polypoid excrescences, or ulcerated lesions may be visualized.

ASSESSMENT

DIFFERENTIAL DIAGNOSIS

Acute cervicitis is an infection of the endocervix caused by a variety of organisms, including gonococci and streptococci. The cervix is reddened and congested with a profuse, purulent discharge. The most common symptom is leukorrhea, which may be accompanied by pelvic pain if the patient has an associated endometritis or salpingitis.

Chronic cervicitis may cause leukorrhea, spotting, or postcoital bleeding. The most common clinical manifestation is *erosion,* a condition characterized by the loss of superficial layers of squamous epithelium and overgrowth of endocervical tissues.

The inflammatory process stimulates a reparative attempt in the form of an upward growth of squamous epithelium that pinches off some of the ducts of endocervical glands. Retained mucus within these glands results in the formation of *Nabothian cysts.*

Eversion is characterized by the rolling out or pouting of the swollen and congested endocervical mucosa.

Polyps are benign, vascular, pedunculated growths that usually arise in the endocervix and project beyond the external cervical os. They are a common cause of cervical bleeding, since the tip tends to bleed easily on contact (douching or intercourse). Polyps also frequently bleed a few days before or after menstruation (Fig. 26-1).

Carcinoma of the cervix is a malignant neoplasm that usually arises in the region of the squamocolumnar junction and invades the cervical stroma. Although the gross appearance is variable, there are essentially three types of lesions: (1) the ulcerative or excavating type, which erodes the cervix and creates an irregular, large crater with infection and discharge; (2) the exophytic or cauliflower type, which may grow to form a large, friable polypoid mass and has a coarsely nodular or papillary appearance; and (3) the infiltrating type, which may grow out on the cervix without ulcerating the cervical mucosa and may extend into the vagina. Symptoms of cervical cancer can vary from none at all to thin, blood-tinged watery discharge to profuse hemorrhage.

Postconization bleeding may be profuse and life-threatening. The diagnosis is established by the history of recent cervical surgery.

Herpetic lesions of the cervix are similar to herpetic lesions on the vulva: groups of multiple vesicles surrounded by a diffuse area of inflammation and edema. The lesions may also appear as multiple small, superficial ulcers with or without vesicles. The diagnosis may be determined from findings on cytologic smear. (See Vulvovaginitis, p. 709.)

Cervical pregnancy is a very rare type of ectopic pregnancy characterized by implantation in the cervical canal below the internal os. Painless bleeding shortly after nidation may be the first sign. Profuse vaginal

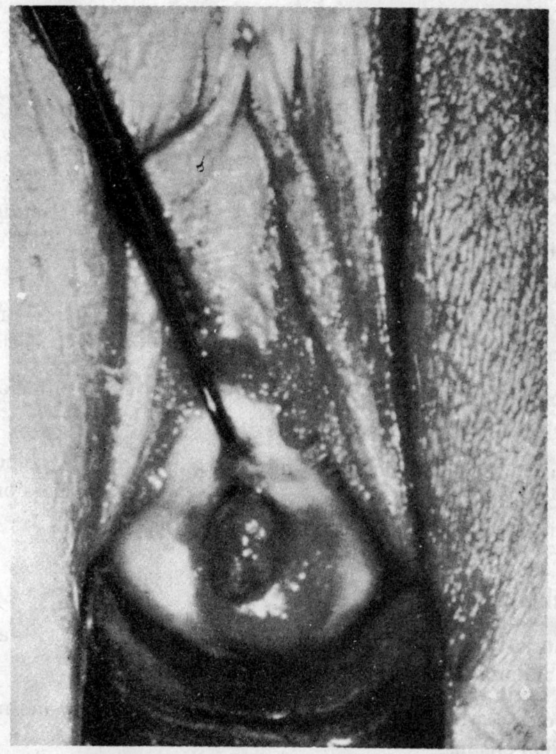

Figure 26-1. A typical cervical polyp, as seen here, is a dark red, soft, pedunculated growth protruding from the cervical canal. (From Huffman JW: Gynecology and Obstetrics. Philadelphia, W.B. Saunders Company, 1962.

bleeding may occur at any time during early pregnancy. Visualization of a hypertrophic, gaping, bleeding cervix with degenerated tissue may create a mistaken impression of carcinoma. (See Ectopic Pregnancy, Cervical Pregnancy, p. 331.)

Endometriosis of the cervix may appear as a slightly raised red area. Dysmenorrhea, dyspareunia, and intermenstrual or postcoital bleeding or both may be associated symptoms. The diagnosis is established by biopsy.

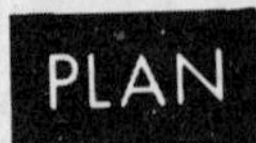

ADDITIONAL DIAGNOSTIC DATA

Cervical Cytologic Test (Pap Smear): A cervical cytologic smear from the squamocolumnar junction and the endocervix is particularly valuable for the evaluation of invisible cervical disease. Findings of dysplasia or possible malignancy indicate the need for additional diagnostic evaluation.

Cervical culture provides a specific bacteriologic diagnosis when gonorrhea is suspected or when a purulent discharge is visualized.

Colposcopy is frequently advised for the evaluation of suspicious cervical lesions or abnormal cytologic smears.

Biopsy provides a definitive histologic diagnosis. A colposcopically directed biopsy plus an endocervical curettage can rule out or confirm a cervical malignancy.

MANAGEMENT

Acute cervicitis due to specific organisms is treated with appropriate antibiotics. (See Gonorrhea, p. 356.)

Chronic cervicitis is frequently treated with cryosurgery and antibacterial vaginal creams.

Polyps can be avulsed by twisting the stalk free from its attachment to the endocervix. With a broad pedicle, the point of attachment is clamped and a ligature tied between the clamp and the cervix. The excised polyp is submitted to the pathology laboratory for microscopic examination. If the stalk is large or there is a history of abnormal bleeding, removal in an operating room may be preferred.

Postconization bleeding may be controlled with Monsel's solution, Avitene, or vaginal packing. Sutures in the bleeding site may be required.

Endometriosis of the cervix may be eradicated with cryosurgery.

Carcinoma of the cervix is treated definitively either by radiation or by radical hysterectomy, depending on the stage of the lesion. Vaginal packing may provide temporary control of the profuse hemorrhage that may occur with recurrent disease. Note: Emergency therapy of hemorrhage always includes intravenous fluids to replace intravascular volume and blood transfusions as necessary.

PATIENT EDUCATION

The importance of follow-up cervical cytologic tests should be emphasized. Often, inflammatory changes that are found on a Pap smear may prevent the cytologist from ruling out cervical dysplasia. After inflammation has been treated, an appropriate follow-up program should be planned.

REFERENCE

DiSaia PJ: The cervix. *In* Romney SL, Gray MJ, Little AB, et al: Gynecology and Obstetrics: The Health Care of Women. New York, McGraw-Hill Book Company, 1975

27 CERVICAL INCOMPETENCE

GENERAL CONSIDERATIONS

Cervical incompetence is a term applied to a rather discrete obstetric condition characterized by *painless, bloodless cervical dilatation* during the second trimester of pregnancy. The cervix appears unable to maintain the products of conception because of injuries or defects of various origins. In spite of the absence of uterine activity and bleeding, the cervix becomes effaced and dilated, and the membranes bulge through it. The bulging membranes rupture, and delivery of the fetus is a rapid and rather painless procedure.

SUBJECTIVE DATA

CURRENT SYMPTOMS

Vaginal mucous discharge may be the first indication of cervical dilatation. Frequently, there are no overt symptoms, although an occasional patient may be aware of lower abdominal discomfort or a sensation of fullness in the vagina.

PRIOR HISTORY

A history of spontaneous rupture of membranes during the second trimester in previous pregnancies followed by short, relatively painless labor with delivery of a live, immature fetus is so characteristic that a presumptive diagnosis of cervical incompetence is often based on the typical history.

Occasional patients give a past history of cervical dilatation, cauterization, or conization.

OBJECTIVE DATA

General examination is normal.

Abdominal examination is normal for gestational age during the second trimester. Fetal heart tones are present.

Pelvic Examination: Speculum examination and digital examination identify the cervical effacement and dilatation. The amniotic sac may be seen bulging through the cervical os.

ASSESSMENT

DIFFERENTIAL DIAGNOSIS

This includes premature labor—premature contractions that may be associated with a uterine anomaly (such as a bicornuate uterus) or uterine myomas.

The diagnosis of cervical incompetence is based on the typical history of prior second trimester abortions, coupled with the findings of painless cervical dilatation during the second trimester.

ETIOLOGIC FACTORS

Etiologic factors that appear to contribute to cervical incompetence are (1) traumatic injuries (cervical cauterization, dilatation, or conization; previous childbirth), (2) congenital defects, and (3) functional disorders involving a physiologic incompetence of the cervical isthmus.

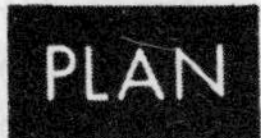

MANAGEMENT

As soon as the diagnosis is suspected, the patient should be hospitalized. As long as the membranes are intact and the patient is not in labor, cervical cerclage—surgical closure of the incompetent cervical os by an encircling suture—should be considered.

Contraindications to cerclage include uterine bleeding, ruptured membranes, amnionitis, and active labor. Potential surgical complications that should be discussed with the patient include hemorrhage, infection, uterine rupture, and cervical stenosis. The patient should also be advised that operative delivery may subsequently be necessary.

Two of the more popular cervical cerclage procedures are the modified Shirodkar and the McDonald.

In a modified Shirodkar procedure an inert tape of nonabsorbable suture material (usually Mersilene) 5 mm wide is used. The vaginal epithelium over the internal os is incised anteriorly and posteriorly. The tissues overlying the cervix are separated from the cervix by undermining the vaginal mucosa. A large aneurysm needle is then used for threading the suture band in a purse-string fashion under the vaginal mucosa and around the cervix, at the level of the internal os. The band is drawn tightly and tied. Anchoring sutures of nonabsorbable material are placed in the band and the cervix in order to keep the band in place. The vaginal epithelium is closed over the supporting suture with absorbable suture.

In the McDonald procedure (Fig. 27-1), the cervix is exposed and grasped at each quadrant with an Allis, Babcock, or ring forceps. A purse-string suture of #4 Mersilene or braided silk is inserted around the exocervix as high as possible at the junction of the rugose vagina and the smooth cervix (the level of the internal os). The suture is started from 11 o'clock to 10 o'clock and then continued around the cervix with two bites posteriorly. The posterior bites should be placed deeply to minimize the possibility of the ligature's subsequently pulling out. Four or five bites are taken. The suture is then pulled tight enough to close the internal os. The knot is tied on the anterior surface, and the ends are left long enough to facilitate subsequent division. The procedure may be done at any time during the second trimester.

After surgery, the patient should remain at bed rest for one or two days. Intravenous alcohol may be considered if uterine contractions ensue.

If ruptured membranes, uterine infection, bleeding, or contractions develop after the cerclage suture has been inserted, it must be released immediately to obviate any risk of serious cervical trauma or sepsis.

In successful cases following the McDonald procedure, the suture is removed at 38 weeks to allow labor to progress. After the Shirodkar procedure, the suture can be left in place if it remains covered by mucosa; in this case, cesarean section is performed near term. Otherwise, the suture could be released and vaginal delivery permitted.

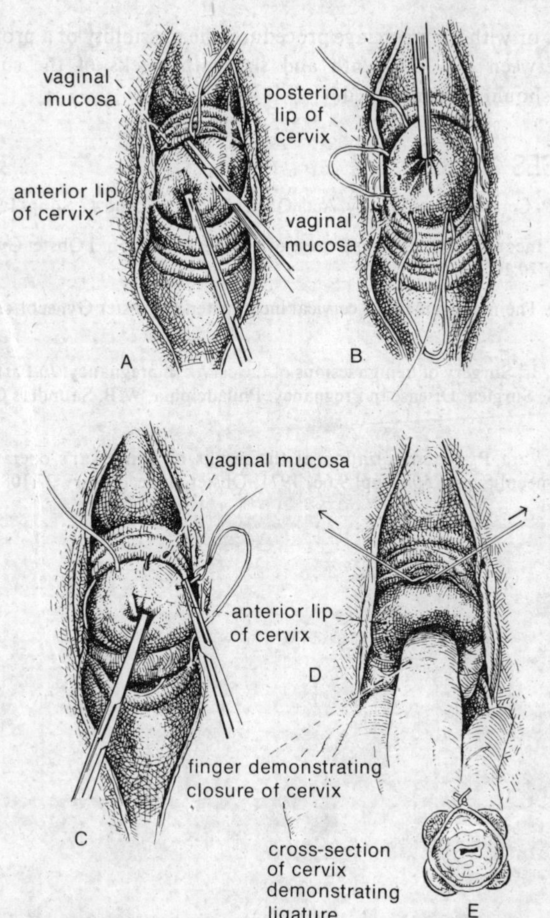

Figure 27-1. The McDonald procedure for cervical cerclage.

PATIENT EDUCATION

The risks of cervical cerclage (cervical trauma, infection, abortion, hemorrhage, uterine rupture, anesthetic risks, and subsequent cesarean section) are reviewed with the patient. If abortion or premature delivery occurs with or without a cerclage procedure, the possibility of a prophylactic cerclage between the fourteenth and sixteenth weeks of the subsequent pregnancy should be considered.

REFERENCES

Bengtsson LP: Cervical insufficiency. Acta Obstet Gynecol Scand *47*:Suppl 1:9-35, 1968

McDonald I: Incompetent cervix as a cause of recurrent abortion. J Obstet Gynaecol Br Commonw *70*:105-109, 1963

Robboy MS: The management of cervical incompetence. Obstet Gynecol *41*:108-112, 1973

Roddick JW, Jr: Surgery of benign lesions of the cervix in pregnancy. *In* Barber HRK, Graber EA: Surgical Disease in Pregnancy. Philadelphia, W.B. Saunders Company, 1974

Seppälä M, Vara P: Standardization of the results of Shirodkar's operation. Acta Obstet Gynecol Scand *50*:Suppl 9:66, 1971; Obstet Gynecol Surv *27*:108-109, 1972

28 CHEST PAIN IN PREGNANCY

GENERAL CONSIDERATIONS

Acute chest pain, a relatively uncommon emergency symptom during pregnancy, may result from the same etiologic factors that would be expected in the nonpregnant patient. (See Dyspnea during Pregnancy, p. 298.)

SUBJECTIVE DATA

The nature of the pain—location, radiation, quality, intensity, duration, and aggravating and alleviating factors—often provides key diagnostic clues.

Sharp, knifelike pain, related to respiratory movements and aggravated by cough or deep inspiration, is characteristically pleural and results from stretching of inflamed parietal pleura.

Sudden anterior chest pain can be caused by a massive pulmonary embolism or pneumothorax. Smaller pulmonary emboli can cause pleuritic chest pain.

Periodic heartburn relieved by antacids or bland food is characteristic of reflux esophagitis and possibly hiatal hernia. Regurgitation of gastric contents as a result of relaxation of the cardioesophageal area and the increasing intra-abdominal pressure caused by the enlarging uterus contribute to gastro-esophageal reflux.

OBJECTIVE DATA

Pulmonary, cardiac, and chest wall examination may disclose a friction rub, tachycardia, pulmonary or cardiac disease, or skin or breast lesions.

ASSESSMENT

DIFFERENTIAL DIAGNOSIS

1. Chest wall, including breast
   a. Injury
   b. Muscle spasm
   c. Infection
   d. Neoplasm
2. Esophagus
   a. Esophagitis, with or without hiatal hernia
3. Lung
   a. Pleuritis
   b. Pulmonary embolism
   c. Pneumothorax
   d. Pneumonia
4. Heart
   a. Coronary thrombosis and ischemic heart disease
   b. Pericarditis
5. Abdominal disorders
   a. Liver and gallbladder disease
   b. Peptic ulcers
   c. Pancreatitis

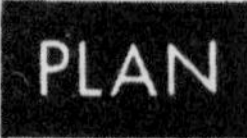

ADDITIONAL DIAGNOSTIC DATA

Chest x-ray is essential when there is any suspicion of pulmonary disease.

Electrocardiogram may aid in the diagnosis of suspected pulmonary embolism or myocardial infarction.

Evaluation of arterial blood gases may be helpful when pulmonary embolism is suspected. A pO_2 of 90 mm Hg or above virtually rules out the diagnosis of pulmonary embolism.

Barium swallow may demonstrate hiatal hernia. During pregnancy, however, x-ray exposure can be avoided, since there is little need to accurately diagnose hiatus hernia.

MANAGEMENT AND PATIENT EDUCATION

Treatment depends on the specific diagnosis:

Pulmonary or Cardiac Disease: Hospitalization may be required for diagnostic evaluation and appropriate management.

Esophagitis and hiatal hernia are among the more common causes of chest discomfort during pregnancy. Symptoms can usually be relieved by 15 to 30 ml of an antacid preparation containing aluminum and magnesium hydroxide. If the magnesium hydroxide produces diarrhea, calcium carbonate or aluminum hydroxide would be preferred.

In addition, the patient should be advised to sleep with the head of the bed slightly elevated and cautioned not to lie down immediately after eating. If stooping and bending over aggravate her symptoms, she should be advised to bend down by squatting.

Fat, orange juice, tomato juice, tomato paste, chocolate, alcohol in large doses, and cigarette smoking should be avoided. Frequent, small meals are advisable.

Anticholinergic drugs are not recommended, since these agents may impair the resting tone of the inferior esophageal sphincter and inhibit gastric emptying, effects that contribute to gastroesophageal reflux.

During pregnancy, surgical therapy is rarely necessary, since improvement often follows delivery. However, complications (massive bleeding, perforation, or obstruction) require surgical consultation.

29 CHOLECYSTITIS DURING PREGNANCY

Acute attacks of gallbladder disease during pregnancy are infrequent, even though gallstones may be present or form during pregnancy.

SUBJECTIVE DATA

CURRENT SYMPTOMS

Abdominal pain may develop gradually or suddenly in the right upper quadrant or epigastric area and may radiate into the right anterior chest or posteriorly to the region of the right scapula. Pain of biliary colic tends to be intermittent and excruciating; usually it is associated with nausea and persistent vomiting. With complete blockage of the cystic duct, the pain becomes constant in character and may be accompanied by chills and fever.

PRIOR HISTORY

A history of gallbladder disease or intolerance to fatty foods is a usual finding.

OBJECTIVE DATA

PHYSICAL EXAMINATION

General Examination: The temperature may be moderately elevated (101°F). Jaundice develops when the common duct is obstructed.

Abdominal Examination: Tenderness in the right upper quadrant is the most characteristic finding.

LABORATORY TESTS

Complete Blood Count with Blood Smear: The white count tends to be moderately elevated.

Urinalysis is normal.

ASSESSMENT

DIFFERENTIAL DIAGNOSIS

The differential diagnosis of acute right upper quadrant pain includes preeclampsia, liver disease (including hepatic rupture), pancreatitis, pyelonephritis, peptic ulcer, esophageal hiatal hernia, and acute appendicitis during the third trimester, when the appendix is displaced into the right upper quadrant.

PLAN

ADDITIONAL DIAGNOSTIC DATA

X-ray Studies: Benefits and risks of cholecystography must be evaluated on an individual basis, depending on the stage of gestation, the nature of the symptoms, and the necessity of radiographic confirmation. An abdominal film of the right upper quadrant may reveal radiopaque calculi. During an acute attack, oral cholecystograms are diagnostically unreliable because of unpredictable absorption and excretion of the contrast agent. Ultrasonic scanning may be helpful.

MANAGEMENT

Medical management is preferred initially, since most patients with acute cholecystitis improve within 48 hours on a conservative regimen. The patient is observed in the hospital, given nothing orally, and placed on nasogastric suction. Fluids and electrolytes are replaced intravenously; meperidine hydrochloride or an equivalent analgesic is given parenterally for pain. If the patient is seen shortly after symptoms begin, and if local signs and symptoms are mild, opinions differ over the need for antibiotic therapy. However, antibiotics are recommended if there is any evidence of suppurative complications.

Biliary tract surgery is rarely necessary during pregnancy unless complications occur. Progressive infection, necrosis, gangrene, perforation, or refractory biliary colic may necessitate surgical intervention.

PATIENT EDUCATION

A patient with known, chronic gallbladder disease should be advised to eat a bland, relatively low-fat diet during pregnancy. If the acute attack subsides spontaneously on medical management, the patient should be advised to have a radiographic study of the biliary tract performed after delivery.

REFERENCE

Hill LM, Johnson CE, Lee RA: Cholecystectomy in pregnancy. Obstet Gynecol *46*:291-293, 1975

30 CHORIOAMNIONITIS

GENERAL CONSIDERATIONS

Chorioamnionitis—infection of fetal membranes—is usually caused by the upward spread of vaginal organisms. Two of the most important predisposing factors are membranes ruptured for over 24 hours and prolonged labor. Bacteria most likely to be responsible include *Escherichia coli,* aerobic and anaerobic Streptococcus, Proteus, Staphylococcus, and Bacteroides.

When membranes are intact, chorioamnionitis may develop from ascending infections; from hematogenous dissemination of viruses, bacteria, fungi, or protozoa (syphilis, toxoplasmosis, rubella, herpes, cytomegalovirus); or as a consequence of diagnostic amniocentesis.

SUBJECTIVE DATA

Fever, chills, and uterine pain are the most typical symptoms. Almost always there is a history of ruptured membranes.

OBJECTIVE DATA

PHYSICAL EXAMINATION

General Examination: Temperature and pulse rate tend to be elevated.

Abdominal Examination: The uterus may be tender and tense upon palpation. Persistent fetal tachycardia may indicate amniotic infection or the fetal response to maternal fever. Since intrauterine death may result from infection, sudden cessation of the fetal heart rate should alert the physician to the possibility of chorioamnionitis.

Pelvic Examination: Speculum examination may reveal malodorous or purulent amniotic fluid.

LABORATORY TESTS

Complete Blood Count and Blood Smear: The white blood count tends to be elevated; there is an increased number of immature cells on the differential smear.

ASSESSMENT

Once chorioamnionitis has developed, the lives of both mother and fetus are in jeopardy.

POTENTIAL COMPLICATIONS

Complications to be anticipated include septicemia, septic shock, renal failure, adrenal hemorrhage, septic pulmonary emboli, disseminated intravascular coagulation, and fetal death.

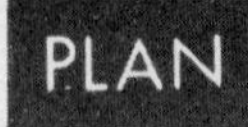

ADDITIONAL DIAGNOSTIC DATA

Bacteriologic examinations should include Gram stain, aerobic cultures of the cervical discharge, and aerobic and anaerobic blood cultures. Cultures should also be taken from the placenta at the time of delivery in order to help determine the responsible organism.

MANAGEMENT AND PATIENT EDUCATION

Antibiotic Therapy: Usually ampicillin (with or without an aminoglycoside) or a cephalosporin is prescribed when there is evidence of chorioamnionitis. The antibiotic chosen may be based on the Gram-stained smear or on knowledge of recent infections.

Delivery: The uterus should be evacuated by the most expeditious route:

Oxytocic induction usually accomplishes delivery without difficulty.

Cesarean section is indicated for fetal malpresentation, fetal distress, or impeded progress of labor (unsatisfactory cervical dilatation or fetal descent). At surgery, aerobic and anaerobic cultures should be taken from the uterine cavity. If abdominal delivery becomes necessary, *cesarean hysterectomy* should be considered when the patient has completed her family, especially when the uterus is grossly infected or traumatized by extensive clostridial infection. (See Pelvic Infection, p. 474.)

REFERENCE

Dudgeon JA: Intrauterine infection. Proc Roy Soc Med *68*:365-374, 1975

31 CIRSOID ANEURYSM OF UTERUS

GENERAL CONSIDERATIONS

Cirsoid aneurysm of the uterus is characterized by multiple abnormal communications between arteries and veins—multiple arteriovenous aneurysms or fistulae with the formation of a mass of dilated arteries and veins. Cirsoid aneurysm has also been defined as a pulsating tumor caused by an anastomosis between small arteries and veins, without the interposition of capillaries.

The condition appears to be congenital in origin and extremely rare.

SUBJECTIVE DATA

Menorrhagia—heavy menses—with or without intermenstrual bleeding is the most characteristic symptom. Menstrual periods can be profuse and gushing.

OBJECTIVE DATA

PHYSICAL EXAMINATION

Pelvic Examination: The uterus is frequently slightly enlarged, soft, and compressible. A palpable thrill, an audible bruit, and parametrial pulsations may be evident.

LABORATORY TESTS

Complete blood count reveals the extent of blood-loss anemia.

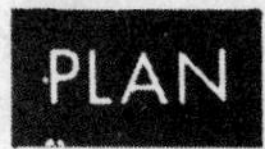

ADDITIONAL DIAGNOSTIC DATA

Arteriogram can provide a specific diagnosis.

MANAGEMENT AND PATIENT EDUCATION

Hysterectomy is the only definitive treatment.

Curettage may be associated with profuse and even uncontrollable bleeding. Consequently, whenever the diagnosis is suspected, either a preoperative arteriogram is indicated or the possibility of hysterectomy anticipated. At least 2 to 4 units of blood should be available for transfusion if necessary.

REFERENCES

Gardner HJ: Cirsoid aneurysm of the uterus. Am J Obstet Gynecol *68*:845-853, 1954

Hibbard BM, Prysor Jones D, Scarrow GD: Cirsoid aneurysm of the uterus as a cause of menorrhagia. J Obstet Gynaecol Br Commonw *79*:855-859, 1972

32 COAGULATION DISORDERS

GENERAL CONSIDERATIONS

Coagulation may be considered to be the final outcome of the interaction between two opposed and normally balanced mechanisms: the conversion of fibrinogen to fibrin, and fibrinolysis. These systems are in dynamic equilibrium and changes altering the activity of either one lead to a tendency toward increased clotting or hemorrhage.

Hemostasis—the process that arrests bleeding from injured blood vessels—may be divided into three phases: vascular, platelet, and coagulation.

The vascular phase is the initial vasoconstriction that reduces the blood flow through an injured area. Escape of blood into normal tissue is also limited by any increased tissue pressure in the extravascular supporting tissue, which tends to collapse venules and capillaries.

The platelet phase becomes active within seconds after injury. Platelets adhere to the surface of the injured vessel and initiate a complex secretory phenomenon, termed the release reaction. This results in further adhesion of platelets to each other—platelet aggregation—a process that becomes self-perpetuating.

A plug or thrombus composed of irreversibly aggregated platelets is rapidly produced. For small injuries, the platelet thrombus alone may be sufficient to arrest bleeding; for larger injuries, the platelet thrombus provides temporary hemostasis.

Various platelet phospholipids, generally termed platelet factor 3 (PF-3), are also essential for at least two steps in blood coagulation: the activation of factor X by factors IX and VIII and the formation of prothrombinase.

The coagulation phase results in permanent hemostasis, with the formation of a firm, impermeable fibrin thrombus.

Two separate pathways lead to the activation of factor X (Table 32-1). In the intrinsic pathway all the factors are present in the

TABLE 32-1. Pathways of Blood Coagulation*

Intrinsic Pathway	*Extrinsic Pathway*
XII —(Negatively charged surface)→ Activated XII (XIIa)	
XI —(XIIa)→ XIa	
IX —(XIa, Ca^{++})→ IXa	
X —(IXa, VIII†, Ca^{++} / Phospholipid)→ Xa	X —(Tissue Factor, VII / Ca^{++})→ Xa

Common Pathway

Prothrombin	Xa, V†, Ca^{++} / Phospholipid →	Thrombin
Fibrinogen†	Thrombin →	Fibrin monomer
Fibrin Monomer	Spontaneous Polymerization →	Loose fibrin gel
Loose Fibrin Gel	XIII† →	Firm clot

*From Zieve PD, Levin J: Disorders of Hemostasis. Philadelphia, W.B. Saunders Company, 1976.

†Proteins modified or activated by thrombin.

circulating blood, whereas in the extrinsic pathway tissue substances or tissue thromboplastin, normally not present in blood, are required.

The intrinsic pathway begins with the activation of factor XII by contact with disrupted vascular endothelium. A sequence of reactions involving factors XI, IX, and VIII and ionic calcium leads to the activation of factor X.

The extrinsic pathway leads to the activation of factor X by tissue factor, factor VII, and calcium ion.

Activated factor X initiates the common pathway of coagulation, converting prothrombin (factor II) into *thrombin.* The reaction is accelerated by a complex formed by factor V, ionic calcium, and phospholipid provided by platelet membranes.

Conversion of Fibrinogen into Fibrin: Conversion of the soluble protein fibrinogen into insoluble fibrin occurs in three stages. (1) The proteolytic action of thrombin removes four polypeptides from the fibrinogen molecule, creating *fibrin monomers.* (2) The fibrin monomers polymerize and ultimately gel to form a loosely structured clot (soluble fibrin). (3) This clot is stabilized by the action of factor XIII (fibrin stabilizing factor).

The effect of pregnancy on the various coagulation factors is summarized in Table 32-2.

TABLE 32-2. Coagulation Factors

	Name	Pregnancy Effect
FACTOR I	Fibrinogen (200-400 mg/100 ml)	Increased 50 per cent (300-600 mg/100 ml)
FACTOR II	Prothrombin	Increased slightly or unchanged
FACTOR III	Tissue thromboplastin	—
FACTOR IV	Calcium	—
FACTOR V	Proaccelerin Labile factor Accelerator globulin (AcG) Thrombogen	Increased slightly or unchanged
FACTOR VI	Activated form of Factor V	—

TABLE 32-2. Coagulation Factors (Continued)

	Name	Pregnancy Effect
FACTOR VII	Proconvertin Stable factor Serum prothrombin conversion accelerator (SPCA) Autoprothrombin I	Increased
FACTOR VIII	Antihemophilic factor (AHF) Antihemophilic globulin (AHG) Thromboplastinogen Platelet cofactor I Plasma thromboplastic factor A	Increased
FACTOR IX	Christmas factor Plasma thromboplstin component (PTC) Platelet cofactor II Autoprothrombin II Plasma thromboplastic factor B	Increased or no change
FACTOR X	Stuart-Prower factor	Increased
FACTOR XI	Plasma thromboplastin antecedent (PTA) Antihemophilic factor C	Decreased
FACTOR XII	Hageman factor	Unchanged
FACTOR XIII	Fibrin-stabilizing factor Laki-Lorand factor Fibrinase	Decreased

Coagulation Inhibitors:

Antithrombin III neutralizes the activity of clotting factor Xa and impedes coagulation. The effectiveness of antithrombin III is enhanced by small amounts of heparin and appears to be inhibited by estrogen. People with an inherited deficiency of antithrombin III have an increased susceptibility to thrombosis.

Fibrinolysis is accomplished by the proteolytic enzyme *plasmin,* which is formed from *plasminogen,* an inert precursor in plasma (Table 32-3). Activation of plasminogen is poorly understood but appears to result when cellular lysosomes are released by a variety of stimuli, including stress, hypoglycemia, anoxia, and even vigorous exercise.

TABLE 32-3. Sequence of Fibrinolysis

Plasminogen	Activators →	Plasmin
Fibrin (or fibrinogen)	Plasmin →	Fibrin (or fibrinogen) breakdown products (FDP-fdp)

*From Zieve PD, Levin J: Disorders of Hemostasis. Philadelphia, W.B. Saunders Company, 1976.

Plasmin breaks down both fibrinogen and fibrin into several degradation products (fibrin-split products). These are large polypeptides that interfere with hemostatis by blocking the polymerization of fibrin.

SUBJECTIVE DATA

CURRENT SYMPTOMS

Vaginal Bleeding: Menorrhagia (prolonged or excessive menstrual bleeding) is the most usual gynecologic symptom. This may be associated with a past history of epistaxis, gastrointestinal bleeding, petechiae, ecchymoses, or excessive bleeding with surgery, delivery, tooth extraction, trauma, or previous menses.

PRIOR HISTORY

A history of ingestion of drugs that can cause bleeding (for example, aspirin) or systemic disease (liver disease, leukemia, renal disease, and so forth), or a family history of bleeding disorders may provide helpful diagnostic clues.

OBJECTIVE DATA

PHYSICAL EXAMINATION

General Examination: Multiple bleeding sites may be evident. Petechiae suggest a vascular or platelet abnormality. Ecchymoses suggest a coagulation factor deficiency or trauma to blood vessels.

Abdominal Examination: Hepatosplenomegaly suggests systemic disease.

Pelvic examination is usually normal.

LABORATORY TESTS

Complete blood count with blood smear may show decreased or absent platelets. Fragmented erythrocytes in addition to thrombocytopenia suggest the possibility of a microangiopathic hemolytic process associated with disseminated intravascular coagulation or thrombotic thrombocytopenic purpura.

ASSESSMENT

CLASSIFICATION OF COAGULATION DISORDERS

1. Inherited disorders of plasma coagulation factors
   a. Von Willebrand's disease (see p. 215)—an abnormality of blood-clotting factors characterized by a dual hemostatic defect: deficiency of factor VIII and a prolonged bleeding time, the latter suggesting an abnormality in the platelet phase of hemostasis. Inherited as an autosomal dominant trait, this disease is the most common clinically significant abnormality of coagulation factors in women.
   b. Factor XI (PTA) deficiency—very rare
2. Thrombocytopenia
   a. Peripheral destruction of platelets
      (1) Immunologic thrombocytopenic purpura (ITP)
      (2) Drug-induced thrombocytopenia
      (3) Disseminated intravascular coagulation
      (4) Thrombotic thrombocytopenic purpura
      (5) Infection

b. Deficient platelet production in bone marrow
   (1) Tumor
   (2) Cytotoxic drugs
   (3) Aplastic anemia
3. Disseminated intravascular coagulation
4. Liver disease
   a. Deficiency of vitamin K-dependent factors: prothrombin and factors VII, IX, and X
   b. Fibrinogen deficiency
   c. Plasminogen and antithrombin III deficiency

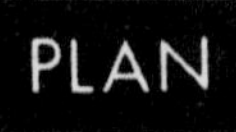

ADDITIONAL DIAGNOSTIC DATA

1. Tests of the vascular and platelet phases
   a. Platelet count: Normal values are 150,000 to 400,000 per cu mm. Functionally normal platelets in numbers greater than 50,000 per cu mm ordinarily prevent hemorrhage during surgical procedures. Spontaneous bleeding is unlikely unless the platelet count is 20,000 per cu mm or less. At these levels, the major threat is intracranial hemorrhage.
2. Tests of the coagulation phase (Tables 32-4 and 32-5)
   a. Prothrombin time: This measures extrinsic pathway and common pathway (factors I, II, V, VII, and X). It is prolonged in liver disease, vitamin K deficiency, intravascular coagulation, hypofibrinogenemia, and therapy with coumarin-like drugs.
   b. Partial thromboplastin time: This measures intrinsic pathway and common pathway (factors I, II, V, VIII, IX, X, XI, and XII). It is prolonged if the level of any of the required factors is below 15 to 20 per cent of normal. The test is also prolonged by heparin.
   c. Fibrinogen
   d. Fibrin-split products
   e. Clot observation for lysis—gross measurement of the fibrinolytic enzyme plasmin.
3. Specific factor assays

TABLE 32-4. Tests of Hemostatic Function: Coagulation*

Test	What Is Tested	How Performed	Normal Value
1. Clotting time of whole blood	Intrinsic and common pathways	Measurement of time for blood to clot in glass tube: observation of clot retraction	5-10 minutes to clot 50 per cent retraction within 1 hour
2. Partial thromboplastin time (PTT)	Intrinsic and common pathways	Recalcification of plasma after addition of phospholipid (plus addition of kaolin for maximum surface activation in activated PTT)	Unactivated: 60-90 seconds Activated: 30-60 seconds
3. Prothrombin time	Extrinsic and common pathways	Recalcification of plasma after addition of tissue factor (thromboplastin)	Varies according to source of thromboplastin: compare to normal control (usually 12-15 seconds)
4. Thrombin time	Fibrinogen concentration: structure of fibrinogen: presence of inhibitors	Addition of thrombin to plasma	Varies according to concentration of thrombin: compare to normal value
5. Specific factor assays	Concentration of functional factor in plasma	Measurement of effect of test plasma on recalcified clotting time of substrate deficient plasma	>50-150% of activity in pooled normal plasma

* From Zieve PD, Levin J: Disorders of Hemostasis. Philadelphia, W.B. Saunders Company, 1976.

TABLE 32-5. What Coagulation Tests Measure*

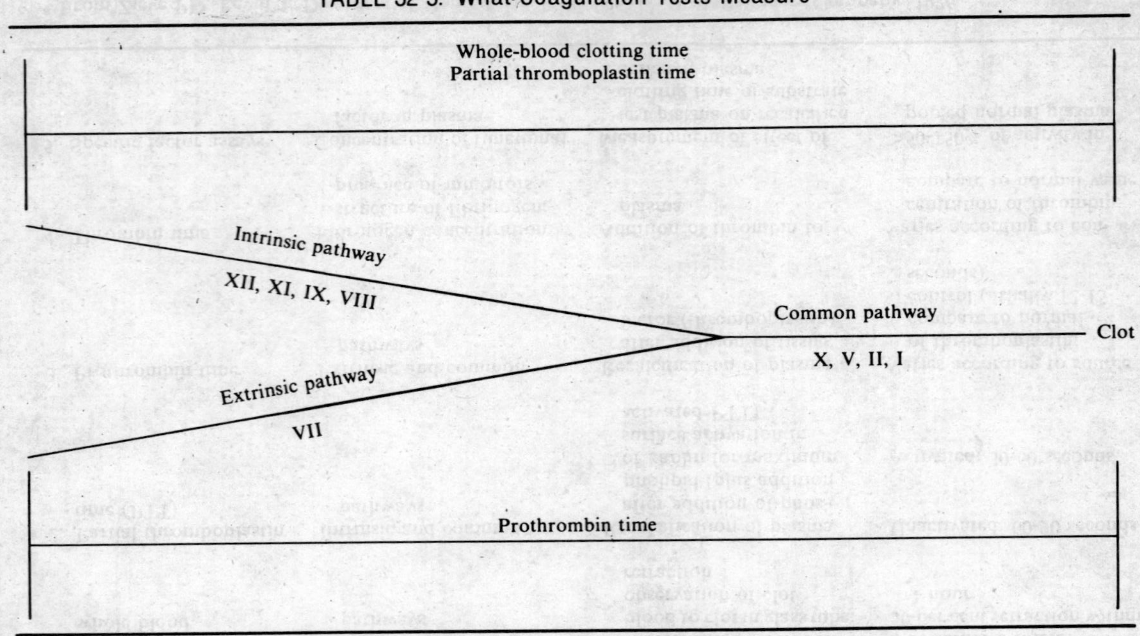

*From Zieve PD, Levin J: Disorders of Hemostasis. Philadelphia, W.B. Saunders Company, 1976.

MANAGEMENT AND PATIENT EDUCATION

Treatment depends on the specific coagulopathy and the extent of the bleeding disorder. When surgery is required or when bleeding is profuse, transfusion with fresh whole blood, platelets, fresh-frozen plasma, or cryoprecipitate may be required. (See Blood Transfusion, p. 750.)

Aspirin and other drugs that interfere with platelet function should be avoided.

Disseminated Intravascular Coagulation (DIC)

GENERAL CONSIDERATIONS

Disseminated intravascular coagulation is a complex disarray of the hemostatic mechanism in which accelerated coagulation and activation of the fibrinolytic system occur simultaneously, with varying degrees of thrombosis and hemorrhage.

Thromboplastic substances released into the circulation provoke a generalized activation of *prothrombin* into *thrombin*. Intravascular clotting causes a reduction in the levels of circulating clotting factors and platelets.

Vasculitis associated with eclampsia or septic abortion causes intimal damage, deposition of platelets, and intravascular clotting in peripheral vessels.

Local activation of the fibrinolytic system—fibrinolysis with a concomitant increase in fibrin-split products—represents the body's attempt to defend itself against the generalized clotting that would occur in the absence of unchecked thrombin activity.

Fibrinogen appears to be altered in such a way that it is no longer able to polymerize and immediately undergoes destruction by plasmin through local lysis, resulting in degradation products. Furthermore, the presence of fibrin degradation products may inhibit the normal conversion of fibrinogen to fibrin, establishing a vicious cycle.

Synonyms for disseminated intravascular clotting are intravascular coagulation and fibrinolysis (ICF), consumption coagulopathy, defibrination, defibrinogenation, and fibrination.

PATHOPHYSIOLOGY

1. Thrombin activities
   a. Fibrinogen (factor I) converted into fibrin
   b. Platelet aggregation
   c. Autocatalytic effect on clotting mechanism
   d. Plasminogen converted into plasmin, the active fibrinolytic agent. (Normally plasminogen is bound in fibrin mesh and the plasmin is released only in fibrin mesh–physiologic proteolysis.)
2. Plasmin in large quantities causes fibrin/fibrinogen degradation products, that is, fibrin-split products. These have anticoagulant effects:
   a. They compete with fibrinogen for available thrombin.
   b. They form insoluble nonclottable complexes with fibrin monomers blocking fibrin gel formation.
   c. They have an antiplatelet effect, inhibiting platelet aggregation.
3. Thrombin's action on fibrinogen results in intravascular deposition of fibrin (DIC) while plasmin activity tends to render the blood nonclottable via the formation of fibrin degradation products. A state of balanced coagulation and anticoagulation may exist at first. With the formation of fibrin thrombi, consumption of clotting factors and platelets occurs; the precarious balance is offset towards a hemorrhagic diathesis. At the same time, fibrin deposition in the small vessels of the kidneys, lungs, liver, and brain may cause tissue anoxia and necrosis. When tissue damage becomes extensive enough, vascular collapse ensues. This sequence of events appears to perpetuate the disordered coagulation process.
4. The end result is either primarily clotting or primarily bleeding, depending on whether the balance is tipped towards the plasmin side (bleeding) or the thrombin side (clotting).
5. Normal mechanisms to prevent generalized coagulation when thrombin is present.
   a. Hepatic clearance—to remove activated factors
   b. Fibrinolysis
   c. Dilution by blood flow
   d. Antifactors to activated products (Antithrombin III)

SUBJECTIVE DATA

Bleeding from multiple sites (vagina, nose, gingival tissues, skin, venipunctures) suggests defective hemostasis. *Hematomas, ecchymoses, or petechiae* may be observed.

ASSESSMENT

TABLE 32-6. Causes of Disseminated Intravascular Coagulation (DIC)*

Obstetric Complications
- Abruptio placentae — Premature placental separation
- Retained dead fetus
- Amniotic fluid embolism†
- Retained placenta
- Preeclampsia or eclampsia
- Intraamniotic injection of hyperosmolar urea or hypertonic saline

Infections and Endotoxins
- Bacterial
- Viral
- Protozoan
- Rickettsial
- Fungal

Hypotension — tissue anoxia, acidosis

Neoplasia
- Acute leukemia
- Carcinoma
- Sarcoma

Heatstroke

*Modified from Zieve PD, Levin J: Disorders of Hemostasis. Philadelphia, W.B. Saunders Company, 1976.

†The manner in which amniotic fluid triggers clotting is obscure. Amniotic fluid does not contain sufficient coagulant activity to produce disseminated intravascular coagulation, even when relatively large quantities are infused (Phillips and Davidson, 1972). Perhaps the "shock lung" resulting from the embolism or the contamination with meconium or squamous cells induces the intravascular coagulation.

TABLE 32-6. Causes of Disseminated Intravascular Coagulation (DIC)* (Continued)

Miscellaneous
Snakebite
Lung surgery
Circulating immune complexes
Massive trauma
Giant hemangioma
Liver disease
Hemolytic transfusion reactions
Trauma (when other predisposing factors are present)

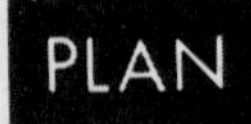

PLAN

ADDITIONAL DIAGNOSTIC DATA

Complete blood count with blood smear indicates the degree of anemia. The morphologic condition of erythrocytes may be abnormal, with fragmented red cells or schistocytes being observable on a smear of peripheral blood.

Urinalysis may disclose hematuria.

Coagulation Tests (Table 32-7):

Clot Observation Test: Blood fails to clot in a test tube, or the initial clot subsequently lyses. When the plasma fibrinogen level falls to 50 mg per 100 ml, the blood clot is flimsy and easily distinguished from normal. In the case of an active fibrinolytic process, the flimsy clot disappears in several minutes' to an hour's time.

Platelet count is decreased.

Fibrinogen is decreased.

Fibrin-split products (fibrin degradation products) are elevated.

Prothrombin time is usually prolonged.

Partial thromboplastin time is usually prolonged.

TABLE 32-7. Tests of Hemostatic Function in Patients with DIC*

Usually Abnormal	*Variably Abnormal*
Platelet count†	Clot observation
Prothrombin time†	Partial thromboplastin time
Fibrinogen concentration†	Assays of factors XI, IX, X, VII, II
Titer of FDP-fdp†§	Red cell morphology
Assay of factors VIII‡, V‡, XIII	Thrombin time

*From Zieve PD, Levin J: Disorders of Hemostasis. Philadelphia, W.B. Saunders Company, 1976.

†These are the important tests to perform to establish diagnosis.

‡Two-stage assays usually are necessary to detect decreased levels of factors V and VIII during DIC.

§(FDP-fdp=Degradation products or fibrinogen and fibrin.)

MANAGEMENT

General Principles:

1. Eliminate the underlying cause.
   a. Evacuate uterus in cases of placental abruption, dead fetus, eclampsia, and septic abortion.
   b. Treat shock.
   c. Treat infection.
2. Correct associated factors.
   a. Hypovolemia
   b. Hypoxia
   c. Acidosis
   d. Vascular stasis
3. Monitor intake and output.
   a. Bladder catheter
   b. Central venous pressure

Specific Measures:

Circulatory Support: With adequate perfusion of vital organs, activated coagulation factors, soluble fibrin, and fibrin degradation products are more promptly removed by the reticuloendothelial system. At the same time, synthesis of procoagulants is promoted.

As soon as the underlying cause can be eradicated or ameliorated, the coagulation defect is rapidly corrected. Transfusion of fresh whole blood, packed red cells, fresh-frozen plasma, platelets, and cryoprecipitate may be indicated (see Blood Transfusion, p. 750). Fresh-frozen plasma replaces most clotting factors. Cryoprecipitate replaces fibrinogen and factor VIII. Each unit of cryoprecipitate contains approximately 1 gm of fibrinogen. After the underlying cause has been eliminated, fibrinogen usually returns to normal levels within 24 hours. (Fibrinogen preparations are not recommended, since they may contain hepatitis virus and lack factor VIII.)

Heparin may be considered when the primary disease cannot be treated or when the maternal circulation is intact (such as in the case of a dead fetus or amniotic fluid embolism). Under these circumstances, heparin may inhibit the effects of thrombin, neutralize tissue thromboplastin, impede pathologic consumption of fibrinogen and other clotting factors, and allow repair of the coagulation mechanism.

A typical course of therapy includes an initial dose of 50 to 100 units of heparin per kg of body weight, followed by 10 to 15 units per kg per hour, administered by intravenous infusion; more may be needed or smaller doses may be appropriate if severe thrombocytopenia is present. This seemingly paradoxical approach to treatment is most effective when the disease is self-limited, as in the case of extensive arterial or venous thrombosis or purpura fulminans, or cases of chronic defibrination, such as instances of metastastic disease.

When hemorrhage predominates, as in cases of premature placental separation, the risk of bleeding from operative wounds or the placental site makes heparin therapy rarely, if ever, advisable.

Epsilon amino caproic acid is *not* recommended because of the danger of its inducing thrombotic disease. Fibrinolysis occurring in an obstetric patient is usually a protective response to the intravascular coagulation. Since the process is self-limited, therapy for fibrinolysis is *not* indicated.

See Specific Precipitating Problems.

Immunologic Thrombocytopenic Purpura (ITP) During Pregnancy

GENERAL CONSIDERATIONS

Immunologic thrombocytopenic purpura is a syndrome characterized by accelerated peripheral platelet destruction. The diagnosis is established by the exclusion of known causes of thrombocytopenia and the demonstration of normal or increased numbers of megakaryocytes on bone marrow examination. The plasma appears to contain an immunoglobulin, a platelet autoantibody, that damages platelets, which are then sequestered and destroyed in the spleen. This condition is often called idiopathic thrombocytopenic purpura.

Treatment of maternal thrombocytopenia and correction of the maternal platelet count does not affect the continuing presence of the circulating antiplatelet factor, which can be transmitted across the placenta.

SUBJECTIVE DATA

Easy bruising, menorrhagia, epistaxis, and a history of bleeding after trauma or minor surgery are the most usual symptoms.

OBJECTIVE DATA

PHYSICAL EXAMINATION

General examination may disclose petechiae or ecchymoses scattered over the body. The spleen is not palpable in most cases.

LABORATORY TESTS

Complete blood count with blood smear is usually normal except for the deficiency of platelets.

ASSESSMENT

POTENTIAL COMPLICATIONS

Complications that must be anticipated include intracranial hemorrhage, bleeding from any site, retroplacental bleeding, postpartum hemorrhage, and increased perinatal mortality.

DIFFERENTIAL DIAGNOSIS

Differential diagnosis includes other causes of thrombocytopenia (see Table 32-8).

TABLE 32-8. Causes of Thrombocytopenia*

Decreased production of platelets
- Generalized diseases of bone marrow
  - Aplasia, congenital and acquired
  - Invasive disease: leukemia, carcinoma, disseminated infection
  - Deficiency states: folate or vitamin B_{12} deficiency
- Diseases affecting megakaryocytes specifically
  - Congenital
    - Deficiency of a thrombopoietin-like substance
    - Reduced or absent megakaryocytes, sometimes in association with other congenital defects
    - Normal numbers of megakaryocytes; defective platelets produced
  - Acquired
    - Infection
    - Drugs: cytotoxic drugs, chloramphenicol, thiazides

Increased destruction of platlets
- Immunologic
  - Autoimmune (ITP)
  - Isoimmune: neonatal and posttransfusion
  - Drug associated
- Infection
- Other drugs: alcohol; gold
- Increased utilization: disseminated intravascular coagulation

*From Zieve PD, Levin J: Disorders of Hemostasis. Philadelphia, W.B. Saunders Company, 1976.

TABLE 32-8. Causes of Thrombocytopenia* (Continued)

Mechanical injury
Prosthetic heart valves
Thrombotic thrombocytopenic purpura
Hemolytic-uremic syndrome
Sequestration of platelets: large spleen syndrome
Dilution of platelets: massive transfusions

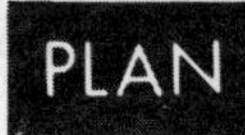

ADDITIONAL DIAGNOSTIC DATA

Platelet count is less than 100,000 per cu mm. (The normal platelet count is usually 150,000 to 400,000.) Spontaneous bleeding is unlikely unless the platelet count is 20,000 per cu mm or less; the major danger is intracranial hemorrhage. In cases of trauma or surgery, functionally normal platelets in numbers greater than 50,000 per cu mm usually prevent hemorrhage.

Bleeding time is usually prolonged when the platelet count is less than 50,000. In cases of ITP, however, the platelets are frequently larger than normal, and the bleeding time may not be prolonged until the platelet count is 20,000 or less.

Bone marrow shows a normal or increased number of megakaryocytes.

Other coagulation tests (prothrombin time, partial thromboplastin time, and fibrinogen) are normal.

MANAGEMENT AND PATIENT EDUCATION

Emergency hospitalization is advised if the platelet count is 20,000 or less because of the danger of spontaneous intracerebral hemorrhage.

Corticosteroid Therapy: Prednisone, 15 mg four times daily, is recommended for initiation of therapy. The dose is then adjusted in accordance with the platelet response. The objective of therapy is a platelet count of 100,000.

This response, at least initially, would be expected in 75 per cent of the patients. The platelet response to prednisone is often not sustained, however.

Splenectomy has been found to produce a sustained remission in 60 to 90 per cent of cases. Although generally postponed until after delivery as long as the patient maintains a satisfactory platelet count with corticosteroid therapy, splenectomy is recommended whenever persistent thrombocytopenia represents a danger to maternal life.

Platelet Transfusions: Transfused platelets are rapidly destroyed by the circulating antiplatelet antibodies. Consequently, platelet transfusions are indicated *only* for the immediate control of severe bleeding or when surgical intervention is required in the face of significant thrombocytopenia.

Salicylates should be avoided, since they interfere with platelet function.

Trauma during pregnancy and delivery should be avoided. The choice of vaginal or abdominal delivery must take into consideration the mother's platelet count and the estimated fetal platelet count. The least traumatic route for both mother and baby should always be selected.

Usually, vaginal delivery is least traumatic to the mother. As far as the baby is concerned, neonatal thrombocytopenia has been reported in 34 to 67 per cent of babies born to mothers with ITP. Perinatal mortality varies from 13 to 25 per cent (Laros, 1975).

Cesarean section has been recommended when the maternal platelet count is less than 100,000, since a large number of these babies may be expected to have thrombocytopenia (Territo, 1973). However, the benefits of cesarean section in the absence of obstetric indications are still not established (Laros, 1975).

Following delivery, each neonate must be carefully evaluated, with the fact that neonatal thrombocytopenia frequently becomes more severe on the second or third day of life borne in mind. When indicated, the newborn may require platelet transfusions or corticosteroid therapy or both.

Thrombotic Thrombocytopenic Purpura (TTP)

GENERAL CONSIDERATIONS

Thrombotic thrombocytopenic purpura, a disorder of unknown cause, is a rare and often fatal syndrome that occurs predominantly in women during their reproductive years. Clinical manifestations include petechiae, purpura, and vaginal bleeding or hematuria. Mental deterioration may progress to convulsions, coma, and death. Diagnostic features include thrombocytopenia, microangiopathic hemolytic anemia, renal disease, neurologic abnormalities, fever, and widespread hyaline occlusions of terminal arterioles. In addition to thrombocytopenia and anemia, hematologic findings include leukocytosis, reticulocytosis, and a negative direct Coombs' test. The peripheral smear shows distorted and fragmented red cells.

Hyalin thrombi in the microvasculature appear to damage platelets and red cells passing through the arterioles and capillaries. These damaged cells and platelets are removed from the circulation by the spleen. Renal and cerebral lesions account for the symptoms of renal failure and neurologic abnormalities.

ASSESSMENT

DIFFERENTIAL DIAGNOSIS

Differential diagnosis of thrombotic thrombocytopenic purpura includes immunologic thrombocytopenic purpura, thrombocytopenia in association with systemic lupus erythematosus, idiopathic autoimmune hemolytic anemia, other "symptomatic" hemolytic anemias, hemolytic uremic syndrome, acute leukemia, eclampsia, and disseminated intravascular coagulation.

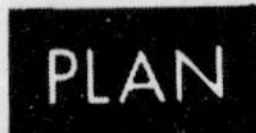

PLAN

MANAGEMENT

Therapy includes corticosteroids and agents to inhibit platelet aggregation. Splenectomy is performed if the patient's condition deteriorates.

Von Willebrand's Disease

GENERAL CONSIDERATIONS

Von Willebrand's disease is a hereditary coagulation disorder characterized by a dual hemostatic defect: a deficiency of factor VIII and a prolonged bleeding time, the latter suggesting an abnormality in the vascular or platelet phase of hemostasis. The disease is transmitted by a dominant autosomal mutant gene and has been detected more often in women than in men. The severity of symptoms varies considerably among affected members of the same family, some of whom may be asymptomatic.

SUBJECTIVE DATA

CURRENT SYMPTOMS

Vaginal bleeding, usually menorrhagia or postpartum bleeding, is the most typical gynecologic symptom.

PRIOR HISTORY

A personal or family history of postoperative bleeding, postpartum bleeding, easy bruising, or epistaxis is typical.

OBJECTIVE DATA

General Examination: Cutaneous ecchymoses or hematomas may be observed.

Pelvic Examination: These findings are usually normal.

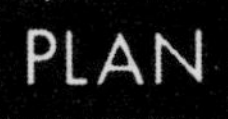

ADDITIONAL DIAGNOSTIC DATA

Bleeding time is prolonged.

Factor VIII is decreased.

Platelet count is normal.

Partial thromboplastin time is usually prolonged.

MANAGEMENT

Treatment of an acute bleeding episode consists of local hemostasis and administration of fresh blood, fresh frozen plasma, or plasma cryoprecipitates in order to elevate factor VIII.

Estrogen-progestin combination hormones may suppress endometrial proliferation and control menorrhagia. Dosages are similar to those used for contraception.

PATIENT EDUCATION

Genetic aspects of the disorder should be discussed with the patient. If pregnancy is desired, the patient may be reassured that factor VIII levels usually rise during pregnancy and term delivery may occur without hemorrhage. However, since factor VIII falls rapidly after delivery, the possibility of postpartum bleeding should be anticipated.

Aspirin and other medications that may interfere with hemostasis should be avoided.

REFERENCES

Baugh R, Brown J, Sargeant R, Hougie C: Separation of human factor VIII activity from the von Willebrand's antigen and ristocetin platelet aggregating activity. Biochim Biophys Acta *371*:360-367, 1974; Obstet and Gynecol Surv *30*:454-455, 1975

Bowie EJW, Fass DN, Olson JD, et al: The spectrum of von Willebrand's disease revisited. Mayo Clin Proc *51*:35-41, 1976

Colman RW, Robboy SJ, Minna JD: Heparin should be used in the therapy of clinically significant disseminated intravascular coagulation. *In* Ingelfinger EJ, Ebert RV, Finland M, Relman AS (eds): Controversy in Internal Medicine II. Philadelphia, W.B. Saunders Company, 1974

Corrigan JJ: Management of disseminated intravascular coagulation: heparin should be used cautiously and selectively. *In* Ingelfinger FJ, Ebert RV, Finland M, Relman AS (eds): Controversy in Internal Medicine II. Philadelphia, W.B. Saunders Company, 1974

Deykin D: The clinical challenge of disseminated intravascular coagulation. N Eng J Med *283*:636-644, 1970

Dixon RE: Disseminated intravascular coagulation. Obstet Gynecol Surv *28*:385-395, 1973

Evans PC: Obstetric and gynecologic patients with von Willebrand's disease. Obstet Gynecol *38*:37-43, 1971

Jacobson RJ, Jackson DP: Erythrocyte fragmentation in defibrination syndromes. Ann Intern Med *81*:207-209, 1974

Laros RK, Sweet RL: Management of idiopathic thrombocytopenic purpura during pregnancy. Am J. Obstet Gynecol *122*:182-191, 1975

Levin J, Algazy KM: Hematologic disorders. *In* Burrow GM, Ferris TF: Medical Complications during Pregnancy. Philadelphia, W.B. Saunders Company, 1975

May HV, Jr, Harbert GM, Thornton WN: Thrombotic thrombocytopenic purpura associated with pregnancy. Am J Obstet Gynecol *126*:452-458, 1976

Mitch WE, Spivak JL, Spangler DB, Bell WR: Thrombotic thrombocytopenic purpura presenting with gynaecologic manifestations. Lancet *1*:849-850, 1973; Obstet Gynecol Surv *29*:75-77, 1974

Murray JM, Harris RE: The management of the pregnant patient with idiopathic thrombocytopenic purpura. Am J. Obstet Gynecol *126*:449-451, 1976

O'Reilly RA: Problems of haemorrhage and thrombosis in pregnancy. Clin Haematol *2*:543-562, 1973

Phillips LL, Davidson EC: Procoagulant properties of amniotic fluid. Am J Obstet Gynecol *113*:911-919, 1972

Pritchard JA: Haematological problems associated with delivery, placental abruption, retained dead fetus and amniotic fluid embolism. Clin Haematol *2*:563-586, 1973

Pugh M: Von Willebrand's disease in gynecologic and obstetric practice. Int J Gynaecol Obstet. *10*:137-143, 1972; Obstet Gynecol Surv *28*:127-129, 1973

Purcell G, Nossel HL: Factor XI (PTA) deficiency. Obstet Gynecol *35*:69-74, 1970

Ratnoff OD: Hemorrhagic disorders: coagulation defects. *In* Beeson PB, McDermott W: Textbook of Medicine. Philadelphia, W.B. Saunders Company, 1975

Territo M, Finklestein J, Oh W, et al: Management of autoimmune thrombocytopenia in pregnancy and in the neonate. Obstet Gynecol *41*:579-584, 1973

Waxman B, Gambrill R: Use of heparin in disseminated intravascular coagulation. Am J Obstet Gynecol *112*:434-438, 1972

33 COMA IN PREGNANCY

GENERAL CONSIDERATIONS

The comatose pregnant patient is one of the most critical emergency problems. When a teenaged patient known to be previously healthy suddenly becomes comatose following a convulsive seizure during the latter half of pregnancy, the obstetrician's first thought is *eclampsia*. Nonobstetric causes must also be considered, however, since coma is only a symptom representing failure of cerebral metabolism, and not a specific disease entity.

Pathophysiologically, there are four causes of coma:

1. Supratentorial mass lesions that by increasing in size distort and compress the brain stem: for example, hemorrhage, abscess, or tumor.
2. Infratentorial lesions that directly compress or destroy the brain stem: for example, basilar artery occlusion or cerebellar hemorrhage.
3. Metabolic encephalopathy, producing unconsciousness by interfering with the metabolism of both brain stem and cerebral cortical structures: for example, anoxia, hypoglycemia, or drug intoxication.
4. Psychogenic "coma," in which the patient is physiologically awake but appears comatose by not responding to her environment.

Metabolic encephalopathy is a term applied to the behavioral changes that result from diffuse or widespread multifocal failure of cerebral metabolism. Causes of metabolic brain disease are listed in Table 33-1.

Delirium describes a state of mental confusion and excitement—a wakeful stage of metabolic encephalopathy. An *obtunded* patient is drowsy but can be coaxed to respond to verbal stimuli. *Stupor* refers to an unconscious condition, in which the patient no longer responds to verbal stimuli but does respond to noxious cutaneous stimuli. *Coma* is complete unresponsiveness to any stimuli.

TABLE 33-1. Causes of Metabolic Brain Disease*

I. Deprivation of oxygen, substrate, or metabolic cofactors
- †A. Hypoxia (interference with oxygen supply to the entire brain—cerebral blood flow normal)
  1. Decreased oxygen tension and content of blood
     - Pulmonary disease
     - Alveolar hypoventilation
     - Decreased atmospheric oxygen tension
  2. Decreased oxygen content of blood—normal tension
     - Anemia
     - Carbon monoxide poisoning
     - Methemoglobinemia
- †B. Ischemia (diffuse or widespread multifocal interference with blood supply to brain)
  1. Decreased cerebral blood flow resulting from decreased cardiac output
     - Stokes-Adams syndrome, cardiac arrest, cardiac arrhythmias
     - Myocardial infarction
     - Congestive heart failure
     - Aortic stenosis
     - Pulmonary embolus
  2. Decreased cerebral blood flow resulting from decreased peripheral resistance in systemic circulation
     - Syncope: orthostatic, vasovagal
     - Carotid sinus hypersensitivity
     - Low blood volume
  3. Decreased cerebral blood flow due to generalized increase in cerebrovascular resistance
     - Hypertensive encephalopathy
     - Hyperventilation syndrome
     - Increased blood viscosity (polycythemia), cryo- and macroglobinemia
  4. Decreased local cerebral blood flow due to widespread small vessel occlusion
     - Disseminated intravascular coagulation
     - Systemic lupus erythematosus
     - Subacute bacterial endocarditis
     - Cardiopulmonary bypass
- †C. Hypoglycemia
  - Resulting from exogenous insulin
  - Spontaneous (endogenous insulin, liver diseases, etc.
- D. Cofactor deficiency
  - Thiamin (Wernicke's encephalopathy)
  - Niacin
  - Pyridoxine
  - B_{12}
  - Folate

II. Diseases of organs other than brain
- †A. Diseases of nonendocrine organs
  - Liver (hepatic coma)
  - Kidney (uremic coma)
  - Lung (CO_2 narcosis)
- †B. Hyper- and/or hypofunction of endocrine organs
  - Pituitary
  - Thyroid (myxedema—thyrotoxicosis)
  - Parathyroid (hyper- and hypoparathyroidism)
  - Adrenal (Addison's disease, Cushing's disease, pheochromocytoma)
  - Pancreas (diabetes, hypoglycemia)

TABLE 33-1. Causes of Metabolic Brain Disease* (Continued)

†C. Other systemic diseases
- Diabetes
- Cancer
- Porphyria
- Sepsis
- Fever

III. Exogenous poisons

†A. Sedative drugs

B. Acid poisons or poisons with acidic breakdown products
- Paraldehyde
- Methyl alcohol
- Ethylene glycol

C. Other enzyme inhibitors
- Heavy metals
- Organic phosphates
- Cyanide
- Salicylates

D. Psychotropic drugs
- Tricyclic antidepressants and anticholinergic drugs
- Amphetamines
- Lithium
- Phenothiazines
- LSD-mescaline
- Monoamine oxidase inhibitors

E. Others
- Penicillin
- Anticonvulsants
- Steroids
- Cardiac glycosides

IV. Diseases producing toxins or enzyme inhibition in CNS

A. Meningitis
B. Encephalitis
C. Subarachnoid hemorrhage

V. Abnormalities of fluid, ionic or acid-base environment of CNS

A. Water and sodium (hyper- and hyponatremia) (hypo- and hyperosmolality)
B. Acidosis (metabolic and respiratory)
C. Alkalosis (metabolic and respiratory)
D. Potassium (hypokalemia)
E. Magnesium (hyper- and hypomagnesemia)
F. Calcium (hyper- and hypocalcemia)

VI. Miscellaneous diseases of unknown cause

A. Seizures and postictal states
†B. "Postoperative" delirium
C. Concussion
†D. "Sensory deprivation"

*From Posner JR: Delirium and exogenous metabolic brain disease. *In* Beeson PB, McDermott W: Textbook of Medicine. Philadelphia, W.B. Saunders Company, 1975.

†Alone or in combination, the most common causes of delirium seen on medical or surgical wards.

SUBJECTIVE DATA

CURRENT SYMPTOMS

Immediately preceding events may provide the essential diagnostic clue. Severe headaches may portend a cerebrovascular accident. Convulsions may be caused by eclampsia. Drug overdosage or withdrawal is significant information.

Associated symptoms of abdominal pain, nausea, and vomiting may occur with diabetic ketoacidosis. Fever may be indicative of overwhelming sepsis.

PRIOR HISTORY

A history of diabetes, convulsive disorders, or systemic disease may clarify an obscure situation.

OBJECTIVE DATA

PHYSICAL EXAMINATION (Table 33-2)

TABLE 33-2. Physical Examination of Patients with Suspected Metabolic Brain Disease*

History (from relatives or friends)
Previous medical illnesses (diabetes, uremia, heart disease)
Previous psychiatric history
Access to drugs (sedative, psychotropic drugs)
Recent complaints (headache, depression)
General physical examination
Evidence of trauma
Evidence of chronic or acute systemic illness
Ventilation

*From Posner JR: Delirium and exogenous metabolic brain disease. *In* Beeson PB, McDermott W: Textbook of Medicine. Philadelphia, W.B. Saunders Company, 1975.

TABLE 33-2. Physical Examination of Patients with Suspected Metabolic Brain Disease* (Continued)

Neurologic examination
- Mental status
  - Affect (agitated, depressed, apathetic)
  - Alertness (delirium, obtundation, stupor, coma)
  - Orientation (time, place, person)
  - Perceptual abnormalities (illusions, delusions, hallucinations)
  - Psychomotor activity
- Motor examination
  - Focal weakness
  - Tremor
  - Asterixis
  - Myoclonus
  - Seizures
- Autonomic examination
  - Pupillary size and responses
  - Temperature
  - Heart rate and rhythm
  - Diaphoresis

General Examination: Heart rate, blood pressure, temperature, respiratory rate, and general state of consciousness must be recorded. Elevated temperature suggests bacterial infection (meningitis, pneumonia, septicemia) or heat stroke. Hypothermia is seen in cases of peripheral circulatory collapse, barbiturate intoxication, phenothiazine overdosage, or alcoholism.

Tachypnea suggests respiratory insufficiency due to pulmonary embolus, or metabolic acidosis due to diabetes or ingested poisons. Respiration may be slow and irregular with a cerebrovascular accident, tumors, or other diseases of the central nervous system.

Blood pressure is elevated with eclampsia and often with cerebrovascular hemorrhage.

The breath may have an odor suggesting alcoholic ingestion or diabetic acidosis (acetone odor).

Neurologic examination includes the sensorium, cranial nerves, cerebellar and meningeal signs, eyes (pupils, reaction, optic fundi, deviation), motor and sensory responses, superficial reflexes (corneal, abdominal, rectal sphincter), deep tendon reflexes (biceps, triceps, patellar, Achilles), and pathologic reflexes (Babinski). Focal neurologic signs (hemiplegia, conjugate ocular deviation, small reactive pupils) suggest cerebral lesions.

Metabolic encephalopathy is characterized by symmetrical motor abnormalities, small but usually reactive pupils, and conjugate eye movements. Exceptions to small and reactive pupils occur when patients have ingested drugs or have been either severely anoxic or ischemic.

LABORATORY TESTS

See Table 33-3.

TABLE 33-3. Laboratory Evaluation of Metabolic Brain Disease*

Test	Reason for Test
Immediate:	
Glucose	Hypoglycemia, hyperosmolar coma
Na^+	Osmolar abnormalities
Ca^{++}	Hyper- or hypocalcemia
BUN	Uremia
pH, Pco_2	Acidosis, alkalosis
Po_2	Hypoxia
Lumbar puncture	Infection, hemorrhage
Later:	
Liver function tests	Hepatic coma
Sedative drug levels	Overdose
Blood and CSF culture	Sepsis, encephalitis, meningitis
Full electrolytes, including Mg^{++}	Electrolyte imbalance
EEG	

*From Posner JR: Delirium and exogenous metabolic brain disease. *In* Beeson PB, McDermott W: Textbook of Medicine, Philadelphia, W.B. Saunders Company, 1975.

ASSESSMENT

DIFFERENTIAL DIAGNOSIS

See Table 33-1.

ETIOLOGIC FACTORS	DIAGNOSTIC FEATURES
Cerebral	
Trauma—Subdural hematoma	Skull or scalp injury Blood or cerebrospinal fluid from nose or ears
Vascular accident Hemorrhage; thrombosis	Hemiplegia, hypertension, nuchal rigidity
Neoplasm	Focal central nervous system signs Papilledema
Infections Brain abscess; meningitis Encephalitis	Fever, nuchal rigidity
Epilepsy	History of convulsions Scarred or bleeding tongue
Metabolic	
Eclampsia	Hypertension, proteinuria, edema, hyperreflexia
Diabetic ketoacidosis	Acetone on breath, dehydration
Hypoglycemia	
Carbon dioxide narcosis	Cyanosis, lung disease
Hepatic	Jaundice, hematemesis
Septicemia	Fever, septic shock
Water intoxication	High doses of oxytocin plus large amounts of electrolyte free fluid administered within a relatively brief time
Hypernatremia	
Drug overdosage	
Alcohol	Breath smell, flushed face
Narcotics	Pinpoint pupils, shallow breathing, cyanosis
Anoxia; ischemia	
Concussion	

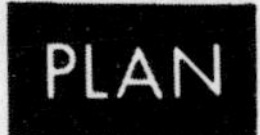

ADDITIONAL DIAGNOSTIC DATA

Blood Tests:

1. Complete blood count with blood smear. An elevated hematocrit usually indicates dehydration.
2. Electrolytes—sodium, potassium, chloride, bicarbonate.
3. Chemistries—glucose, blood urea nitrogen, calcium, acetone, ketone. Blood glucose is one of the most critical diagnostic tests, since both diabetic acidosis and hypoglycemia can cause coma. The values of blood glucose will differentiate these two entities.
4. Type—Rh and antibody screen. (Blood should be crossmatched if there is evidence of hypovolemic hemorrhage.)
5. Blood cultures (aerobic and anaerobic) if bacteremia is suspected.

Urinalysis—specific gravity, pH, color, protein, sugar, acetone, and microscopic examination—may provide essential diagnostic clues. Four-plus sugar and acetone is evidence of diabetic ketoacidosis. Proteinuria in association with hypertension is indicative of eclampsia.

Gastric analysis may be helpful when poisoning or drug overdosage is suspected.

Arterial blood gases may reveal acidosis or alkalosis (see Table 33-4).

Lumbar puncture provides valuable diagnostic information when meningitis or subarachnoid hemorrhage is suspected. The cerebrospinal fluid is examined for pressure, color, turbidity, protein, sugar, and cells. Whenever infection is suspected, a Gram stain and bacteriologic culture are essential.

Grossly bloody fluid suggests fresh subarachnoid bleeding. Xanthochromic (yellow-tinged) fluid is found in patients with previous hemorrhage (chronic subdural hematoma). Cloudy fluid may result from an infectious process (meningitis). White blood cells indicate infection. Elevated protein levels may be found with a neoplasm.

In the case of intracranial mass lesions, lumbar puncture carries a potential risk of fatal herniation of the brain. Neurologic consultation is recommended.

TABLE 33-4. A Differential Analysis of Hyperventilation and Hypoventilation in Delirious Patients*

Clinical and Laboratory Findings	Probable Diagnosis
I. Hyperventilation:	
A. Metabolic acidosis (arterial pH <7.30, $Pco_2 < 35$, $HCO_3^- < 10$ mEq per liter)	
1. BUN $>$ 60 mg per 100 ml	Uremic encephalopathy
2. Hyperglycemia (blood sugar $>$250 mg per 100 ml)	Diabetic coma
a. 4+ Serum acetone	Diabetic ketoacidosis
b. No acetonemia	Diabetic lactic acidosis
3. Cyanosis ($Po_2 < 50$ mm Hg)—shock	Anoxic lactic acidosis
4. History: diarrhea; hyperchloremia, ±hypokalemia	Diarrheal acidosis
5. Hyponatremia, hyperkalemia, ±hypoglycemia	Addison's disease
6. BUN, sugar, oxygen, blood pressure—normal	Exogenous poisoning
a. Paraldehyde odor on breath	Acidosis secondary to paraldehyde ingestion
b. Hyperemic optic discs, dilated sluggish pupils	Methyl alcohol poisoning
c. Oxalate crystals in urine	Ethylene glycol poisoning
7. None of the abnormal findings above	Spontaneous lactic acidosis
B. Respiratory alkalosis (arterial pH >7.45, $Pco_2 < 35$, $HCO_3^- > 15$ mEq per liter)	
1. $Po_2 > 50$, hepatomegaly, serum NH_3 elevated	Hepatic encephalopathy
2. $Po_2 < 50$, cyanosis	Cardiopulmonary disease
a. Rales, elevated venous pressure, cardiomegaly	Pulmonary edema
b. No heart disease	Pneumonia, alveolar-capillary block, pulmonary emboli
3. Absent pupillary and oculovestibular responses, decerebrate rigidity	Central neurogenic hyperventilation
4. Nystagmus on caloric testing, normal examination	Psychogenic hyperventilation

C. Mixed respiratory alkalosis and metabolic acidosis (arterial pH $>$7.35, P_{CO_2} $<$35, HCO_3^- $<$15 mEq per liter)	
1. Fever, tachycardia, hypotension	Gram-negative sepsis
2. Hyperthermia, positive urine $FeCl_3$ test	Salicylate poisoning
3. Abnormal liver function tests	Hepatic encephalopathy
II. Hypoventilation:	
A. Respiratory acidosis (arterial pH $<$7.30, P_{CO_2} $>$45, HCO_3^- $>$20 mEq per liter)	
1. Serum HCO_3^- $>$20 mEq per liter but $<$30 mEq per liter	
a. Normal lungs	Depressant drug poisoning
b. Rales, emphysema, P_{O_2} $<$40 mm Hg	Chronic pulmonary disease with acute CO_2 retention
2. Serum HCO_3^- $>$35 mEq per liter	
a. Normal lungs	
(1) Obesity	Pickwickian syndrome
(2) Not obese	"Central alveolar hypoventilation"
b. Rales, emphysema, P_{O_2} $<$40 mm Hg	Chronic pulmonary disease with slowly developing CO_2 retention
B. Metabolic alkalosis (arterial pH $>$7.45, P_{CO_2} $<$55, HCO_3^- $>$35 mEq per liter)	
a. Alkali ingestion	
(1) History of peptic ulcer	$NaHCO_3$ ingestion alkalosis
b. Gastric acid losses	
(1) Vomiting, hypotension, hypovolemia	Gastric HCl depletion
c. Renal acid losses	
(1) Edema, heart disease	Diuretic therapy
(2) Hypokalemia, moon face, truncal obesity	Cushing's syndrome secondary to adrenal hyperfunction, steroid therapy, hormone-secreting lung neoplasms
(3) Hypertension, hypokalemia	Primary hyperaldosteronism

*From Posner JR: Delirium and exogenous metabolic brain disease. *In* Beeson PB, McDermott W: Textbook of Medicine. Philadelphia, W.B. Saunders Company, 1975.

Skull films may reveal a skull fracture.

Brain scan, angiography or computerized axial tomography (CAT) may localize a mass lesion.

X-rays of chest or any areas of suspected injury.

Electrocardiogram provides an evaluation of cardiac status and the possibility of potassium imbalance.

Electroencephalogram may be useful in the diagnostic evaluation.

Coagulation studies—fibrinogen, fibrin-split products and platelet count—are indicated if a coagulopathy such as disseminated intravascular coagulation is suspected.

MANAGEMENT AND PATIENT EDUCATION

General Measures:

Oxygenation must be assured. The airway must be clear, oxygen administered, and adequate ventilation maintained. If the patient is deeply unconscious, a cuffed endotracheal tube and a mechanical respirator may be necessary. Endotracheal suctioning often improves oxygenation. For patients with metabolic coma, a semiprone, head-down position with frequent turning from side to side assures pulmonary drainage and tends to avoid long-term complications.

Circulation must be maintained. An intravenous line is inserted, blood drawn for laboratory screening, and fluid infusion begun with dextrose or saline. Blood volume loss should be replaced. In cases of drug overdose, cardiac rhythm should be monitored.

Glucose is administered. After blood is drawn for laboratory evaluation 25 gm of glucose (50 ml of 50 per cent solution) is given intravenously to any comatose patient when the diagnosis is unclear. The glucose tends to prevent hypoglycemic brain damage while results of laboratory tests are awaited.

Elevated intracranial pressure is lowered. Three approaches may be used:

1. Patients are passively hyperventilated to achieve a pCO_2 of 25 to 30 mm Hg. Lowering the pCO_2 decreases cerebral blood flow and cerebral volume, thus lowering intracranial pressure.

2. Mannitol, 50 grams in a 20 per cent solution, may be given intravenously over 10 to 20 minutes in order to increase osmolar pressure and pull water from the brain.
3. Steroids (dexamethasone, 10 mg intravenously, or the equivalent) may decrease cerebral edema.

Convulsive seizures must be controlled. Magnesium sulfate or diazepam (Valium) may be administered intravenously. Respiratory assistance should be available, since these drugs may produce respiratory depression. (See Convulsive Seizures and Eclampsia, p. 268.)

Infection must be treated if present.

Acid-base balance must be restored. Arterial blood gases and serum electrolytes provide the basis for specific therapy.

Body temperature must be controlled. Both hyperthermia and hypothermia may exacerbate abnormalities of cerebral metabolism.

Naloxone (Narcan) (0.4 mg intravenously) reverses the effects of an acute narcotic overdose. The action of naloxone lasts only two or three hours. Thus, patients who have taken an overdose of methadone and whose toxic reactions are reversed by naloxone may relapse over a period of four or five hours and need retreatment.

Urinary bladder is catheterized with a Foley catheter for an initial specimen. The catheter is then left in the bladder in order to record urine output every 15 to 60 minutes.

Gastric lavage is indicated when toxic dosages of drugs have been ingested.

Specific Measures: Definitive therapeutic efforts must be directed toward the underlying disease: surgical evacuation of a subdural hematoma, or hydration and insulin for diabetic ketoacidosis.

(See Cerebrovascular Accident during Pregnancy, p. 185; Convulsive Seizures in Pregnancy, p. 268; Diabetic Emergencies in Pregnancy, p. 276; Eclampsia, p. 303.)

REFERENCES

Petito F, Plum F: The lumbar puncture. N Engl J Med *290*:225-226, 1974

Posner JB: The comatose patient. JAMA *233*:1313-1314, 1975

34 CONSTIPATION, SEVERE, IN PREGNANCY

GENERAL CONSIDERATIONS

Constipation—a common complaint during pregnancy—may be due to irregular bowel habits, generalized smooth-muscle hypotonia, compression of the lower bowel by the enlarging uterus or all of these.

SUBJECTIVE DATA

Defecation is difficult and infrequent. Fecal material tends to be hard and dry. Anorexia, nausea, and abdominal cramps may cause severe discomfort.

OBJECTIVE DATA

Abdominal Examination: There is no evidence of abdominal disease. Bowel sounds are normal.

Rectal Examination: Feces may be impacted in the rectum. Anal fissures or hemorrhoids may inhibit defecation.

ASSESSMENT

PREDISPOSING FACTORS

These include inadequate fluid intake, inadequate dietary roughage, and poor bowel habits. If a patient postpones defecation from the time that she first feels the sensation, the stool may become hard and impacted.

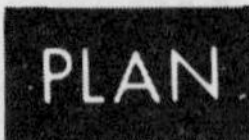

MANAGEMENT AND PATIENT EDUCATION

Adequate fluid intake should include five to seven glasses of water or liquids per day. The diet should contain substantial amounts of bulk food and cooked fruits and vegetables, particularly prune juice.

Stool softeners, such as dioctyl sodium sulfosuccinate (Colace), 100 to 200 mg per day or dioctyl calcium sulfosuccinate (Surfak), 240 mg per day, may be helpful.

Psyllium hydrophilic mucilloid (Metamucil) provides bland nonirritating bulk and promotes natural elimination. Usual dosage is one rounded teaspoonful stirred into a glass of cool water or other suitable liquid and taken orally one to three times daily.

Milk of magnesia (one tablespoon at bedtime), a glycerin suppository or a bisacodyl (Dulcolax) suppository may be necessary if the preceding measures are ineffective. The persistent use of mineral oil should be avoided because of possible interference with the absorption of fat-soluble vitamins.

With very severe symptoms and fecal impaction, enemas may become necessary; infrequently, manual release of the impacted feces is required.

35 CONTRACEPTIVE EMERGENCIES

GENERAL CONSIDERATIONS

Problems that develop while a woman is using a contraceptive method may be associated with the method per se; the consequence of unrelated, predisposing factors; or spontaneous, coincidental occurrences. Extensive prospective and retrospective epidemiologic studies have attempted to answer this question: Which problems are fortuitous occurrences and which problems are caused or exacerbated by the contraceptive method? Although many of the conclusions remain controversial, emergency personnel must be aware of the adverse reactions associated with each contraceptive method in order to appraise and elucidate specific symptoms.

Oral Contraception

GENERAL CONSIDERATIONS

Two types of oral contraceptives are available. The type most widely prescribed contains a combination of estrogen and progestin in each tablet. These pills are taken for 21 consecutive days; no tablets or inert tablets are taken for the next seven days. Withdrawal bleeding usually occurs during the medication-free interval. By consistently suppressing ovulation, combination pills are highly effective in preventing pregnancy (1 or less per 100 woman-years of use).

The other type of oral contraceptive medication is the progestin-only tablet that is taken every day without interruption. The effectiveness of the progestin-only method is less than that of the combined pills (approximately 2 to 4 pregnancies, both intrauterine and extrauterine, per 100 woman-years).

ASSESSMENT

POTENTIAL PROBLEMS

Thromboembolic Disorders: An increased risk of thromboembolic disease (peripheral thrombophlebitis, pulmonary embolism, cerebral thrombosis, coronary thrombosis, retinal thrombosis, and mesenteric thrombosis) has been reported. Although these conditions are most likely to occur in women with predisposing factors (hypertension, varicose veins, diabetes, obesity, chronic disease, cancer, advancing age, localized trauma or infection, surgery, prolonged immobilization of a limb, or a history of vascular disorder), they may also occur suddenly and spontaneously.

The risk of thrombotic stroke is estimated to be four to nine times greater in oral contraceptive users; hemorrhagic stroke is estimated to be two times greater in this group. Hypertension increases the risk of both thrombotic and hemorrhagic stroke. The presence of migraine increases the incidence of thrombotic stroke, and hemorrhagic stroke is increased by smoking (one pack or more per day). The total occurrence of all types of cerebral vascular disease is low in the reproductive age group; the estimated incidence of thrombotic stroke in oral contraceptive users is 1 per 10,000 woman-years.

If thromboembolic disorders occur, or are even suspected, the oral contraceptive medication should be discontinued immediately. Symptoms that warrant discontinuation include severe headaches, visual disturbances, chest pain, leg pain or swelling, calf tenderness, and shortness of breath.

Detailed diagnostic evaluation is essential.

Hypertension: An elevation in blood pressure has been reported in approximately 5 per cent of women taking oral contraceptives and may develop at any time during the administration of the pill. When detected, the oral contraceptives should be discontinued. Usually the hypertension is promptly reversed.

Liver adenoma with intraabdominal hemorrhage is a rare condition that may present as an "acute abdomen." Sudden abdominal pain and hypovolemic shock are the characteristic symptoms and signs. A right upper quadrant mass may be palpable. Immediate surgical repair is essential.

Gallbladder disease may occur more frequently in users of oral contraceptives. Abdominal pain or jaundice requires appropriate diagnostic studies.

COMMON HORMONAL SIDE EFFECTS

Breakthrough bleeding is most likely to occur during the first few cycles, and it usually decreases with continuing use. Irregular bleeding is often associated with missed tablets and usually resolves spontaneously without specific therapy unless there is underlying endometrial disease.

In users of the progestin-only pill, persistent irregular and unpredictable vaginal bleeding may necessitate discontinuation.

In users of combination pills, bleeding early in the cycle usually indicates inadequate stromal support. Frequently, this can be managed by the substitution of an oral contraceptive formula containing an increased concentration of estrogen in relation to the progestin. If bleeding develops on or after the nineteenth or twentieth day of the cycle (14 or 15 days of combined estrogen-progestin medication), the pills are discontinued and endometrial shedding permitted as a result of hormonal withdrawal. A new cycle of pills is then initiated five days later.

Breakthrough bleeding associated with the prolonged use of birth control pills or with depot forms of progesterone derivatives may denote an endometrium composed almost exclusively of pseudodecidual stroma and blood vessels with minimal glands. Since this condition usually signifies insufficient endogenous and exogenous estrogen, the most appropriate therapy is supplemental estrogen—either 20 mcg of ethinyl estradiol or 2.5 mg of conjugated estrogens—prescribed in addition to the birth control pill or intermittently in the case of depot progestin administration.

Amenorrhea or Oligomenorrhea: Most patients on combined oral contraceptives experience a reduction in the length and quantity of menstrual flow. Amenorrhea may be expected in 4 to 6 per cent of pill cycles, with the incidence being slightly higher on the lower dose pills. If amenorrhea occurs in two consecutive cycles, pregnancy must be ruled out.

Breast changes, particularly breast soreness and breast enlargement, may be associated with the more estrogenic pills.

Note: A detailed listing of all side effects reported with oral contraceptive medications is contained in the product package insert.

The Food and Drug Administration in the United States has required the following information to be included with all oral contraceptive preparations:*

CONTRAINDICATIONS

1. Known or suspected pregnancy (see warning No. 5).
2. Oral contraceptives should not be used in women who have or have had any of the following conditions:
   a. Thrombophlebitis or thromboembolic disorders.
   b. Cerebral vascular or coronary artery disease.
   c. Markedly impaired liver function.
   d. Known or suspected carcinoma of the breast.
   e. Known or suspected estrogen dependent neoplasia.
   f. Undiagnosed abnormal genital bleeding.

WARNINGS

The use of oral contraceptives is associated with increased risk of several serious conditions including thromboembolism, stroke, myocardial infarction, hepatic adenoma, gallbladder disease, hypertension. Practitioners prescribing oral contraceptives should be familiar with the following information relating to these risks.

1. *Thromboembolic Disorders and Other Vascular Problems.* An increased risk of thromboembolic and thrombotic disease associated with the use of oral contraceptives is well established. Three principal studies in Great Britain and three in the United States have demonstrated an increased risk of fatal and nonfatal venous thromboembolism and stroke, both hemorrhagic and thrombotic. These studies estimate that users of oral contraceptives are 4 to 11 times more likely than nonusers to develop these diseases without evident cause (Tables 1 and 4) than are nonusers. Overall excess mortality due

*Federal Register *41*:53634-53642, December 7, 1976

to pulmonary embolism or stroke is on the order of 1 to 3.5 deaths annually per 100,000 users and increases with age (Table 2). In a collaborative American study of cerebrovascular disorders in women with and without predisposing causes, it was estimated that the risk of hemorrhagic stroke was 2.0 times greater in users than nonusers and the risk of thrombotic stroke was 4 to 9.5 times greater in users than in nonusers (Table 4).

TABLE 1. Hospitalization Rates Due to Venous Thromboembolic Disease

	Admissions Annually per 100,000 Women, Age 20-44
Users of oral contraceptives	45
Nonusers	5

TABLE 2. Death Rates Due to Pulmonary Embolism or Cerebral Thrombosis—Deaths Annually per 100,000 Nonpregnant Women

	Age 20 to 34	**Age 35 to 41**
Users of oral contraceptives	1.6	3.9
Nonusers	.2	.5

An increased risk of myocardial infarction associated with the use of oral contraceptives has been reported, confirming a previously suspected association (Tables 3 and 4). These studies, conducted in the United Kingdom, found, as expected, that the greater the number of underlying risk factors for coronary artery disease (cigarette smoking, hypertension, hypercholesterolemia, obesity, diabetes, history of preeclamptic toxemia) the higher the risk of developing myocardial infarction, regardless of whether the patient was an oral contraceptive user or not. Oral contraceptives, however, were found to be an additional risk factor. The annual excess case rate of myocardial infarction (fatal and nonfatal) in oral contraceptive users was estimated to be approximately 7 cases per 100,000 women users in the 30 to 39 year age group and 67 cases per 100,000 women users in the 40 to 44 age group.

TABLE 3. Myocardial Infarction Rates in Users and Nonusers of Oral Contraceptives in Britain—Cases Annually per 100,000 Women

	Nonfatal		Fatal	
	Age 30 to 39	*Age 40 to 44*	*Age 30 to 39*	*Age 40 to 44*
Users of oral contraceptives	5.6	56.9	5.4	32
Nonusers of oral contraceptives	2.1	9.9	1.9	12
Relative risk	2.7	5.7	2.8	2.8

In an analysis of data derived from several national adverse reaction reporting systems, British investigators concluded that the risk of thromboembolism including coronary thrombosis is directly related to the dose of estrogen used in oral contraceptives. Preparations containing 100 mcg or more of estrogen were associated with a higher risk of thromboembolism than those containing 50 to 80 mcg of estrogen. Their analysis did suggest, however, that the quantity of estrogen may not be the sole factor involved. This finding has been confirmed in the United States. Careful epidemiological studies to determine the degree of thromboembolic risk associated with progestin-only oral contraceptives have not been performed. Causes of thromboembolic disease have been reported in women using these products, and they should not be presumed to be free of excess risk.

The risk of thromboembolic and thrombotic disorders, in both users and nonusers of oral contraceptives, increases with age. Oral contraceptives are, however, an independent risk factor for these events.

TABLE 4. Summary of Relative Risk of Thromboembolic Disorders and Other Vascular Problems in Oral Contraceptive Users Compared to Nonusers

	Relative Risk, Times Greater
Idiopathic thromboembolic disease	4-11
Post-surgery thromboembolic complications	4-6
Thrombotic stroke	4-9.5
Hemorrhagic stroke	2
Heart attack (fatal) (age 30-39)	2.8
Heart attack (fatal) (age 40-44)	2.8
Heart attack (nonfatal) (age 30-39)	2.7
Heart attack (nonfatal) (age 40-44)	5.7

The available data from a variety of sources have been analyzed to estimate the risk of death associated with various methods of contraception. The estimates of risk of death for each method include the combined risk of the contraceptive method (e.g., thromboembolic and thrombotic disease in the case of oral contraceptives) plus the risk attributable to pregnancy or abortion in the event of method failure. This latter risk varies with the effectiveness of the contraceptive method. The study concluded that the mortality associated with all methods of birth control is low compared to the risk of childbirth, with the exception of oral contraceptives in women over 40, and that the lowest mortality is associated with the condom or diaphragm backed up by early abortion.

The risk of thromboembolic and thrombotic disease associated with oral contraceptives increases with age after approximately age 30 and, for myocardial infarction, is further increased by cigarette smoking, hypertension, hypercholesterolemia, obesity, diabetes, or history of preeclamptic toxemia. The risk of myocardial infarction in oral contraceptive users is substantially increased in women age 40 and over, especially those with other risk factors. The use of oral contraceptives in women in this age group is not recommended.

The physician and the patient should be alert to the earliest manifestations of thromboembolic and thrombotic disorders (e.g., thrombophlebitis, pulmonary embolism, cerebrovascular insufficiency, coronary occlusion, retinal thrombosis, and mesenteric thrombosis). Should any of these occur or be suspected, the drug should be discontinued immediately.

A four- to sixfold increased risk of post-surgery thromboembolic complications has been reported in oral contraceptive users. If feasible, oral contraceptives should be discontinued at least four weeks before surgery of a type associated with an increased risk of thromboembolism or prolonged immobilization.

2. *Ocular Lesions.* There have been reports of neuro-ocular lesions such as optic neuritis or retinal thrombosis associated with the use of oral contraceptives. Discontinue oral contraceptive medication if there is unexplained, sudden or gradual, partial or complete loss of vision; sudden onset of proptosis or diplopia; papilledema; or retinal vascular lesions, and institute appropriate diagnostic and therapeutic measures.

3. *Carcinoma.* Long-term continuous administration of either natural or synthetic estrogen in certain animal species increases the frequency of carcinoma of the breast, cervix, vagina, and liver. Certain synthetic progestins, none currently marketed, have been noted to increase the incidence of mammary nodules, benign and malignant, in dogs.

In humans, three case control studies have reported an increased risk of endometrial carcinoma associated with the prolonged use of exogenous estrogen in postmenopausal women. One publication reported on the first 21 cases submitted by physicians to a registry of cases of adenocarcinoma of the endometrium in women under 40 on oral contraceptives. Of the cases found in women without predisposing risk factors for adenocarcinoma of the endometrium (e.g., irregular bleeding at the time oral contraceptives were first given, polycystic ovaries), nearly all occurred in women who had used a sequential oral contraceptive. These products are no longer marketed. No evidence has been reported suggesting an increased risk of endometrial cancer in users of conventional combination or progestin-only oral contraceptives.

Several studies have found no increase in breast cancer in women taking oral contraceptives or estrogens. One study, however, while also noting no overall increased risk of breast cancer in women treated with oral contraceptives, found an excess risk in the subgroups of oral contraceptive users with documented benign breast disease. A reduced occurrence of benign breast tumors in users of oral contraceptives has been well-documented.

In summary, there is at present no confirmed evidence from human studies of an increased risk of cancer associated with oral contraceptives. Close clinical surveillance of all women taking oral contraceptives is, nevertheless, essential. In all cases of undiagnosed persistent or recurrent abnormal vaginal bleeding, appropriate diagnostic measures should be taken to rule out malignancy. Women with a strong family history of breast cancer or who have breast nodules, fibrocystic disease, or abnormal mammograms should be monitored with particular care if they elect to use oral contraceptives instead of other methods of contraception.

4. *Hepatic Adenoma.* Benign hepatic adenomas appear to be associated with the use of oral contraceptives. Although benign, and rare, hepatic adenomas may rupture and may cause death through intraabdominal hemorrhage. This has been reported in short-term as well as long-term users of oral contraceptives, although one study relates risk with duration of use of the contraceptive. While hepatic adenoma is a rare lesion, it should be considered in women presenting abdominal pain and tenderness, abdominal mass, or shock.

A few cases of hepatocellular carcinoma have been reported in women taking oral contraceptives. The relationship of these drugs to this type of malignancy is not known at this time.

5. *Use in Pregnancy, Birth Defects in Offspring, and Malignancy in Female Offspring.* The use of female sex hormones—both estrogenic and progestational agents—during early pregnancy may seriously damage the offspring. It has been shown that females exposed *in utero* to diethylstilbestrol, a nonsteroidal estrogen, have an increased risk of developing in later life a form of vaginal or cervical cancer that is ordinarily extremely rare. This risk has been estimated at not greater than 4 per 1000 exposures. Although there is no evidence at the present time that oral contraceptives further enhance the risk of developing this type of malignancy, such patients should be monitored with particular care if they elect to use oral contraceptives instead of other methods of contraception. Furthermore, a high percentage of such exposed women (from 30 to 90%) have been found to have epithelial changes of the vagina and cervix. Although these changes are histologically benign, it is not known whether this condition is a precursor of vaginal malignancy. Although similar data are not available concerning the use of other estrogens, it cannot be presumed that they would not induce similar changes.

Several reports suggest an association between intrauterine exposure to female sex hormones and congenital anomalies, including congenital heart defects and limb-reduction defects. One case control study has estimated a 4.7-fold increase in risk of limb-reduction defects in infants exposed *in utero* to sex hormones (oral contraceptives, hormonal withdrawal tests for pregnancy, or attempted treatment for threatened abortion). Some of these exposures were very short and involved only a few days of treatment. The data suggest that the risk of limb-reduction defects in exposed fetuses is somewhat less than 1 in 1000 live births.

In the past, female sex hormones have been used during pregnancy in an attempt to treat threatened or habitual abortion. There is considerable evidence that estrogens are ineffective for these indications, and there is no evidence from well-controlled studies that progestins are effective for these uses.

There is some evidence that triploidy and possibly other types of polyploidy are increased among abortuses from women who become pregnant soon after ceasing oral contraceptives. Embryos with these anomalies are virtually always aborted spontaneously. Whether there is an overall increase in spontaneous abortion of pregnancies conceived soon after stopping oral contraceptives is unknown.

It is recommended that for any patient who has missed two consecutive periods, pregnancy should be ruled out before continuing the contraceptive regimen. If the patient has not adhered to the prescribed schedule, the possibility of pregnancy should be considered at the time of the first missed period, and further use of oral contraceptives should be withheld until pregnancy has been ruled out. If pregnancy is confirmed, the patient should be apprised of the potential risks to the fetus, and the advisability of continuation of the pregnancy should be discussed in the light of these risks.

It is also recommended that women who discontinue oral contraceptives with the intent of becoming pregnant use an alternate form of contraception for a period of time before attempting to conceive. Many clinicians recommend three months.

The administration of progestin-only or progestin-estrogen combinations to induce withdrawal bleeding should not be used as a test of pregnancy.

6. *Gallbladder Disease.* Studies report a doubling of the risk of surgically confirmed gallbladder disease in users of oral contraceptives or estrogen for two or more years.

7. *Carbohydrate and Lipid Metabolic Effects.* A decrease in glucose tolerance has been observed in a significant percentage of patients on oral contraceptives. For this reason, prediabetic and diabetic patients should be carefully observed while receiving oral contraceptives.

An increase in triglycerides and total phospholipids has been observed in patients receiving oral contraceptives. The clinical significance of this finding remains to be defined.

8. *Elevated Blood Pressure.* An increase in blood pressure has been reported in patients receiving oral contraceptives. In some women, hypertension may occur within a

few months of beginning oral contraceptive use. In the first year of use, the prevalence of women with hypertension is low in users and may be no higher than that of a comparable group of nonusers. The prevalence in users increases, however, with longer exposure and in the fifth year of use is two and a half to three times the reported prevalence in the first year. Age is also strongly correlated with the development of hypertension in oral contraceptive users. Women who previously have had hypertension during pregnancy may be more likely to develop elevation of blood pressure when given oral contraceptives.

9. *Headache.* The onset or exacerbation of migraine or development of headache of a new pattern which is recurrent, persistent, or severe requires discontinuation of oral contraceptives and evaluation of the cause.

10. *Bleeding Irregularities.* Breakthrough bleeding, spotting, and amenorrhea are frequent reasons for patients discontinuing oral contraceptives. In breakthrough bleeding, as in all cases of irregular bleeding from the vagina, nonfunctional causes should be borne in mind. In undiagnosed persistent or recurrent abnormal bleeding from the vagina, adequate diagnostic measures are indicated to rule out pregnancy or malignancy. If pathology has been excluded, time or a change to another formulation may solve the problem. Changing to an oral contraceptive with a higher estrogen content, while potentially useful in minimizing menstrual irregularity, should be done only if necessary since this may increase the risk of thromboembolic disease.

Following paragraph to be inserted for progestin-only oral contraceptives:

An alteration in menstrual patterns is likely to occur in women using progestin-only oral contraceptives. The amount and duration of flow, cycle length, breakthrough bleeding, spotting, and amenorrhea will probably be quite variable. Bleeding irregularities occur more frequently with the use of progestin-only oral contraceptives than with the combinations and the dropout rate due to such conditions is higher.

Women with a past history of oligomenorrhea or secondary amenorrhea or young women without regular cycles may have a tendency to remain anovulatory or to become amenorrheic after discontinuation of oral contraceptives. Women with these preexisting problems should be advised of this possibility and encouraged to use other contraceptive methods.

11. *Ectopic Pregnancy.* Ectopic as well as intrauterine pregnancy may occur in contraceptive failures. However, in oral contraceptive failures, the ratio of ectopic to intrauterine pregnancies is higher than in women who are not receiving oral contraceptives since the drugs are more effective in preventing intrauterine than ectopic pregnancies. The higher ectopic-intrauterine ratio has been reported with both combination products and progestin-only oral contraceptives.

12. *Breast Feeding.* Oral contraceptives given in the postpartum period interfere with lactation. There may be a decrease in the quantity and quality of the breast milk. Furthermore, a small fraction of the hormonal agents in oral contraceptives has been identified in the milk of mothers receiving these drugs. The effects, if any, on the breast-fed child have not been determined. If feasible, the use of oral contraceptives should be deferred until the infant has been weaned.

PRECAUTIONS

General

1. A complete medical and family history should be taken prior to the initiation of oral contraceptives. The pretreatment and periodic physical examinations should include special reference to blood pressure, breasts, abdomen, and pelvic organs, including Papanicolaou smear and relevant laboratory tests. As a general rule, oral contraceptives should not be prescribed for longer than 1 year without another physical examination being performed.

2. Under the influence of estrogen-progestogen preparations, preexisting uterine leiomyomata may increase in size.

3. Patients with a history of psychic depression should be carefully observed and the drug discontinued if depression recurs to a serious degree. Patients becoming significantly depressed while taking oral contraceptives should stop the medication and use an alternate method of contraception in an attempt to determine if the symptom is drug related.

4. Oral contraceptives may cause some degree of fluid retention. They should be prescribed with caution, and only with careful monitoring, in patients with conditions which might be aggravated by fluid retention, such as convulsive disorders, migraine syndrome, or cardiac or renal insufficiency.

5. Patients with a past history of jaundice during pregnancy have an increased risk of recurrence of jaundice while receiving oral contraceptive therapy. If jaundice develops in any patient receiving such drugs, the medication should be discontinued.

6. Steroid hormones may be poorly metabolized in patients with impaired liver function and should be administered with caution in such patients.

7. Oral contraceptive users may have disturbances in normal tryptophan metabolism which may result in a relative pyridoxine deficiency. The clinical significance of this is yet to be determined.

8. Serum folate levels may be depressed by oral contraceptive therapy. Since the pregnant woman is predisposed to the development of folate deficiency and the incidence of folate deficiency increases with increasing gestation, it is possible that if a woman becomes pregnant shortly after stopping oral contraceptives, she may have a greater chance of developing folate deficiency and complications attributed to this deficiency.

9. The pathologist should be advised of oral contraceptive therapy when relevant specimens are submitted.

10. Certain endocrine and liver function tests and blood components may be affected by estrogen-containing oral contraceptives:

a. Increased sulfobromophthalein retention.

b. Increased prothrombin and factors VII, VIII, IX, and X; decreased antithrombin 3; increased norepinephrine-induced platelet aggregability.

c. Increased thyroid binding globulin (TBG) leading to increased circulating total thyroid hormone, as measured by protein-bound iodine (PBI), T4 by column, or T4 by radioimmunoassay. Free T3 resin uptake is decreased, reflecting the elevated TBG; free_T4 concentration is unaltered.

d. Decreased pregnanediol excretion.

e. Reduced response to metyrapone test.

Adverse Reactions

An increased risk of the following serious adverse reactions has been associated with the use of oral contraceptives (see Warnings):

Thrombophlebitis.
Pulmonary embolism.
Coronary thrombosis.
Cerebral thrombosis.
Cerebral hemorrhage.
Hypertension.
Gallbladder disease.
Congenital anomalies.

There is evidence of an association between the following conditions and the use of oral contraceptives, although additional confirmatory studies are needed:

Mesenteric thrombosis.
Benign hepatomas.
Neuro-ocular lesions, e.g., retinal thrombosis and optic neuritis.

The following adverse reactions have been reported in patients receiving oral contraceptives and are believed to be drug related:

Nausea
Vomiting } Usually the most common adverse reactions, occurring in approximately 10% or less of patients during the first cycle. Other reactions, as a general rule, are seen much less frequently or only occasionally.

Gastrointestinal symptoms (such as abdominal cramps and bloating).
Breakthrough bleeding.
Spotting.
Change in menstrual flow.
Dysmenorrhea.
Amenorrhea during and after treatment.
Temporary infertility after discontinuance of treatment.
Edema.
Chloasma or melasma, which may persist.
Breast changes: tenderness, enlargement, and secretion.
Change in weight (increase or decrease).
Change in cervical erosion and cervical secretion.
Possible diminution in lactation when given immediately post partum.
Cholestatic jaundice.
Migraine.
Increase in size of uterine leiomyomata.

Rash (allergic):

Mental depression.

Reduced tolerance to carbohydrates.

Vaginal candidiasis.

The following adverse reactions have been reported in users of oral contraceptives, and the association has been neither confirmed not refuted:

Premenstrual-like syndrome.

Intolerance to contact lenses.

Change in corneal curvature (steepening).

Cataracts.

Changes in libido.

Chorea.

Changes in appetite.

Cystitis-like syndrome.

Headache.

Nervousness.

Dizziness.

Hirsutism.

Loss of scalp hair.

Erythema multiforme.

Erythema nodosum.

Hemorrhagic eruption.

Vaginitis.

Porphyria.

Impaired renal function.

Intrauterine Device (IUD)

GENERAL CONSIDERATIONS

The intrauterine device is an effective contraceptive method with the particular advantage that once the device is in place, no further motivation, effort, or equipment is required for continuing contraception. Devices most commonly used are either inert (Lippes Loop, Saf-T-Coil) or bioactive (copper or progesterone). Net pregnancy rates range from 1 to 3 per hundred woman-years.

ASSESSMENT

POTENTIAL PROBLEMS

Syncope associated with insertion is usually a vasovagal effect and rarely a serious problem. The reaction is treated by keeping the patient recumbent until recovered. Inhalations of aromatic spirits of ammonia are traditional.

Uterine bleeding, that is, increased quantity and duration of menstrual flow, frequently occurs. Many women can be reassured that this is a common effect without serious significance. Serial hemoglobin or hematocrit determinations help in the evaluation of potential iron-deficiency anemia. Persistent, profuse, or irregular bleeding may necessitate removal of the device.

Uterine pain may be due to uterine contraction stimulated by the intrauterine device. Mild analgesia and reassurance are adequate therapy for many patients; for others the discomfort necessitates removal of the device.

Pelvic infection, including unilateral tuboovarian abscess, is one of the most serious complications of the intrauterine device. The mechanism is unclear, but many believe that the device somehow alters the uterine resistance to bacterial invasion.

Whenever pelvic infection is evident, antibiotic therapy is prescribed (see Pelvic Infection, p. 474). The device is removed; a Gram stain and bacteriologic culture are taken from the device in order to identify the offending bacteria.

Pelvic pain and increased vaginal bleeding may be the earliest symptoms of pelvic infection.

Uterine Perforation: If the string of the intrauterine device is not visualized in the cervical canal, the following possibilities must be considered: the device has been expelled spontaneously; the string has become detached from the device; the string has migrated into the uterine cavity; uterine perforation has occurred.

Ultrasound B-scan or abdominal x-ray or both usually can localize the device (Fig. 35-1). Each type of intrauterine device gives a characteristic echo pattern within the echo-free space of the uterus. Consequently, if the device is not within the uterus and a plain radiograph shows the device in the pelvis, intraperitoneal perforation is assumed. An x-ray with a sound in the uterus or hysterography may facilitate localization when the diagnosis is doubtful.

A device in the peritoneal cavity is usually removed; copper devices should be removed as soon as feasible because of the predisposition to adhesion formation. Many times the device can be removed by laparoscopy; laparotomy is necessary if there is any evidence of intestinal injury or if the device has become imbedded.

Ectopic Pregnancy: The intrauterine device does not prevent ovulation or extrauterine implantation. Consequently, ectopic pregnancy must always be suspected when irregular bleeding or pelvic pain develops in a patient with an intrauterine device. Four to five per cent of all pregnancies occurring in women with IUDs are likely to be extrauterine.

(For the treatment plan see Ectopic Pregnancy, p. 311.)

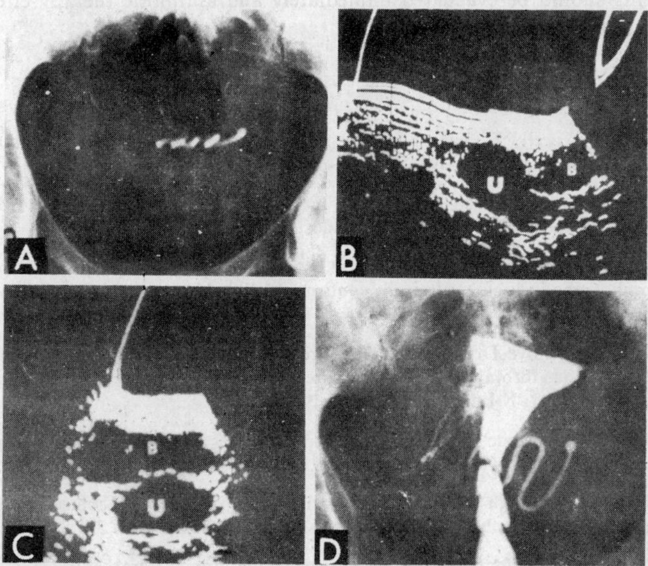

Figure 35-1. *A*, A plain radiograph shows an intrauterine device in the pelvis. *B*, Longitudinal scan showing empty uterus. *C*, Transverse scan showing empty uterus. *D*, Extrauterine position of intrauterine device is confirmed by hysterography. (From Cochrane WJ: Ultrasound in gynecology. Radiol Clin North Am *13*:457-466, 1975.

INTRAUTERINE DEVICE AND PREGNANCY

When an intrauterine device is encountered in a patient in early pregnancy and the string is visible, the device should be removed in order to avoid risks of ascending intrauterine infection during the course of the pregnancy. If the string is not visible, it is important to determine whether the pregnancy occurred as a result of spontaneous, unnoticed expulsion or the device is still present. After 10 to 12 or more weeks' gestation, the string of the device may be drawn up inside the enlarging uterus. Ultrasonography for IUD identification is preferred, particularly when the patient wishes the pregnancy to continue.

If the device is present, the patient should be advised of associated risks—abortion, premature labor, and especially, the increased hazard of intrauterine sepsis. Patients who elect to continue the pregnancy should be instructed to report all abnormal symptoms: fever, abdominal cramping, pain, or bleeding. If symptoms suggestive of midtrimester septic abortion develop, uterine contents should be evacuated immediately and antibiotic therapy effective against anaerobes prescribed.

REFERENCES

Arthes FG, Sartwell PE, Lewison EF: The pill, estrogens, and the breast. Epidemiologic aspects. Cancer *28*:1391-1394, 1971

Baum J, Holtz F, Bookstein JJ, Klein EW: Possible association between benign hepatomas and oral contraceptives. Lancet *2*:926-928, 1973

Boston Collaborative Drug Surveillance Program: Oral contraceptives and venous thromboembolic disease, surgically confirmed gallbladder disease and breast tumors. Lancet *1*:1399-1404, 1973

Boston Collaborative Drug Surveillance Program: Surgically confirmed gallbladder disease, venous thromboembolism and breast tumors in relation to postmenopausal estrogen therapy. N Engl J Med *290*:15-19, 1974

Carr DH: Chromosome studies in selected spontaneous abortions: I Conception after oral contraceptives. Can Med Assoc J *103*:343-348, 1970

Collaborative Group for the Study of Stroke in Young Women: Oral contraception and increased risk of cerebral ischemia or thrombosis. N Engl J Med *228*:871-878, 1973

Collaborative Group for the Study of Stroke in Young Women: Oral contraceptives and stroke in young women; associated factors. JAMA *231*:718-722, 1975

Edmonson HA, Henderson B, Benton B: Liver cell adenomas associated with use of oral contraceptives. N Engl J Med *294*:470-472, 1976

Fasal E, Paffenbarger RS: Oral contraceptives as related to cancer and benign lesions of the breast. J Natl Cancer Inst *55*:767-773, 1975

Faulkner WL, Ory HW: Intrauterine devices and acute pelvic inflammatory disease. JAMA *235*:1851-1853, 1976

Gal I, Kirman B, Stern J: Hormone pregnancy tests and congenital malformation. Nature *216*:83, 1967

Greene GR, Sartwell PE: Oral contraceptive use in patients with thromboembolism following surgery, trauma, or infection. Am J Public Health *62*:680-685, 1972

Greenwald P, Barlow JJ, Nasca PC, Burnett W: Vaginal cancer after maternal treatment with synthetic estrogens. N Engl J Med *285*:390-392, 1971

Herbst AL, Kurman RJ, Scully RE: Vaginal and cervical abnormalities after exposure to stilbestrol in utero. Obstet Gynecol *40*:287-298, 1972

Herbst AL, Poskanzer DC, Robboy SJ, Friedlander L, Scully RE: Prenatal exposure to stilbestrol; a prospective comparison of exposed female offspring with unexposed controls. N Engl J Med *292*:334-339, 1975

Herbst AL, Robboy SJ, MacDonald GJ, Scully RE: The effects of local progesterone on stilbestrol-associated vagina adenosis. Am J Obstet Gynecol *118*:607-615, 1974

Herbst AL, Ulfelder H, Poskanzer DC: Adenocarcinoma of the vagina. N Engl J Med *284*:878-881, 1971

Inman, WHW, Vessey MP: Investigation of deaths from pulmonary, coronary and cerebral thrombosis and embolism in women of childbearing age. Br Med J *2*:193-199, 1968

Inman WHW, Vessey MP, Westerholm B, Engelund A: Thromboembolic disease and the steroidal content of oral contraceptives. A report to the Committee on Safety of Drugs. Br Med J *2*:203-209, 1970

Janerich DT, Piper JM, Glebetis DM: Oral contraceptives and congenital limb-reduction defects. N Engl J Med *291*:697-700, 1974

Kahn HS, Tyler CW: IUD-related hospitalizations, United States and Puerto Rico, 1973. JAMA *234*:53-56, 1975; Obstet Gynecol Surv *31*:155-157, 1976

Kahn HS, Tyler CW: Mortality associated with use of IUDs. JAMA *234*:57-59, 1975

Kirkpatrick D, Schneider J, Peterson EP: Large bowel perforation by intrauterine contraceptive devices. Obstet Gynecol *46*:610-612, 1975

Lanier AP, Notter KL, Decker DG, Elveback L, Kurland LT: Cancer and stilbestrol. A follow-up of 1719 persons exposed to estrogens in utero and born 1943-1959. Mayo Clin Proc *48*:793-799, 1973

Laumas KR, Malkani PK, Bhatnagar S, Laumas V: Radioactivity in the breast milk of lactating women after oral administration of 3 H-norethynodrel. Am J Obstet Gynecol *98*:411-413, 1967

Levy EP, Cohen A, Fraser FC: Hormone treatment during pregnancy and congenital heart defects. Lancet *1*:611, 1973

Mack TN, Pike MC, Henderson BE, Pfeffer RI, Gerkins VR, Arthur M, Brown SE: Estrogens and endometrial cancer in a retirement community. N Engl J Med *294*:1262-1267, 1976

MacKay DHW, Mowat J: Translocation of intrauterine contraceptive devices. Lancet I: 652-653, 1974

Mann JI, Inman WHW: Oral contraceptives and death from myocardial infarction. Br Med J *2*:245-248, 1975

Mann JI, Inman WHW, Thorogood M: Oral contraceptive use in older women and fatal myocardial infarction. Br Med J *2*:445-447, 1976

Mann JI, Vessey MP, Thorogood M, Doll R: Myocardial infarction in young women with special reference to oral contraceptive practice. Br Med J *2*:241-245, 1975

Mays ET, Christopherson WM, Mahr MM, Williams HC: Hepatic changes in young women ingesting contraceptive steroids. Hepatic hemorrhage and primary hepatic tumors. JAMA *235*:730-732, 1976

Mead PB, Beecham JB, Maeck JV: Incidence of infections associated with intrauterine contraceptive device in an isolated community. Am J Obstet Gynecol *125*:79-82, 1976; Obstet Gynecol Surv *31*:752-754, 1976

Nora JJ, Nora AH: Birth defects and oral contraceptives. Lancet *1*:941-942, 1973

Novak ER (ed): Textbook of Gynecology. Baltimore, The Williams and Wilkins Company, 1975

Ory H, Cole P, MacMahon B, Hoover R: Oral contraceptives and reduced risk of benign breast diseases. N Engl J Med *294*:419-422, 1976

Royal College of General Practitioners: Oral Contraception and thromboembolic disease. J Coll Gen Pract *13*:267-279, 1967

Royal College of General Practitioners: Oral Contraceptives and Health. London, Pitman Publishing Ltd, 1974

Sartwell PE, Masi AT, Arthes FG, Greene GR, Smith HE: Thromboembolism and oral contraceptives: an epidemiological case control study. Am J Epidemiol *90*:365-380, 1969

Sherman AI, Goldrath M, Berlin A, Vakhariya V, Banooni F, Michaels W, Goodman P, Brown S: Cervical-vaginal adenosis after in utero exposure to synthetic estrogens. Obstet Gynecol *44*:531-545, 1974

Silverberg SG, Makowski EL: Endometrial carcinoma in young women taking oral contraceptive agents. Obstet Gynecol *46*:503-506, 1975

Smith DS, Prentice R, Thompson DJ, Herrmann WL: Association of exogenous estrogen and endometrial carcinoma. N Engl J Med *293*:1164-1167, 1975

Stafl A, Mattingly RF, Foley DV, Fetherston W: Clinical diagnosis of vaginal adenosis. Obstet Gynecol *43*:118-128, 1974

Stolley PD, Tonascia JA, Tockman MS, Sartwell PE, Rutledge AH, Jacobs MP: Thrombosis with low-estrogen oral contraceptives. Am J Epidemiol *102*:197-208, 1975

Targum SD, Wright NH: Association of the intrauterine device and pelvic inflammatory disease: a retrospective pilot study. Am J Epidemiol *100*:262-271, 1974

Taylor ES, McMillan JH, Greer BE, Droegemueller W, Thompson HE: The intrauterine device and tubo-ovarian abscess. Am J Obstet Gynecol *123*-338-348, 1975; Obstet Gynecol Surv *31*:154-155, 1976

Tietze C, Bongaarts J, Schearer B: Mortality associated with the control of fertility, Family Planning Perspectives *8*:6-14, 1976

Vessey MP, Doll R: Investigation of relation between use of oral contraceptives and thromboembolic disease. A further report. Br Med J *2*:651-657, 1969

Vessey MP, Doll R, Fairbairn AS, Glober G: Post-operative thromboembolism and the use of oral contraceptives. Br Med J *3*:123-126, 1970

Vessey MP, Doll R, Jones K: Oral contraceptives and breast cancer. Progress report of an epidemiological study. Lancet *1*:941-943, 1975

Vessey MR, Doll R, Peto R, Johnson B, Wiggins P: A long-term follow-up study of women using different methods of contraception—an interim report. J. Biosoc Sci *8*:373-427, 1976

Vessey MP, Doll R, Sutton PM: Oral contraceptives and breast neoplasia: a retrospective study. Br Med J *3*:719-724, 1972

Wynn V, Doar JWH, Mills GL: Some effects of oral contraceptives on serum-lipid and lipoprotein levels. Lancet *2*:720-723, 1966

Ziel HK, Finkle WD: Increased risk of endometrial carcinoma among users of conjugated estrogens. N Engl J Med *293*:1167-1170, 1975

36 CONVULSIVE SEIZURES IN PREGNANCY

GENERAL CONSIDERATIONS

Convulsive seizures are a life-threatening medical emergency. If seizures occur for the first time during the latter half of pregnancy, the obstetrician's first suspicion should be of eclampsia, particularly if there is associated hypertension, proteinuria, and edema. However, nonobstetric causes must also be considered. If generalized or one-sided seizures suddenly develop in a patient not known to have been epileptic, diagnostic possibilities include drug intoxication, infection, and metabolic and endocrine diseases.

SUBJECTIVE DATA

CURRENT SYMPTOMS

Convulsive Seizure: A grand mal generalized convulsion begins with a sudden loss of consciousness, a cry, a fall to the ground, and tonic, then clonic, movements of muscles of the tongue and limbs, and sometimes with sphincteric incontinence and other autonomic disorders. When the motor activity terminates, the patient is left in a state of postictal coma, which may last up to a half hour. As the coma recedes, mental confusion, drowsiness, and headache supervene.

Severe seizures may cause hypoxia, acidosis, and an accumulation of lactic acid secondary to respiratory spasm, airway obstruction, and excessive muscular activity. A violent seizure can cause respiratory arrest or cardiac standstill.

Associated symptoms may include headache, visual disturbances, speech disturbances, muscle weakness, and disorientation.

PRIOR HISTORY

A history of epilepsy, drug intake, or trauma may provide the clue to the correct diagnosis.

OBJECTIVE DATA

PHYSICAL EXAMINATION

General Examination: Examination of blood pressure, pulse, respiration, and general appearance aid in the initial diagnosis and management. Hypertension and edema (with proteinuria) are characteristic of eclampsia.

Neurologic Examination: Examination for motor activity, sensory disturbances, reflexes, and nuchal rigidity, and a retinal examination provide a base-line assessment of the patient's problem.

LABORATORY TESTS

Urinalysis is often particularly helpful. Proteinuria points to eclampsia. Four-plus sugar and acetone indicate diabetic ketoacidosis.

ASSESSMENT

DIFFERENTIAL DIAGNOSIS

Differential diagnosis of convulsive seizures includes

1. Alkalosis
2. Cerebral infection
3. Cerebral trauma (head injury)
4. Cerebral tumor
5. Cerebrovascular accident* (hemorrhage, thrombosis, embolism)
6. Drug intoxication (local anesthetics)

---

*Cerebral venous thrombosis: Associated symptoms are severe headaches, paresis, speech disorders, visual disturbances, disorientation, and confusion. Neurologic examination may disclose localizing signs.

Cerebral arterial thrombosis: Predominant symptom is paresis. The most common site is the middle cerebral artery. The diagnosis is suggested by localizing signs.

Subarachnoid hemorrhage: Associated symptoms are suboccipital headache, nuchal rigidity, nausea, vomiting, syncope, coma, focal convulsions, and hemiplegia.

7. Drug withdrawal (barbiturates, alcohol)
8. Eclampsia
9. Epilepsy
10. Hepatic disease
11. Hypernatremia
12. Hyponatremia† (water intoxication)
13. Hypertensive encephalopathy
14. Hyperventilation
15. Porphyria, acute
16. Renal failure
17. Sickle cell crisis
18. Thrombotic thrombocytopenic purpura

(See Coma in Pregnancy, p. 234; Eclampsia, p. 303; Syncope in Pregnancy, p. 633.)

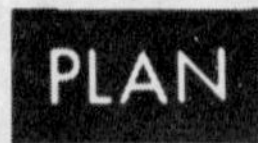

ADDITIONAL DIAGNOSTIC DATA

Blood glucose should be determined initially, since both hypoglycemia and hyperglycemia can cause convulsive seizures.

Blood calcium provides the clue to hypocalcemia.

Blood urea nitrogen elevation indicates renal disease.

Sodium and potassium levels may disclose metabolic disturbances (hyponatremia or hypernatremia).

Arterial blood gases aid in the diagnosis of alkalosis or acidosis. Serial values are important in assessing the patient's response to therapy.

X-rays of the skull may reveal a fracture line, hyperostoses, abnormal vascular markings, or intracranial calcifications.

Angiography may locate the source of bleeding in the case of an aneurysm or angiomatous tumor.

Brain scan or computerized axial tomography can be valuable when the diagnosis is obscure.

---

†Hyponatremia (water intoxication) can be caused by high doses of oxytocin plus large quantities of electrolyte-free fluids administered within relatively brief periods of time. The risk appears to be compounded if hypertonic saline solution is also injected into the amniotic fluid in order to induce abortion. Symptoms include nausea, vomiting, stupor, and convulsions.

Lumbar puncture is particularly helpful when subarachnoid hemorrhage or infection is suspected. (See Coma in Pregnancy, p. 234.)

Electroencephalogram may disclose a characteristic pattern of epilepsy.

MANAGEMENT AND PATIENT EDUCATION

Immediate emergency treatment is fourfold:

1. **Patent airway** for adequate *oxygenation* is essential. Mucus secretions are removed with a suction catheter, and oxygen is administered. Aspiration of vomitus must be prevented.

2. **Protection from Physical Harm:** The patient should be placed supine on a flat surface with her head turned to one side. Gentle restraints may be necessary. A padded tongue blade is inserted between the teeth to prevent trauma to the tongue and oral mucous membranes.

3. **Intravenous fluids** should be given.

4. **Anticonvulsant Medications:**

   Magnesium sulfate is usually preferred for eclampsia (see Eclampsia, p. 303).

   Diazepam (Valium): Ten mg may be given intravenously over a period of two minutes. Repeat, if necessary, two or three times at 20-minute intervals.

   Phenobarbital: A dose of 120 to 240 mg may be given slowly intravenously, at a rate of 60 mg per minute. Repeat, if necessary, two or three times at 20-minute intervals. (Maximal dosage is 1000 mg.)

   Sodium Amobarbital (Amytal): A dose of 120 to 250 mg may be given intravenously at a rate not to exceed 30 mg per minute.

   Phenytoin (Dilantin): A dose of 200 to 300 mg may be given intravenously at a rate no faster than 50 mg per minute. Total dosage should not exceed 1 gm.

Facilities for managing respiratory depression must be readily available.

Specific Measures depend on the underlying diagnosis:

Eclampsia: See Eclampsia, p. 303.

Epilepsy: Phenytoin (Dilantin) (200 to 400 mg per day) may be prescribed orally for maintenance therapy. Therapeutic blood levels are 10 to 25 mcg per ml.

Hypoglycemia: Fifty per cent glucose should be given intravenously. See Diabetic Emergencies, p. 276.

Hyponatremia: Three per cent sodium chloride solution may be given intravenously.

Cerebral Disease: Neurologic or neurosurgical consultation may be helpful.

Some epileptic patients may discontinue their medications during pregnancy because of concern over potential fetal defects. The risk of recurrent seizures, however, particularly of maternal and fetal anoxia, usually necessitates anticonvulsant therapy despite the risk of congenital anomalies. Neurologic consultation is advisable.

REFERENCES

Gupta DR, Cohen NH: Oxytocin, "salting out" and water intoxication. JAMA *220*:681-683, 1972; Obstet Gynecol Surv *28*:39-41, 1973

Nicol CF: Status epilepticus. JAMA *234*:419-420, 1975

37 CYSTITIS

GENERAL CONSIDERATIONS

Cystitis—bladder infection—is one of the most common problems of pregnant and nonpregnant women. The source is usually colon bacteria, which colonize the vaginal introitus and then ascend through the urethra into the bladder.

SUBJECTIVE DATA

Dysuria, burning on urination, urgency, frequency, suprapubic discomfort, hematuria, or passage of cloudy urine are the symptoms most usually observed. Fever is unlikely unless there is an associated renal infection.

OBJECTIVE DATA

PHYSICAL EXAMINATION

Abdominal Examination: These findings are usually normal, with the possible exception of suprapubic tenderness.

Pelvic Examination: A purulent discharge may be expressed from the urethra or Skene's glands. On bimanual examination, bladder tenderness may be palpable. Frequently, the pelvic examination is completely normal.

LABORATORY TESTS

Complete blood count and blood smear are normal unless there is an associated upper urinary tract infection.

Urinalysis reveals white cells, red cells, and bacteria. Ten or more leukocytes and many bacteria per high-power field in a centrifuged specimen signify pyuria and correlate with bacterial colony counts of 100,000 or more.

ASSESSMENT

DIFFERENTIAL DIAGNOSIS

This includes *trigonitis,* a noninfectious inflammatory process. Although the patient may complain of dysuria and frequency, the urine is usually devoid of clumps of white blood cells or bacteria. Cystoscopy may disclose mild trigonal hyperemia. Since trigonitis may be caused by vigorous penile thrusts against the base of the bladder, analgesics such as phenazopyridine (Pyridium) (200 mg three times daily) and modifications of coital position are frequently beneficial.

PREDISPOSING FACTORS

These include coitus, urethral catheterization, bladder overdistention, trauma to the base of the bladder during labor and delivery, poor perineal hygiene, cystocele, and suburethral diverticula.

ETIOLOGIC FACTORS

Etiologic bacteria are usually *Escherichia coli* or other enteric bacilli.

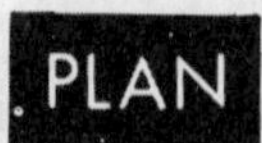

ADDITIONAL DIAGNOSTIC DATA

Bacterial cultures and sensitivity studies should be performed on any purulent discharge expressed from the urethra or Skene's glands and on a clean-catch midstream urine specimen. After the urethral orifice is cleansed with an antiseptic solution, the patient voids and a sterile container is used to catch the middle of the stream. A fixed volume of urine, usually 0.01 ml, is then inoculated on agar plates; after incubation the colonies are counted and the number of colony-forming units (bacteria) in the original specimen calculated. Colony counts of 100,000 or more are considered to represent "significant bacteriuria."

Cystoscopy may be indicated when cystitis is persistent and recurrent.

MANAGEMENT

Antimicrobial therapy is initiated as soon as the diagnosis of bacterial infection is established. The species of bacteria most likely to be recovered depends upon previous history of infection, previous antimicrobial therapy, hospitalization, surgical procedures, and instrumentation of the urinary tract. Gram-negative coliform bacilli are the usual organisms identified; *Escherichia coli* accounts for more than 80 per cent of the bacteria identified from uncomplicated cases.

The most frequently prescribed antimicrobials include sulfisoxazole (Gantrisin) 2 gm initially, followed by 1 gm four times daily) and ampicillin (500 mg orally four times daily for ten days). During pregnancy, ampicillin is preferred.

When infections are recurrent, complicated by underlying genitourinary disease, or resistant to commonly used antimicrobial agents, therapy must be based on sensitivity studies, which often indicate alternative agents. Carbenicillin, for example, has demonstrated clinical efficacy in urinary tract infections caused by susceptible strains of *Proteus, Pseudomonas,* Enterobacteriaceae, *Escherichia coli,* and enterococcus.

PATIENT EDUCATION

Since cystitis can be caused by fecal bacteria, patient instruction in perineal hygiene is advisable. After a bowel movement, stools should be wiped from the anus in a posterior direction and the tissue discarded. A second fold of tissue is then used to pat the urethral meatus. Increased cleansing of the vaginal introitus with soap and water or povidone-iodine solution may be beneficial.

Cystitis associated with coitus may be prevented by modifications of coital position as well as by voiding immediately after intercourse.

Follow-up urine cultures are recommended one week after therapy, in order to be certain that bladder bacteria have been eradicated.

REFERENCES

Bailey RR, Gower PE, Roberts AP, et al: Urinary-tract infection in non-pregnant women. Lancet *2*:275-277, 1973; Obstet Gynecol Surv *29*:296-297, 1974

Fass RJ, Klainer AS, Perkins RL: Urinary tract infection. JAMA *225*:1509-1513, 1973

38 DIABETIC EMERGENCIES IN PREGNANCY

GENERAL CONSIDERATIONS

Diabetes mellitus is one of the more common medical complications of pregnancy. Either hyperglycemia with or without ketoacidosis or hypoglycemia can create an acute emergency problem requiring immediate attention.

During early pregnancy, nausea, vomiting, and liver glycogen depletion may combine to predispose toward ketoacidosis.

As pregnancy progresses, insulin requirements usually increase; with an intercurrent infection or other stress, diabetic acidosis may develop rapidly.

The classification of diabetes in pregnancy proposed by White is widely employed:

Class A: Abnormal glucose tolerance test only

Class B: Onset of clinical diabetes after age 20, duration less than 10 years, no demonstrable vascular disease

Class C: Onset between ages 10 and 19, duration 10 to 19 years, no evidence of vascular disease

Class D: Onset before age 10, duration over 20 years, vascular lesions of benign retinopathy

Class F: Diabetic nephropathy

Class R: Proliferating retinopathy

Diabetic Ketoacidosis

GENERAL CONSIDERATIONS

Diabetic Ketoacidosis is a state of severe insulin deficiency characterized by hyperglycemia, systemic acidosis, and hyperketonemia. Acidosis and osmotic diuresis cause a large total body deficit of sodium, potassium, and body water. (The sodium deficit may be greater than 7 mEq/kg body weight, the potassium deficit greater than 5 mEq/kg, and the total body water decreased 4 to 10 liters.) Fluid loss leads to hemoconcentration and dehydration.

Infection should always be suspected as a possible precipitating factor.

SUBJECTIVE AND OBJECTIVE DATA

The patient may be flushed, dehydrated, comatose, and hypotensive with dry, cold skin. Breathing tends to be rapid and deep (Kussmaul respiration). The breath may have an odor of acetone. The heart rate is usually rapid. The abdomen may be tender with guarding.

Typical laboratory values are blood glucose greater than 300 mg/100 ml, glucosuria—usually 4+, decreased carbon dioxide, and metabolic acidosis. Serum sodium is usually within the normal range; potassium may be elevated. An elevated hematocrit indicates hemoconcentration.

ASSESSMENT

DIFFERENTIAL DIAGNOSIS

See Table 38-1.

TABLE 38-1. Differential Diagnosis of Diabetic Ketoacidosis*

	Hyperglycemia with Ketosis (Diabetic Coma)	Hyperinsulinism (Insulin Shock or Reaction)
History	Known diabetes; increasing thirst, air hunger, sleepiness; nausea and vomiting	Rapid onset following insulin; may not have eaten usual meal before or after dose; may have taken too much insulin
Diet	Too much food	Not enough food
Nausea and vomiting	Often present	Seldom present
Fever	May be present	Seldom present
Thirst	Intense	Absent
Facies	Looks toxic	Looks pale and weak
Vision	Dim	Diplopia
Eyeballs	Soft	Normal
Mouth	Dry; ketotic fruity odor	Drooling
Skin	Dry and flushed	Moist and pale
Blood pressure	Low	Normal or low
Respiration	Rapid and deep	Normal
Abdominal pain	Common; may simulate an acute surgical abdomen	Absent
Tremor	Absent	Frequent
Mental state	Gradual development of coma	Sudden onset of delirium, deep coma and bizarre neurologic picture
Convulsions	None	Late
Infection	May bring on symptoms	No effect
Insulin	May have omitted usual dose	Always has taken dose; sometimes too much
Urine	Sugar and diacetic acid present	Sugar may be present and diacetic acid absent in first specimen; in second specimen, both absent
Blood sugar (normal, 80-120 mg/100 ml)	Above normal (also serum acetone present)	Below normal

*From Flint T, Cain HD: Emergency Treatment and Management. Philadelphia, W.B. Saunders Company, 1975.

TABLE 38-1. Differential Diagnosis of Diabetic Ketoacidosis* (Continued)

	Hyperglycemia with Ketosis (Diabetic Coma)	Hyperinsulinism (Insulin Shock or Reaction)
CO_2 combining power (normal, 21-30 mEq/L)	10 mEq/L or less	Normal
Response to treatment	Slow	Rapid (may be delayed if protamine zinc or NPH insulin overdosage)

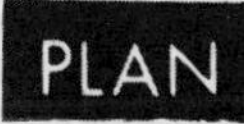

ADDITIONAL DIAGNOSTIC DATA

1. Blood glucose, ketones, BUN
2. Serum electrolytes—sodium, chloride, potassium, carbon dioxide
3. Arterial blood gases—pO_2, pCO_2, pH
4. Complete blood count
5. Urinalysis—sugar, acetone

MANAGEMENT

If there is the slightest question of hypoglycemia, one or two ampules or 50 ml of 50 per cent dextrose is administered intravenously, since this cannot harm the patient with ketoacidosis and is essential therapy for the patient with hypoglycemia.

Therapeutic Principles:

1. Insulin is provided to correct the endogenous insulin deficiency and enable the patient to incorporate glucose into the normal metabolic pathways.
2. Water and electrolyte losses are restored in order to reestablish the circulating plasma volume.
3. Precipitating factors (infection, medication errors, psychosocial stresses) are identified.

Specific Measures:

Insulin: An initial dose of 50 to 100 units of regular insulin is given half intravenously and half subcutaneously. The blood glucose level is measured hourly, and 25 to 50 units of regular insulin are given subcutaneously or intravenously each hour until the blood glucose has fallen to 250 mg/100 ml. (If hyperglycemia occurs without severe hyperketonemia or severe acidosis, treatment may be initiated with smaller insulin doses.)

During the next 24 hours, insulin dosage is determined by blood glucose levels, measured at five-hour intervals (7 AM, noon, 5 PM, 10 PM). Usually, 10 to 15 units of regular insulin are given subcutaneously during the day, with a similar dose of semilente insulin being given at 10 PM. Glucose is administered intravenously at a rate of 10 gm per hour. If the blood glucose level fails to fall, insulin dosage is increased. During pregnancy, preprandial glucose levels in the range of 100 mg per 100 ml appear to be a desirable goal.

Intravenous Fluids and Electrolytes: Two liters of normal saline should be administered during the first two or three hours. This serves to expand intravascular volume, correct severe dehydration and hypotension, and reestablish urinary output. Alternatively, half normal saline (0.45 per cent) has been recommended, since water loss is greater than sodium loss in osmotic diuresis (Felig, 1974).

As soon as the blood glucose level reaches 250 mg/100 ml, the intravenous infusion is changed to 5 per cent glucose in 0.45 per cent saline. The glucose is administered not only to prevent hypoglycemia but also to reduce the likelihood of cerebral edema, which may accompany rapid, insulin-induced reductions in blood glucose to levels below 250 mg/100 ml.

During the first 24 hours, approximately 50 to 75 per cent of the calculated fluid and electrolyte deficits should be replaced (usually, 5 or 6 liters of fluid and 350 to 400 mEq of sodium).

Potassium is replaced as soon as urinary output is well-established and acidosis is corrected. Although ketoacidosis causes a severe depletion of total body potassium, the initial serum potassium level is often normal or elevated because of the potassium shift from the intracellular to extracellular fluid. As acidosis is corrected, cellular uptake of glucose resumes and serum potassium levels may decline rapidly. Consequently, frequent determinations of serum potassium are essential to evaluate the need for and rate of potassium supplementation. Before hypokalemia becomes evident, 40 mEq of potassium chloride are added to 1000 ml of intravenous fluid and infused over a two-hour period. During the first 24 hours, a total of 100 to 200 mEq of potassium is usually required.

Sodium bicarbonate is rarely needed even though the patient is acidotic and serum carbon dioxide levels are decreased. The majority of patients respond to insulin therapy and volume replacement. In severe cases of acidosis (pH<7.1), 44 mEq of sodium bicarbonate can be added to the intravenously administered solution and given over a period of one to two hours. Additional bicarbonate is given until the pH is more than 7.1.

Close monitoring of glucose, electrolytes, and pH is essential.

Once the patient has become responsive, and the blood pressure and urinary output have stabilized, oral feedings of broth, fruit juices, and potassium can be initiated.

PATIENT EDUCATION

A thorough understanding of diabetic management during pregnancy (diet, activity, insulin therapy, and so forth) is vital in order to avoid maternal complications and minimize perinatal morbidity and mortality. After the initial crisis is corrected, a palatable and practical diet must be planned. Consultation with a dietician is helpful. A caloric intake of 30 to 35 calories per kg is usually recommended, consisting of 200 gm of carbohydrate, 100 gm of protein, and the remainder of fat. Insulin requirements tend to increase progressively during pregnancy and then decrease markedly after delivery.

Close medical supervision is essential in order to maintain glucose control and minimize complications. The patient is instructed to maintain a daily record of urine sugar and acetone in order to report immediately any marked fluctuations.

The optimal time for delivery is based on multiple factors including previous obstetric history, fetal maturity, uteroplacental function, and development of maternal complications.

Hypoglycemia

GENERAL CONSIDERATIONS

Hypoglycemia is characterized by tachycardia, sweating, pallor, tremor, and hunger. In cases of severe chronic hypoglycemia, symptoms may range from headache, change in affect, anorexia, irritability, or lethargy to seizures, psychotic behavior, or coma. The blood glucose level is below 50 mg/100 ml.

PLAN

MANAGEMENT AND PATIENT EDUCATION

Specific therapy is an intravenous bolus of 50 ml of 50 per cent dextrose. As soon as the patient is conscious, she should be given orange juice or other fruit juice orally. If the patient is receiving insulin, she should be instructed concerning the importance of proper diet in order to prevent hypoglycemic reactions.

REFERENCES

Felig P: Body fuel metabolism and diabetes mellitus in pregnancy. Med Clin North Am *61*:43-66, 1977

Felig P: Diabetic ketoacidosis. N Engl J Med *290*:1360-1363, 1974

Karlsson K, Kjellmer I: The outcome of diabetic pregnancies in relation to the mother's blood sugar level. Am J Obstet Gynecol *112*:213-220, 1972; Obstet Gynecol Surv *27*:418-420, 1972

Newmark SR, Himathongkam T, Shane JM: Hyperglycemic and hypoglycemic crises. JAMA *231*:185-187, 1975

White P: Classification of obstetric diabetes. Am J Obstet Gynecol *130*:228-230, 1978

39 DRUG HYPERSENSITIVITY REACTIONS

GENERAL CONSIDERATIONS

Drug hypersensitivity refers to a variety of reactions ranging from a slight rash to acute anaphylaxis.

Immediate hypersensitivity reactions resulting from the interaction of antigen with circulating antibody may appear as anaphylaxis, urticaria, or serum sickness.

Anaphylaxis: See Anaphylaxis, p. 125.

Serum sickness is a systemic allergic reaction produced by circulating immune complexes and characterized by fever, rash, lymphadenopathy, arthritis, nephritis, edema, and neuritis. The syndrome is produced by antigens that remain in the circulation for prolonged periods, so that at the time antibody is first formed, intravascular antigen is still present. Drugs that produce serum sickness include penicillin, sulfonamides, phenytoin, aminosalicylic acid, and streptomycin. Symptoms of serum sickness may develop after a latent period of six days or more after initial exposure to one of these drugs (the latent period reflects the time needed to synthesize appreciable amounts of antibody).

Delayed hypersensitivity is characterized by the interaction of a drug-protein conjugate with sensitized cells, causing a release of various biologically active materials which lead to perivascular accumulation of mononuclear cells and the development of induration. In this form of immunity, circulating antibody is not important. An example of delayed hypersensitivity is skin sensitization resulting from direct contact with a variety of medications.

Hypersensitivity reactions should be distinguished from two other untoward effects of drugs. The first is *intolerance,* the occurrence of toxic effects at dosages well below the levels that would be expected to produce toxicity in the general population. The second is *idiosyncrasy,* the reaction of a patient to a drug that is qualitatively different from the reaction expected. An example of idiosyncrasy is the hemolytic anemia that results from treatment with phenacetin or sulfonamides in patients with glucose-6-phosphate dehydrogenase deficiency.

Hypersensitivity reactions always follow a prior sensitizing exposure. Topical application to the skin or mucous membrane is most apt to cause sensitization, parenteral administration causes intermediate sensitization, and oral administration produces the least sensitization. Intermittent courses of drug therapy may increase the risk of sensitization. Once an allergy has developed, very minute amounts of the drug may precipitate a reaction in highly sensitive people.

SUBJECTIVE AND OBJECTIVE DATA

CURRENT SYMPTOMS

Fever may develop immediately after administration of a drug or, more commonly, may increase after the seventh or eighth day of therapy. The fever tends to be in the range of 38 to 39° C (100 to 102° F). Penicillin, sulfonamides, phenytoin, and barbiturates are some of the drugs that can cause fever.

Skin rash may take several forms: maculopapular with confluent erythroderma and subsequent exfoliative dermatitis; urticarial rashes with prutitus; and erythema multiforme-like eruptions characterized by sharply circumscribed, usually symmetrical lesions.

Hematologic disorders include thrombocytopenic purpura, hemolytic anemia, and agranulocytosis.

PRIOR HISTORY

Patients with a history of an allergic reaction to one drug appear to be more prone to the development of a subsequent additional hypersensitivity reaction.

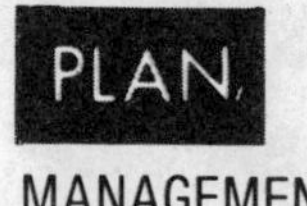

MANAGEMENT

Discontinuance: Allergic reactions usually subside promptly after discontinuance of the drug. Treatment of a specific reaction is directed against the altered physiologic condition.

Epinephrine—0.5 to 1 ml of a 1:1000 dilution administered subcutaneously—is the drug of choice for treatment of an acute anaphylactic reaction (sudden vascular collapse, severe pruritus and bronchospasm). (See Anaphylaxis, p. 125.)

Antihistamines: Diphenhydramine (Benadryl)—50 mg or the equivalent—may be beneficial.

Corticosteroids such as methylprednisolone sodium succinate (Solu-Medrol)—10 to 40 mg or the equivalent—may be administered intravenously or intramuscularly for the management of the pruritus, skin rash, and edema of serum sickness. Short-term tapered therapy with 4 mg tablets of methylprednisolone (Medrol) usually relieves the symptoms of severe allergic drug reactions. (The Medrol Dosepak contains 21 4-mg tablets, with patient instructions for six days of countdown therapy.)

PATIENT EDUCATION

Patients who have had a hypersensitivity reaction should always inform all medical personnel of their previous reaction. Since skin testing for drug sensitivity can be unreliable, decisions for future drug therapy must be based on past experiences. Patients should also be encouraged to wear an identification tag that would be readily apparent in an emergency situation.

REFERENCES

Parker CW: Drug allergy. N Engl J Med *292*:511-514, 732-736, 957-960, 1975

40 DYSFUNCTIONAL UTERINE BLEEDING

GENERAL CONSIDERATIONS

Dysfunctional uterine bleeding may be defined as abnormal endometrial bleeding not associated with an organic condition—pregnancy, tumor, inflammation, or systemic disease. Prolonged menses may alternate with periods of amenorrhea, producing complete irregularity of the menstrual cycle. Bleeding results from disturbances in the hormonal and vascular mechanisms that normally initiate and terminate menstrual flow. The endometrium tends to be proliferative in approximately 85 per cent of the cases, indicating ovarian dysfunction and anovulation.

Anovulatory dysfunctional uterine bleeding occurs most commonly during the extremes of a woman's reproductive years. Persistent estrogenic stimulation in the absence of growth-limiting progesterone causes abnormal endometrial thickness without concomitant structural support. The intensely vascular, abnormally fragile, endometrium tends to bleed spontaneously. As one site heals, another site breaks down. Bleeding may persist for days and weeks.

Normal endometrial control mechanisms are missing. Tissue breakdown involves random portions of the endometrium in a variable and irregular pattern; bleeding does not occur simultaneously throughout the entire endometrium. The large quantity of tissue combined with the disorderly, abrupt, random tissue breakdown *without* vasoconstrictive rhythmicity, tight coiling of spiral vessels, or the orderly collapse necessary to induce stasis accounts for the prolonged and excessive bleeding.

Irregular shedding of secretory endometrium is a less common type of dysfunctional bleeding associated with ovulatory cycles.

SUBJECTIVE DATA

Vaginal bleeding associated with anovulation is usually irregular, acyclic, and painless. The quantity of bleeding varies from scanty to profuse.

OBJECTIVE DATA

PHYSICAL EXAMINATION

General Examination: Findings are usually normal unless excessive blood loss has caused hypovolemia or anemia. Petechiae or ecchymoses can be the first clue to a possible coagulation disorder.

Abdominal and Pelvic Examinations: These findings are normal.

LABORATORY TESTS

Complete blood count with blood smear provides an evaluation of blood-loss anemia as well as of any possible hematologic condition (aplastic anemia, leukemia, red-cell fragmentation). Leukocytosis suggests the possibility of an associated infection. The finding of adequate platelets in the blood smear virtually excludes the possibility of thrombocytopenia. When platelets are inadequate, a platelet count should be ordered.

ASSESSMENT

DIFFERENTIAL DIAGNOSIS

This must rule out tumor, pregnancy, infection, hormonal therapy, intrauterine device, and coagulation disorders. (See Vaginal Bleeding, p. 686.)

Ovulatory bleeding tends to be predictable and cyclic in nature. Heavier-than-normal bleeding associated with an ovulatory cycle may be the result of submucous leiomyoma, endometrial polyp, persistent corpus luteum, coagulation disorders, or irregular shedding.

Progestin breakthrough bleeding is associated with prolonged use of birth control pills or with depot forms of progesterone derivatives. In the absence of sufficient endogenous and exogenous estrogen, the endometrium shrinks to a shallow height and is composed almost exclusively of pseudodecidual stroma and blood vessels with minimal glands. Variable vaginal spotting may occur during the month, with no bleeding occurring during the nontreatment interval.

Coagulation disorders are suggested by the history of bleeding from other sites, personal history of coagulation disorders, or family history of bleeding disorders. (See Coagulation Disorders, p. 210.)

PREDISPOSING FACTORS

Predisposing factors to anovulation include the perimenarchal years, the perimenopausal years, chronic disease, thyroid or adrenal dysfunction, exogenous steroid hormones, obesity, malnutrition, ovarian cysts or tumors, psychotropic drugs, and psychogenic factors.

Although anovulatory bleeding can occur at any age, dysfunctional bleeding is one of the most common gynecologic problems during the perimenarchal and perimenopausal years.

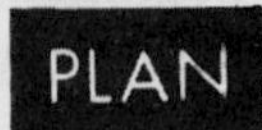

ADDITIONAL DIAGNOSTIC DATA

Endometrial biopsy or curettage is always indicated whenever there is any question of endometrial disease. Histologic identification of the bleeding endometrium (proliferative, atrophic, or secretory) aids in the selection of rational hormonal therapy.

In the case of dysfunctional bleeding, the endometrium is almost always proliferative or hyperplastic, indicating excessive estrogenic stimulation without the progesterone effect associated with ovulation.

Endometrial curettage is not only diagnostic but also therapeutic, since curettage usually terminates excessive endometrial bleeding promptly.

Pregnancy Test for HCG: A negative test helps rule out the possibility of pregnancy. When bleeding is associated with abdominal pain, however, ectopic pregnancy must *always* be considered, since the pregnancy test may be negative in the case of ectopic pregnancy.

Coagulation Tests: Platelet count or bleeding time or both are indicated if there is any suspicion of thrombocytopenia or von Willebrand's disease. (See Coagulation Disorders, p. 210.)

Serum gonadotropins—follicle stimulating hormone and luteinizing hormone—are not usually included with an emergency diagnostic evaluation. However, persistent dysfunctional bleeding during the reproductive years often requires follow-up diagnostic procedures. Elevated luteinizing hormone levels and depressed follicle stimulating hormone may be associated with the polycystic ovary syndrome (Stein-Leventhal syndrome).

Thyroid function tests are indicated if there is any suspicion of associated hypo- or hyperthyroidism.

MANAGEMENT

Factors Governing Therapy:

1. Age of patient
2. Bleeding—quantity, duration
3. Possibility of an organic pathologic condition (pregnancy, tumor, infection, systemic disease)
4. Desire for future childbearing

Adolescent Age Group: During the perimenarchal years, anovulation is so frequently the cause of excessive endometrial bleeding that biopsy or curettage is often deferred.

Progestational Therapy: Acute bleeding episodes from a persistently proliferative endometrium can usually be initially controlled by converting the endometrium into the secretory phase and suppressing endometrial proliferation. For this purpose, 100 mg of progesterone in oil may be injected intramuscularly. Alternative oral therapy is either 10 mg of medroxyprogesterone acetate (Provera) daily for five days or 1 mg of norethindrone with 0.050 mg of mestranol four times a day for five to seven days.

Failure to control bleeding within 12 to 36 hours is usually an indication for curettage.

When anovulatory bleeding responds to progestational therapy, withdrawal bleeding resulting from declining values of the progestational hormone must be anticipated within two to six days after the intramuscular injection or the termination of oral therapy. This bleeding episode tends to be self-limited as a result of the vasomotor rhythmicity associated with secretory endometrium. However, to assure limited bleeding, particularly for patients who do not desire pregnancy immediately, a combination estrogen-progestin medication (0.5 mg of norgestrel plus 50 mcg ethinyl estradiol or 1 mg of norethindrone with 50 mcg of mestranol) is initiated on the fifth day of progesterone withdrawal flow. The estrogen-progestin hormones suppress ovarian follicular activity and prevent excessive endometrial regrowth. The combination estrogen-progestin hormones are prescribed for 21-day intervals punctuated by seven-day withdrawal-flow intervals. Treatment is usually continued for three to six cycles.

An alternative method of treatment is synthetic progestin daily for five to seven days every four weeks in order to produce a secretory endometrium and regular endometrial desquamation. Since these patients almost always have sufficient endogenous estrogen, the use of the progestin alone at four-week intervals has the advantage of not inhibiting spontaneous ovulation, which can be detected by the determination of basal body temperature.

[An exception with regard to progestational therapy is the young anovulatory patient with *prolonged hemorrhagic desquamation,* a minimal residual endometrium, and severe anemia. If this patient is treated with 25 mg of conjugated estrogens intravenously every four hours, bleeding should be controlled within 12 hours. After 24 hours of high-dose estrogen therapy, oral estrogen-progestin combination medication is initiated (2 mg of norethindrone with 0.1 mg of mestranol or the equivalent for 21 days).]

Iron therapy is always indicated whenever there is any evidence of iron deficiency anemia.

Ovulation induction with clomiphene citrate beginning on the fifth day of the cycle following induced bleeding may be indicated for the patient who desires to become pregnant. The initial dose is 50 mg daily for five days.

Reproductive Age Group:

Curettage: Whenever bleeding is likely to result from an endometrial pathologic condition, curettage (suction or sharp) is both diagnostic and therapeutic.

Follow-up hormonal therapy is based on the endometrial histologic condition and the patient's childbearing desires. Women requesting contraception are usually treated with the estrogen-progestin combination preparations that suppress ovulation and prevent persistent endometrial proliferation. Oral contraceptives are administered for 21 days, followed by a seven-day medication-free interval. For the patient who wishes to become pregnant, ovulation induction with clomiphene citrate may be beneficial.

Hysterectomy may be preferred for definitive management of persistent dysfunctional bleeding when the patient declines hormonal therapy and desires permanent sterilization.

Estrogen Therapy: Bleeding associated with an atrophic endometrium, the prolonged use of birth control pills, or depot forms of progesterone derivatives does not respond to progestin therapy, since the tissue base on which the progestin would exert its effect is lacking. Under these circumstances, 20 mcg of ethinyl estradiol or 2.5 mg of conjugated estrogens daily for ten days stimulates endometrial proliferation. The estrogen is then followed by estrogen and progestin in combination for five to seven days unless the patient has previously received a depot progestin.

Although high doses of intravenous estrogen *temporarily* suppress endometrial bleeding from a hyperplastic, proliferative endometrium, bleeding *recurs* as soon as the exogenous hormonal support declines.

Perimenopausal Age Group:

Biopsy or Curettage: Since the possibility of endometrial hyperplasia or malignancy increases with age, a thorough endometrial suction biopsy or curettage is recommended in order to establish a histologic diagnosis.

As long as the endometrium is benign, a progestin (10 mg of medroxyprogesterone acetate or 2 mg of norethindrone) may be given at monthly intervals for five to seven days to induce regular withdrawal periods and prevent recurrence of abnormal bleeding episodes. Alternatively, periodic courses of an estrogen-progestin oral contraceptive may be effective, although the possibility of an increased risk of thromboembolic disease in women over age 40 must be considered.

Hysterectomy may be required when bleeding is recurrent and persistent or when hormone therapy is contraindicated.

PATIENT EDUCATION

In the adolescent age group, anovulatory, dysfunctional bleeding tends to resolve with the onset of ovulatory cycles. Consequently, the adolescent patient can usually be reassured that her problem is likely to be self-limited and corrected by the onset of regular ovulation.

During the perimenopausal years, dysfunctional bleeding may resolve spontaneously with the gradual decline in ovarian activity associated with the climacteric.

Periodic follow-up examinations are always essential.

REFERENCES

Aksel S, Jones GS: Etiology and treatment of dysfunctional uterine bleeding. Obstet Gynecol *44*:1-13, 1974

Bryner JR, Greenblatt RB: Dysfunctional uterine bleeding: causes and management. Contemp OB/GYN *7*:65-69, 1976

Shane JM, Naftolin F, Newmark SR: Gynecologic endocrine emergencies. JAMA *231*:393-395, 1975

Speroff L, Glass RH, Kase NG: Clinical gynecologic endocrinology and infertility. Baltimore, The Williams & Wilkins Company, 1973

41 DYSMENORRHEA

GENERAL CONSIDERATIONS

Dysmenorrhea—pain during the menstrual period—is one of the most common gynecologic symptoms. Even though women with dysmenorrhea tend to have periodically recurrent menstrual pain, the severity of an individual episode may cause the patient to seek emergency care.

Primary dysmenorrhea, with its onset a few months to a few years after menarche, appears to be associated with ovulatory cycles. The pelvic organs are normal, and the dysmenorrhea often improves following pregnancy. The mechanism of painful menses is not certain and may vary with different women. Possibilities include retrograde menstruation, uterine spasm, and uterine ischemia.

Secondary dysmenorrhea is caused by a specific pelvic pathologic condition and may occur at any time during the reproductive life of the patient.

SUBJECTIVE DATA

CURRENT SYMPTOMS

Abdominal pain may commence a few hours to a day prior to menstrual flow. The pain is usually greatest about 12 hours after the onset of flow, at the time when endometrial shedding is maximal. The pain tends to be sharp and colicky in nature and is usually felt in the suprapubic area. The pain may also involve the lumbosacral area and the inner and anterior aspects of the thighs—areas of ovarian and uterine nerve innervation referred to the body surface.

Usually the pain persists only through the first menstrual day; pain may persist, however, throughout the entire menstrual period. The pain may be so intense that the patient requests emergency care.

Menstrual Symptoms: Menses are usually regular. The amount and duration of bleeding are variable. Many patients associate pain with the passage of blood clots or an endometrial cast.

Other Symptoms: Nausea, vomiting, and diarrhea may be associated with the painful menses. These symptoms may possibly indicate increased circulating prostaglandin stimulating hyperactivity of intestinal smooth muscle.

PRIOR HISTORY

Patients with dysmenorrhea are likely to recount a history of similar pain occurring with each menstrual period. Primary dysmenorrhea usually begins shortly after menarche and often terminates after the first pregnancy. At times, patients give a history of excessive fatigue and nervous tension.

OBJECTIVE DATA

PHYSICAL EXAMINATION

Abdominal Examination: The abdomen is soft without any evidence of peritoneal irritation or a localized pathologic condition. Bowel sounds are normal.

Pelvic Examination: In cases of primary dysmenorrhea the pelvic examination is normal. In cases of secondary dysmenorrhea the pelvic examination may disclose the underlying pathologic condition, for example, endometriotic nodules in the cul-de-sac, or tuboovarian disease or leiomyomata.

LABORATORY TESTS

Complete blood count is normal.

Urinalysis is normal.

ASSESSMENT

DIFFERENTIAL DIAGNOSIS

This may include virtually all the causes of abdominal pain (see Abdominal Pain, p. 70).

ETIOLOGIC FACTORS

Etiologic factors that may be responsible for *primary dysmenorrhea* include

Inherent hyperactivity of uterine smooth muscle: Under the influence of progesterone, the secretory endometrium synthesizes prostaglandin F_2 alpha, a hormone that causes smooth-muscle contraction. This substance is released when the endometrium breaks down at menstruation and may act on the uterine muscle and vasculature to cause contraction and associated pain.

Psychogenic Factors: Emotional stress and tension associated with school or work may accentuate the severity of the pain.

Etiologic factors that may be responsible for *secondary dysmenorrhea* include

Congenital Uterine Anomalies: A blind pouch of the uterus may be lined with endometrium, which cycles and sheds. Since there is no opening, the menstrual fluids cause the cavity to become swollen, creating severe pain. On pelvic examination the uterus may feel irregular. Occasionally a dimple will be seen in the vagina where the incomplete cervix ends. The pain tends to be colicky in nature, starting near menarche and occurring toward the end rather than the beginning of the menstrual flow.

Submucous Leiomyoma: Painful, profuse menses may be caused by the uterine contractions attempting to expel a submucous leiomyoma. On occasion the submucous leiomyoma may be visualized in the cervical os. (See Leiomyoma of Uterus, p. 419.)

Intrauterine or Intracervical Polyps: The uterus may respond to a polyp as it would to a foreign body and contract forcefully in the attempt to expel the polyp.

Endometriosis is a frequent cause of secondary dysmenorrhea. The location of the pain varies depending on the site of the endometrial implants and whether there is any associated rectal or ureteral involvement. (See Endometriosis, p. 334.)

Adenomyosis: The uterus may be slightly enlarged. (See Adenomyosis, p. 119.)

Acute and Chronic Pelvic Infection: Although pelvic pain may occur at any time during the menstrual cycle, some patients report exacerbation of pain at the time of menses.

Cervical Stenosis: Obstruction of the menstrual flow causes severe colicky pain.

Intrauterine device may stimulate painful uterine contractions.

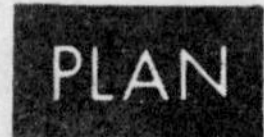

MANAGEMENT

Emergency therapy is usually limited to oral analgesic medications, oral tranquilizers, and oral sedatives. The patient should be advised to avoid any imminent stressful situation and to obtain adequate rest and sleep. Often a glass of wine or an alcoholic beverage is helpful.

When nausea, vomiting, or gastrointestinal colic are associated symptoms, promethazine hydrochloride (Phenergan) rectal suppositories (25 mg) or oral anticholinergic medications may be helpful. Adiphenine hydrochloride is an antispasmodic medication that may be prescribed before meals. Prostaglandin inhibitors, such as indomethacin and naproxen have been reported to be beneficial.

Ovulation Suppression: Oral contraceptive medications containing combined low-dose estrogen and progestin may be prescribed from days 5 to 25 of the next menstrual cycle. This regimen usually alleviates or at least modifies the anticipated recurrent primary dysmenorrhea.

Specific Pelvic Pathologic Conditions require definitive therapy. (See specific diagnoses.)

PATIENT EDUCATION

The various factors that may contribute to dysmenorrhea are reviewed with the patient. Often, menstrual pain is exacerbated by emotional stress, tension, or fatigue. The importance of adequate rest is emphasized, since uterine contractions associated with menses tend to be more uncomfortable when a woman is tired or tense. Many patients are reassured by the absence of pelvic disease.

When oral contraceptive hormones are prescribed for ovulatory suppression, the benefits and risks of these medications must be discussed in detail.

REFERENCES

Halbert DR, Demers LM, Darnell Jones DE: Dysmenorrhea and prostaglandins. Obstet Gynecol Surv *31*:77-81, 1976

Lundstrom V, Green K: Endogenous levels of prostaglandin $F_2\alpha$ and its main metabolites in plasma and endometrium of normal and dysmenorrheic women. Am J Obstet Gynecol *130*:640-646, 1978

42 DYSPNEA DURING PREGNANCY

GENERAL CONSIDERATIONS

Dyspnea, or shortness of breath, may be defined as an undue awareness of respiratory effort. Although dyspnea during exercise or at rest is a common manifestation of many forms of pulmonary and cardiovascular disease, shortness of breath is a subjective symptom that can also have a psychologic origin.

During pregnancy, many women become aware of their breathing for the first time and may interpret the "normal" hyperventilation of pregnancy as shortness of breath suggestive of cardiac or pulmonary disease.

As pregnancy advances, tidal volume, minute ventilatory volume, and minute oxygen uptake increase, while respiratory rate remains unchanged. The increased tidal volume lowers the blood pCO_2 to levels of 30 to 32 mm Hg, causing a transient respiratory alkalosis, which is well compensated by the renal excretion of bicarbonate. The hyperventilation of pregnancy appears to be due to a central effect of progesterone, which lowers the respiratory center's threshold to carbon dioxide. The dyspnea of pregnancy tends to be noted at rest, rather than during exertion, and may be episodic in nature.

ASSESSMENT

DIFFERENTIAL DIAGNOSIS

Pulmonary Disease (Disease of the Bronchi, Alveoli, Pleura, or Thoracic Cage, see Table 42-1): Dyspnea is usually brought on by exertion and is a prominent symptom in those conditions in which the lungs or thorax is

TABLE 42-1. Causes of Respiratory Failure*

I. Disorders of the central nervous system:
  A. Drug intoxication
    Sedatives (barbiturates, glutethimide)
    Tranquilizers (phenothiazines, meprobamate)
    Analgesics (opiates, e.g., morphine, heroin, methadone)
    Anesthetic gases
  B. Vascular disorders and hypoperfusion states
    Brainstem infarction
    Brainstem hemorrhage
    Postcardiac arrest
    Shock
  C. Trauma to the brainstem
    Head injury
    Increased intracranial pressure
  D. Infection
    Encephalitis (viral)
    Bulbar poliomyelitis
  E. Miscellaneous
    Primary alveolar hypoventilation (with or without obesity)
    Myxedema
    Status epilepticus

II. Disorders of the peripheral nervous system and respiratory muscles:
  A. Anterior horn cell and peripheral nerve disorders
    Guillain-Barré syndrome
    Poliomyelitis
    Amyotrophic lateral sclerosis
    Other polyneuritides
  B. Myoneural junction disorders
    Myasthenia gravis
    Tetanus
    Curariform drugs (succinylcholine, curare, polymyxin, colistimethate, streptomycin, kanamycin)
    Anticholinesterase drugs (insecticides, neostigmine)
  C. Muscular disorders
    Polymyositis
    Muscular dystrophies
    Myotonia

*From Smith JP: Respiratory failure and its management. *In* Beeson PB, McDermott W: Textbook of Medicine. Philadelphia, W.B. Saunders Company, 1975.

TABLE 42-1. Causes of Respiratory Failure* (Continued)

III. Disorders of the chest wall and pleura:
  A. Scoliosis
    Congenital
    Idiopathic
    Paralytic (post polio)
    Miscellaneous (post-thoracic surgery, post-tubercular, Marfan's syndrome, von Recklinghausen's disease)
  B. Chest trauma
    Flail chest
    Multiple rib fractures
    Post-thoracotomy
  C. Pleural disorders
    Massive effusions
    Tension pneumothorax
    Massive fibrosis

IV. Intrinsic pulmonary disorders:
  A. Airway obstruction
    Chronic obstructive pulmonary disease (chronic bronchitis, emphysema, asthma)
    Acute obstruction (foreign body, acute epiglottitis and laryngitis, inhalation burns, noxious gases)
  B. Alveolar and interstitial disorders
    Pneumonia (lobar, aspiration, interstitial)
    The granulomatoses and fibroses
    Pulmonary edema (left ventricular failure)
    Lymphangitic metastases
  C. Vascular disorders
    Embolic disease (thrombo-, fat, tumor)
    Obliterative vasculitis (primary pulmonary hypertension, scleroderma)

V. Extrapulmonary disorders leading to pulmonary disease:
    Hepatic failure, shock, renal failure, acute pancreatitis, peritonitis, sepsis, postcardiopulmonary bypass, and post-traumatic states (extrathoracic injuries and surgery)

stiffer than normal because the inspiratory muscles have to develop greater tension to produce the same tidal volume.

Dyspnea developing suddenly at rest suggests pulmonary embolism or spontaneous pneumothorax. Associated symptoms may include cough and pleuritic pain.

In cases of obstructive airway disease, asthma, and chronic bronchitis, patients breathe near their maximal inspiratory level and tend to use accessory inspiratory muscles.

Restrictive lung disease includes pulmonary resections, space-occupying lesions, pleural effusion, and spontaneous pneumothorax.

Pulmonary infections include lobar pneumonia and acute bronchitis. Vascular congestion and the accumulation of secretions cause an increased airway resistance. Hypoxemia resulting from variations in the ventilation-perfusion ratio throughout the lungs combined with pyrexia stimulates ventilation. If the infection is complicated by pleurisy, vital capacity can be further reduced when impaired coughing leads to the accumulation of bronchial secretions and breathing is restricted by pain.

Pulmonary edema is most commonly caused by increased pulmonary capillary pressure. The usual mechanism is left ventricular failure. Rapid, shallow breathing is characteristic of developing pulmonary edema and is believed to be related to neurogenic stimuli arising from receptors in the alveolar septa. Cyanosis can be present when edema is severe.

Weakness of respiratory muscles (polio, polyneuropathy, myasthenia gravis, muscular dystrophies, and potassium depletion) can be another cause of respiratory impairment.

Cardiac Failure: Dyspnea is usually present when the patient is supine, since gravitational effects increase lung congestion.

Hypoxia, acidosis, and fever stimulate central receptors to increase respiratory demand.

Psychogenic Factors: Any chest discomfort may be interpreted as breathlessness by a nervous patient. Responsible factors include anxiety about cardiac or pulmonary disease, muscular symptoms, or gastric flatulence. Often there is a desire to take frequent deep breaths with sighing respiration. Hyperventilation lowers pCO_2, creating a respiratory alkalosis with symptoms of dizziness, paresthesia, and tetanic hand and leg cramps.

Abdominal Distention caused by hydramnios can also lead to dyspnea.

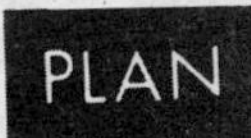

ADDITIONAL DIAGNOSTIC DATA

Complete Blood Count with Blood Smear: Decreased hemoglobin or hematocrit may indicate anemia. Increased white blood count suggests infection.

Chest x-ray is usually essential for an initial assessment of cardiac and pulmonary disease.

Arterial blood gases—pO_2, pCO_2, and pH—provide the best assessment of pulmonary ventilation.

Electrocardiogram is advisable when cardiac disease is suspected.

MANAGEMENT AND PATIENT EDUCATION

An adequate airway, ventilation and oxygenation must be assured. The upper airway is cleared by suctioning or manual removal of debris and secretions from the nose and mouth.

Endotracheal intubation is indicated when the oropharyngeal airway is inadequate or when the patient is comatose.

Emergency tracheostomy may be required if the airway is obstructed at or above the level of the larynx.

Specific therapy depends on the specific diagnosis. (See Asthma, p. 148; Pulmonary Aspiration, p. 577; Pulmonary Edema, p. 582; Pulmonary Embolism, p. 585; and Hydramnios, p. 379.)

The dyspnea of pregnancy or hyperventilation syndrome requires no specific therapy other than reassurance. If hyperventilation has produced faintness or light-headedness, it is almost always a manifestation of acute anxiety. The patient may be reassured by the fact that she can control the symptoms by breath holding or breathing into a paper bag. A prescription for an ataraxic medication, such as hydroxyzine (Atarax, Vistaril) may be helpful. (Note: Hydroxyzine is contraindicated in early pregnancy because fetal abnormalities have been induced in the rat at doses substantially above the human therapeutic range.)

43 ECLAMPSIA

GENERAL CONSIDERATIONS

Eclampsia: One of the most serious emergency problems during the latter half of pregnancy, this is an acute disorder characterized by one or more convulsions not attributable to other cerebral conditions, such as epilepsy or cerebral hemorrhage, in a woman in whom hypertension, with proteinuria, edema, or both, has developed as the result of pregnancy. Although eclampsia usually occurs after the twentieth week of gestation, it may develop earlier in the presence of trophoblastic disease (molar pregnancy).

Arteriolar vasospasm with impaired circulation of the blood vessels themselves as well as of the organs they supply is basic to the disease process of preeclampsia and eclampsia. Vascular damage, together with local hypoxia of the surrounding tissues, leads to edema, hemorrhage, and necrosis of various organs, including the liver, lung, and brain.

The most common findings are extravascular fluid retention and intravascular dehydration or hemoconcentration. Renal changes characteristic of preeclampsia and eclampsia are glomerular capillary endothelial swelling with narrowing of the capillary lumens. Fibrinoid changes in the walls of cerebral vessels may be responsible for the prodromal neurologic symptoms and convulsions.

SUBJECTIVE DATA

CURRENT SYMPTOMS

Convulsive Seizures: The patient may be seen during the convulsive phase or in a comatose state following one or more convulsions. Dyspnea and cyanosis may be associated findings.

Other Symptoms: During the late second trimester or the third trimester of pregnancy, the following symptoms may portend an eclamptic convulsion: sudden weight gain resulting from fluid retention, puffiness of the face and hands, headache, visual disturbances, epigastric or right upper quadrant pain with or without nausea and vomiting, and decreased urine output.

PRIOR HISTORY

The typical patient with eclampsia is nulliparous and teenaged. The prenatal record may disclose sudden or gradual development of hypertension, edema, weight gain, and albuminuria.

OBJECTIVE DATA

PHYSICAL EXAMINATION

General Examination: The patient is usually unconscious or semiconscious immediately after an eclamptic convulsion.

The typical seizure is characterized by the occurrence of generalized tonic contractions followed by a clonic phase progressing to coma. Convulsive movements usually begin about the mouth in the form of facial twitchings. Within a few seconds all the muscles of the body are rigidly contracted (the face is distorted, the eyes protrude, the arms are flexed, the hands are clenched, and the legs are drawn up). After 15 to 20 seconds the muscles alternately contract and relax in rapid succession. The muscular movements may be so violent that the tongue may be bitten by the violent action of the jaws. When the patient regains consciousness, she is usually disoriented and restless for a variable period of time. Blood pressure is elevated, and respiration is usually increased in rate and may be stertorous. In the case of severe respiratory distress the patient is cyanotic.

Generalized fluid retention is frequently obvious. Facial edema as well as peripheral edema of the hands and legs is a common finding.

Retinal examination may disclose arteriolar narrowing and retinal edema.

Chest examination may disclose basilar rales that are indicative of pulmonary edema.

The patellar and ankle reflexes are usually hyperactive. Ankle clonus is a frequent finding.

Abdominal Examination: Measurement of the uterine height provides an estimate of the fetus' gestational age. Fetal presentation must be determined in order to plan for delivery. Resting uterine tone is normal unless there is an associated placental separation. Intermittent uterine contractions suggest that labor may have ensued. Fetal heart tones are usually present unless placental separation or the convulsion has caused fetal anoxia.

Vaginal Examination: The station of the presenting part as well as the status of the cervix is evaluated.

LABORATORY TESTS

Complete Blood Count with Blood Smear: Hematocrit is frequently elevated, indicating hemoconcentration. If the hematocrit is lower than anticipated, the possibility of pre-existing anemia or hemolysis must be considered. Examination of the peripheral blood smear may reveal the target cells, helmet cells, or schistocytes associated with a hemolytic process.

Urinalysis: A Foley catheter should be inserted into the bladder in order to obtain an initial urine specimen and to monitor the urine output. Usually the bladder contains a relatively small amount of dark urine that contains 3+ or 4+ protein.

Blood Type and Rh: Blood should be sent to the blood bank to be crossmatched in the event that cesarean section is necessary and the patient requires blood transfusions.

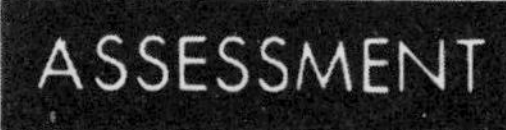

DIFFERENTIAL DIAGNOSIS

See Convulsive Seizures in Pregnancy, p. 268.

PREDISPOSING FACTORS

These include teenaged nulliparity, poor nutrition, a family history of preeclampsia or eclampsia, preexisting hypertensive vascular disease, multiple pregnancy, diabetes mellitus, and hydatidiform mole.

POTENTIAL COMPLICATIONS

These include placental separation (abruptio), cerebral thrombosis or hemorrhage, perinatal mortality (10 to 30 per cent), disseminated intravascular coagulation, microangiopathic hemolytic anemia, renal cortical necrosis, renal tubular necrosis, hepatic failure with periportal necrosis, hepatic rupture, cardiac failure, pulmonary edema, and maternal mortality.

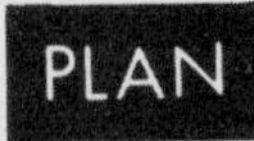

ADDITIONAL DIAGNOSTIC DATA

Blood electrolytes are usually normal unless the patient has previously received diuretics. The plasma bicarbonate may be reduced as a consequence of lactic acidemia.

Blood Chemistry Tests: Blood urea nitrogen (BUN), creatinine, and uric acid tests evaluate renal function. Uric acid may be elevated, whereas BUN and creatinine are within the normal range.

Plasma magnesium levels may be helpful in the evaluation of therapy with magnesium sulfate.

Coagulation Tests: Coagulation abnormalities may be associated with eclampsia. The platelet count may be decreased; fibrinogen may be decreased and fibrin-split products may be elevated.

Platelet counts of less than 150,000 were observed in 29 per cent of cases by Pritchard, Cunningham, and Mason (1976). These authors conclude that these findings reflect platelet adherence at sites of vascular endothelial damage. Others believe that disseminated intravascular coagulation may be a characteristic feature of preeclampsia and eclampsia.

MANAGEMENT AND PATIENT EDUCATION

General Principles:

1. Clear the patient's airway and initiate intravenous fluids.
2. Control convulsions.
3. Prevent hypertensive complications.
4. Monitor the vital signs of patient closely: blood pressure, pulse, respiration, temperature, urinary output, and reflexes.
5. Terminate pregnancy within 6 to 12 hours.

Specific Measures

Clearing of Airway and Initiation of Intravenous Fluids: Adequate ventilation is essential. The airway must be clear. Oxygen is administered by mask or nasal catheter. Any secretions in the airway should be suctioned, and the patient should be positioned to avoid aspiration of vomitus.

Intravenous fluids, usually 5 per cent dextrose in water at a rate of 100 ml per hour, are initiated immediately. The amount of fluid infused is based on the urine output and the estimated insensible fluid loss.

Control of Convulsions:

Magnesium sulfate is the anticonvulsant medication preferred by many obstetricians. Magnesium acts upon both the peripheral and central nervous systems. The curare-like action on the neuromuscular junction and the central depressant effect practically always arrest eclamptic convulsions and prevent recurrence.

The usual initial dose is 4 gm intravenously (either a 20 ml injection of a 20 per cent solution over a period of not less than three minutes or an injection of magnesium sulfate diluted into 100 ml of 5 per cent dextrose infusion and administered over a period of 15 to 30 minutes). This is immediately followed by intramuscular injections or a continuous intravenous infusion.

Intramuscular dosage is 20 ml of 50 per cent magnesium sulfate solution, one half (5 gm, 10 ml) injected deeply in the upper outer quadrant of each buttock through a three-inch long 20-gauge needle. To minimize the discomfort of the intramuscular injection, 1 ml of 1 or 2 per cent lidocaine may be added to the syringe containing the magnesium sulfate.

Every four hours thereafter 10 ml of 50 per cent magnesium sulfate solution (5 gm) is injected intramuscularly into alternate buttocks after it has been ascertained that the patellar reflex is present, urine flow has been 100 ml or more during the previous four hours, and respirations are not depressed (Pritchard, 1975).

For continuous intravenous infusion, 10 gm of magnesium sulfate are added to 1000 ml of 5 per cent dextrose and infused at a rate of 100 ml (1 gm) per hour. The therapeutic effect of magnesium sulfate is estimated clinically by the patellar reflex activity and the dosage titrated by reflexes. Hyperactive reflexes indicate the need for increased medication, whereas absent reflexes indicate that the infusion rate should be slowed or stopped.

The patellar reflex, urine flow, and respiratory rate must be carefully monitored. If respiratory depression develops, 10 ml of 10 per cent calcium gluconate is administered intravenously over three minutes.

Emergency plasma magnesium levels should be obtained if there is any question of magnesium toxicity. The therapeutic range is 3.5 to 7.0 mEq/l. The patellar reflex usually disappears at about 8 mEq/l; respiratory depression is likely to occur when the plasma levels reach 10 to 11 mEq/l.

Since the magnesium ion is eliminated by the kidney, toxic levels of magnesium are most apt to develop when patients are anuric or oliguric.

Amobarbital (Amytal) may be administered if convulsions persist despite therapy with magnesium sulfate or if magnesium sulfate is not immediately available. As many as 250 mg are injected slowly intravenously, over a period of not less than three minutes. Transplacental passage can cause fetal respiratory depression.

Phenobarbital is another alternative anticonvulsant. A dose of 200 to 300 mg may be required intravenously. Transplacental passage can cause fetal respiratory depression.

Diazepam (Valium) is considered an excellent anticonvulsant for status epilepticus. Five to 10 mg should be injected slowly intravenously, at a rate of at least one minute for each 5 mg. Hypotonia has been reported in infants who have been given a high dosage, Diazepam may be preferred for the prevention or treatment of postpartum convulsions.

Protection against Trauma: The patient must be protected against trauma during current and subsequent convulsions. A padded tongue blade should be readily available for insertion between the teeth to prevent injury to the tongue.

Antihypertensive Therapy: Antihypertensive therapy is indicated when the blood pressure is greater than 180 systolic or 110 to 120 diastolic in order to prevent cerebral vascular hemorrhage. Precipitous or marked lowering of the blood pressure may decrease placental perfusion and increase fetal jeopardy.

Hydralazine (Apresoline) is usually preferred, since it is a direct-acting vasodilator, reduces peripheral vascular resistance, and tends to cause a reflex increase in cardiac output and renal blood flow.

The initial dose is 5 mg intravenously; the blood pressure is monitored every five minutes. If the diastolic pressure has not been lowered to 100 mm Hg within 20 minutes, a second dose of 10 mg is injected intravenously. The desired effect is usually achieved with 5 to 20 mg of hydralazine. The medication is repeated whenever the diastolic blood pressure exceeds 110 to 120 mm Hg.

Close Monitoring of Patient's Condition: A special flow sheet may be helpful for following the patient's progress. Blood pressure, pulse, respiration, and reflexes are checked every 15 minutes. Fluid intake and output are recorded hourly. A Foley catheter in the bladder provides a precise measure of urinary output.

Diuretic therapy is rarely beneficial or advisable unless there is evidence of pulmonary edema, which may respond to 20 mg of furosemide intravenously. (See Pulmonary Edema, p. 582.)

Central venous pressure determinations may be helpful in fluid replacement therapy, particularly to minimize the risk of pulmonary edema associated with fluid overloading.

Appropriate fluid therapy is based on electrolyte values and urine output.

The patient should be under constant attendance and observation in order to prevent any trauma from a subsequent convulsion. The quantity of urine produced each hour, the amount of albumin, and the specific gravity reflect the severity of the disease process. Changes in the patient's pulse, blood pressure, and respiration reflect the patient's response to therapy.

Delivery within 6 to 12 Hours: Once the patient has been stabilized and has regained consciousness, preparations for delivery should be initiated. If there are no obstetric contraindications, labor is induced with an intravenous oxytocin infusion. Amniotomy is performed at the same time unless the vertex is high and the cervix closed.

During labor, the fetal heart rate and uterine contractions should be monitored closely. Uterine hyperstimulation must be avoided, since the uterus may be unusually responsive to oxytocin.

As soon as the cervix is fully dilated, the second stage should be shortened with forceps delivery if possible.

Delivery by cesarean section is indicated when

1. Oxytocin induction fails.
2. There is any evidence of fetopelvic disproportion.
3. The fetus is in breech presentation or other abnormal lie.
4. There is any evidence of fetal distress.
5. The patient has had a previous cesarean section.

REFERENCES

McKay DG: Hematologic evidence of disseminated intravascular coagulation in eclampsia. Obstet Gynecol Surv *27*:399-417, 1972

Newcombe DS: The hyperuricemia of preeclampsia and eclampsia. Obstet Gynecol Surv *27*:543-551, 1972

Pritchard JA, Cunningham FG, Mason RA: Coagulation changes in eclampsia: their frequency and pathogenesis. Am J Obstet Gynecol *124*:855-864, 1976

Pritchard JA, Pritchard SA: Standardized treatment of 154 consecutive cases of eclampsia. Am J Obstet Gynecol *123*:543-552, 1975

44 ECTOPIC PREGNANCY

GENERAL CONSIDERATIONS

DEFINITIONS

Ectopic pregnancy—gestation outside the uterine cavity. Ectopic pregnancy is a broader term than extrauterine pregnancy, since it includes gestations in the interstitial portion of the tube, cornual pregnancy (gestation in a rudimentary uterine horn), and cervical pregnancy (gestation in the cervical canal) as well as abdominal pregnancy, ovarian pregnancy, and tubal pregnancy. See Figure 44-1 for sites of implantation.

Abdominal pregnancy—gestation occurring within the peritoneal cavity. (Synonym: intraperitoneal pregnancy.)

Ampullar pregnancy—an ectopic pregnancy in the ampullar portion of the fallopian tube. It generally ends in tubal abortion.

Cervical pregnancy—gestation that develops when the fertilized ovum becomes implanted in the cervical canal of the uterus.

Cornual pregnancy—gestation that has developed in a rudimentary horn of the uterus.

Interstitial pregnancy—pregnancy in the interstitial portion of the fallopian tube.

Intraligamentous pregnancy—growth of the fetus and placenta between the folds of the broad ligament, after rupture of a tubal pregnancy through the floor of the fallopian tube.

Isthmic pregnancy—a gestation in the narrow portion of the fallopian tube.

Ovarian pregnancy—a rare form of ectopic pregnancy in which the blastocyst implants on the surface of the ovary.

Tubal pregnancy—an ectopic pregnancy in any portion of the fallopian tube. It is the commonest type of extrauterine gestation, accounting for 95 per cent of ectopic pregnancies.

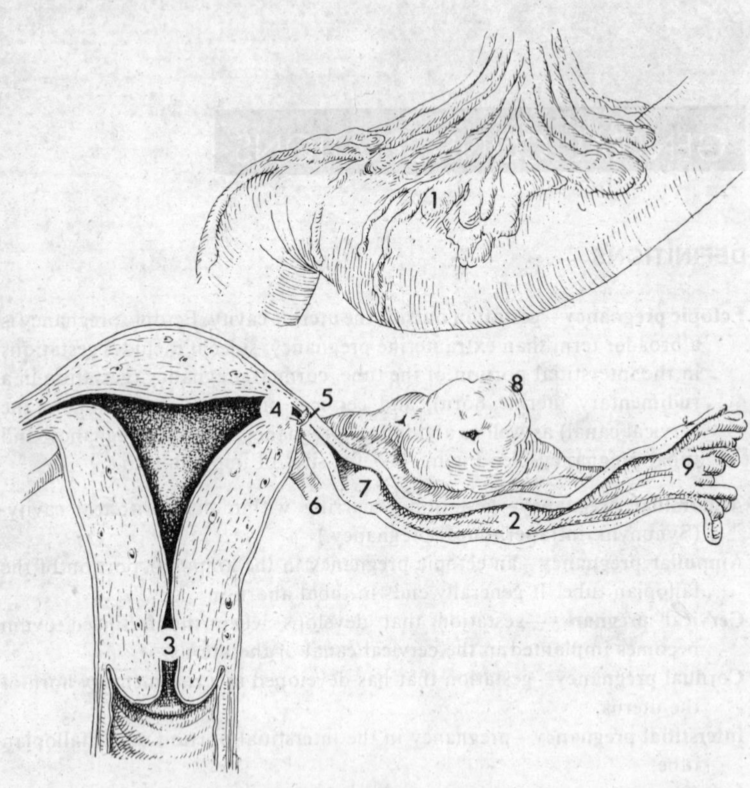

Figure 44-1. Sites of implantation of ectopic pregnancies. *1*, On the peritoneum covering the bowel or elsewhere in the pelvis, creating an abdominal pregnancy; *2*, in the ampulla; *3*, in the cervix; *4*, in the cornual angle of the uterus; *5*, in the interstitial part of the uterine tube; *6*, in the round ligament; *7*, in the isthmic part of the tube; *8*, in the ovary; *9*, in the infundibulum of the tube. (Modified from Huffman JW: Gynecology and Obstetrics: Philadelphia, W.B. Saunders Company, 1962.)

Tubal Pregnancy

GENERAL CONSIDERATIONS

Although the incidence of tubal pregnancy varies widely among different hospital populations, approximately three to ten ectopic pregnancies may be expected per 1000 infant births.

SUBJECTIVE DATA

CURRENT SYMPTOMS

Abdominal pain, particularly unilateral pelvic pain, is the most characteristic symptom of patients with tubal pregnancy. However, pain may also be bilateral in the lower abdomen, in the upper abdomen, or generalized.

Some patients are aware of a unilateral cramplike pain localized to one side of the uterus, which may be due to tubal distention by an enlarging pregnancy. Sudden, sharp, stabbing pain in the lower abdomen is usually caused by acute rupture of the tube with intraabdominal bleeding.

A third variety of pain may be dull, aching pain associated with an organized hematoma around a "chronic ruptured ectopic." Trickling blood, more or less walled off by adhesions, collects in the pelvis, and a *pelvic hematocele* results.

Many patients give a history of one or more episodes of sudden, severe pain over the preceding few days. Between these intermittent painful episodes, the patient may be relatively comfortable and able to attend to normal duties.

Pain due to ectopic pregnancy is usually aggravated by body motion, such as bending over, rising, or riding in an automobile.

Shoulder pain suggests intraperitoneal bleeding with diaphragmatic irritation. This may be expected in 15 to 20 per cent of patients.

Vaginal Bleeding or Spotting: Abnormal vaginal bleeding or spotting is noted by approximately 75 per cent of patients with an ectopic pregnancy. This abnormal bleeding frequently occurs a week or two after a delayed menstrual period. In some instances, however, the spotting may

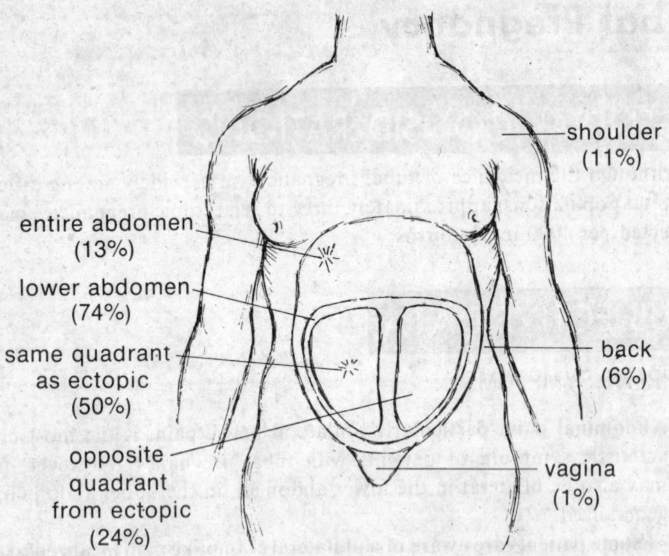

Figure 44-2. Pain in an ectopic pregnancy. (Adapted from Breen JL: A 21 year survey of 654 ectopic pregnancies. Am J Obstet Gynecol *106*:1004-1019, 1970.)

coincide with the time of the expected menses so closely that the patient is not even aware of any menstrual delay. [This is the case in 53 per cent of patients according to Hallatt (1975).]

The nature of the bleeding is not diagnostic, since bleeding of any character may occur—continuous or intermittent spotting, moderate flow for many days, or even recurrent vaginal hemorrhage. Compared with the patient's normal menses, however, the bleeding is abnormal.

Menstrual History: The last normal menstrual period is likely to have occurred six to eight weeks prior to the onset of abdominal pain and vaginal spotting. The triad of missed menses, abdominal pain, and vaginal bleeding should always suggest the possibility of an ectopic pregnancy.

Not all patients, however, are aware of a missed menstrual period; the last period may have occurred at the usual time but may have been shorter or lighter than normal.

Interstitial pregnancies are apt to rupture 8 to 16 weeks after the last menstrual period.

Syncope or orthostatic changes may be associated with acute intraperitoneal bleeding and consequent hypovolemia. Some patients report sudden pain followed by faintness and weakness; others report the occurrence of an episode of fainting a few days previously, which may be explained by formation of a peritubal hematoma around the bleeding site, limiting the intraperitoneal hemorrhage. Repeated episodes of fainting occurring with attempts to assume a seated or standing position are symptomatic of hypovolemia from intraperitoneal hemorrhage.

Other Symptoms: Nausea, vomiting, and breast engorgement are nonspecific symptoms that may be associated with early pregnancy. Rectal pressure or an urge to defecate may be caused by the presence of blood in the cul-de-sac.

PRIOR HISTORY

Once a patient has experienced an ectopic pregnancy she has a 10 to 25 per cent chance of having another. Consequently, some patients report a previous ectopic pregnancy and recognize the similarity of their current symptoms.

Approximately one third to one half of patients with an ectopic pregnancy have a history of prior pelvic infection. This history may not be particularly helpful, however, since ectopic pregnancy must be distinguished from recurrent pelvic infection.

Contraceptive history aids in the assessment of pregnancy probability. In cases of contraceptive failure in women using oral contraceptives or intrauterine devices, the ratio of ectopic to intrauterine pregnancies is higher than in women not using these contraceptive methods. (Both oral contraceptives and intrauterine devices are more effective in preventing intrauterine than ectopic pregnancies.)

OBJECTIVE DATA

PHYSICAL EXAMINATION

General Examination: Overt manifestations of hypovolemic shock (hypotension; tachycardia; pale, cold, clammy skin) are seen in 15 to 20 per cent of patients.

Orthostatic (postural) hypotension and tachycardia may be the earliest signs of hypovolemia resulting from intraperitoneal bleeding.

As long as blood loss is not profuse, vital signs remain normal.

The temperature is usually within a normal range, rarely exceeding 101°F.

Abdominal Examination: Unilateral lower quadrant tenderness is the most characteristic finding. With more extensive intraperitoneal bleeding, tenderness tends to be more diffuse. Signs of peritoneal irritation include rebound tenderness, rigidity, guarding, and possibly, decreased bowel sounds. With chronic intraabdominal bleeding, there may be distention, with a doughy feeling on palpation.

Prior to rupture, the findings of the abdominal examination are often normal.

Pelvic Examination: The most characteristic finding is unilateral pelvic pain and tenderness localized to one adnexal area. The cervix often feels soft; cervical motion almost invariably precipitates or aggravates the adnexal pain.

The uterus may be tender, softened, and of normal size or slightly enlarged. An intrauterine device may be present in the uterus.

A feeling of fullness or an indefinite tender mass in the adnexal area may indicate clotted blood associated with a peritubal hematoma. Frequently, exquisite tenderness and guarding prevent the examiner from detecting an adnexal mass, unless the pelvic examination is performed under anesthesia or after the patient has received systemic analgesia. The adnexal mass associated with a tubal pregnancy is usually ill-defined, whereas an ovarian cyst tends to have a more circumscribed outline.

Frequently an ectopic pregnancy will bleed from the fimbriated end of the tube into the cul-de-sac. Under these circumstances, the organized blood clot in the cul-de-sac is very tender. A soft, indefinite fullness or bulging of the cul-de-sac may be palpable on vaginal or rectovaginal examination.

LABORATORY TESTS

Complete Blood Count and Blood Smear: Hemoglobin and hematocrit values are an indication of prior blood loss. In the case of acute bleeding, the initial hematocrit value does not indicate the extent of blood loss.

In the absence of overt bleeding, however, a decline in hemoglobin or hematocrit from previous determinations suggests occult, intraperitoneal bleeding.

White blood counts are usually within the normal range. (Approximately 75 per cent of patients with ectopic pregnancy have white counts of less than 15,000, and 50 per cent of patients with ectopic pregnancy have white counts of less than 10,000.)

Urinalysis is normal.

Blood Type and Rh: Blood is sent to the blood bank for type, Rh, and crossmatching in order that blood replacement may be administered as indicated.

ASSESSMENT

DIFFERENTIAL DIAGNOSIS (Table 44-1)

TABLE 44-1. Differential Diagnosis of Ectopic Pregnancy

	Ectopic Pregnancy	Pelvic Infection	Uterine Abortion
SUBJECTIVE SYMPTOMS			
Menses	Missed or decreased followed by spotting	Normal or increased	Missed, followed by spotting, followed by brisk bleeding
Pain	Unilateral cramps before rupture	Bilateral	Midline cramps
Syncope	Possible	Rare	Rare
Vaginal Discharge	Brownish, bloody	Purulent	Bloody

TABLE 44-1. Differential Diagnosis of Ectopic Pregnancy (Continued)

	Ectopic Pregnancy	Pelvic Infection	Uterine Abortion
OBJECTIVE FINDINGS			
Abdominal Tenderness	Unilateral	Bilateral	Midline or none
Pelvic Exam	Unilateral tenderness especially on cervical motion; possible unilateral mass	Bilateral tenderness accentuated with cervical motion.	Cervix slightly patulous; uterus enlarged, irregularly softened
White Blood Count	Up to 15,000	15,000 to 30,000	Up to 15,000
Hematocrit	Decreased or dropping	Normal, stable	Normal or decreased, reflecting vaginal bleeding
Temperature	Normal	Elevated	Normal unless infected
Blood Pressure	Normal or decreased	Normal	Normal
Sedimentation Rate	Normal	Elevated	Normal

Threatened Abortion or Incomplete Abortion of an Intrauterine Pregnancy: When the patient's history and physical examination suggest pregnancy, particularly when this is confirmed by a positive pregnancy test for human chorionic gonadotropin (HCG), the possibility of an intrauterine pregnancy threatening to abort or in the process of aborting must be considered.

One possible differentiating feature between intrauterine abortion and extrauterine pregnancy is the time interval between the last menstrual period and the onset of the abdominal pain or vaginal bleeding. In tubal pregnancy, symptoms may occur as early as six to seven weeks after the last menstrual period, whereas in intrauterine abortion symptoms may not become evident until 10 to 12 weeks after the last period.

The uterus containing an intrauterine pregnancy is more likely to be larger and softer than the uterus associated with an extrauterine pregnancy. In cases of threatened abortion the pain tends to be less severe and located in the midline rather than in the adnexal area.

Vaginal bleeding associated with an incomplete abortion is generally more profuse than vaginal bleeding associated with an ectopic pregnancy. Furthermore, in an abortion all bleeding is external and the degree of anemia reflects the external blood loss. In an ectopic pregnancy there may be extensive intraperitoneal bleeding and minimal external blood loss. Whenever the severity of anemia cannot be explained by external blood loss, concealed bleeding, either intraperitoneal or retroperitoneal, must be suspected.

Pelvic Infection: In cases of pelvic infection, pain and tenderness are commonly bilateral. In cases of acute infection, findings of elevated temperature, leukocytosis, and an increased sedimentation rate aid in diagnosis. A palpable tuboovarian abscess is usually much larger than the adnexal fullness associated with an ectopic pregnancy.

Persistent Corpus Luteum with Intraabdominal Hemorrhage: A persistent corpus luteum (Halban's disease) may cause menstrual delay followed by persistent slight bleeding—symptoms identical to those of an ectopic pregnancy. The enlarged ovary is a unilateral mass that may be difficult to distinguish from a tubal gestation. If the corpus luteum bleeds profusely into the peritoneal cavity, differentiation from a ruptured ectopic pregnancy can be made only when the ovary is directly visualized at laparoscopy, colpotomy, or laparotomy.

Ovarian Cyst with Torsion or Adnexal Torsion: The sudden onset of pain, often combined with nausea and vomiting, may resemble the severe pain of tubal rupture.

A definite adnexal mass is usually palpable.

Acute Appendicitis: Ectopic pregnancy in the right tube may be mistaken for appendicitis, although the history of the two conditions is usually dissimilar. In appendicitis the initial pain is characteristically periumbilical, followed by anorexia, nausea or vomiting, and a shifting of the pain into the right lower quadrant. Pain due to ectopic pregnancy is usually pelvic in origin.

In appendicitis, the temperature and white count are more likely to be slightly elevated; the uterus is not tender nor is cervical motion likely to accentuate the pelvic pain; uterine bleeding does not occur unless the patient is menstruating coincidentally.

ETIOLOGICAL FACTORS

Any condition that interferes with tubal structure or function may delay the passage of the fertilized egg into the uterine cavity. Included among these conditions are the following:

1. Chronic salpingitis, which may cause partial obstruction of the tube, either by impairing tubal motility or by creating diverticula that entrap the fertilized ova
2. Surgery of the fallopian tube, including tubal sterilization procedures
3. Congenital abnormalities of the tube, especially diverticula and accessory ostia
4. Transmigration of the ovum from the opposite ovary
5. Intrauterine devices and low-dose progestogen contraception.

Since these contraceptive methods do not necessarily inhibit ovulation, they are effective mainly as intrauterine contraceptives and cannot prevent ectopic gestations.

POTENTIAL COMPLICATIONS

Usual complications of tubal pregnancy are tubal rupture or tubal abortion. Erosive action of the trophoblast may cause sudden disruption of the tubal wall; rupture is most likely to occur when the pregnancy implants in the narrow isthmic portion of the tube. Expulsion of the products of gestation from the ampullary portion of the tube into the peritoneal cavity is called tubal abortion. A local inflammatory reaction and secondary infection may develop in the tissue adjacent to the organized clot.

SEVERITY OF DISEASE PROCESS

The duration and quantity of intraperitoneal bleeding associated with ectopic pregnancy can be variable. Some patients bleed slowly and intermittently, whereas others have sudden, profuse intraperitoneal hemorrhage with hypovolemic shock.

Interstitial pregnancy, accounting for 2 to 3 per cent of all tubal gestations, is the gravest type of ectopic pregnancy. Since the myometrium is more distensible than the tubal wall, patients often remain asymptomatic prior to cornual rupture, which causes profuse intraabdominal hemorrhage and is most likely to occur between the second and fourth gestational months.

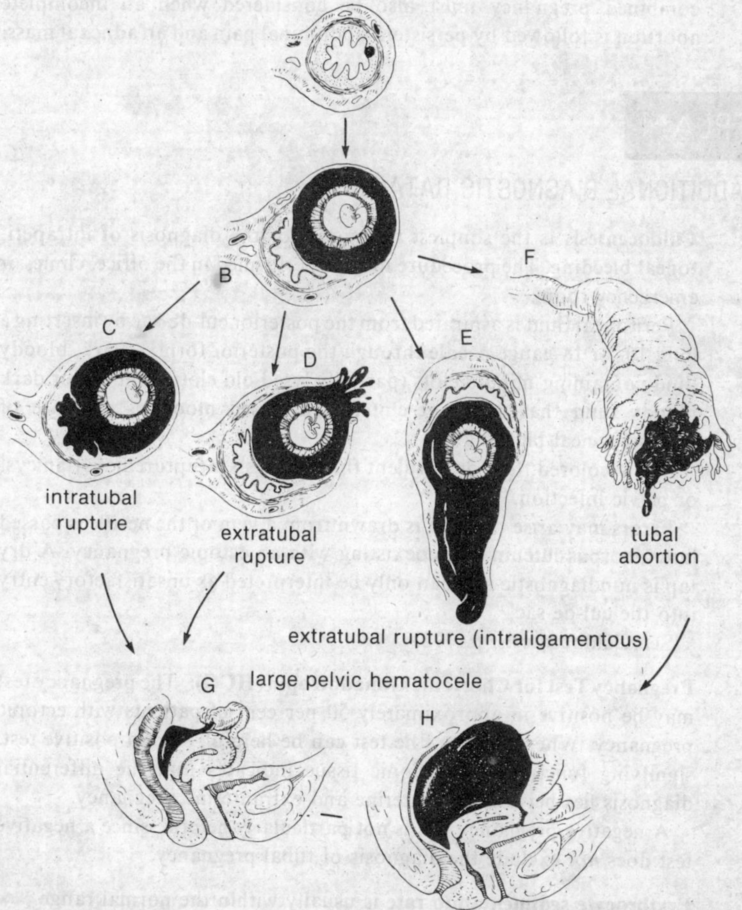

Figure 44-3. Tubal pregnancy, showing development and possible methods of termination. (Modified from Danforth DN [ed.]: Textbook of Obstetrics and Gynecology. New York, Harper and Row, 1966.)

Combined pregnancy, that is, tubal pregnancy complicated by a coexisting intrauterine gestation, is a very rare event. The diagnosis should be considered when the uterus is enlarged, the cervix is closed with minimal bleeding, and there are clinical signs of ectopic pregnancy. A combined pregnancy must also be considered when an incomplete abortion is followed by persistent abdominal pain and an adnexal mass.

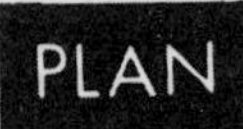

ADDITIONAL DIAGNOSTIC DATA

Culdocentesis is the simplest technique for the diagnosis of intraperitoneal bleeding. The procedure may be performed in the office, clinic, or emergency room.

Peritoneal fluid is aspirated from the posterior cul-de-sac by inserting a long 16- or 18-gauge needle through the posterior fornix. Dark, bloody fluid containing minute clots (partially lysed old clotted blood) or dark bloody fluid that does not clot (totally lysed blood) is evidence of intraperitoneal bleeding.

Straw-colored fluid or purulent fluid suggests a ruptured ovarian cyst or pelvic infection.

Errors may arise if blood is drawn from a vein or the needle is passed into a corpus luteum cyst coexisting with an ectopic pregnancy. A dry tap is nondiagnostic and can only be interpreted as unsatisfactory entry into the cul-de-sac.

See Culdocentesis, p. 772.

Pregnancy Test for Chorionic Gonadotropin (HCG): The pregnancy test may be positive in approximately 50 per cent of patients with ectopic pregnancy. When positive, the test can be helpful, since a positive test, signifying functioning chorionic tissue indicates that the differential diagnosis lies between intrauterine and extrauterine pregnancy.

A negative pregnancy test is not particularly helpful, since a negative test does *not* exclude the diagnosis of tubal pregnancy.

Erythrocyte sedimentation rate is usually within the normal range.

Serial Hematocrit Determinations: At times, the symptoms and findings are so ambiguous that the patient is observed over a period of time. A declining hematocrit on serial determinations may provide the clue to occult blood loss.

Ultrasound B-Scan: When a patient is not bleeding actively and does not wish to have an intrauterine pregnancy disturbed, an ultrasound B-scan can often show whether the gestational sac is normally situated within the uterus.

Demonstration of a normal-appearing intrauterine gestational sac virtually rules out the possibility of ectopic pregnancy and suggests an alternative diagnosis, possibly threatened abortion with a tender or bleeding corpus luteum. (The intrauterine gestational sac can be seen when it reaches a diameter of 1 cm, at five to six weeks of amenorrhea. It appears as an echo-free zone, representing the amniotic fluid, surrounded by a ring of moderately strong echoes from the chorionic villi invading the uterine wall. A few echoes can be seen from the fetus within the gestational sac.)

Failure to demonstrate an intrauterine gestational sac in the presence of clinical and laboratory signs of pregnancy makes the probability of ectopic gestation high.

Abdominal X-rays may reveal free fluid in the peritoneal cavity. X-rays may be particularly helpful when culdocentesis has been unsuccessful and the pregnancy test is negative.

Laparoscopy provides excellent visualization of pelvic structures and is one of the most valuable aids in the evaluation of an adnexal pathologic condition. Ectopic pregnancy, pelvic infection, and ovarian cysts can be clearly differentiated. Not only can a definite diagnosis of tubal pregnancy be made, even prior to rupture, but also the diagnosis can be clearly ruled out and laparotomy obviated.

Endometrial Curettage: When a patient is bleeding actively, endometrial curettage may be indicated. If the uterus contains obvious placental tissue, the likelihood of a coexisting ectopic pregnancy is remote. When the uterus does not contain chorionic villi, however, the possibility of ectopic pregnancy must be considered. In cases of ectopic pregnancy, endometrium may be scanty, particularly if the patient has been bleeding for a number of days. Stromal decidual changes may be observed in only approximately one third of patients with tubal pregnancy, since fetal death and subsequent passage of decidua may have allowed the reestablishment of ovulation and renewed endometrial proliferation.

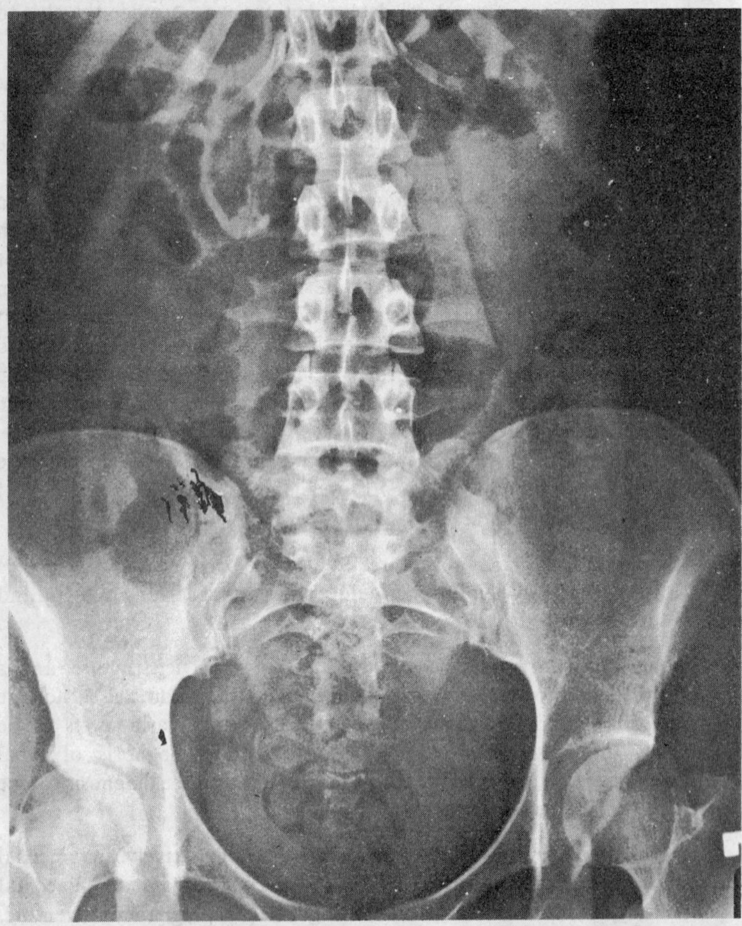

Figure 44-4. History of sudden onset of abdominal pain, most prominent in the left lower quadrant, and two missed periods. The abdomen is diffusely tender and tense with left lower quadrant guarding. On pelvic examination, there is a boggy, ill-defined, tender mass to the left of a normal-sized uterus. Hct 28; WBC 8000; T 98; Pulse 90. The abdominal film shows "dog ears" shadows on either side above the urinary bladder, indicating free fluid in the pelvic recesses. The diagnosis of left ruptured tubal pregnancy was confirmed at surgery. (From Squire LF, Colaiace WM, Strutynsky N: Exercises in Diagnostic Radiology. Vol. 2, The Abdomen. Philadelphia, W.B. Saunders Company, 1971.)

A reaction consisting of endometrial glandular changes associated with the presence of chorionic tissue, whether intra- or extrauterine, has been described by Arias-Stella. Known as the Arias-Stella reaction, these changes are characterized by enlarged endometrial glandular cells with swollen, clear cytoplasm and hyperchromatic, pleomorphic nuclei, which tend to extrude into the gland lumen. These changes may be associated with a stromal decidual change, a hypersecretory glandular pattern, or a proliferative endometrium.

If the decidual cells undergo retrogressive changes, becoming small and spindly, the glands lined by large, clear epithelial cells may be the only evidence of the antecedent pregnancy. Since the Arias-Stella reaction generally develops focally, the incidence of this finding in conjunction with an ectopic or other pregnancy varies in different laboratories from less than 5 per cent to nearly 75 per cent. It has been observed as early as 22 days after the last missed period.

- **Colpotomy or Culdoscopy:** Some clinicians prefer colpotomy or culdoscopy for direct visualization of the tubes and ovaries.

MANAGEMENT

General Principles:

1. Immediate hospitalization
2. Surgery as soon as the diagnosis is established
3. Blood replacement as indicated for hypovolemia or anemia

Specific Measures:

1. Preoperative orders
   a. Intravenous fluids—1000 ml of 5 per cent dextrose in lactated Ringer's solution.
   b. Blood crossmatching—2 to 4 units
   c. Blood transfusion as required for anemia and hypovolemia
   d. Anesthesia evaluation for surgery
   e. Nothing by mouth
   f. No enemas or cathartics
2. Surgery
   a. Salpingectomy
   b. Salpingo-oophorectomy
   c. Salpingotomy (removal of ectopic pregnancy and preservation of the tube)

3. Postoperative orders for day of surgery
   a. Nothing by mouth
   b. Connect Foley catheter for continuous bladder drainage.
   c. Record intake and output.
   d. Correct any blood volume deficit.
   e. Serial hematocrits at four-hour intervals (two times if stable)
   f. Monitor vital signs every 15 minutes until stable for two hours.
   g. Meperidine (Demerol) 50 mg q3h prn for pain
   h. Promethazine (Phenergan) 25 mg q4h prn for nausea
   i. Pentobarbital (Nembutal) 100 mg for sleep
   j. Intravenous fluids—1000 ml of 5 per cent dextrose in lactated Ringer's solution alternating with 1000 ml of 5 per cent dextrose in water every eight hours
   k. Rh immune globulin if patient is Rh-negative and unsensitized

Surgical Decisions: Approaching an ectopic pregnancy, the surgeon is faced with a number of choices: He must decide whether to (1) make a colpotomy or laparotomy incision, (2) resect or preserve the tube, (3) include cornual resection with salpingectomy, and (4) remove or conserve the ovary on the involved side.

Laparotomy is usually preferred for the best evaluation of the pathologic process. With adequate exposure, reparative or ancillary pelvic surgery may be performed if indicated. Removal of an ectopic pregnancy through a colpotomy incision may be feasible at times, particularly when colpotomy has been performed for diagnosis.

Decisions concerning the extent of the surgical procedure must take into consideration the patient's desire for future childbearing balanced against the risk of a repeat ectopic pregnancy. Three situations may be encountered: the ectopic pregnancy may exist in the patient's sole remaining tube, the other tube may be present and apparently normal, or the other tube may be present but apparently diseased.

When the opposite tube appears normal, it is usually best to remove the involved tube. Cornual resection is also advocated by many in order to minimize the risk of recurrent pregnancy in the tubal stump. However, interstitial pregnancy is rare after ipsilateral salpingectomy and has even been reported following cornual resection. Furthermore, cornual resection carries with it the risk of increased surgical blood loss and the possibility of uterine rupture during a subsequent intrauterine pregnancy. If cornual resection is performed, only the outer third of the interstitial portion of the tube is excised. Care should be taken *not* to enter the endometrial cavity.

Removal of the ovary on the affected side may be necessary when it is involved in the pathologic process. It has also been suggested that ipsilateral oophorectomy be performed to improve subsequent fertility and to prevent future ectopic pregnancies that might result from external migration of the ovum (Schenker et al., 1972). Despite these theoretical considerations, a normal ovary is usually *not* removed.

Finally, the surgeon may elect to preserve the involved tube, particularly when it is the patient's only tube and she wishes to bear children. Under these circumstances the risk of a subsequent ectopic pregnancy must be balanced against the possibility of a future intrauterine pregnancy (Stromme, 1973). In the case of an unruptured tubal pregnancy a linear salpingotomy may be performed, the gestational sac shelled out, bleeding points ligated, and the incision closed. Stangel et al. (1976) reported two patients treated with excision and reanastomosis that subsequently successfully established intrauterine gestations.

In the case of a ruptured tubal pregnancy partial salpingectomy with reanastomosis may also be considered. In cases of tubal abortion and nidation in the fimbriated ostium, the abortus may be expressed or "milked out" of the tube and bleeding points ligated (Stromme, 1973).

In a ruptured interstitial pregnancy, hysterectomy is often required. Repair of the uterine defect may be attempted, however, when the patient desires to bear children.

Pregnancy Prognosis: Approximately one half of all women with an ectopic pregnancy fail to conceive subsequently (Schenker et al., 1972). Furthermore, the possibility of a second ectopic pregnancy is approximately 10 to 25 per cent.

PATIENT EDUCATION

Whenever there is any possibility of ectopic pregnancy, the patient should be warned about specific symptoms—*severe abdominal pain, shoulder pain, weakness and faintness*—that necessitate *immediate* medical reevaluation.

Abdominal Pregnancy

GENERAL CONSIDERATIONS

Abdominal pregnancy is gestation occurring within the peritoneal cavity. Almost all cases are secondary to early rupture or abortion of a tubal pregnancy into the peritoneal cavity. The incidence is approximately one in 3000 births.

The incidence of perinatal loss ranges from 75 to 95 per cent, with a high incidence of congenital malformations.

SUBJECTIVE DATA

CURRENT SYMPTOMS

Abdominal Pain: Lower abdominal pain, constant or intermittent, is the most consistent symptom of abdominal pregnancy. The pain results from peritoneal irritation. If the baby is alive, fetal movements may be very painful.

Menstrual History: The duration of amenorrhea usually correlates with the gestational age. Abdominal pregnancies are most apt to become symptomatic between 12 and 40 weeks of gestation (Clark, 1975).

Other Symptoms: Nausea, vomiting, constipation, and diarrhea are variable symptoms.

PRIOR HISTORY

A history of spotting, irregular bleeding, or pain during the early months of pregnancy can be suggestive of a tubal pregnancy that has ruptured into the peritoneal cavity.

OBJECTIVE DATA

General Examination: These findings are frequently normal unless there has been an acute intraabdominal accident.

Abdominal Examination: The abdomen may be more tender than normal. Fetal parts may be palpable extremely close to the abdominal wall. The fetus may lie in an abnormal presentation (oblique, transverse). At times, no specific findings are present (Maas, 1975).

Fetal heart tones are frequently absent. Uterine contractions are not palpable and the uterine souffle is absent.

Pelvic Examination: The cervix is frequently displaced anteriorly and superiorly. Often the cervix feels firmer than would be expected in an intrauterine pregnancy. The uterus may be displaced upward and identified separately from the fetus. Palpation of the fornices may distinguish fetal small parts or the fetal head outside the uterus.

ASSESSMENT

DIFFERENTIAL DIAGNOSIS

Abdominal pregnancy must be distinguished from intrauterine pregnancy.

POTENTIAL COMPLICATIONS

These include intraabdominal hemorrhage from placental separation and intestinal obstruction.

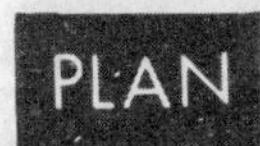

ADDITIONAL DIAGNOSTIC DATA

Ultrasound B-scan may be able to display an empty uterus. Demonstration of the uterine wall surrounding an intrauterine pregnancy rules out the diagnosis of abdominal pregnancy.

Oxytocin Challenge Test: Palpation of a uterine contraction also rules out the diagnosis of abdominal pregnancy.

Abdominal X-ray: Radiologic signs of abdominal pregnancy include the intimate application of the fetus to the maternal abdominal wall without any evidence of uterine soft tissue around the fetus, high fetal position with a bizarre lie, and fetal parts overlapping the maternal vertebral column (Cockshott, 1972). Abdominal x-ray may also confirm a suspected fetal death.

Hysterogram may demonstrate an empty uterine cavity. This procedure is used only if the fetus is known to be dead.

Pelvic angiography can provide information about the state of the placental circulation and evidence of an abdominal pregnancy. In a normal intrauterine pregnancy both uterine vessels are enlarged; after approaching the cervix, they spread laterally around the uterus, giving off large branches to the myometrium, particularly near the placental bed. In an extrauterine pregnancy, the vessels are small, do not ascend, and are closely applied to the lateral walls of the small uterus, giving off small myometrial branches (Cockshott, 1972).

MANAGEMENT

As soon as the diagnosis is suspected, the patient should be hospitalized. Procrastination is dangerous, since placental separation with intraabdominal hemorrhage can occur at any time. The perinatal loss associated with abdominal pregnancies is so great that efforts at fetal salvage are virtually fruitless.

As soon as the diagnosis has been established exploratory laparotomy is indicated. Prior to surgery 4 to 6 units of blood should be available for possible transfusion, since surgery may precipitate violent hemorrhage.

The incision is made to avoid the placenta if possible. The amniotic sac should be opened well away from the edge of the placenta and the fetus carefully removed. The umbilical cord is tied close to the placenta.

Massive hemorrhage from the placental site is the greatest danger. Only *if* the placental blood supply can be clearly identified and effectively ligated is the placenta removed, in order to minimize postoperative complications—infection, abscesses, adhesions, and intestinal obstruction.

In general, it is safest to avoid unnecessary exploration of the surrounding organs and to leave the placenta *in situ*. Unless the placental blood supply can be completely controlled, any attempt to remove the placenta could result in massive uncontrollable hemorrhage.

Postoperative care requires a careful watch for continued intraabdominal bleeding. The Rh-negative unsensitized patient should receive Rh immune globulin.

Cervical Pregnancy

GENERAL CONSIDERATIONS

Cervical pregnancy is a very rare form of ectopic gestation in which the ovum implants within the cervix at or below the internal os. The endocervix is eroded by trophoblast, and the pregnancy invades the fibrous cervical wall.

SUBJECTIVE DATA

Vaginal bleeding, usually painless, is the earliest symptom appearing shortly after nidation.

Fever and chills are rare symptoms that may indicate infection of necrotic placental tissue.

OBJECTIVE DATA

Pelvic Examination: The cervix may be distended and thin-walled, with the external os partially dilated. The uterine fundus may be slightly enlarged.

ASSESSMENT

DIFFERENTIAL DIAGNOSIS

This includes threatened abortion, incomplete abortion, septic abortion, cervical malignancy, and placenta previa.

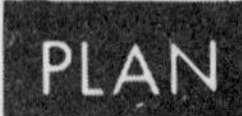

MANAGEMENT

Surgical intervention is necessitated by hemorrhage or signs of septic abortion. Although curettage may be attempted, hysterectomy may be required to control bleeding, since hemorrhage can result from chorionic invasion into the fibromuscular tissue and vasculature of the cervix.

REFERENCES

Arias-Stella J: Atypical endometrial changes associated with the presence of chorionic tissue. Arch Pathol *58*:112-128, 1954

Beral V: Epidemiologic study of recent trends in ectopic pregnancy. Br J Obstet Gynaecol *82*:775-782, 1975

Breen JL: A 21 year survey of 654 ectopic pregnancies. Am J Obstet Gynecol *106*:1004-1019, 1970

Clark JFJ, Jones SA: Advanced ectopic pregnancy. J Reprod Med *14*:30-33, 1975

Cockshott WP, Lawson J: Radiology of advanced abdominal pregnancy. Radiology *103*:21-29, 1972; Obstet Gynecol Surv *27*:667-675, 1972

Franklin EW, Zeiderman AM: Tubal ectopic pregnancy: etiology and obstetric and gynecologic sequelae. Am J Obstet Gynecol *117*:220-225, 1973

Gabbe SG, Kitzmiller JL, Kosasa TS, et al: Cervical pregnancy presenting as septic abortion. Am J Obstet Gynecol *123*:212-213, 1975

Hallatt JG: Repeat ectopic pregnancy: a study of 123 consecutive cases. Am J Obstet Gynecol *122*:520-523, 1975

Hallatt JG: Ectopic pregnancy associated with the intrauterine device: a study of seventy cases. Am J Obstet Gynecol *125*:754-758, 1976

Kalchman GG, Meltzer RM: Interstitial pregnancy following homolateral salpingectomy. Am J Obstet Gynecol *96*:1139-1143, 1966

Katz J, Marcus RG: The risk of Rh isoimmunization in ruptured tubal pregnancy. Br Med J *3*:667-669, 1972

Kosasa TS, Taymor ML, Goldstein DP, Levesque LA: Use of radioimmunoassay specific for human chorionic gonadotropin in diagnosis of early ectopic pregnancy. Obstet Gynecol *42*:868-871, 1973

Maas DA, Slabber CF: Diagnosis and treatment of advanced extrauterine pregnancy. S Afr Med J *49*:2007, 1975; Obstet Gynecol Surv *31*:541-543, 1976

Paterson WG, Grant KA: Advanced intraligamentous pregnancy. Obstet Gynecol Surv *30*:715-726, 1975

Schenker JG, Eyal F, Polishuk WZ: Fertility after tubal pregnancy. Surg Gynecol Obstet *135*:74-76, 1972; Obstet Gynecol Surv *28*:105-107, 1973

Schoen JA, Nowak RJ: Repeat ectopic pregnancy. Obstet Gynecol *45*:542-546, 1975

Stangel JJ, Reyniak JV, Stone ML: Conservative surgical management of tubal pregnancy. Obstet Gynecol *48*:241-244, 1976

Stromme WB: Conservative surgery for ectopic pregnancy. A 20 year review. Obstet Gynecol *41*:215-223, 1973

45 ENDOMETRIOSIS

GENERAL CONSIDERATIONS

Endometriosis—a relatively common problem during the reproductive years—is characterized by the presence and proliferation of endometrial tissue in various sites outside the endometrial cavity. Although the ovaries, uterosacral ligaments, rectovaginal septum, and pelvic peritoneum are more frequently involved, endometriosis may also affect the intestinal tract (rectosigmoid colon) and the urinary tract.

The ectopic endometrium, composed of the same epithelial and stromal elements as normal endometrium, responds to estrogen and progesterone stimulation with cyclic changes—periodic proliferation, necrosis, and menstrual-type bleeding. Destructive by local extension, ectopic endometrial tissue can distort, kink, obstruct, and even devitalize adjacent organs. Fibrotic reactions incident to the recurrent cyclic bleeding may cause adhesions and scar tissue formation.

No single theory explains the histogenesis of all cases of endometriosis. Possible etiologic factors include retrograde menstruation, direct invasion, traumatic seeding, mesothelial metaplasia, lymphatic spread, hematogenous spread, or a combination of influences.

Although most frequently encountered during the later reproductive years, endometriosis can be responsible for acute symptoms in teenaged patients.

Endometrioma is a cystic lesion, usually found in the ovary, lined by functioning endometrium, and filled with material that looks like chocolate syrup but is composed of blood and blood pigment (chocolate cyst of the ovary). In addition to symptoms of endometriosis, an endometrioma may produce symptoms and findings similar to those of other ovarian cysts and tumors.

SUBJECTIVE DATA

Abdominal (Pelvic) Pain: Dysmenorrhea and dyspareunia are the most characteristic symptoms. Dysmenorrhea beginning in the late twenties or early thirties tends to increase in severity. Pelvic discomfort, particularly pelvic or sacral pain, is frequently chronic in nature, periodic, recurring, and aggravated by menstruation. Pelvic pain and dysmenorrhea may be related to the hemorrhagic distention of an endometrial cyst or to the escape of bloody fluid into the peritoneal cavity.

Sudden, severe pelvic pain can be caused by peritoneal irritation resulting from a ruptured endometrioma or hemoperitoneum. Nausea, vomiting, and shoulder pain may be associated symptoms.

Menstrual symptoms may include premenstrual staining, hypermenorrhea, or irregular bleeding, in addition to dysmenorrhea.

Pregnancy history often reveals involuntary infertility.

Other Symptoms: Pain with defecation during menstruation may be caused by lesions involving the rectovaginal septum. Constipation, diarrhea, and rectal bleeding exacerbated by menstruation may indicate intestinal endometriosis.

Dysuria, frequency, urgency, hematuria, and suprapubic pain, exaggerated by menstruation, are suggestive of vesical endometriosis. Flank pain or renal colic exacerbated by menstruation may signify ureteral endometriosis.

OBJECTIVE DATA

PHYSICAL EXAMINATION

General Examination: Although temperature, pulse, and blood pressure are usually normal, hypotension, and tachycardia may signify intra-abdominal bleeding from a ruptured endometrioma.

Abdominal Examination: These findings are also normal unless an acute accident has occurred. Generalized abdominal tenderness with guarding and rebound tenderness suggests intraperitoneal rupture. Abdominal distention may suggest intestinal endometriosis or adhesions that are causing bowel obstruction. Tenderness in the costovertebral angle can be an indication of ureteral obstruction.

Pelvic examination tends to be variable. Frequently the uterus is fixed in retroversion and very sensitive to motion owing to pelvic adhesions. Ovaries containing endometriomas are enlarged (up to 12 cm), painful, rarely moveable, and often closely adherent to the uterus. Tender, blue-domed nodules may be visualized or palpated in the posterior vaginal fornix.

Beading, nodularity, tenderness, and induration along the uterosacral ligaments or in the rectovaginal septum are characteristic findings of endometriosis. These may be evaluated best with rectovaginal examination.

LABORATORY TESTS

Complete blood count and blood smear are usually normal unless there is intraperitoneal bleeding.

Urinalysis may disclose hematuria at the time of menses in cases of urinary tract endometriosis.

ASSESSMENT

DIFFERENTIAL DIAGNOSIS

This includes primary dysmenorrhea, pelvic inflammatory disease, pelvic adhesions, ovarian cysts and neoplasms, gastrointestinal lesions, and urinary tract disorders.

The differential diagnosis of a ruptured endometrioma includes other acute abdominal emergencies such as appendicitis, ectopic pregnancy, and rupture or torsion of other types of ovarian cysts or neoplasms.

In primary dysmenorrhea, the pain generally begins immediately before the flow, reaches a crescendo in the first few hours after its onset, and is generally gone within a day or two. In endometriosis, pelvic pain often starts a few days before the onset of flow, increases more gradually in intensity, and tends to persist throughout the menstrual period or even for several days beyond the menses. In primary dysmenorrhea, the pain may be more cramping in nature and localized in the midline. In endometriosis, the pain is often of a dull, persistent character, possibly radiating to the back and rectum, worsened on defecation, or even localized outside of the uterine area.

PREDISPOSING FACTORS

Associated factors predisposing to the development of teenage endometriosis include congenital obstructive uterine anomalies favoring the retrograde flow of menstrual fluid (Schifrin, 1973).

Whether retroversion of the uterus plays any role in the production of endometriosis, contributes to preexisting lesions by facilitating retrograde flow, or is merely secondary to pelvic adhesions remains uncertain.

POTENTIAL COMPLICATIONS

These include infertility, intraperitoneal rupture of an endometrioma, and intestinal and ureteral obstruction.

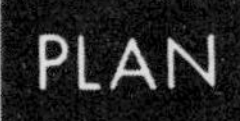

ADDITIONAL DIAGNOSTIC DATA

X-ray of the abdomen with barium enema or excretory urogram or both may show a pelvic mass, displaced or enlarged organs, adhesions, or fibrosis.

Lesions of the colon include polypoid filling defects, long, funnel-shaped lesions simulating an inflammatory process, and a long, scalloped intramural lesion in the antimesenteric margin of the colon (Fagan, 1974).

Findings on excretory urograms may include extrinsic or intrinsic ureteral obstruction, an extrinsic pelvic mass, or a small intramural vesical defect (Fagan, 1974).

Culdocentesis may disclose intraabdominal bleeding associated with spontaneous rupture of an endometrial cyst.

Laparoscopy with visualization and biopsy of typical lesions confirms the diagnosis of endometriosis.

MANAGEMENT

Hospitalization is advised whenever intraperitoneal bleeding is suspected. Observation over a period of 6 to 24 hours may clarify the diagnosis of a self-limited process. If symptoms persist or worsen and an adnexal mass cannot be palpated, laparoscopy may be helpful, permitting direct visualization of the tubes and ovaries.

Laparotomy is indicated for

1. Ruptured endometrioma
2. Active intraperitoneal bleeding
3. Intestinal or ureteral obstruction
4. Ovarian cysts 6 to 8 cm in diameter or larger
5. Progressively increasing lesions
6. Women who desire improvement of fertility in the childbearing years
7. Severe intractable pain

Conservative surgical procedures (excision or cauterization of endometriotic lesions, uterine suspension, or presacral neurectomy) may be recommended for patients interested in future fertility. The extent of surgery depends on the extent and location of the lesions, as well as the surgeon's judgment concerning the safety of surgical removal. When future fertility is desired all functional tissue is preserved.

Oophorectomy becomes necessary when the ovary is completely destroyed by an endometrioma. However, even fairly large endometrial cysts may be resected from one or both ovaries and normal, adequately functioning ovarian tissue conserved.

Hysterectomy with or without oophorectomy can be curative, but is recommended only for those patients with extensive or recurrent endometriosis who have no desire for future childbearing.

Hormonal therapy is recommended for patients who desire subsequent pregnancy when symptoms are not relieved by reassurance and mild analgesia and when surgery is either contraindicated or not acceptable to the patient. Hormonal therapy may also benefit the patient with recurrent symptoms following conservative surgery.

Norethindrone (10 mg) with mestranol (0.060 mg) suppresses ovulation and endogenous ovarian hormonal stimuli to the endometrium. In addition, these hormones produce a decidual reaction in the endometrial stroma and atrophy of endometrial glands. One tablet is prescribed daily as long as amenorrhea persists. If bleeding occurs, the daily dose is increased to 20 mg and eventually to 30 mg. Therapy is continued for three to nine months, as long as symptoms are improved.

Danazol, a synthetic steroid with antigonadotropic properties, may provide symptomatic relief and possibly enhance the fertility potential of previously infertile patients. Administered orally, 400 mg twice daily, Danazol is continued for three to six months without interruption. Since the endometrium tends to become static and atrophic without proliferative activity, cyclic alterations, withdrawal bleeding, and the repeated insults of intraperitoneal bleeding are prevented.

PATIENT EDUCATION

Endometriosis is a complex disease with protean manifestations, the most common being pelvic pain and infertility. Appropriate management will depend on the age of the patient, her desire for children, and the extent of the pathologic condition. The pros and cons of observation, surgery, and hormonal therapy must be carefully analyzed in order to prepare a management plan best suited for the individual patient.

REFERENCES

Andrews WC, Larsen GD: Endometriosis: treatment with hormonal pseudopregnancy and/or operation. Am J Obstet Gynecol *118*:643-651, 1974

Bullock JL, Massey FM, Gambrell RD: Symptomatic endometriosis in teen-agers. Obstet Gynecol *43*:896-900, 1974

Fagan CJ: Endometriosis—clinical and roentgenographic manifestations. Radiol Clin North Am *12*:109-125, 1974

Greenblatt RB, Borenstein R, Hernandez-Ayup S: Experiences with Danazol (an antigonadotropin) in the treatment of infertility. Am J Obstet Gynecol *118*:783-787, 1974

Ranney B: Endometriosis. II. Emergency operations due to hemoperitoneum. Obstet Gynecol *36*:437-441, 1970

Schifrin BS, Erez S, Moore JG: Teen-age endometriosis. Am J Obstet Gynecol *116*:973-980, 1973

46 FACE PRESENTATION

GENERAL CONSIDERATIONS

Face presentation is a longitudinal presentation of the fetus in which the head becomes extended so that the face becomes the presenting part.

The mentum (chin) is the designated point on the face used to determine the position of the fetus in the maternal pelvis.

The incidence of face presentation is approximately 1 in 500 deliveries.

DEFINITIONS OF POSITIONS (Fig. 46-1)

Mentum right anterior (MRA)—a position of the fetus in which the chin is located in the right anterior quadrant of the maternal pelvis.

Mentum right posterior (MRP)—a position of the fetus in which the chin is located in the right posterior quadrant of the maternal pelvis.

Mentum Left Anterior (MLA)—a position of the fetus in which the chin is located in the left anterior quadrant of the maternal pelvis.

Mentum left posterior (MLP)—a position of the fetus in which the chin is located in the left posterior quadrant of the maternal pelvis.

Mentum right transverse (MRT)—a position of the fetus in which the chin is located in the transverse position midway between the right anterior and posterior quadrants.

Mentum left transverse (MLT)—a position of the fetus in which the chin is located in the transverse position midway between the left anterior and posterior quadrants.

OBJECTIVE DATA

Abdominal Examination: The fetal back is extended, with the cephalic prominence on the same side as the back.

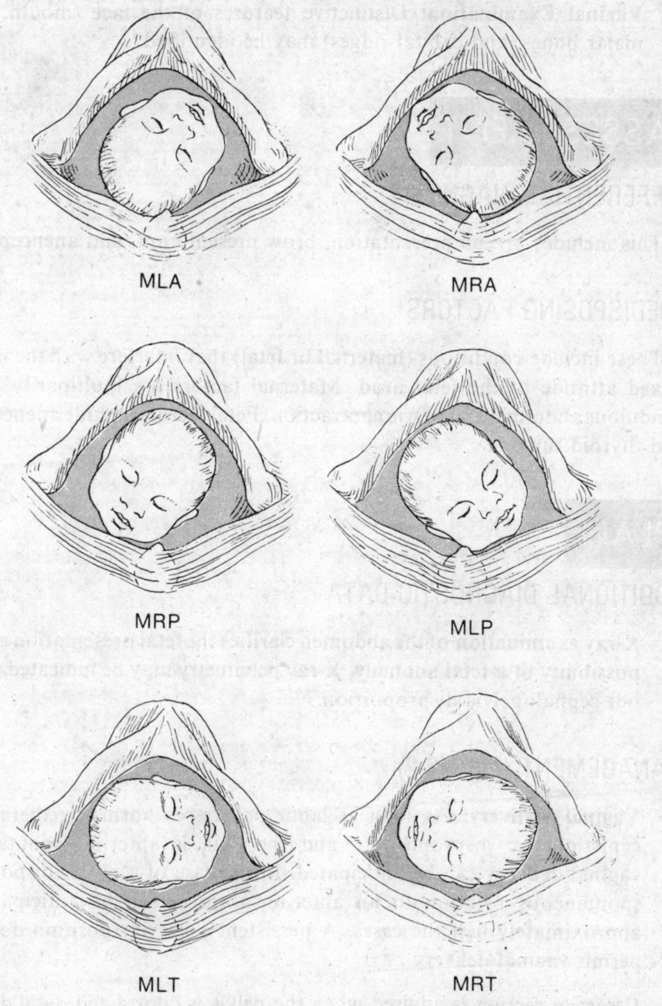

Figure 46-1. Face presentations. The chin, or mentum, is the designated point for determining the position of the fetus. See the text for definitions of positions. (Modified from Huffman JW: Gynecology and Obstetrics. Philadelphia, W.B. Saunders Company, 1962.)

Vaginal Examination: Distinctive features of the face (mouth, nose, malar bones, and orbital ridges) may be identified.

ASSESSMENT

DIFFERENTIAL DIAGNOSIS

This includes breech presentation, brow presentation, and anencephalus.

PREDISPOSING FACTORS

These include conditions (maternal or fetal) that interfere with the normal flexed attitude of the fetal head. Maternal factors are multiparity with a pendulous abdomen and pelvic contraction. Fetal factors include anencephaly and thyroid tumors.

PLAN

ADDITIONAL DIAGNOSTIC DATA

X-ray examination of the abdomen clarifies the fetal presentation and the possibility of a fetal anomaly. X-ray pelvimetry may be indicated to rule out cephalopelvic disproportion.

MANAGEMENT (Fig. 46-2)

Vaginal Delivery: As long as labor progresses normally, there is no cephalopelvic disproportion, and the chin is anterior, spontaneous vaginal delivery can be anticipated. In the case of a posterior position, spontaneous rotation to an anterior position can be anticipated in approximately half the cases. A persistent posterior position does not permit vaginal delivery.

Cesarean section is advised when the pelvis is contracted, fetal distress develops, or the chin persists in a posterior position.

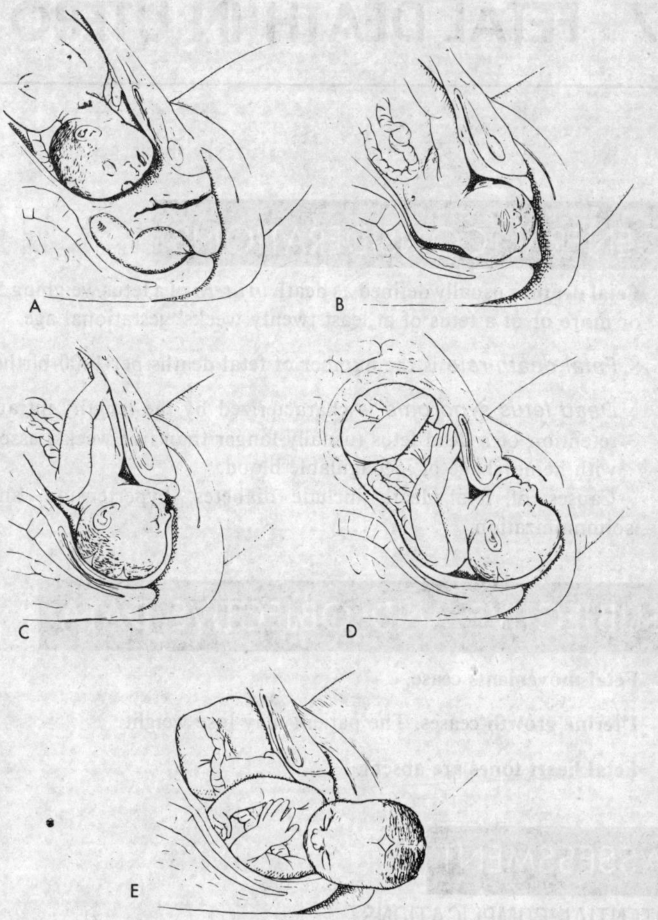

Figure 46-2. The mechanism of labor in face presentations. *A*, The head engages, the chin descends ahead of the back part of the head, and the deflection increases progressively. *B*, Continuation of descent and deflection; the face is in a transverse position. *C*, Internal rotation proceeds; the chin turns to an anterior position. *D*, The chin passes under the symphysis, and the face is delivered by flexion. *E*, External rotation follows the delivery of the head. (Modified from Huffman JW: Gynecology and Obstetrics. Philadelphia, W.B. Saunders Company, 1962.)

47 FETAL DEATH IN UTERO

GENERAL CONSIDERATIONS

Fetal death is usually defined as death *in utero* of a fetus weighing 500 gm or more or of a fetus of at least twenty weeks' gestational age.

Fetal death rate is the number of fetal deaths per 1000 births.

Dead fetus syndrome is characterized by the lengthy intrauterine retention of a dead fetus (usually longer than five weeks) associated with hemorrhage of incoagulable blood.

Causes of fetal death include diabetes, hypertension, and Rh isoimmunization.

SUBJECTIVE AND OBJECTIVE DATA

Fetal movements cease.

Uterine growth ceases. The patient may lose weight.

Fetal heart tones are absent.

ASSESSMENT

POTENTIAL COMPLICATIONS

These include disseminated intravascular coagulation, sepsis, postpartum hemorrhage, and amniotic fluid embolism.

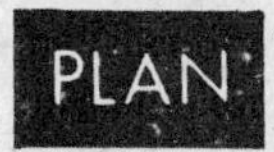

ADDITIONAL DIAGNOSTIC DATA

Ultrasound B-scan may reveal collapse of the fetal skull. With a real-time scanner, no fetal heart motion is discernible.

Abdominal x-ray findings include overlapping of fetal skull bones (Spalding's sign) caused by liquefaction of the brain, exaggerated curvature of the fetal spine, abnormal fetal position, and fetal gas.

Amniocentesis: Amniotic fluid is red, brown, or turbid. Methemoglobin may be identified. The fluid should be sent to the bacteriology laboratory for Gram stain and culture in order to detect intrauterine infection.

Coagulation tests—fibrinogen, platelet count, prothrombin time, and partial thromboplastin time—may identify or rule out a coagulation disorder.

MANAGEMENT AND PATIENT EDUCATION

Labor is induced as long as the fibrinogen level is above 150 mg/100 ml in order to avoid potential coagulation defects, sepsis, and the depressing psychologic problems that can be associated with the knowledge that the intrauterine fetus is dead.

When the uterus is larger than 16 weeks' size, laminaria may be inserted into the cervix to facilitate cervical dilatation. Prostaglandin F_2 alpha (40 mg) is injected into the amniotic cavity, followed in six hours by intravenous oxytocin (50 units diluted into 1000 ml of lactated Ringer's solution). Prostaglandin vaginal suppositories (Prostin E2) provide an alternative method of management. Antibiotics are initiated if there is any evidence of infection. Emotional support is extremely important.

(If the fibrinogen level is less than 150 mg/100 ml and there is no vaginal bleeding, 5000 units of heparin administered intravenously every four hours blocks further pathologic consumption of fibrinogen and other clotting factors, allowing the coagulation mechanism to repair itself. Serial fibrinogen values are obtained and pregnancy is terminated as soon as the fibrinogen level is above 200 mg/100 ml.)

REFERENCES

Courtney LD, Boxall RR, Child P: Permeability of membranes of dead fetus. Br Med J *1*:492-493, 1971; Obstet Gynecol Surv *26*:750-751, 1971

Pritchard JA: Haematological problems associated with delivery, placental abruption, retained dead fetus and amniotic fluid embolism. Clin Haematol *2*:563-586, 1973

Ursell W: Induction of labour following fetal death. J Obstet Gynaeol Br Commonw *79*:260-264, 1972; Obstet Gynecol Surv *27*:722-724, 1972

48 FETAL DISTRESS PRIOR TO LABOR

GENERAL CONSIDERATIONS

Fetal distress refers to a state of relative jeopardy to the fetus that may seriously threaten fetal health. *Chronic* distress may occur over a prolonged period of time during the antenatal period when the ideal, normal, physiologic state of the maternal-fetal-placental unit is disturbed. *Acute* fetal distress is caused by a sudden catastrophic event that interferes with fetal oxygenation.

SUBJECTIVE AND OBJECTIVE DATA

Fetal movements may be decreased. The patient may fail to gain weight, and the uterus may fail to increase in size. A uterus smaller than expected for the gestational age is suggestive of intrauterine growth retardation or oligohydramnios.

A history of one or more high-risk factors, obstetric problems, premature labors, or stillbirths may suggest an increased risk of fetal distress.

ASSESSMENT

PREDISPOSING FACTORS

High-risk factors include hypertensive disorders, diabetes mellitus, heart disease, postmaturity, maternal malnutrition, anemia, Rh isoimmunization, and renal disease.

FETAL MOVEMENTS

	Mon.	Tues.	Wed.	Thurs.	Fri.	Sat.	Sun.
Date: ______							
Morning							
Afternoon							
Evening							
Night							
Date: ______							
Morning							
Afternoon							
Evening							
Night							
Date:							
Morning							
Afternoon							
Evening							
Night							

0 = no fetal movements
1 = minimal fetal movements
2 = average fetal movements
3 = more-than-average fetal movements
4 = excessive fetal movements

Figure 48-1.

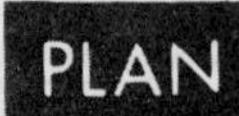

ADDITIONAL DIAGNOSTIC DATA

Fetal heart rate monitoring rules out fetal distress as long as (1) the baseline rate is within the normal range; (2) beat-to-beat variability is normal, (3) accelerations occur with fetal movement, and (4) there are no late decelerations with uterine contractions.

Fetal Movement Chart: Normal fetal movements are generally a sign of fetal well-being. Consequently, a daily record of fetal movements may be helpful in the evaluation of high-risk pregnancies (see Fig. 48-1).

Ultrasound B-Scan: Serial measurements of the biparietal diameter may disclose early evidence of intrauterine growth retardation. The B-scan may also reveal fetal anomalies or multiple pregnancy.

Estriol levels in maternal blood or urine provide a measure of fetal and placental function, since estriol formation requires the activity of enzymes in the fetal adrenal glands and liver as well as in the placenta. As pregnancy advances, estriol values rise. Normal estriol values are an indicator of a normally functioning fetoplacental unit and are reassuring evidence of fetal well-being.

Abnormally low estriol values or a decline of 50 per cent or more from previously normal values suggests placental insufficiency and a failing fetoplacental unit. Other causes for low estriol values are fetal adrenal hypoplasia (anencephaly) and placental sulfatase deficiency. Patients receiving ampicillin therapy may have abnormally low estriol values. This appears to be due to the loss through the feces of steroids secondary to inhibition of hydrolysis of biliary estriol conjugates in the intestinal tract.

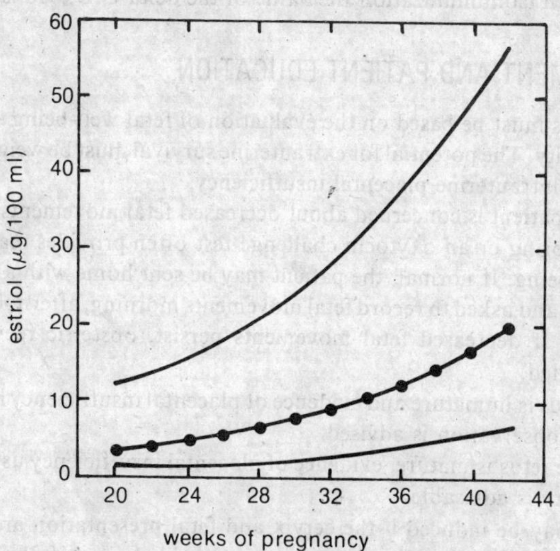

Figure 48-2. Estriol levels in pregnancy. The black dotted line represents average normal values. The upper and lower lines designate the range of values for various weeks of pregnancy.

Human Placental Lactogen (HPL) in Maternal Blood: Values of 4 mcg/ml or less after 30 weeks' gestation suggest abnormal placental function and fetal danger. This test appears to be of value primarily in the assessment of pregnancies complicated by hypertensive vascular disease.

Abdominal x-ray may disclose fetal anomalies.

Oxytocin challenge test (oxytocin stress test) provides an assessment of placental function, detecting uteroplacental insufficiency by the response of the fetal heart rate to spontaneous or induced contractions (see Oxytocin Challenge Test, p. 820).

Amniocentesis: The significance of meconium is uncertain and controversial. Many believe that meconium in the amniotic fluid indicates a pathologic or physiologic stress to the fetus, whereas others believe that intrauterine passage of meconium denotes only temporary vagal stimulation without inevitable jeopardy.

A determination of the lecithin:sphingomyelin (L/S) ratio and creatinine values provide an estimate of fetal maturity.

In Rh isoimmunization the value of the delta O.D. 450 is important.

MANAGEMENT AND PATIENT EDUCATION

Decisions must be based on the evaluation of fetal well-being *in utero* and fetal maturity. The potential for extrauterine survival must be weighed against the risk of intrauterine placental insufficiency.

When a patient is concerned about decreased fetal movements, fetal heart rate monitoring or an oxytocin challenge test often provides reassurance of fetal well-being. If normal, the patient may be sent home with a fetal movement chart and asked to record fetal movements morning, afternoon, evening, and night. If decreased fetal movements persist, obstetric reevaluation is recommended.

If the fetus is immature and evidence of placental insufficiency is equivocal, additional observation is advised.

Once the fetus is mature, evidence of placental insufficiency usually means that delivery is advisable.

Labor may be induced if the cervix and fetal presentation are favorable. During induction the fetal heart rate should be carefully monitored; determination of scalp pH may be indicated. Cesarean section is performed if fetal distress develops. Cesarean section is also preferred for the delivery of a breech presentation, or if the patient has had prior uterine surgery.

The combination of persistently low or falling estriol values and a positive oxytocin challenge test signifies a failing fetoplacental unit. Delivery is usually indicated even if the L/S ratio is not mature, since the intrauterine environment appears to offer greater risk than intensive neonatal care in a high-risk premature nursery. Cesarean section may be necessary, since conditions for induced labor are rarely favorable.

REFERENCES

Adlercreutz H, Martin F, Tikkanen MJ, Pulkkinen M: Effect of ampicillin administration on the excretion of twelve Oestrogens in pregnancy urine. Acta Endocrinol *80*:551, 1975; Obstet Gynecol Surv *31*:530-531, 1976

Aickin DR, Smith MA, Brown JB: Comparison between plasma and urinary Oestrogen measurements in predicting fetal risk. Aust NZ J Obstet Gynaecol *14*:59-76, 1974

Beischer NA, Brown JB: Current status of estrogen assays in obstetrics and gynecology. Part 2: Estrogen assays in late pregnancy. Obstet Gynecol Surv *27*:303-343, 1972

Fairbrother PF, van Coeverden de Groot HA, Coetzee EJ, Shardlow JP: The significance of prelabour type II deceleration of fetal heart rate in relation to Braxton Hicks-contractions. Report on four patients. S Afr Med J *48*:2391-2393, 1974; Obstet Gynecol Surv *30*:598-600, 1975

Fliegner JRH, Schindler I, Brown JB: Low urinary oestriol excretion during pregnancy associated with placental sulphatase deficiency or congenital adrenal hypoplasia. J Obstet Gynaecol Br Commw *79*:810-815, 1972

Hobel CJ, Hyvarinen MA, Okada DM, Oh W: Prenatal and intrapartum high-risk screening I. Prediction of the high-risk neonate. Am J Obstet Gynecol *117*:1-9, 1973

Perkins RP: Antenatal assessment of fetal maturity. Obstet Gynecol Surv *29*:369-384, 1974

Sadovsky E, Yaffe H: Daily fetal movement recording and fetal prognosis. Obstet Gynecol *41*:845-850, 1973

Spellacy WN: Peptide hormones in assessing fetal status. Clin Perinatol *1*:65-72, 1974

Spellacy WN, Buhi WC, Birk SA: The effectiveness of human placental lactogen measurements as an adjunct in decreasing perinatal deaths. Am J Obstet Gynecol *121*:835-844, 1975

Tabei T, Heinrichs WL: Diagnosis of placental sulfatase deficiency. Am J Obstet Gynecol *124*:409-414, 1976

49 FETAL DISTRESS DURING LABOR

GENERAL CONSIDERATIONS

Fetal distress during labor implies fetal hypoxia. Without adequate oxygen, the fetal heart rate loses normal baseline variability and shows late decelerations with uterine contractions. When hypoxia persists, anaerobic glycolysis produces lactic acid with a resultant fall in fetal pH.

SUBJECTIVE AND OBJECTIVE DATA

Decreased or excessive *fetal movements* may portend fetal distress. Usually, however, there are *no* subjective symptoms. Often the first indicator of fetal distress is an alteration in the fetal heart rate pattern (bradycardia, tachycardia, absent variability, or late decelerations).

Maternal hypotension, elevated temperature, or hypertonic uterine contractions or all three may contribute to fetal asphyxia.

ASSESSMENT

ETIOLOGIC FACTORS

1. Acute uteroplacental insufficiency
   a. Excessive uterine activity—uterine hypertonus—may be associated with oxytocin administration.
   b. Maternal hypotension—epidural anesthesia, vena caval compression, supine position, maternal hemorrhage
   c. Placental separation—abruptio
   d. Placenta previa with hemorrhage

2. Chronic uteroplacental insufficiency
   a. Hypertensive disease
   b. Diabetes mellitus
   c. Rh isoimmunization
   d. Postmaturity or dysmaturity
3. Umbilical cord compression
4. Paracervical block anesthesia

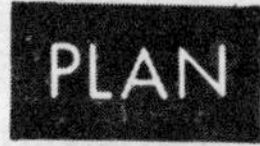

ADDITIONAL DIAGNOSTIC DATA

Fetal Heart Rate Monitoring: Continuous, instantaneous recording of the fetal heart rate provides the most readily available method for the evaluation of fetal well-being (see Fetal Heart Rate Monitoring, p. 786).

Periodic accelerations with fetal movements are reassuring evidence of normal fetal reactivity.

Indications of possible fetal distress are

1. Bradycardia—fetal heart rate less than 120 beats per minute
2. Tachycardia. Prolonged accelerations of the fetal heart rate (>160) may be associated with maternal fever secondary to intrauterine infection. Prematurity and atropine are also associated with an increased baseline heart rate.
3. Decreased baseline variability, which can signify depression of the fetal autonomic nervous system by hypoxia or maternal medications (atropine, scopolamine, diazepam, phenobarbital, magnesium, and narcotic analgesics).
4. Deceleration patterns. *Late* decelerations signify fetal hypoxia due to uteroplacental insufficiency. *Variable* decelerations unrelated to uterine contractions are much more common and appear to represent transient compression of umbilical vessels. As long as the duration of bradycardia is brief and the baseline is normal with good beat-to-beat variability, fetal acidosis is unlikely and the fetal pH remains within the normal range. The significance of deceleration patterns depends on the type, the degree of deceleration, and the duration of the pattern.

Fetal blood sampling provides objective information regarding the fetal acid-base status. Electronic fetal monitoring can be so sensitive to changes in the fetal heart rate that fetal distress may be suspected even when the fetus is healthy and merely reacting to the stress of uterine contractions during labor. Therefore, fetal capillary pH determinations combined with fetal heart rate monitoring provide a more reliable estimate of fetal well-being than heart rate monitoring alone.

Fetal blood sampling is indicated whenever abnormal or confusing fetal heart rate patterns require clarification.

When the fetus is hypoxic, anaerobic glycolysis causes fetal acidosis; fetal pH is less than 7.20. (See Fetal Blood Sampling, p. 782.)

Meconium in Amniotic Fluid: The significance of meconium in amniotic fluid is uncertain and controversial. Whereas some believe that the intrauterine passage of meconium is a sign of fetal stress and possibly distress, others feel that the presence of meconium without other evidence of fetal asphyxia does not indicate fetal danger. However, the combination of fetal asphyxia and meconium does appear to enhance the potential for meconium aspiration and a poor neonatal outcome.

MANAGEMENT AND PATIENT EDUCATION

General Principles:

1. Remove any umbilical cord compression.
2. Improve uteroplacental blood flow.
3. Assess whether labor can proceed safely or immediate delivery is indicated. Delivery plans (vaginal or abdominal) are based on etiologic factors, fetal condition, the patient's obstetric history, and the progress of labor.

Specific Measures:

Maternal position is changed from supine to lateral in order to relieve aortocaval compression and improve venous return, cardiac output, and uteroplacental blood flow. The change in position may also relieve umbilical cord compression.

Oxygen is provided by face mask at 6 liters per minute in order to increase maternal-fetal oxygen transfer.

Oxytocin is discontinued, since uterine contractions may be impairing the blood flow to the intervillous space.

Hypotension is corrected with an intravenous infusion of 5 per cent dextrose in lactated Ringer's solution. Blood transfusion may be indicated for hemorrhagic shock.

Vaginal examination rules out umbilical cord prolapse and determines the progress of labor. (See Prolapsed Umbilical Cord, p. 568.) Gentle elevation of the fetal head may be a salutary procedure.

Fetal scalp pH often can clarify the significance of confusing or abnormal fetal heart rate patterns (p. 782). Scalp pH greater than 7.25 is normal. Repeat determinations (at 15 minute intervals) may be indicated as long as fetal heart rate abnormalities persist.

Scalp pH less than 7.20 indicates fetal hypoxia with acidosis. Immediate delivery preparations are made. Unless vaginal delivery is imminent, cesarean section is usually advisable.

REFERENCES

Bretscher J, Saling E: pH values in the human fetus during labor. Am J Obstet Gynecol *97*:906-911, 1967

Goodlin RC, Lowe E: A functional umbilical cord occlusion heart rate pattern. Obstet Gynecol *43*:22-30, 1974

Goodlin RC, Lowe EW: Multiphasic fetal monitoring. Am J Obstet Gynecol *119*:341-357, 1974

Hon EH: Biophysical intrapartal fetal monitoring. Clin Perinatol *1*:149-159, 1974

Hon EH, Petrie RH: Clinical value of fetal heart rate monitoring. Clin Obstet Gynecol *18*:1-23, 1975

McCrann DJ, Schifrin BS: Fetal monitoring in high risk pregnancy. Clin Perinatol *1*:229-252, 1974

Miller F, Sacks D, Yeh S, Paul RH, Schifrin BS, Martin CB, Hon EH: Significance of meconium during labor. Am J Obstet Gynecol *122*:573-580, 1975

Ott WJ: Current status of intrapartum fetal monitoring. Obstet Gynecol Surv *31*:339-364, 1976

Saling E, Schneider D: Biochemical supervision of the foetus during labor. J Obstet Gynaecol Br Commonw *74*:799-811, 1967

Tejani N, Mann LI, Bhakthavathsalan A, Weiss RR: Correlation of fetal heart rate-uterine contraction patterns with fetal scalp blood pH. Obstet Gynecol *46*: 392-396, 1975

50 GONORRHEA

GENERAL CONSIDERATIONS

Gonorrhea is an infection of the mucous membrane of the urethra and genital tract caused by *Neisseria gonorrhoeae*.

The pharynx and rectal mucosa may also be involved. Infection is almost always the result of sexual contact. After invasion of mucosal sites, gonococci may spread and cause arthritis, tenosynovitis, perihepatitis, endocarditis, and meningitis.

N. gonorrhoeae is a gram-negative coccus (Fig. 50-1). In stained smears of exudates the organisms appear as diplococci within polymorphonuclear leukocytes.

Thayer-Martin selective medium permits growth of *N. gonorrhoeae* but inhibits growth of many other bacteria frequently found in specimens from urethra, cervix, rectum, and pharynx.

SUBJECTIVE DATA

Dysuria, urgency, and frequency may be symptomatic of urethritis or infection of Skene's paraurethral ducts or glands.

Mucopurulent vaginal discharge may be associated with cervicitis, although many patients who harbor gonococci are asymptomatic.

Acute onset of fever and lower abdominal pain may be indicative of gonococcal salpingitis.

Abnormal uterine bleeding, usually menorrhagia, may be an associated symptom.

OBJECTIVE DATA

Abdominal Examination: Tenderness in the lower abdomen is suggestive of bilateral salpingitis.

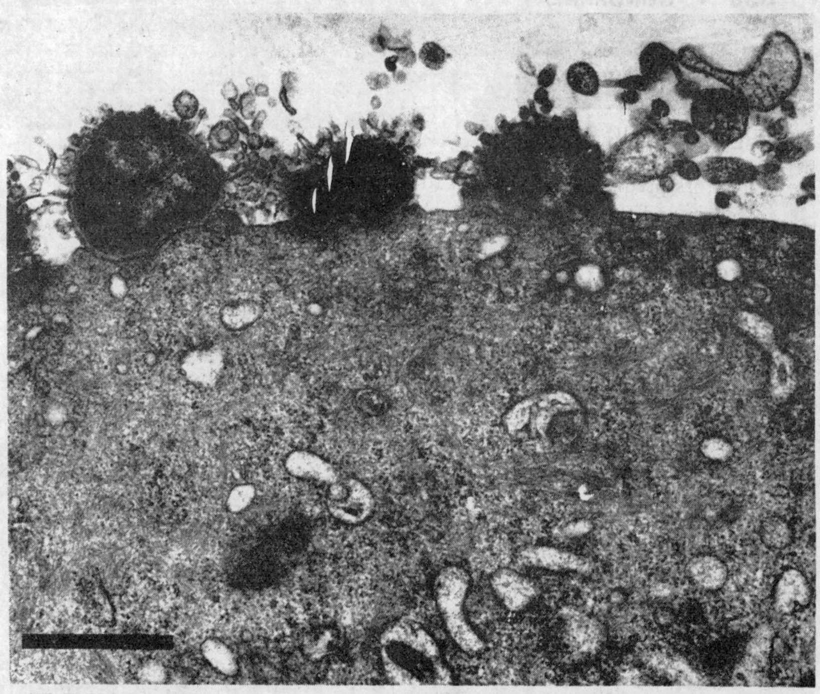

Figure 50-1. Electron micrograph showing gonococci closely attached to the surface of a urethral epithelial cell. The membrane of the host cell appears pushed up around the gonococcus to form cushion-like structures. The bar represents 500 nm (× 46,000). (From Ward ME, Watt PJ: Adherence of Neisseria gonorrhoeae to urethral mucosal cells: an electron-microscopic study of human gonorrhea. J. Infect. Dis., *126*:601, 1972. The University of Chicago Press, © 1972 by the Journal of Infectious Diseases.)

Pelvic Examination: Purulent discharge from the urethra, Skene's ducts, or Bartholin's glands may be caused by gonorrhea.

On speculum examination a purulent discharge may be seen in the cervical os.

Pain on cervical motion and bilateral adnexal pain are associated with salpingitis.

ASSESSMENT

PREDISPOSING FACTORS

Factors predisposing a patient to salpingitis include previous gonococcal infection and the presence of an intrauterine device.

POTENTIAL COMPLICATIONS

Complications of gonococcal cervicitis include ascending infection into the fallopian tubes with acute salpingitis or disseminated intravascular infection such as bacteremia, arthritis, endocarditis, or perihepatitis.

Gonococcemia is characterized by fever, polyarthralgia, maculopapular cutaneous lesions, and possibly, pericarditis. Gonococcemia seems to be more likely to develop in pregnant women during the late second and third trimester, labor, and the immediate postpartum period.

Perihepatitis (Fitz-Hugh-Curtis Syndrome): Gonococcal perihepatitis may be a sequela of acute gonococcal pelvic infection, even when gonorrhea assumes a latent and asymptomatic form. In perihepatitis the initial symptom is usually dramatic—a sudden onset of sharp pain, most intense at the right lower rib margin over the area of the gallbladder. The pain tends to be pleuritic and is exaggerated by deep breathing, coughing, laughing, and movement of the trunk. Hiccups, nausea, chills, fever, and headache may be present.

Physical examination in the acute phase discloses tenderness and rigidity of the anterior abdominal wall, particularly in the right upper quadrant.

The gonococci are thought to pass from the fallopian tubes into the paracolic gutters of the abdominal cavity and then to the subphrenic spaces. The pathologic picture is characterized by "violin string" or band adhesions between the anterior surface of the liver and the anterior abdominal wall.

The white blood count may be elevated up to 15,000/cu mm, and the erythrocyte sedimentation rate may also be elevated.

The differential diagnosis includes pyelonephritis, cholecystitis, hepatitis, peptic ulcer disease, pneumonia, and pleurisy. Laparoscopy may offer a definite diagnosis.

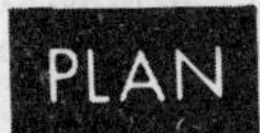

ADDITIONAL DIAGNOSTIC DATA

Cervical Culture: A sterile cotton-tipped swab is inserted into the endocervical canal after removing the mucus from the external os. The swab is then moved from side to side to sample the crypts and allowed to remain in the endocervix several seconds for absorption. The swab is then rolled in a large "Z" pattern onto modified Thayer-Martin medium in culture plates. The primary inoculation is then cross-streaked immediately with a sterile wire loop or the tip of the swab. The culture is placed in a carbon dioxide–enriched atmosphere (for example, a candle jar) within 15 minutes and delivered to the laboratory as soon as possible.

Rectal Culture: A sterile cotton-tipped swab is inserted approximately 1 inch into the anal canal. The swab is moved from side to side to sample the crypts and allowed to remain in place 10 to 30 seconds for absorption of organisms onto the swab. If the swab is inadvertently pushed into feces, the exam should be repeated with a clean swab.

This culture is indicated prior to treatment only for rectal symptoms.

Throat Culture: The posterior pharynx and tonsillar crypts are swabbed. This is indicated for patients who have had oral sexual contact.

RECOMMENDED TREATMENT SCHEDULES*

Uncomplicated Gonococcal Infections in Men and Women:

Drug Regimen of Choice: Aqueous procaine penicillin G (APPG), 4.8 million units intramuscularly divided into at least two doses and injected at different sites at one visit, together with 1 gram of probenecid by mouth just before the injections.

Alternative Regimens:

A. Patients in whom oral therapy is preferred, ampicillin, 3.5 gm by mouth, together with 1 gm probenecid by mouth administered at the same time. There is evidence that this regimen may be slightly less effective than the recommended APPG regimen.

*Center for Disease Control, U.S. Department of Health, Education and Welfare, Public Health Service, Atlanta, Georgia.

B. Patients who are allergic to the penicillins or probenecid (allergy to penicillin, ampicillin, probenecid, or previous anaphylactic reaction):

1. Tetracycline hydrochloride, 1.5 gm initially by mouth, followed by 0.5 gm by mouth four times per day for four days (total dosage: 9.5 gm). Other tetracyclines are not more effective than tetracycline hydrochloride. All tetracyclines are ineffective as single-dose therapy. (Tetracyclines should not be administered during pregnancy.) (Food and some dairy products interfere with absorption. Oral tetracycline should be given one hour before or two hours after meals.)
2. Spectinomycin hydrochloride, 2 grams intramuscularly in one injection

Treatment of Sexual Partners: Men and women with known recent exposure to gonorrhea should receive the same treatment as those known to have gonorrhea. Male sex partners of persons with gonorrhea must be examined and treated because of the high prevalence of nonsymptomatic urethral gonococcal infection in such men.

Follow-up: Follow-up urethral and other appropriate cultures should be obtained from men, and cervical, anal, and other appropriate cultures should be obtained from women, 7 to 14 days after completion of treatment.

Treatment Failures: Most recurrent infection after treatment with the recommended schedules is due to reinfection. True treatment failure after therapy with penicillin, ampicillin, or tetracycline should be treated with 2 gm of spectinomycin intramuscularly.

Postgonococcal Urethritis. Tetracycline, 0.5 gm four times a day by mouth for at least seven days.

Pharyngeal Infection: Pharyngeal gonococcal infections may be more difficult to treat than anogenital gonorrhea. Post-treatment cultures are essential follow-up for pharyngeal infection. The schedules of ampicillin and spectinomycin recommended for anogenital gonorrhea are ineffective in pharyngeal gonorrhea. Patients whose infection is not eradicated after treatment with 4.8 million units of APPG plus one gram of probenecid may be treated with 9.5 grams of tetracycline in the dosage schedule outlined above (Alternative Regimens).

Syphilis: All patients with gonorrhea should have a serologic test for syphilis at the time of diagnosis. Seronegative patients without clinical signs of syphilis who are receiving the recommended parenteral penicillin schedule need not have follow-up serologic tests for syphilis. Patients treated with ampicillin, spectinomycin, or tetracycline should have a follow-up serologic test after 3 months to detect inadequately treated syphilis.

Patients with gonorrhea who also have syphilis should be given additional treatment appropriate to the stage of syphilis.

Not Recommended: Although long-acting forms of penicillin (such as benzathine penicillin G) are effective in syphilotherapy, they have *no* place in the treatment of gonorrhea. Oral penicillin preparations such as penicillin V are not recommended for the treatment of gonococcal infection.

Treatment of Uncomplicated Gonorrhea in Pregnant Patients:

A. For women who are not allergic to penicillin:
   Use the regimen of APPG plus probenecid or use ampicillin plus probenecid as defined above.
B. For pregnant patients who are allergic to penicillins (Note: There are several possible alternative regimens, each of which has potential disadvantages):
   1. Erythromycin, 1.5 gm orally, followed by 0.5 gm 4 times a day for 4 days for a total of 9.5 gm. This regimen is safe for mother and fetus, but its efficacy has not been established. Erythromycin estolate should not be used in patients with underlying liver disease.
   2. Cefazolin, 2 gm intramuscularly, with 1 gm of probenecid. Because of the possibility of cross-allergenicity between penicillins and cephalosporins, this regimen should not be used in patients with a history of penicillin anaphylaxis.
   3. Spectinomycin, 2 gm intramuscularly, is an effective dose, but safety for the fetus has not been established.

Contraindicated: Tetracycline should not be used for uncomplicated gonococcal infection in pregnant women because of potential toxic effects for mother and fetus.

Acute Salpingitis (Pelvic Inflammatory Disease): The diagnosis of acute salpingitis should be considered in women with acute lower abdominal pain and adnexal tenderness on pelvic examination. Since there are no completely reliable clinical criteria on which to distinguish gonococcal from nongonococcal salpingitis, endocervical cultures for *Neisseria gonorrhoeae* are essential in such patients. Therapy, however, should be initiated immediately, without waiting for the results of the cultures.

A. *Hospitalization* should be strongly considered for women with suspected salpingitis in these situations:
   1. Uncertain diagnosis, where surgical emergencies must be excluded
   2. Suspicion of pelvic abscess
   3. Pregnant patients with salpingitis
   4. Inability of the patient to follow an outpatient regimen of oral medication, especially because of nausea and vomiting
   5. Failure to respond to outpatient therapy

B. *Antimicrobial Agents.* Controlled studies of the treatment of acute salpingitis are not available. Initial management must *at least* be adequate for gonococcal infection. These regimens are known to be adequate for the treatment of gonococcal salpingitis:
   1. Outpatients
      a. 1.5 gm tetracycline hydrochloride given as a single oral loading dose, followed by 500 mg taken orally 4 times a day for 10 days.
      b. APPG 4.8 million units intramuscularly, divided into at least 2 doses and injected at different sites at one visit or 3.5 gm of oral ampicillin. One gm of oral probenecid is given along with either penicillin or ampicillin, and both are followed by 500 mg of ampicillin taken orally 4 times a day for 10 days.
   2. Hospitalized patients
      a. Aqueous crystalline penicillin G, 20 million units given intravenously each day until *clear-cut* improvement occurs, followed by 500 mg of ampicillin taken orally 4 times a day to complete 10 days of therapy. The need for additional or alternative antibiotics for the treatment of nongonococcal salpingitis requires further study. Since it is impossible to distinguish gonococcal from nongonococcal salpingitis clinically, many physicians also use an aminoglycoside in addition to penicillin and/or antibiotics which are effective against *Bacteroides fragilis* as initial therapy.
      b. Tetracycline hydrochloride, 500 mg given intravenously 4 times a day until improvement occurs, followed by 500 mg taken orally 4 times a day to complete 10 days of therapy. This

regimen should not be used for pregnant women or for patients with renal failure.

3. Failure to improve on the recommended regimens does not necessarily indicate the need for stepwise additional antibiotics, but requires reassessment of the possibility of other diagnoses and of the specific microbial etiology.

C. The effect of the removal of an intrauterine device on the response of acute salpingitis to antimicrobial therapy and on the risk of recurrent salpingitis requires further study.

D. Adequate treatment of women with acute gonococcal salpingitis must include examination and appropriate treatment of their male sex partners because of the high prevalence of nonsymptomatic urethral gonococcal infection in such men. Failure to treat male sex partners is a major cause of recurrent gonococcal salpingitis.

E. Follow-up of patients with acute salpingitis is essential. All patients should receive repeat pelvic examinations and cultures for *N. gonorrhoeae* after treatment.

Disseminated Gonococcal Infection:

A. Equally effective treatment schedules in the arthritis-dermatitis syndrome include:

1. Aqueous crystalline penicillin G, 10 million units intravenously per day for 3 days or until there is significant clinical improvement. This may be followed with ampicillin, 500 mg 4 times a day orally to complete 7 days of antibiotic treatment.
2. Ampicillin, 3.5 gm orally, plus probenecid, 1 gm, followed by ampicillin, 500 mg 4 times a day orally for at least 7 days.

B. In penicillin- and/or probenecid-allergic patients:

1. Tetracycline, 1.5 gm orally followed by 500 mg 4 times a day orally for at least 7 days. Tetracycline should not be used for complicated gonococcal infection in pregnant women because of potential toxic effects for mother and fetus.
2. Erythromycin, 0.5 gm intravenously every 6 hours for at least 3 days.

C. Additional measures:

1. Hospitalization is indicated in patients who are unreliable, have uncertain diagnosis, or have purulent joint effusions or other complications.

2. Immobilization of the affected joint(s) appears helpful. Repeated aspirations and saline irrigations appear beneficial, but controlled studies of these procedures have not been performed. Open drainage of joints other than the hip is now generally discouraged in patients with gonococcal arthritis.
3. Intra-articular injection of penicillin is unnecessary, since penicillin levels in the synovial fluid of inflamed joints approximate serum levels; furthermore, intra-articular injection per se may produce a toxic synovitis.

D. Meningitis and endocarditis due to the gonococcus require high-dose intravenous penicillin therapy (at least 10 million units per day) for longer periods: usually at least 10 days for meningitis and 3-4 weeks for endocarditis.

Gonococcal Infection in Pediatric Patients: Pediatric patients encompass those from birth to adolescence. When a child is postpubertal and/or over 100 pounds, he or she should be treated with dosage regimens as defined above for adults.

The efficacy of therapeutic regimens for uncomplicated and complicated gonococcal infections of childhood is unproven at present.

With gonococcal infection in children, the possibility of child abuse must be considered.

Prevention of Neonatal Infection: All pregnant women should have endocervical cultures examined for gonococci as an integral part of prenatal care.

Prevention of Gonococcal Ophthalmia:

A. One per cent silver nitrate (do not irrigate with saline, as this may reduce efficacy).
B. Ophthalmic ointments containing tetracycline, erythromycin, or neomycin are also probably effective.
C. Not Recommended: Bacitracin ointment (not effective) and penicillin drops (sensitizing).

Management of Infants Born to Mothers with Gonococcal Infection: Orogastric and rectal cultures should be taken from all patients. Blood cultures should be taken if septicemia is suspected. Aqueous crystalline penicillin G, 50,000 units/kg/day should be administered in 2 daily doses intravenously if cultures or Gram-stained smears reveal gonococci. The duration of therapy should be determined by clinical response. In suspected septicemia, an aminoglycoside should also be given.

Neonatal Disease:

A. Gonococcal ophthalmia: Patient should be hospitalized. Antimicrobial agents: Aqueous crystalline penicillin G, 50,000 units/kg/day in 2 or 3 doses intravenously for 7 days *plus* frequent saline irrigations and instillation of penicillin, tetracycline, or chloramphenicol eyedrops.
B. Complicated infection: Arthritis and septicemia should be treated by hospitalization and administration of aqueous crystalline penicillin G, 75,000-100,000 units/kg/day in 4 doses, or procaine penicillin G, 75,000-100,000 units/kg/day in 2 doses for 7 days. Meningitis should be treated with aqueous crystalline penicillin G, 100,000 units/kg/day divided into 2 or 3 intravenous doses a day and continued for at least 10 days.

Childhood Disease: Gonococcal ophthalmia should be treated with hospitalization and by the administration of aqueous crystalline penicillin G intravenously, 75,000-100,000 units/kg/day in 4 doses, or procaine penicillin G intramuscularly, 75,000-100,000 units/kg/day in 2 doses for 7 days, *plus* saline irrigations and instillation of penicillin, tetracycline, or chloramphenicol eyedrops. Topical antibiotics alone are *not* recommended in therapy of gonococcal ophthalmitis. The source of the infection must be identified.

Uncomplicated vulvovaginitis and urethritis usually do not require hospitalization. Both may be treated at one visit with APPG, 75,000-100,000 units/kg intramuscularly, and probenecid, 25 mg/kg by mouth. Topical and systemic estrogen therapy are of no benefit in vulvovaginitis. All patients should have follow-up cultures, and the source of infection should be identified, examined, and treated.

Infection complicated by peritonitis or arthritis should be treated by hospitalization and administration of aqueous crystalline penicillin G intravenously, 75,000-100,000 units/kg/day in 4 doses, or procaine penicillin G, 75,000-100,000 units/kg/day intramuscularly in 2 doses for 7 days.

Treatment of patients with allergy to penicillin: Patients under 6 years of age should be treated with erythromycin, 40 mg/kg/day in 4 doses by mouth for 7 days, for uncomplicated disease. Complicated disease should be treated with cephalothin, 60-80 mg/kg/day in 4 doses intravenously for 7 days. Patients older than 6 may be treated with an oral regimen of tetracycline, 25 mg/kg as an initial dose followed by 40-60 mg/kg/day in 4 doses for 7 days, or an intravenous regimen of tetracycline, 15-20 mg/kg/day in 4 doses for 7 days.

REFERENCES

Curran JW, Rendtorff RD, Chandler RW, Wiser WL, Robinson H: Female gonorrhea. Obstet Gynecol *45*:195-198, 1975

Genadry RR, Thompson BH, Niebyl JR: Gonococcal salpingitis in pregnancy. Am J Obstet Gynecol *126*:512-513, 1976

Gonorrhea: Recommended treatment schedules—1974. Part I: Uncomplicated gonococcal infections in men and women; uncomplicated gonorrhea in pregnant patients; and acute salpingitis. Obstet Gynecol *45*:596-598, 1975

Henderson R: Recommended treatment schedules for gonorrhea—1974. Arch Dermatol *111*:317-320, 1975

Reichert JA, Valle RF: Fitz-Hugh-Curtis syndrome. JAMA *236*:266-268, 1976

Watring WG, Vaughn DL: Gonococcemia in pregnancy. Obstet Gynecol *48*:428-430, 1976

51 HEADACHE DURING PREGNANCY

GENERAL CONSIDERATIONS

Headache during pregnancy is a frequent symptom. For the most part, headaches result from the tensions of life, eye strain, or allergic sinusitis. Nonetheless, persistent headache may be a premonitory sign of preeclampsia or eclampsia, or a presenting symptom of a catastrophic neurologic disorder (such as brain tumor, cerebral hemorrhage, meningitis).

SUBJECTIVE DATA

Mode of Onset: Circumstances preceding or surrounding the onset of headache often provide key diagnostic clues. A history of generalized edema and sudden weight gain suggests preeclampsia. A preceding convulsion may signify eclampsia or a cerebral disorder. (See Convulsive Seizures in Pregnancy, p. 268.)

A severe headache of sudden onset followed by impaired consciousness or focal neurologic signs may be the first indication of intracranial bleeding. (See Cerebrovascular Accident during Pregnancy, p. 185.)

Chills and fever suggest the possibility of meningitis or cerebral infection.

A history of trauma, migraine, rhinorrhea, or allergy may elucidate the cause of the current symptoms.

Headaches resulting from hypertension are usually present on wakening. The onset of tension headache tends to be gradual and variable. Often the tension headache is related to stress or depression.

Headache due to migraine may be preceded by a prodromal stage with sharply defined visual, sensory, or motor symptoms.

Localization: Bilateral generalized headache, more intense in the occipital-nuchal area, is frequently caused by tension. Unilateral or localized pain is more characteristic of migraine, tumor, and sinus headaches. Disease of the paranasal sinuses, teeth, eyes, or upper cervical vertebrae induces pain that is referred in a regional, fairly constant, but not sharply localized, distribution.

Quality of Pain: Migraine and hypertensive headaches tend to be throbbing in nature. Tension, muscular, and sinus headaches are frequently described as producing continuous band-like pressure.

Aggravating Factors: An intracranial vascular lesion, whether caused by fever, tumor, or bleeding, tends to be aggravated by sudden jarring, head movements, coughing, sneezing, or straining. Changes in barometric pressure may increase the pain of sinusitis. Headache associated with cervical spondylosis is aggravated by neck movements, and muscle-contraction headache due to eye strain is aggravated by reading or close work. A correlation between the occurrence of tension headache and periods of worry, anger, or excitement can often be seen.

Relieving Factors: The patient with migraine prefers to lie quietly in a darkened room, whereas the patient with intracranial bleeding is relieved of pain only slightly by bed rest. The pain of sinusitis may be reduced when the patient sits up or moves around or when the sinuses are cleared of nasal obstruction.

OBJECTIVE DATA

PHYSICAL EXAMINATION

General Examination: Elevated blood pressure, edema, and proteinuria usually denote preeclampsia or eclampsia (see Preeclampsia, p. 552, and Eclampsia, p. 303). Elevated temperature may be an indication of meningitis.

Disorientation or altered consciousness or both may be associated with an acute vascular accident, meningitis, or metabolic brain disease. (See Coma in Pregnancy, p. 234.)

Meningismus is an indication of meningitis or subarachnoid hemorrhage. Irritation of the meninges causes reflex spasm of neck muscles.

Pain in cervical muscles is usually due to muscle spasm.

Neurologic examination may identify generalized or focal abnormalities that are indicative of an organic lesion. Mental status, cranial nerves, deep tendon reflexes, motor strength, gait, sensory responses and speech may provide important diagnostic clues.

LABORATORY TESTS

Complete Blood Count with Blood Smear: Leukocytosis may be seen in cases of meningeal infection. Lymphocytosis may be indicative of a viral illness.

Urinalysis: Proteinuria is usually associated with preeclampsia or eclampsia.

ASSESSMENT

DIFFERENTIAL DIAGNOSIS

This includes three major groups (See Table 51-1):

Vascular Headache (migraine, cluster, toxic, and hypertensive): Common to this group is the tendency toward vascular dilatation.

Classic migraine is a symptom complex, a whole spectrum of body alterations of which headache is only a single part. In classic migraine nonpainful sensory experiences (usually scotomas or visual field defects) precede the headache phase. The pain is usually described as aching and throbbing, frequently coincides with the pulse beat, and is often associated with nausea and vomiting. The patient usually tries to avoid sensory stimuli of all types, especially light. Pain tends to last from 8 to 24 hours and then subsides spontaneously, usually after a period of sleep.

Toxic vascular headache is evoked by systemic vasodilatation secondary to fever, alcohol, and carbon dioxide retention.

Hypertensive headache may be symptomatic of severe preeclampsia and portend an eclamptic convulsion.

Muscle contraction (tension) headache—the most frequent type of headache—results from chronic muscular contraction about the head and neck.

TABLE 51-1. Classification and Treatment of Headache in Pregnancy*

Vascular Headache	Muscle Contraction (Psychogenic) Headache	Traction and Inflammatory Headache
Migraine	Cervical osteoarthritis	Mass lesions (tumors, edema, hematomas, cerebral hemorrhage)
Classic	Chronic myositis	
Common	Depressive equivalents and conversion reactions	
Complicated		Diseases of the eye, ear, nose, throat, teeth
Hemiplegic		
Ophthalmoplegic		Allergy
Cluster (histamine)		Infection
Toxic (vascular)		Arteritis, phlebitis
Hypertensive		Cranial neuralgias
		Occlusive vascular disease
Suggested treatment		
Sedation	Mild analgesics	Appropriate consultation
Cyproheptadine	Sedation	Therapy of underlying disease
Analgesics	Amitriptyline	Allergy therapy (as indicated)
Antihypertensives	Physical therapy	Antibiotics (as indicated)
		Anticonvulsants (as indicated)
		Corticosteroids (as indicated)
		Miotics (as indicated)
		Surgery (as indicated)

*From Burrow GN, Ferris TF: Medical Complications during Pregnancy. Philadelphia, W.B. Saunders Company, 1975.

Traction and inflammatory headache is evoked by organic disease of the skull or its components, including the brain, meninges, arteries, veins, eyes, ears, teeth, nose, and paranasal sinuses. Brain tumors, hematomas, abscesses, edema, hemorrhage, thromboses, and meningitis are possible causes.

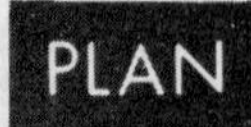

MANAGEMENT AND PATIENT EDUCATION

Migraine during pregnancy is treated with analgesics and sedatives, much as any other self-limited pain syndrome. Ergotamine is avoided during pregnancy.

Dietary Suggestions (Dalessio, 1975):

1. Avoid alcohol, particularly red wines and champagne.
2. Avoid aged or strong cheese, particularly cheddar cheese.
3. Avoid chicken livers, pickled herring, canned figs, and pods of broad beans.
4. Use monosodium glutamate sparingly.
5. Avoid cured meats such as hot dogs, bacon, ham, and salami if it has been demonstrated that they evoke vascular headache.
6. Eat three well-balanced meals per day. Do not skip meals and avoid prolonged fasting and excessive ingestion of carbohydrates at any single sitting.

Muscle Contraction (Tension) Headaches: Analgesic medications, such as acetaminophen with codeine, are usually effective. During late pregnancy hydroxyzine (Vistaril or Atarax) may be helpful.

Attempts to minimize stressful situations are advisable.

Traction and Inflammatory Headache: Treatment involves specific therapy for the associated underlying disease.

REFERENCES

Dalessio DJ: Neurologic complications. *In* Burrow GN, Ferris TF: Medical Complications during Pregnancy. Philadelphia, W.B. Saunders Company, 1975

Somerville BW: A study of migraine in pregnancy. Neurology *22*:824-828, 1972

52 HEMATOCOLPOS

GENERAL CONSIDERATIONS

Hematocolpos is an accumulation of menstrual blood in the vagina resulting from an imperforate hymen or other obstruction.

SUBJECTIVE DATA

CURRENT SYMPTOMS

Abdominal Pain: Periodic suprapubic cramps may develop with the onset of puberty. Expected menses are absent.

Fever and chills may be an indication of an associated pyometra.

PRIOR HISTORY

A history of absent menses in an adolescent girl may provide the key diagnostic clue to a congenital abnormality. In older patients scar tissue from previous surgery or irradiation may obstruct endometrial bleeding.

OBJECTIVE DATA

PHYSICAL EXAMINATION

General Examination: These findings are usually normal. An elevated temperature may indicate an associated infection, for example, endometrial obstruction caused by tumor.

Abdominal Examination: The lower abdomen is often tender over the distended uterus. At times the distended uterus may be palpable abdominally as a lower midline mass.

Pelvic Examination: On inspection the hymen may appear bulging and imperforate.

LABORATORY TESTS

Complete Blood Count with Blood Smear: Leukocytosis is usually indicative of an associated infection.

ASSESSMENT

ETIOLOGIC FACTORS

Etiologic factors include an imperforate hymen or a transverse vaginal septum in the adolescent patient and postsurgical or postirradiation scarring in the older patient.

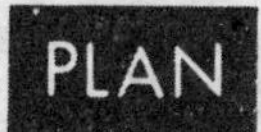

MANAGEMENT

Cruciate incision of an imperforate hymen or a transverse vaginal septum permits blood to escape. No further therapy is usually required.

When hematocolpos develops after irradiation, the cervix may have to be dilated to permit drainage. Since pyometra is often an associated finding, systemic antibiotic therapy may be indicated.

53 HEMATURIA IN PREGNANCY

GENERAL CONSIDERATIONS

Hematuria in pregnancy usually results from urinary tract trauma, calculi, or infection. The possibility of contamination of the urine specimen with vaginal blood must always be considered.

As pregnancy progresses, the urinary bladder becomes an abdominal organ, vulnerable to trauma, particularly from injuries to the adjacent bony pelvis.

SUBJECTIVE DATA

CURRENT SYMPTOMS

Lumbar pain is the most characteristic symptom of an impacted ureteral calculus. Severe colicky pain in the costovertebral angle tends to radiate down the ureter into the groin. Urgency, frequency, dysuria, hematuria, nausea, vomiting, and fever may be associated symptoms.

Inability to void combined with urinary retetention may result from urethral or bladder trauma. A history of recent traumatic injury provides the key diagnostic clue. (Possible causes include forceps delivery, cesarean surgery, uterine rupture, and prolonged obstructed labor.)

PRIOR HISTORY

History of anticoagulant therapy may be significant.

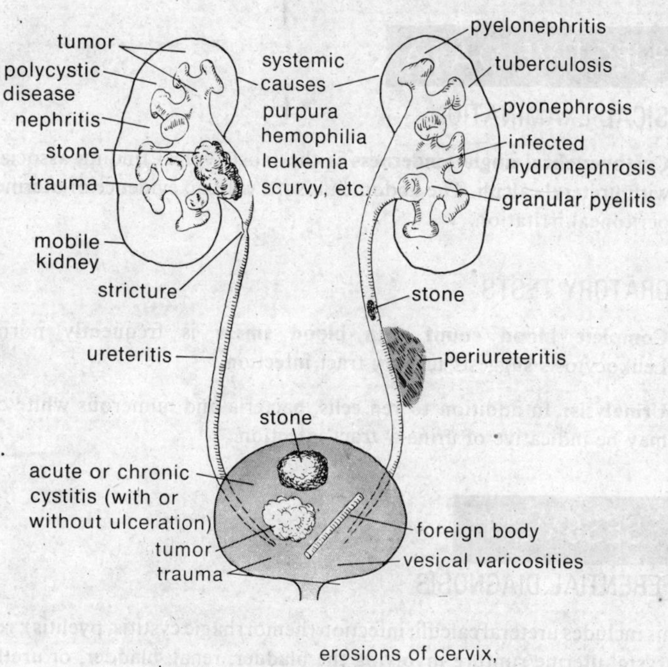

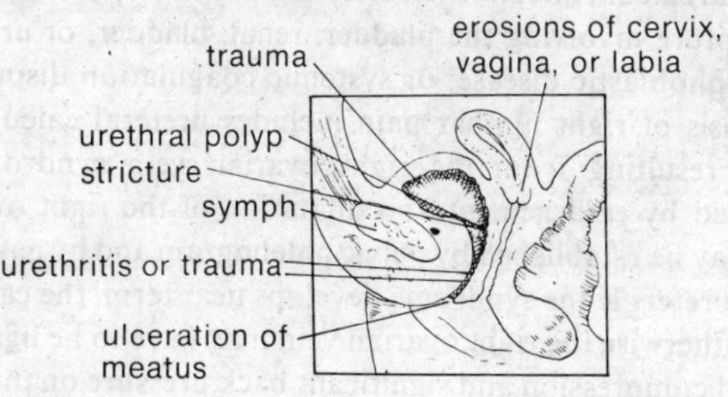

Figure 53-1. Causes of hematuria. (Modified from Harrison JH, et al.: Campbell's Urology. 3rd ed. Philadelphia, W.B. Saunders Company, 1963.)

OBJECTIVE DATA

PHYSICAL EXAMINATION

Costovertebral angle tenderness is the most typical finding associated with ureteral calculi. The abdomen is soft, with no evidence of uterine or peritoneal irritation.

LABORATORY TESTS

Complete blood count with blood smear is frequently normal. Leukocytosis suggests urinary tract infection.

Urinalysis: In addition to red cells, bacteria and numerous white cells may be indicative of urinary tract infection.

ASSESSMENT

DIFFERENTIAL DIAGNOSIS

This includes ureteral calculi; infection (hemorrhagic cystitis, pyelitis); renal aneurysm; uterine rupture involving the bladder; renal, bladder, or urethral trauma; recurrent trophoblastic disease; or systemic coagulation disorders.

Differential diagnosis of right lumbar pain includes ureteral calculi and ureteral obstruction resulting from the right ovarian vein syndrome, a condition characterized by enlargement and dilatation of the right ovarian vein. The diagnosis may be established by pelvic phlebogram and by passing a catheter up the right ureter. If the syndrome develops near term, the catheter may be left in place; otherwise the right ovarian vein may have to be ligated if there is undue ureteral compression and significant back pressure on the right kidney.

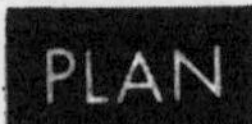

ADDITIONAL DIAGNOSTIC DATA

Abdominal x-ray may reveal a radiopaque stone. Intravenous urography may be indicated for the evaluation of ureteral obstruction. Radiologic consultation is advisable.

Cystoscopy may disclose bladder calculi, trauma, or metastatic trophoblastic disease.

Coagulation studies (platelet count, fibrinogen, prothrombin time, and partial thromboplastin time) may identify a coagulopathy.

MANAGEMENT AND PATIENT EDUCATION

Ureteral Calculi: The patient should be hospitalized. Usually it is desirable to await spontaneous passage of the stone. Persistent, severe symptoms with deterioration may necessitate operative intervention.

Urethral Injury: In cases of urethral injury, a catheter is inserted into the bladder cautiously in order to slowly release the accumulated urine. The urethra can then be repaired over the catheter. In order to prevent trauma and pressure on the suture line, a suprapubic catheter is inserted into the bladder.

Bladder Rupture: A ruptured bladder requires bladder drainage per urethra immediately and exploratory laparotomy for control of bleeding. An extraperitoneal, transvesical approach may identify the injury site and permit evacuation of the hematoma and extravasated urine from the paravesical spaces. The retroperitoneal space should be drained through separate incisions in the lower abdomen. The bladder is usually drained with a suprapubic catheter.

REFERENCES

Mattingly RF, Borkowf HI: Lower urinary tract injuries in pregnancy. *In* Barber HRK, Graber EA: Surgical Disease in Pregnancy. Philadelphia, W.B. Saunders Company, 1974

54 HEMORRHOIDS AND PREGNANCY

GENERAL CONSIDERATIONS

Hemorrhoids—dilated veins of the internal and external hemorrhoidal plexus—are common during pregnancy. The increased pressure in the hemorrhoidal veins results from venous obstruction by the enlarged uterus as well as from a tendency toward constipation during pregnancy.

SUBJECTIVE AND OBJECTIVE DATA

Rectal bleeding, pruritus, and pain are the most common symptoms. Acute, severe pain may be caused by thrombosis or prolapse. Constipation may be secondary to painful defecation.

Tender, swollen hemorrhoidal veins are obvious to both patient and physician. A thrombosed vein can be exquisitely painful.

PLAN

MANAGEMENT AND PATIENT EDUCATION

Pain and swelling are usually relieved by bed rest, topically applied anesthetics, and cold witch hazel packs, and possibly, by warm soaks. In addition, medications that provide a soft, bulky stool are usually beneficial. When a thrombosed hemorrhoidal vein causes considerable pain, the clot can be evacuated by incising the vein wall under local anesthesia.

When rectal bleeding is persistent and anemia develops, hemorrhoidectomy may be necessary. After delivery, hemorrhoids frequently become asymptomatic, although they do tend to recur during succeeding pregnancies.

55 HYDRAMNIOS

GENERAL CONSIDERATIONS

Hydramnios (or polyhydramnios) is an excessive quantity of amniotic fluid (more than 2000 ml). By 36 weeks' gestation the normal volume of amniotic fluid is approximately 1000 ml.

The incidence of hydramnios varies widely, from one to seven cases per 1000 deliveries; minor degrees are more common.

Rarely, the volume of amniotic fluid increases very suddenly; the uterus becomes immensely distended within a few days as a result of *acute hydramnios.*

The incidence of hydramnios is especially high in pregnancies complicated by diabetes and erythroblastosis. Excessive amniotic fluid is also common in twin pregnancies.

Fetal malformations, particularly central nervous system and gastrointestinal tract defects, are often associated with hydramnios; approximately half the cases of anencephalus and nearly all cases of esophageal atresia are accompanied by hydramnios.

SUBJECTIVE DATA

Dyspnea, edema of the lower extremities due to compression of the venous system by the very large uterus, and abdominal pain are the most frequent symptoms. The patient can be extremely uncomfortable from the pressure exerted by the overdistended uterus upon adjacent organs.

OBJECTIVE DATA

Abdominal Examination: Uterine size is greatly increased, and the uterine wall is very tense. Fetal parts are not easily palpable, and the fetal presentation is frequently abnormal.

ASSESSMENT

DIFFERENTIAL DIAGNOSIS

This includes twins, ovarian cyst, and leiomyoma of the uterus.

POTENTIAL COMPLICATIONS

Complications to be anticipated include fetal malformation, abnormal fetal presentation, premature labor, premature rupture of membranes, and prolapsed cord, all of which contribute to an increased perinatal mortality. Maternal complications include premature placental separation, uterine dysfunction, and postpartum hemorrhage.

PLAN

ADDITIONAL DIAGNOSTIC DATA

Sonography facilitates the diagnosis of hydramnios.

Ultrasound B-scan or abdominal x-ray may identify fetal abnormalities (particularly anencephaly), multiple fetuses, or an abnormal presentation.

MANAGEMENT

Minimal degrees of hydramnios rarely require treatment.

Dyspnea, abdominal pain, or difficult ambulation may necessitate hospitalization. Excess amniotic fluid is removed by abdominal amniocentesis. Fluid is withdrawn slowly, at a rate of approximately 500 ml over a period of an hour. As much as 1500 to 2000 ml may have to be removed to provide symptomatic relief.

PATIENT EDUCATION

The perinatal mortality associated with hydramnios is approximately 50 per cent. Causative factors include prematurity, fetal malformation, prolapsed umbilical cord, erythroblastosis, and diabetes.

REFERENCES

Queenan JT, Gadow EC: Polyhydramnios: chronic versus acute. Am J Obstet Gynecol *108*:349-355, 1970

56 HYPEREMESIS GRAVIDARUM

GENERAL CONSIDERATIONS

Hyperemesis gravidarum (pernicious vomiting in pregnancy) is nausea and vomiting in pregnancy that have progressed to such an extent that systemic effects, dehydration, and substantial weight loss have resulted.

The onset is usually during the second month of pregnancy; the disease may last several weeks and then disappear during the third or fourth gestational month. Persistent severe nausea and vomiting may accompany 15 to 30 per cent of molar pregnancies.

SUBJECTIVE DATA

Nausea and vomiting are the cardinal symptoms. The patient is unable to retain any food and loses weight. Some patients complain of excessive salivation.

Menstrual History: Most patients are aware of missed periods and know that they are pregnant. An occasional patient, however, may not provide this essential information, thereby obscuring the diagnosis.

OBJECTIVE DATA

PHYSICAL EXAMINATION

General Examination: Skin and mucous membranes often appear dry and lack normal turgor. The patient may be emaciated. The irritating vomitus may erode the lips and lower part of the face; the tongue is red, dry, and cracked. The pharynx is dry and red, and the breath is fetid, with a fruity odor characteristic of ketoacidosis.

Tachycardia and hypotension may indicate dehydration hypovolemia. With severe and prolonged disease, mental aberration, delirium, headache, somnolence, stupor, and coma can occur.

Abdominal Examination: These findings are usually normal, although liver tenderness may be noted.

Pelvic Examination: The uterus is softened and enlarged consistent with the gestational age.

LABORATORY TESTS

Complete Blood Count with Blood Smear: Elevated hemoglobin and hematocrit values indicate hemoconcentration associated with dehydration. Anemia may be a consequence of malnutrition.

Urinalysis: Urine is usually scanty and highly concentrated as a result of dehydration. Acetone indicates starvation acidosis.

ASSESSMENT

DIFFERENTIAL DIAGNOSIS

The possibility of an organic cause for the vomiting coexisting with pregnancy must be excluded. Possible diagnoses to be considered are appendicitis, cholecystitis, diabetic ketoacidosis, drug toxicity, gastroenteritis, hepatitis, intestinal obstruction, pancreatitis, peptic ulcer, pyelonephritis, and twisted ovarian cyst.

PREDISPOSING FACTORS

Factors predisposing the patient to hyperemesis include chorionic gonadotropin levels higher than normal (molar pregnancy, twin pregnancy) and an emotional psychopathologic condition. The cause of hyperemesis gravidarum remains unknown, however.

POTENTIAL COMPLICATIONS

These include fluid and electrolyte depletion, acid-base disturbance, malnutrition, aspiration pneumonia, mucosal tears at the gastroesophageal junction causing severe hemorrhage (Mallory-Weiss syndrome), esophageal rupture, liver damage, and renal damage.

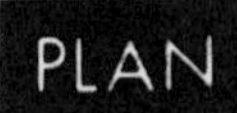

ADDITIONAL DIAGNOSTIC DATA

Serum electrolyte determinations may detect hyponatremia, hypokalemia, hypochloremia, and metabolic alkalosis.

Liver function tests may indicate hepatic disease.

Amylase determinations are of value when pancreatitis is suspected.

MANAGEMENT

Principles of management include rest, reassurance, and restoration of fluid, electrolyte, and nutritional balance. Psychologic and social problems should be evaluated.

Hospitalization permits vigorous parenteral therapy and, in addition, separates the patient from any stressful psychosocial problems in her home environment.

Intravenous fluids are administered for parenteral alimentation. Oral foods and fluids are avoided. The starvation and dehydration are treated initially with 5 to 10 per cent dextrose in normal saline solution. Two thousand five hundred to 3500 ml are administered over a period of 24 hours. The dextrose furnishes calories and combats acidosis. The saline restores the electrolytes lost by vomiting, and the water corrects dehydration. Postassium supplementation is provided if the serum potassium value indicates hypokalemia. Parenteral vitamins are usually added to the intravenous fluids.

Antiemetic or sedative medication may be necessary. Promethazine hydrochloride may be given intravenously, intramuscularly, or by rectal suppository. The usual dose is 25 mg every four to six hours. Some patients may require 50 mg for satisfactory sedation. When the patient is able to retain oral medications, doxylamine combined with pyridoxine may be helpful.

Visitors should be restricted initially and the patient encouraged to rest as much as possible.

After 48 hours the patient's condition has usually improved and bland foods may be tried. At first, only small amounts of fluid are given between meals and intravenous fluid supplementation is continued.

Psychiatric or social service consultation may be helpful in order to evaluate underlying psychopathologic conditions and support to relieve environmental stress factors.

Termination of pregnancy is rarely necessary unless the patient fails to respond to therapy; jaundice, tachycardia, pyrexia, or delirium develop; or the patient personally desires the pregnancy to be aborted.

The best guide to recovery is the weight chart. Once weight loss has ceased and weight gain has begun, the patient is well on the way to recovery.

PATIENT EDUCATION

Morning nausea and vomiting are common symptoms of early pregnancy. Since these symptoms can be most troublesome when the stomach is empty, pregnant women tend to feel better if there is some food in the stomach most of the time. Many prefer to eat six small meals per day rather than three large meals. Dry crackers or toast by the bedside may be helpful.

Greasy foods and disagreeable cooking smells should be avoided.

57 HYPERTENSION DURING PREGNANCY

GENERAL CONSIDERATIONS

Hypertension is one of the most serious complications of pregnancy. Consequently, whenever acute hypertension develops during pregnancy, the patient must have a complete diagnostic evaluation.

During normal pregnancy, peripheral vascular resistance is decreased as a result of a dilated vasculature. For this reason, diastolic blood pressure is slightly decreased during normal gestation, reaching its nadir at about the thirtieth week. If peripheral resistance becomes increased, hypertension results. The actual cause of the increased peripheral resistance and the mechanism by which pregnancy causes hypertension remain unknown.

DEFINITIONS

The Committee on Terminology of the American College of Obstetricians and Gynecologists has suggested the following definitions of the hypertensive states of pregnancy:

Hypertension—a rise in the systolic pressure of at least 30 mm Hg, or a rise in the diastolic pressure of at least 15 mm Hg, or the presence of a systolic pressure of at least 140 mm Hg, or a diastolic pressure of at least 90 mm Hg. Hypertension may also be determined by a *mean arterial pressure** of 105 mm Hg or more or by a rise of 20 mm Hg or more. The levels cited must be manifest on at least two occasions six or more hours apart and should be based on previously known blood pressure levels.

*Mean Arterial Pressure = $\frac{(2 \times \text{Diastolic}) + \text{Systolic}}{3}$

Proteinuria—the presence of urinary protein in concentrations greater than 0.3 gm per l in a 24-hour urine collection or in concentrations greater than 1 gm per l (1+ to 2+ by standard turbidimetric methods) in a random urine collection on two or more occasions at least six hours apart. The specimens must be clean—either voided midstream or obtained by catheterization.

Edema—a general and excessive accumulation of fluids in the tissues, commonly demonstrated by swelling of the extremities and face.

ASSESSMENT

CLASSIFICATION

The Committee on Terminology of the American College of Obstetricians and Gynecologists has suggested the following classification of the hypertensive states of pregnancy:

Gestational hypertension is the development of hypertension during pregnancy or within the first 24 hours post partum in a previously normotensive woman. No other evidence of preeclampsia or hypertensive vascular disease is present. The blood pressure returns to normotensive levels within ten days following parturition. Some patients with gestational hypertension may, in fact, have preeclampsia or hypertensive vascular disease, but they do not satisfy the criteria for either of these diagnoses.

Preeclampsia is the development of hypertension with proteinuria or edema or both due to pregnancy or the influence of a recent pregnancy. It usually occurs after the twentieth week of gestation, but it may develop before this time in the presence of trophoblastic disease. Preeclampsia is predominantly a disorder of primigravidas.

Eclampsia is the occurrence of one or more convulsions not attributable to other cerebral conditions such as epilepsy or cerebral hemorrhage in a patient with preeclampsia.

Superimposed preeclampsia or eclampsia is the development of preeclampsia or eclampsia in a patient with chronic hypertensive vascular or renal disease. When the hypertension antedates the pregnancy, as established by previous blood pressure recordings, a rise in the systolic pressure of 30 mm Hg or a rise in the diastolic pressure of 15 mm Hg, and the development of proteinuria, edema, or both must occur during pregnancy to establish the diagnosis.

Chronic hypertensive disease is the presence of persistent hypertension, of any cause, before pregnancy or before the twentieth week of gestation, or beyond the forty-second postpartum day. (Diagnoses include essential hypertension, renal disease, coarctation of the aorta, primary aldosteronism, and pheochromocytoma.)

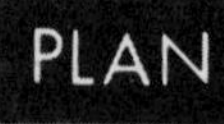

MANAGEMENT AND PATIENT EDUCATION

Any pregnant patient in whom hypertension develops should be hospitalized for diagnosis and evaluation. During the latter half of pregnancy the most probable diagnosis is preeclampsia or eclampsia or superimposed preeclampsia or eclampsia. (See Preeclampsia, p. 552; and Eclampsia, p. 303.)

58 INTESTINAL OBSTRUCTION IN PREGNANCY

GENERAL CONSIDERATIONS

Intestinal obstruction caused by extrinsic blockage of the intestinal lumen is a relatively rare but extremely serious emergency problem during pregnancy, with a high potential for fetal and maternal morbidity and mortality. The reported incidence is 1 in 3000 to 60,000 deliveries, with approximately 50 per cent of the cases occurring during the third trimester.

SUBJECTIVE DATA

CURRENT SYMPTOMS

Abdominal pain tends to be severe, intermittent, and colicky in cases of mechanical obstruction. The rhythmic periodicity characteristic of obstructive pain differentiates it from the cramps of minor intestinal disturbances and the constant pain of peritonitis. The interval between the bouts of pain may suggest the location of the obstruction. In cases of small bowel obstruction, the interval tends to be about four or five minutes; in cases of lower obstruction, the interval is more likely to be 10 to 15 minutes.

Nausea and vomiting can be variable symptoms. Vomiting is most typical of small bowel obstruction; it is frequently absent initially in low obstruction.

Distention, constipation, and obstipation may be associated symptoms.

PRIOR HISTORY

A history of abdominal surgery suggests the possibility of adhesive bands.

OBJECTIVE DATA

PHYSICAL EXAMNATION

General Examination: These findings depend on the underlying cause and severity of obstruction. Often the patient is dehydrated from vomiting or third space losses into the intestinal lumen. The presence of shock suggests decreased intravascular volume resulting from massive fluid and electrolyte loss into a segment of strangulated bowel.

Abdominal Examination: Distention is usually evident. A surgical scar on the abdomen may provide an important diagnostic clue to the presence of an adhesive band from previous surgery.

Bowel sounds in cases of mechanical obstruction are loud, metallic, high-pitched, and hyperperistaltic. In adynamic ileus and peritonitis, bowel sounds are either hypoactive or absent.

LABORATORY TESTS

Complete Blood Count with Blood Smear: The hematocrit may be elevated, indicating dehydration. The white count is often elevated, as well as shifted to the left. If obstruction has compromised the intestinal blood supply, the white blood cell count is likely to be markedly elevated.

Urinalysis: The specific gravity may provide a clue to the patient's hydration. Urinary ketones suggest starvation ketosis.

ASSESSMENT

DIFFERENTIAL DIAGNOSIS

The differential diagnosis of mechanical intestinal obstruction includes labor, threatened abortion, gastroenteritis, cholecystitis, pancreatitis, appendicitis, pyelonephritis, and premature placental separation.

During the third trimester, labor may be ruled out by abdominal auscultation, and by palpation of the uterus during an attack. In cases of mechanical obstruction, the bowel sounds become loud and high pitched, occurring in rushes, whereas the uterus remains relaxed.

Mechanical obstruction must be distinguished from *adynamic ileus* (absent peristaltic activity of the small bowel), which is characterized by abdominal distention with absent bowel sounds. Ileus appears to be a reflex response to injury that decreases parasympathetic stimulation of the gut and increases sympathetic stimulation of the gut. Causes range from sepsis and metabolic problems such as hypokalemia to vascular compromise of the intestinal blood supply. Ordinarily, ileus occurs after abdominal surgery as well as in the presence of peritonitis.

PREDISPOSING FACTORS

Predisposing factors to mechanical intestinal obstruction are adhesive bands from previous surgery, volvulus, intussusception, and hernias (particularly diaphragmatic). In the presence of any of these factors an enlarging uterus may precipitate an acute intestinal obstruction.

POTENTIAL COMPLICATIONS

Complications of mechanical obstruction include strangulation, closed loop obstruction, and marked distention of the colon. These can cause ischemic necrosis of the bowel, bowel perforation, and bacteremia. Strangulation is suspected whenever the patient notes a change in the abdominal pain pattern from intermittent cramps to a severe, steady pain. Associated changes in physical and laboratory findings may also point to the diagnosis of peritonitis.

SEVERITY OF DISEASE PROCESS

Mechanical intestinal obstruction implies obstruction without major impairment of the intestinal blood supply. It is usually due to postoperative bands or adhesions.

Strangulation signifies an impairment of the vascular supply and is usually due to an incarcerated hernia or volvulus. Mesenteric vascular occlusion is another possible rare cause.

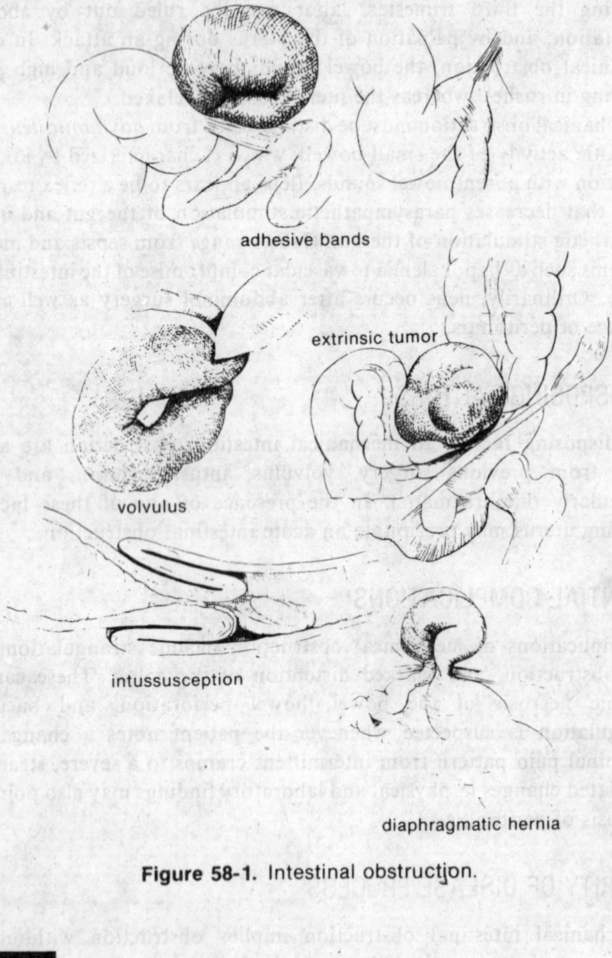

adhesive bands

extrinsic tumor

volvulus

intussusception

diaphragmatic hernia

Figure 58-1. Intestinal obstruction.

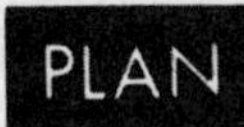

ADDITIONAL DIAGNOSTIC DATA

Abdominal x-rays (flat, upright, and decubitus) reveal distended loops of air and fluid-filled bowel, multiple air-fluid levels on the upright or decubitus views, and increasing amounts of air or fluid in one part of the bowel with decreasing amounts of gas in more distal bowel on serial films.

Serum electrolytes are an important guide to fluid replacement therapy.

MANAGEMENT

Cardinal principles of therapy include

1. Replacement of metabolic losses
2. Decompression of the intestine
3. Removal of the cause of obstruction

The patient is hospitalized, oral intake is suspended, and intravenous fluids and electrolytes are initiated. The intestine is decompressed with nasogastric suction. If strangulation is suspected, antibiotic therapy is prescribed. Exploratory laparotomy is indicated as soon as the diagnosis is established and the patient is adequately prepared for surgery.

Surgical procedures depend on the findings at laparotomy, particularly on the viability of the bowel. Lysis of adhesions may be adequate therapy if the intestinal blood supply is unimpaired; otherwise, resection and anastomosis may be indicated.

PATIENT EDUCATION

The necessity and risks of surgery must be discussed in detail, since the longer the intestinal obstruction remains untreated, the more likely the development of significant complications, and the greater the maternal and fetal risks.

REFERENCES

Beck WW: Intestinal obstruction in pregnancy. Obstet Gynecol *43*:374-378, 1974

Hill LM, Symmonds RE: Small bowel obstruction in pregnancy. Obstet Gynecol *49*:170-173, 1977

Kesseler HJ: Hernias in pregnancy. *In* Barber HRK, Graber EA: Surgical Disease in Pregnancy. Philadelphia, W.B. Saunders Company, 1974

59 LABOR AND DELIVERY

GENERAL CONSIDERATIONS

Labor (parturition) is the physiologic process by which the uterus expels or attempts to expel the fetus and placenta after 20 weeks or more of gestation. Labor is divided into three stages:

First stage of labor refers to the period from the onset of labor to the complete dilatation of the cervix. (This may be subdivided into two phases: *latent* and *active*. The latent, prodromal, or preparatory phase is an interval during which uterine contractions are oriented and the cervix is softened and effaced in preparation for subsequent active dilatation. In nulliparas the latent phase averages 8.6 hours and normally does not exceed 20 hours; in multiparas it averages 5.3 hours and usually does not go beyond 14 hours. The active dilatational phase, characterized by continuous cervical dilatation, terminates when the cervix is fully dilated and effaced. The slope of active-phase dilatation in nulliparas averages 3 cm per hour and is not less than 1.2 cm per hour under normal circumstances; in multiparas it averages 5.7 cm per hour and is rarely less than 1.5 cm per hour.)

Second stage of labor refers to the period from complete cervical dilatation to the birth of the fetus.

Third stage of labor refers to the period from birth of the fetus to the expulsion or extraction of the placenta and membranes.

Labor may also be divided into three divisions; *preparatory, dilatation*, and *pelvic* (Friedman, 1971). The pelvic division is characterized by descent of the fetal presenting part (see Table 59-1).

TABLE 59-1. Principal Clinical Features of the Functional Divisions of Labor*

Characteristics	Preparatory Division	Dilatational Division	Pelvic Division
Functions fulfilled	Contractions coordinated, cervix prepared	Cervix actively dilated	Pelvis negotiated by mechanisms of labor, descent and delivery
Interval included	From onset of contractions to end of acceleration phase	Phase of maximal slope	From onset of deceleration phase to delivery of infant
Measured by	Duration of time elapsed (hr)	Rate of dilatation, linear (cm/hr)	Rate of descent, linear (cm/hr)
Adversely affected by	Excessive sedation, unprepared cervix	Myometrial dysfunction, disproportion	Disproportion
Secondary adverse factors	Myometrial dysfunction, false labor, anesthesia	Excessive sedation, anesthesia†	Malposition, anesthesia†
Pathology manifest by	Prolonged latent phase, prolonged acceleration phase (?)	Protracted active phase Secondary arrest of descent	Prolonged deceleration phase, protracted descent
Aberrations benefited by	Therapeutic rest	Support or stimulation‡	Stimulation‡

*From Friedman EA: The functional divisions of labor. Am J Obstet Gynecol *109*: 274-280, 1971.

†Continuous caudal or epidural anesthesia when improperly administered, i.e., too early, too high level, or with coexisting adverse factor.

‡Oxytocin stimulation indicated only in absence of cephalopelvic disproportion for arrested progress.

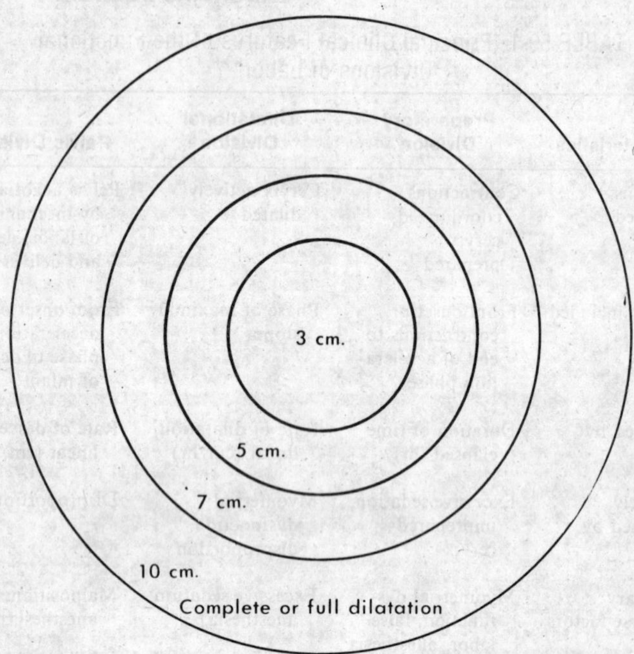

Figure 59-1.

SUBJECTIVE DATA

Abdominal pain, intermittent and rhythmic, coincides with uterine contractions. Initially, the pain may be perceived in the back. As labor progresses the contractions become stronger, more frequent, and increasingly painful.

Vaginal Discharge or Bleeding: As the cervix dilates, a vaginal discharge of thick, blood-streaked mucus—"bloody show"—may be noted.

Rupture of the Membranes: A gush of amniotic fluid from the vagina may precede the onset of labor or may occur during labor.

Bearing-down sensation is often symptomatic of the second stage of labor. As the baby's head descends, rectal pressure gives the patient the sensation that she needs to have a bowel movement. Increased bloody show and bulging of the perineum presage imminent delivery.

OBJECTIVE DATA

Abdominal Examination: Intermittent uterine contractions are usually palpable abdominally. Initially, contractions may occur 5 to 15 minutes apart; they gradually become more frequent as labor progresses. During the latter part of the first stage and during the second stage, contractions frequently recur every two or three minutes. The duration of the contractions also increases from 30 to 45 and 60 seconds as labor progresses.

Vaginal Examination: The cervix becomes effaced and dilated (see (Fig. 59-1). If membranes are intact, the amniotic sac may bulge through the cervical os. After membranes are ruptured, amniotic fluid may be expressed with each contraction.

ASSESSMENT

DIFFERENTIAL DIAGNOSIS

Differential diagnosis of true labor includes false labor and dysfunctional labor.

False labor contractions are usually not progressive, whereas true labor contractions tend to become stronger. The pain of false labor is more likely to be irregular and may be localized to the abdomen rather than to the back. False labor represents intrinsic uterine contractions that become perceptible or even painful toward the end of gestation. The contractions effect neither effacement nor dilatation of the cervix.

Dysfunctional labor can be very painful, but it does not effect the progressive cervical dilatation and effacement characteristic of true labor.

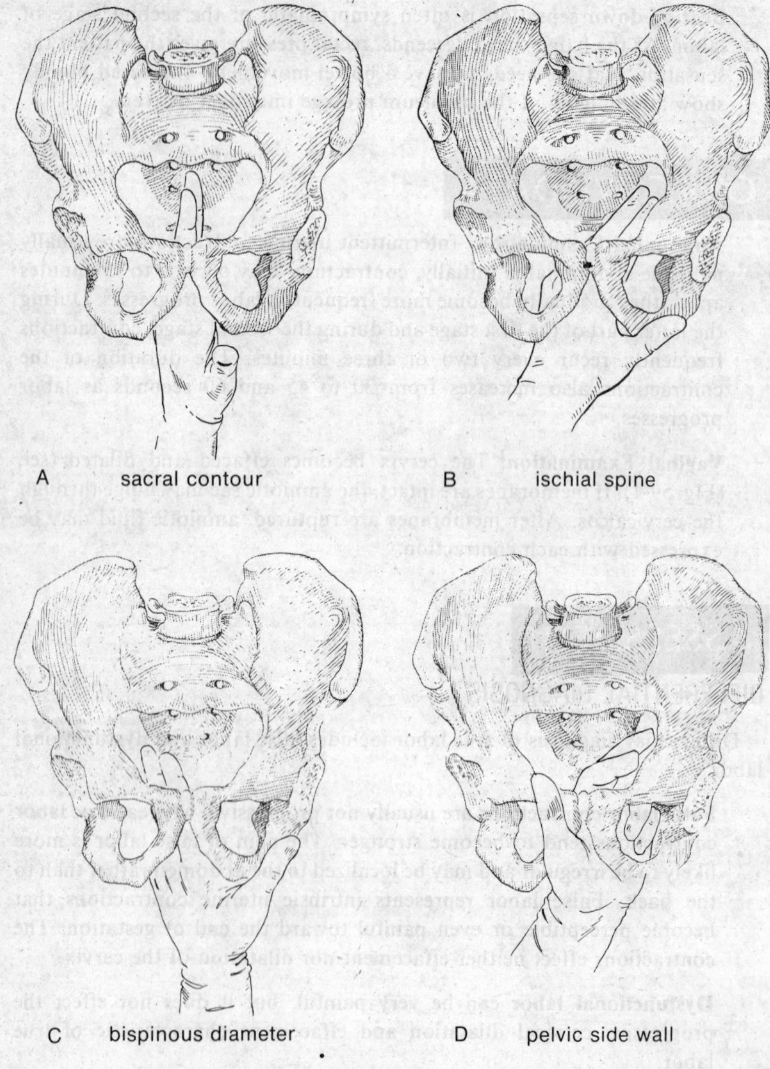
A sacral contour
B ischial spine
C bispinous diameter
D pelvic side wall

Figure 59-2.

PROGRESS OF LABOR

Progress of labor may be evaluated in terms of "powers," "passengers," and "passages."

"Powers" refers to the uterine contractions responsible for cervical dilatation as well as to the abdominal muscular contractions that contribute to fetal descent and delivery. In normal labor, contractions occur with increasing frequency and intensity as labor progresses.

"Passengers" refers to the fetus, placenta, and membranes. Fetal size, heart tones, presentation, and position and the station of the presenting part must be evaluated. In normal labor, the fetal heart rate is normal and the presenting part descends as labor progresses.

"Passages" refers to the cervix and bony pelvis. At the onset of labor, the cervix may be posterior. With effacement, the cervix comes into a mid-position. As labor progresses, the cervix becomes softer, effaces, and dilates. The bony pelvis may be evaluated clinically and radiologically. On vaginal examination, the diagonal conjugate, the distance between the ischial spines and the sacral curvature, may be evaluated. Outlet evaluation includes an estimate of the subpubic angle and the intertuberous diameter. For normal labor to occur, there can be no fetopelvic disproportion. (See Fig. 59-2.)

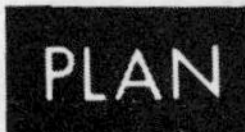

ADDITIONAL DIAGNOSTIC DATA

X-ray pelvimetry may be helpful when there is any clinical suspicion of fetopelvic disproportion.

MANAGEMENT

If the patient is seen in early labor, an enema may be given to evacuate the lower bowel. Because of the risk of the patient's vomiting during labor, she should not receive any foods orally. To prevent dehydration, intravenous fluids are recommended. Oral antacids may reduce the risk of aspiration pneumonitis.

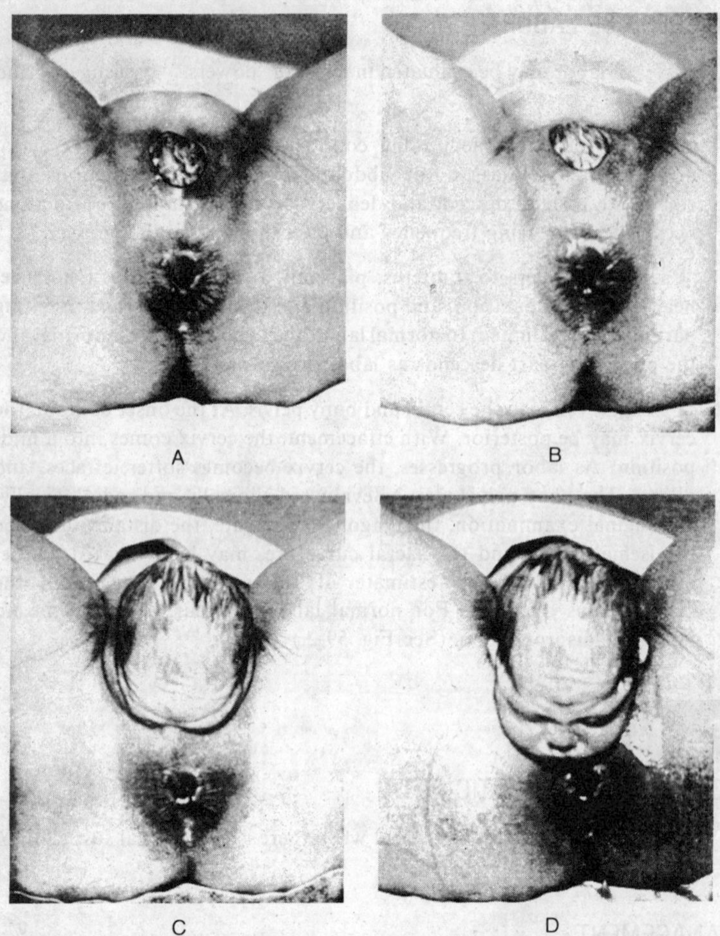

Figure 59-3. *A*, Head beginning to distend perineum, a process called "crowning." Note anus is flattened. *B*, Perineum much distended and thinned. Note glistening surface of the stretched perineal skin. Anus is opened, showing anterior wall of rectum. *C*, Perineum slipping back over face. Fetal head in process of being delivered by extension as the perineum slips back over the face of the fetus. *D*, Fetal head is delivered and the perineum is retracted under the chin. Greenhill JP, Friedman EA: Biological principles and modern practice of Obstetrics. W.B. Saunders Company, 1974.

When delivery is imminent, no attempt should ever be made to forcibly restrain the natural mechanism of fetal descent. If the patient is pushing excessively, however, she should be encouraged to cease bearing down and to breathe rapidly through her mouth (pant) during uterine contractions.

Meanwhile, delivery preparations are expedited. Whenever time permits, the perineum is cleansed with soap and water. In emergency situations, spontaneous delivery is often inevitable.

As the head distends the perineum and vulva, the perineal skin may be slipped back over the face (Fig. 59-3). If a perineal tear appears likely, a well-placed *episiotomy* (median or mediolateral) can avoid paraurethral and vaginal lacerations, as well as provide protection for the rectal sphincter. A clean surgical incision is preferred to a jagged tear wherever possible. (See Episiotomy, p. 779.)

If the child is delivered with the amniotic sac intact over the head, the child is said to be born with a *caul*. The caul must be removed as soon as the head is delivered, to allow the infant to breathe.

Once the head has been delivered, the mouth and nasopharynx should be suctioned with a bulb syringe.

At this point, the infant's neck should be examined to determine whether the umbilical cord is wrapped around the neck. If so, a gentle attempt should be made to slip the cord over the head or the shoulder. If this fails, the tight umbilical cord may have to be doubly clamped and cut before the shoulders are delivered. Tension on the umbilical cord is avoided in order to prevent tearing, with consequent fetal blood loss.

After the head has been delivered, the shoulders usually follow with the next contraction. The patient is asked to bear down until the anterior shoulder is delivered. This may be aided by gently depressing the head. This is followed by delivery of the posterior shoulder aided by gentle elevation of the head. The remainder of the baby's body then slips from the vagina without difficulty, the sole manipulation required of the obstetric attendant being support of the infant as it emerges from the introitus. The umbilical cord is then doubly clamped and cut (unless this was done previously). (Although the optimal time for clamping the umbilical cord is still a subject of discussion, the cord is generally clamped as soon as is reasonably convenient. The infant is never elevated above the introitus nor depressed below the introitus before the cord is clamped. With premature infants, particularly, the risk of circulatory overloading from placental transfusion may be formidable.)

A newborn infant normally cries and breathes spontaneously within one minute after birth. If necessary, respirations may be stimulated by gently rubbing the infant's back or patting the soles of the feet. The airway must be cleared of all mucus and fluid with gentle bulb suction and the infant placed into a warm environment.

If the infant does not breathe spontaneously, active resuscitation is required (see Resuscitation of the Newborn, p. 845).

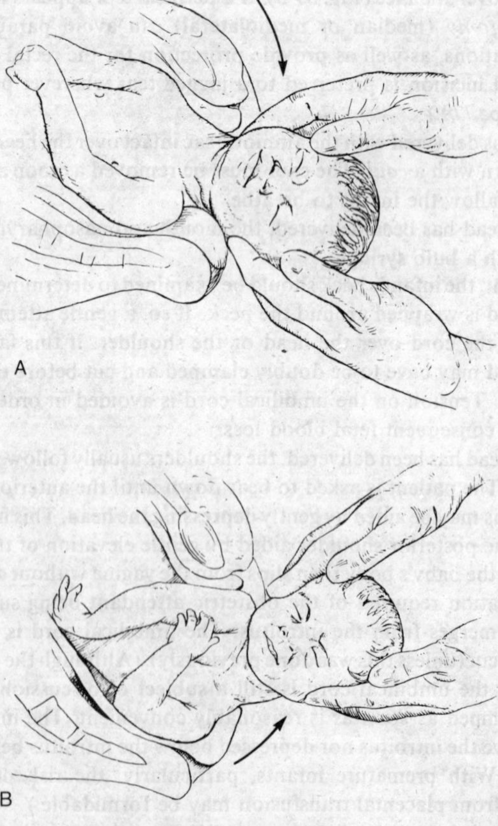

Figure 59-4A and B.

If the amniotic fluid is meconium stained, immediate laryngeal visualization and direct tracheal suction appear to decrease the risk of meconium aspiration (Ting, 1975).

Following delivery of the infant, uterine contractions often cease for several minutes as the uterus accommodates to its markedly diminished intracavitary volume. Once rhythmic uterine contractions resume, the placenta is expelled (usually within 20 minutes). As long as bleeding is minimal, spontaneous placental separation is awaited. (If bleeding is excessive, however, or if the placenta fails to separate after 30 minutes, the placenta may have to be removed manually under appropriate anesthesia.)

The Brandt-Andrews maneuver may aid in the management of the third stage of labor (Fig. 59-5). The umbilical cord is held in one hand while the fingertips of the other hand are pressed between the symphysis pubis and the contracted uterine fundus. When the uterus is elevated, there is no increase in umbilical cord tension if the placenta has separated. The placenta is then delivered with gentle traction on the cord while the fundus is elevated. (If the cord moves upward with the uterus, the placenta is still in the upper uterine segment and has not separated; further cord traction is deferred.)

As soon as the placenta has been delivered, oxytocin (10 units) is added to 500 ml of an intravenous infusion or administered intramuscularly to aid uterine contractions and minimize postpartum blood loss. Ergonovine (0.2mg) may be given intramuscularly unless the mother's blood pressure is elevated.

The placenta is carefully examined for completeness; the maternal surface is checked for the presence of all cotyledons. Interrupted blood vessels on the fetal surface of the placenta may be indicative of a missing succenturiate lobe. Whenever there is any question of retained placental fragments, the uterine cavity is explored.

The vulva and vagina are examined for injuries and undue bleeding. Actively bleeding lacerations are repaired.

Rh immune globulin is recommended for every Rh-negative unsensitized mother.

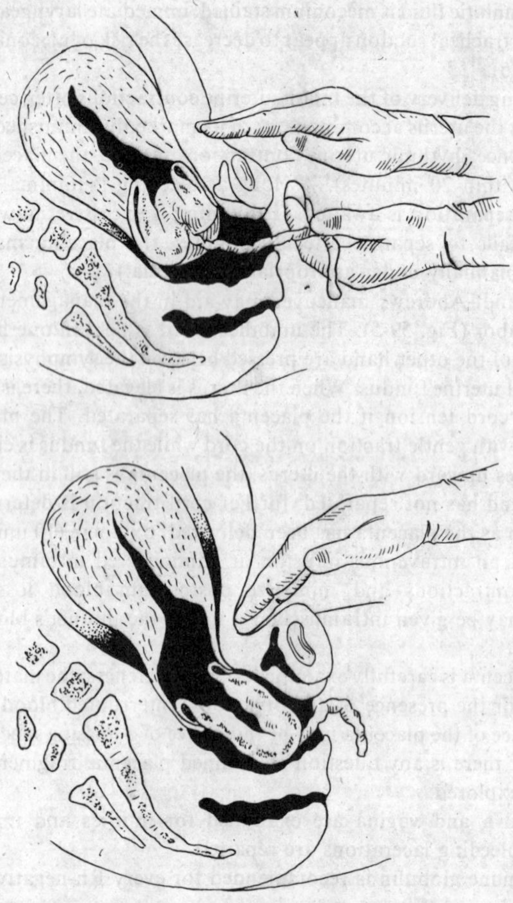

Figure 59-5. Brandt method of expressing the separated placenta. The cord is grasped in the left hand and the right hand is placed above the symphysis in order to elevate the uterus with a backward and upward pressure. If the placenta is separated, no increase in tension on the cord is felt. If the cord becomes taut and moves upward, the placenta is not completely separated. Further cord traction is postponed until upward pressure on the uterus fails to increase the cord tension. When placental separation is complete, the placenta is expressed by backward and downward pressure with the hand above the symphysis. Following delivery of the placenta the uterus is again elevated out of the pelvis.

Dysfunctional Labor

GENERAL CONSIDERATIONS

Dysfunctional labor (dystocia) may be defined as abnormal labor resulting from any variation of the normal patterns in the latent or active phases of cervical dilatation, such as a prolonged latent phase, protracted active phase, or secondary arrest of cervical dilatation.

Owing to the increasing interest in natural childbirth and home deliveries, some pregnant patients may seek medical care only after prolonged labor or prolonged rupture of the membranes or both. Evaluation of these patients requires consideration of possible abnormalities of

Powers (uterine and abdominal muscles): Uterine contractions may be hypotonic or hypertonic.

Passages: The bony pelvis or maternal soft tissues may obstruct fetal descent.

Passenger: Fetal malpresentation or abnormal development may impede normal delivery.

SUBJECTIVE AND OBJECTIVE DATA

Uterine contractions may be irregular and variable with respect to frequency, duration, and intensity.

The pelvis may feel contracted, and the presenting part may or may not be well engaged (Fig. 59-6). The possibility of fetal malpresentation (cephalic deflexion, breech, or transverse lie) must be excluded.

Fetal station and cervical dilatation are determined and then plotted on a graph with time on the horizontal axis.

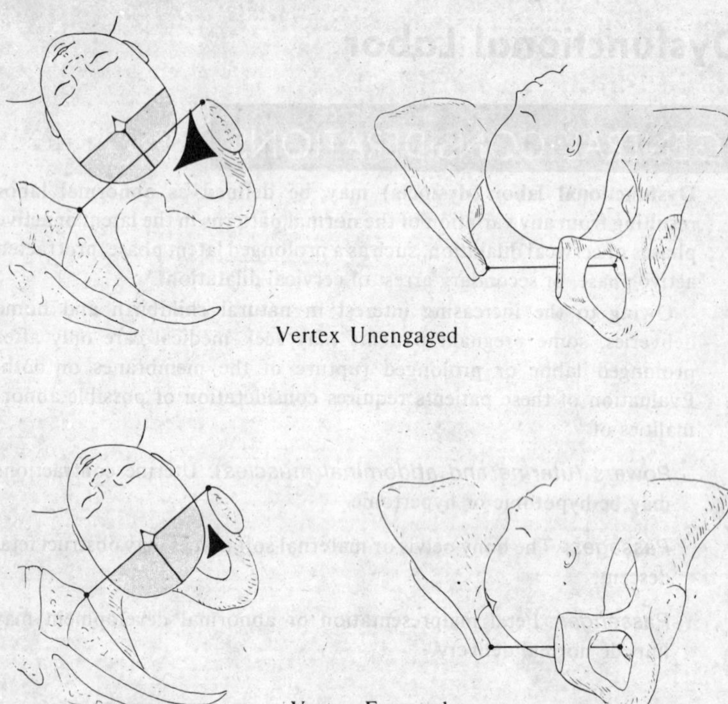

Figure 59-6. Engagement is indicated by descent of the vertex to the level of the interspinous line (zero station).

ASSESSMENT

DIFFERENTIAL DIAGNOSIS

The differential diagnosis of dysfunctional labor patterns includes (1) a prolonged latent phase, (2) protraction disorders, and (3) arrest disorders.

Prolonged latent phase (uterine contractions without active cervical dilatation) is defined by Friedman (1971) as 20 hours or more in nulliparas or 14 hours or more in multiparas (Figure 59-7, line 1).

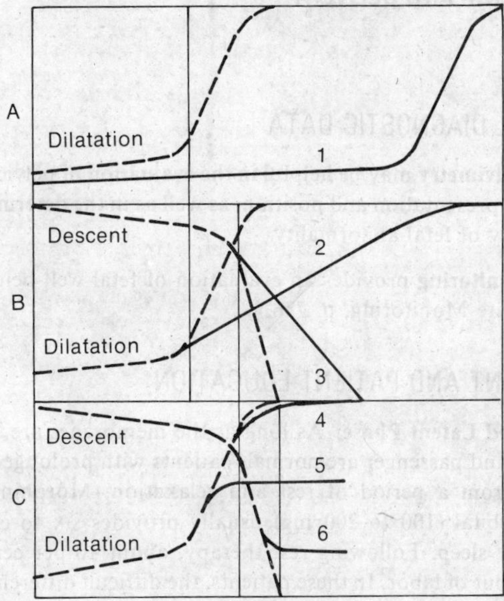

Figure 59-7.

Protraction Disorders:

Protracted active-phase dilatation is defined as a rate of cervical dilatation less than 1.2 cm per hour in nulliparas and less than 1.5 cm per hour in multiparas (Fig. 59-7, line 2).

Protracted descent occurs when the rate of descent is under 1 cm per hour in nulliparas and 2 cm per hour in multiparas, based on station determinations in centimeters above or below the plane of the ischial spines (Fig. 59-7, line 3).

Arrest Disorders:

Secondary arrest of dilatation is apparent when the expected linear progression of cervical dilatation in the active phase ceases for at least two hours (Fig. 59-7, line 5).

Arrest of descent is recognized by descent interrupted, usually in the second stage, for at least one hour (Fig. 59-7, line 6).

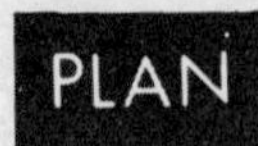

ADDITIONAL DIAGNOSTIC DATA

X-ray pelvimetry may be helpful in the evaluation of pelvic architecture, and fetal presentation and position, as well as in the determination of the possibility of fetal abnormality.

Fetal monitoring provides an evaluation of fetal well-being. (See Fetal Heart Rate Monitoring, p. 786.)

MANAGEMENT AND PATIENT EDUCATION

Prolonged Latent Phase: As long as the membranes are intact and the passage and passenger are normal, patients with prolonged latent phase benefit from a period of rest and relaxation. Morphine (15 mg) or pentobarbital (100 to 200 mg) usually provides six to eight hours of necessary sleep. Following rest therapy, about 10 per cent of patients awaken out of labor. In these patients, the difficult differential diagnosis of false labor has been established in retrospect.

If ineffective, uncoordinated contractions persist or recur, amniotomy and oxytocin stimulation may be effective in producing active-phase progression. If a normal labor pattern fails to develop or if fetal distress occurs, cesarean section becomes necessary.

Protraction Disorders (Passenger and Passage Normal): If uterine contractions are hypotonic, oxytocin augmentation and amniotomy may be beneficial. Close fetal monitoring is essential.

If uterine contractions are of normal intensity and frequency, amniotomy is usually performed. Continued progress should be expected with the administration of emotional support, intravenous fluids, and appropriate sedation. Evidence of fetal distress or arrest of descent necessitates cesarean section.

Arrest Disorders (Passenger and Passage Normal): If uterine contractions are hypotonic and ineffectual, oxytocin augmentation and amniotomy often are successful in effecting resumption of progress. The optimal duration of stimulation is between three and seven hours.

Cesarean section is indicated whenever the arrest persists or fetal distress develops.

Cephalopelvic Disproportion or Fetal Malpresentation: Cesarean section is recommended for delivery.

Fetal Dystocia

GENERAL CONSIDERATIONS

Fetal dystocia is defined as abnormal labor due to an anomaly, abnormal size, or abnormal position of the fetus. Fetal malformations include hydrocephalus; abdominal distention from ascites, tumors, and congenital cystic kidneys; and conjoined twins.

Shoulder Dystocia: After the infant's head has been delivered, impaction of the shoulder girdle against the symphysis pubis (shoulder dystocia) is an urgent emergency requiring immediate corrective action. Although predisposing factors include macrosomia associated with diabetes mellitus, and fetal abnormalities, the problem often arises suddenly and unexpectedly. Immediately after the head has been delivered the condition becomes apparent when the head is pulled back tightly against the perineum and the shoulders do not follow with gentle traction. Potential complications include brachial plexus damage, fractured fetal clavicle, and fetal anoxia.

The treatment objective is release of the anterior shoulder from its impacted position without injury to the cervical nerve roots (brachial plexus). Unnecessary haste and overly aggressive force must be avoided, since excessive lateral flexion of the neck and overly vigorous traction of the head or neck increases the probability of damage to the brachial plexus. Excessive fundal pressure may aggravate the shoulder impaction.

Management: The two methods most frequently recommended are rotation of the shoulder girdle and delivery of the posterior arm. Both are facilitated by an adequate episiotomy and anesthesia.

Rotation: The bisacromial diameter must be dislodged from the impacted position against the symphysis pubis and rotated into an oblique diameter of the pelvis. With the fingers of one hand inside

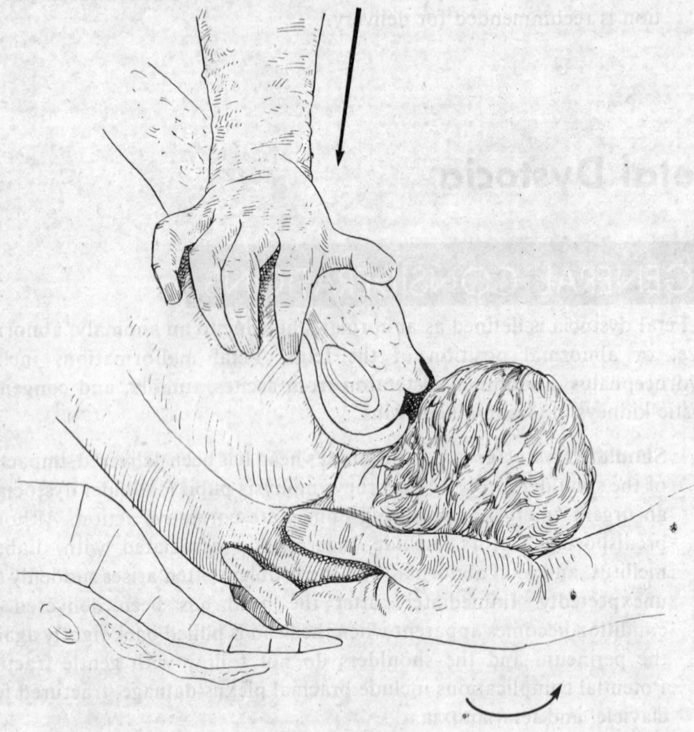

Figure 59-8.

the vagina and the opposite hand outside, light suprapubic pressure is exerted against the anterior shoulder while the posterior shoulder is being pulled downward and into the left posterior quadrant. At times it may be necessary to rotate the shoulder girdle through 180°, utilizing the screw principle of Woods. The posterior shoulder is rotated anteriorly and downward in a corkscrew fashion (Fig. 59-9).

Delivery of Posterior Arm: The obstetrician's hand is inserted along the hollow of the sacrum in order to grasp the infant's posterior arm and hand, which are pulled downward across the baby's chest and delivered. The shoulder girdle is then rotated into one of the oblique

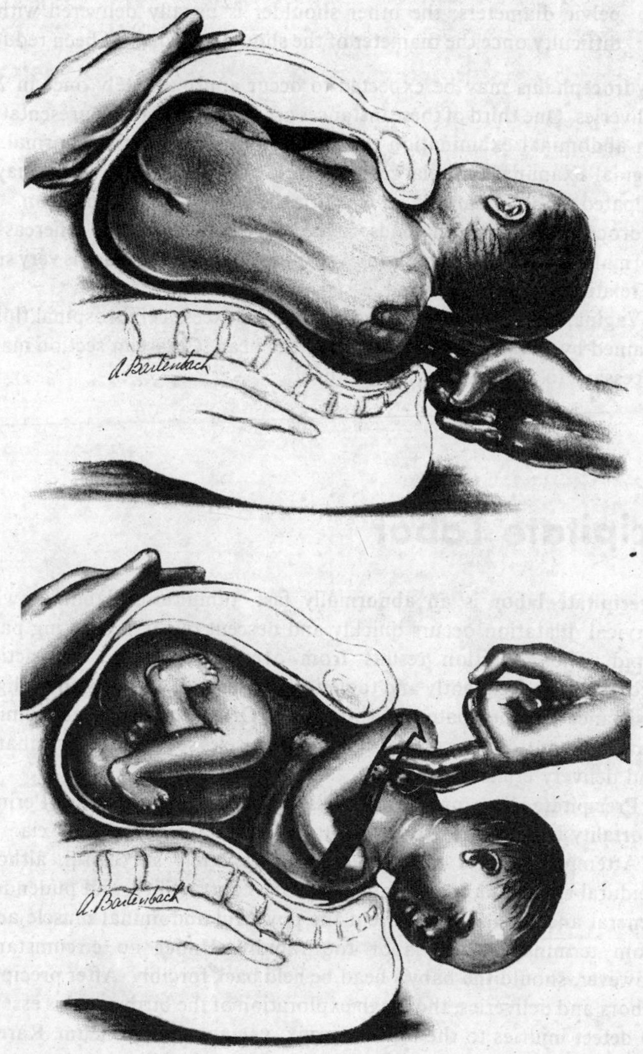

Figure 59-9A and B. Shoulder Dystocia. The posterior shoulder is rotated with lateral, clockwise pressure.

pelvic diameters; the other shoulder is usually delivered without difficulty once the diameter of the shoulder girdle has been reduced.

Hydrocephalus may be expected to occur approximately once in 2000 deliveries. One third of these instances are in cases of breech presentation. On abdominal examination the head may feel larger than normal. On vaginal examination enlarged fontanels and wide suture lines may be palpated. The diagnosis is confirmed by x-ray examination. The hydrocephalic cranium tends to be large and globular, whereas the normal head is ovoid. The cranial outline is thin, and the face is very small in relation to the large head.

Vaginal delivery is usually possible if the excess cerebrospinal fluid is drained by spinal needle puncture of the head. Cesarean section may be necessary to prevent uterine rupture.

Precipitate Labor

Precipitate labor is an abnormally fast, tumultuous labor in which cervical dilatation occurs quickly and descent of the presenting part is rapid. The condition results from overactive uterine contractions, occurring too frequently and too intensely, in conjunction with negligible resistance of the maternal soft parts. Often there are concomitant powerful contractions of the abdominal muscles so that labor is enhanced and delivery effected quickly.

Precipitate labor may be injurious to both mother and fetus. Perinatal mortality is increased from both trauma and associated hypoxia.

Attempts to treat this dysfunction are rarely successful, although epidural anesthesia may diminish uterine contractility, and pudendal or general anesthesia may prevent the powerful abdominal muscle action from terminating the labor too rapidly. Under no circumstances, however, should the baby's head be held back forcibly. After precipitate labors and deliveries, thorough exploration of the birth canal is essential to detect injuries to the uterus, cervix, vagina, and perineum. Rare but serious consequences that should be anticipated include uterine rupture, amniotic fluid embolism, and postpartum hemorrhage.

Premature Labor

GENERAL CONSIDERATIONS

Premature labor may be defined as regular uterine contractions with progressive dilatation of the cervix after the twentieth week of gestation and prior to the thirty-seventh week.

SUBJECTIVE AND OBJECTIVE DATA

Uterine contractions are regular and rhythmic.

Vaginal examination determines the degree of cervical effacement and dilatation as well as the status of the amniotic sac (intact or ruptured).

Fetal maturity is assessed by one or more of the following measures:

1. Gestational age based on menstrual history
2. Fetal weight estimated by abdominal palpation
3. Biparietal diameter on ultrasound examination
4. Amniocentesis—lecithin-sphingomyelin ratio values of 2:1 or more suggest fetal lung maturity. Creatinine values of 2 or more suggest a fetal weight greater than 2500 gm.

ASSESSMENT

PREDISPOSING FACTORS

These include uterine anomalies (bicornuate uterus and so forth), urinary tract infection, hypertensive disease, amnionitis, maternal smoking, and previous premature labor.

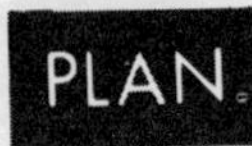

ADDITIONAL DIAGNOSTIC DATA

Amniocentesis: Amniotic fluid analysis provides an estimate of fetal lung maturity as well as of the possibility of intrauterine infection or Rh isoimmunization. (See Amniocentesis, p. 731.)

MANAGEMENT AND PATIENT EDUCATION

Whether premature labor should be suppressed, if possible, depends on the answer to the question, Is further intrauterine stay more likely to benefit or harm the fetus? In the case of placental insufficiency, for example, fetal growth may be retarded; the fetus may be expected to fare better in the high-risk nursery than in a hostile intrauterine environment.

Furthermore, none of the treatment regimens proposed for labor suppression have proven to be consistently effective and safe for both mother and fetus. Methods under investigation include ethanol, beta adrenergic stimulators, antiprostaglandin agents, and long-acting progestational hormones. Bed rest and reassurance are traditional methods that may be beneficial in decreasing maternal anxiety.

If the gestational age is greater than 34 weeks, if the amniotic sac is ruptured, or if there is evidence of fetal lung maturity (L/S ratio of 2 or more), labor is allowed to proceed spontaneously. In addition, when conditions are present that may be life endangering to the fetus or mother (placental separation, intrauterine infection, severe preeclampsia, hypertensive cardiovascular disease, fetal distress), termination of pregnancy may be advantageous to both. In the case of fetal anomalies or fetal death there is no reason to inhibit normal labor.

However, when there is no evidence of a maternal or fetal pathologic condition and membranes are intact, labor is inhibited, if possible, to allow the fetus to remain *in utero* as long as the intrauterine environment remains favorable. This grants the fetus as much development endowment as feasible.

Ethanol administered intravenously has inhibited labor and delayed delivery in some patients (Zlatnik and Fuchs, 1972). A loading dose of 10 per cent ethanol in 5 per cent dextrose in water is initiated at a rate of 15 ml/kg over *two* hours. This is followed by a maintenance dose of 1.5 ml/kg each hour over the next *ten* hours. After 12 hours the alcohol is tapered off gradually.

Although ethanol appears to suppress endogenous oxytocin, it has several disadvantages; patients must be watched very closely. Under the influence of ethanol patients become inebriated and are often restless and crying. Increased gastric acid production plus the sedation and nausea may increase the risk of pulmonary aspiration. (A dose of 15 to 30 ml of antacids should be given orally every two or three hours to neutralize gastric pH and reduce the risk of aspiration pneumonitis.)

Corticosteroids appear to accelerate fetal lung maturity. Both betamethasone and dexamethasone have been reported to decrease the incidence of respiratory distress syndrome (RDS) among infants born prior to 34 weeks' gestation. (Liggins, 1972; Ballard, 1976). Although the optimal dosage, optimal duration of therapy, and long-term risks are still unknown, an initial intramuscular dose of 12 mg of dexamethasone or betamethasone may be followed by a second dose after 12 to 24 hours. Labor is suppressed, if possible, for 24 to 48 hours.

Inevitable Premature Delivery: When premature delivery is inevitable, the optimal neonatal outcome would be anticipated when the mother can be delivered in a hospital prepared for intensive care of premature, immature infants. During labor, analgesic medications are minimized to avoid neonatal respiratory depression; epidural or pudendal block anesthesia is preferred. A generous episiotomy is recommended to prevent cranial trauma. Although gentle delivery with low forceps is advocated by many to protect the fragile fetal head, opinions differ over the merits of spontaneous delivery versus those of forceps delivery. The cord is promptly clamped to avoid placental transfusion, which is poorly tolerated by the premature cardiovascular and hepatobiliary systems. The premature neonate must be handled very gently and protected from heat loss.

Cesarean section is frequently recommended for the delivery of a premature infant in a breech presentation.

Childbirth Outside the Hospital

The virtues and risks of delivery outside a hospital environment have been the subject of acrimonious debates. Regardless of one's opinion in this matter, and despite the most careful plans, the first stage of labor may progress so rapidly that delivery occurs before the woman can reach the hospital. Under such circumstances, the basic principle must be delivery of the mother with minimal trauma and without injury to the child.

When the woman is straining as if to have a bowel movement, the vagina is bulging, and the fetal head is visible at the vaginal opening, delivery is imminent. *No attempt should be made to restrain or delay delivery.* The mother should lie on her back with her knees flexed and widely separated. A pillow or firm pad may be placed under the buttocks to facilitate the delivery of the baby's head and shoulders. In an automobile, the mother may be placed flat on the seat with one leg bent and resting on the seat while the other foot rests on the floorboard.

The attendant stands at the patient's side and places the palm of the hand over the advancing head in order to assist with extension of the head and, at the same time, prevent the head from popping out of the vagina (Fig. 59-10).

As the head emerges, the mother is constantly reassured and encouraged *not* to push, in order to minimize the trauma associated with expulsive delivery. The most satisfactory method for inhibiting the desire to push, which is involuntary and overwhelmingly strong when the head is distending the perineum, is for the mother to breathe through her mouth as deeply as she can.

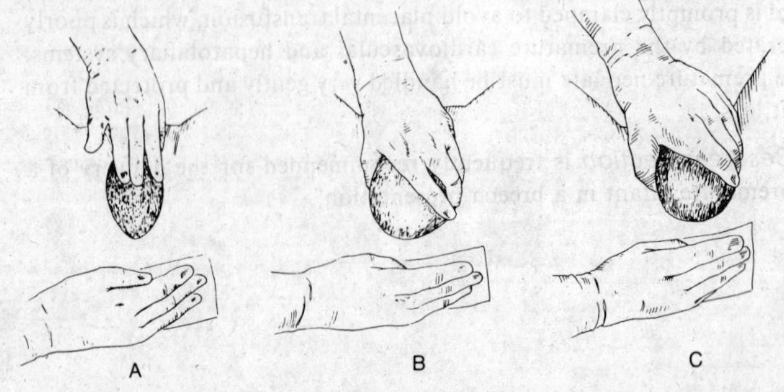

Figure 59-10.

Uterine contractions are sufficient force for delivery of the head. If the mother protests that she has to move her bowels, she must be reassured that the sensation is a normal one, resulting from the pressure of the baby's head on her rectum. If necessary, the baby's chin is freed by slipping the index finger under the side of the jaw and sweeping the finger below the chin. Mucus is wiped from the baby's mouth and nostrils; the air passages must be clear. If a bulb syringe is available, the tip is inserted into the baby's mouth in order to aspirate mucus and fluids. This procedure is repeated three or four times to clear the baby's mouth and nose.

If the umbilical cord is wrapped around the baby's neck, it can usually be slipped over the anterior shoulder, which is born during the contraction following birth of the head. Expulsion of the anterior shoulder may be facilitated by gentle depression of the head toward the anus. Traction on the head, however, must be minimal. After the anterior shoulder is free, the baby's head is guided in an upward direction toward the mother's abdomen so that the posterior shoulder can escape over the perineum slowly and smoothly. The uterine contraction is usually sufficient to accomplish the expulsion of the body.

When the feet have been born, the baby should be held at the level of the vaginal introitus until the cord is clamped. The baby is very slippery and may be placed on the bed or surface between the mother's legs. The baby should not be held with its head straight down.

The umbilical cord is doubly clamped or tied with plastic clamps, rubber bands, or linen or tape ligatures; the cord is cut between the two clamps or ties.

By this time the baby is usually breathing on its own. The baby should be kept warm with a blanket or towel arranged so that only the baby's face is exposed.

Emergency vehicles should carry a sterile delivery pack containing the following items:

1. Surgical scissors
2. Three hemostats or cord clamps
3. Umbilical tape or sterilized cord
4. Ear syringe, rubber bulb-type, for aspiration of the baby's mouth and airway
5. Five towels
6. One dozen, 4×4-inch gauze sponges
7. Three or four pairs of rubber gloves
8. Baby blanket
9. Sanitary napkins

REFERENCES

Ballard RA, Ballard PL: Use of prenatal glucocorticoid therapy to prevent respiratory distress syndrome. Am J Dis Child *130*:982-987, 1976

Brown BJ, Gabert HA, Stenchever MA: Respiratory distress syndrome. Obstet Gynecol Surv *30*:71-90, 1975

Dignam WJ: Difficulties in delivery, including shoulder dystocia and malpresentations of the fetus. Clin Obstet Gynecol *19*:577-585, 1976

Friedman EA: The functional divisions of labor. Am J Obstet Gynecol *109*:274-280, 1971

Fuchs F: Prevention of prematurity. Am J Obstet Gynecol *126*:809-820, 1976

Gluck L: Administration of corticosteroids to induce maturation of fetal lung. Am J Dis Child *130*:976-978, 1976

Greenhill JP, Friedman EA: Biological principles and modern practice of obstetrics. Philadelphia, W.B. Saunders Company, 1974

Hendricks CH, Brenner WE, Kraus G: Normal cervical dilatation pattern in late pregnancy and labor. Am J Obstet Gynecol *106*:1065-1082, 1970

Hibbard LT: Shoulder dystocia. Obstet Gynecol *34*:424-429, 1969

Johnson JWC, Austin KL, Jones GS, et al: Efficacy of 17 alpha hydroxyprogesterone caproate in the prevention of premature labor. N Engl J Med *293*:675-680, 1975; Obstet Gynecol Surv *31*:114-115, 1976

Liggins GC: Adrenocortical related maturational events in the fetus. Am J Obstet Gynecol *126*:931-941, 1976

Liggins GC, Howie RN: A controlled trial of antepartum glucocorticoid treatment for prevention of the respiratory distress syndrome in premature infants. Pediatrics *50*:515-525, 1972

Perkins RP: Antenatal assessment of fetal maturity. Obstet Gynecol Surv *29*:369-384, 1974

Ting P, Brady JP: Tracheal suction in meconium aspiration. Am J Obstet Gynecol *122*:767-771, 1975

Zlatnik FJ, Fuchs F: A controlled study of ethanol in threatened premature labor. Am J Obstet Gynecol *112*:610-612, 1972

60 LEIOMYOMA

GENERAL CONSIDERATIONS

Leiomyoma of the uterus is a well-circumscribed but nonencapsulated benign uterine tumor composed mainly of muscle but with a variable fibrous connective tissue element. Grossly, leiomyomas may occur anywhere within the uterus: subserosal (sometimes pedunculated), intramural, or submucosal, encroaching on the uterine cavity. Usually they are multiple, although they may be single. Leiomyomas are well demarcated from the surrounding muscle, which they may flatten to form a false capsule, but they have no true capsule. Microscopically, the leiomyoma is composed of groups and bundles of smooth muscle fibers in a twisted, whorled pattern.

Commonly asymptomatic, leiomyomas can on occasion be responsible for acute problems. Degeneration or hemorrhage within a leiomyoma is especially likely to occur during pregnancy. Torsion of a pedunculated tumor may cause acute tissue necrosis.

Leiomyomas, commonly called *fibroids or myomas*, are the most common uterine tumor.

SUBJECTIVE DATA

CURRENT SYMPTOMS

Abdominal pain can be caused by torsion, degeneration, or hemorrhage within the tumor. Cramping pain may be due to uterine contractions attempting to deliver a fibroid polyp through the cervical canal.

Vaginal Bleeding: Prolonged, excessive menstrual periods may be associated with submucous leiomyomas. Profuse, gushing bleeding can be caused by a submucous fibroid polyp. Endometrium covering a leiomyoma is often thin and atrophic as a result of congestion, necrosis, and ulceration. Furthermore, the endometrial surface area is increased by tumors that enlarge and distort the endometrial cavity.

Submucous and intramural leiomyomas may affect uterine hemostatic mechanisms by mechanical interference with the endometrial blood supply, causing endometrial venule ectasia or impairing normal vascular occlusion at the times of menses. Associated anovulation may cause bleeding from a persistently proliferative endometrium.

Other Symptoms: Syncope and weakness may be caused by hypovolemia or anemia.

PRIOR HISTORY

There may be a history of asymptomatic uterine leiomyomas or heavy menses.

OBJECTIVE DATA

PHYSICAL EXAMINATION

Abdominal Examination: A much enlarged uterus may be palpable abdominally. The tumors are felt as firm, irregular nodules; tender areas suggest degenerative changes.

Leiomyomas are more likely to be palpable abdominally during pregnancy.

Abdominal tenderness with rebound tenderness may be caused by intraperitoneal bleeding from ruptured veins on the surface of the tumor.

Pelvic Examination: The cervix is usually normal. On occasion, however, a pedunculated submucous leiomyoma may initiate cervical dilatation and be visible in the cervical os.

The uterus tends to be irregularly enlarged and nodular. Tenderness depends on the degree of degeneration and vascular compromise. Unless there is a coexisting adnexal pathologic condition, the uterus is frequently mobile. The endometrial cavity may be enlarged by submucous tumors. The possibility of leiomyomas coexisting with pregnancy must always be considered.

LABORATORY TESTS

Complete Blood Count with Blood Smear: Leukocytosis may be caused by necrosis resulting from torsion or degeneration. Decreased hemoglobin and hematocrit values indicate chronic blood loss.

ASSESSMENT

DIFFERENTIAL DIAGNOSIS

This must always consider the possibilities of pregnancy, an adnexal pathologic condition, and a coexisting uterine or abdominal pathologic condition. (See Abdominal Pain, p. 70, and Vaginal Bleeding, p. 686.)

POTENTIAL COMPLICATIONS

In addition to degeneration and torsion, other possible complications include abortion, premature labor, obstructed labor, and intraperitoneal hemorrhage.

PLAN

ADDITIONAL DIAGNOSTIC DATA

Pregnancy test for chorionic gonadotropin is frequently helpful in the evaluation of an enlarged uterus. Leiomyomas may cause symmetrical uterine enlargement simulating pregnancy or may coexist with pregnancy.

Ultrasound B-Scan: When uncertainty exists concerning a pelvic mass, an ultrasound B-scan may be helpful (see Fig. 60-1).

Intravenous pyelogram may also be helpful in the diagnostic evaluation (Birnholz, 1972).

Cervical Pap smear is always indicated to rule out cervical neoplasia prior to hysterectomy.

Hysterosalpingogram may be advisable when the patient desires future children in order to evaluate uterine cavity distortion and the patency of the fallopian tubes.

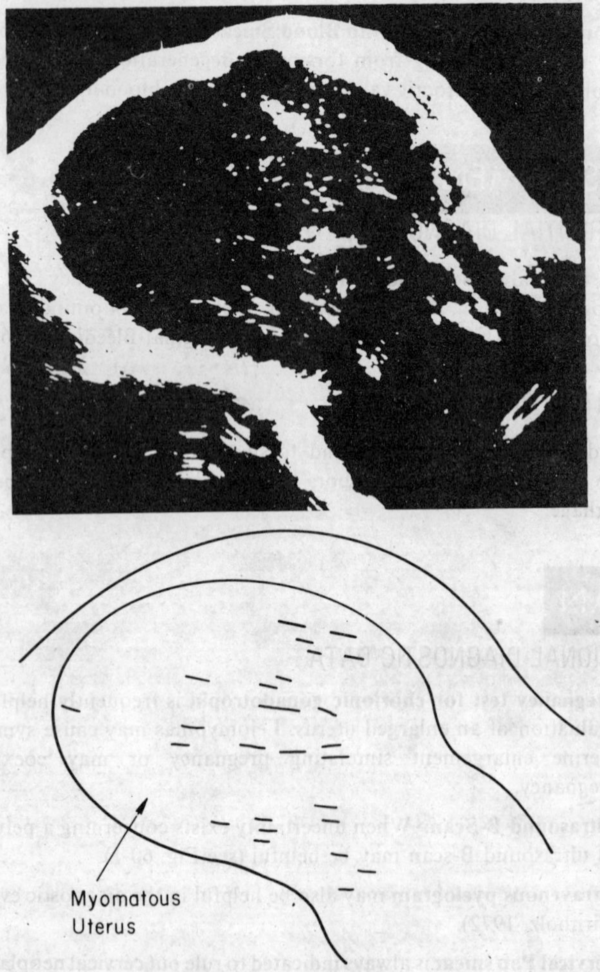

Figure 60-1. Sagittal scan of large solid pelvic mass made at high receiver sensitivity (gain). The presence of multiple small internal echoes indicates the complex nature of the mass. No uterus could be identified separate from the mass, which at surgery proved to be a leiomyoma. (From Schreiber MH (ed.): Symposium on obstetric and gynecologic radiology. Radiol Clin North Am 12:131, 1974.)

MANAGEMENT AND PATIENT EDUCATION

Emergency hospitalization is indicated whenever bleeding is life-threatening or acute abdominal pain must be differentiated from an acute surgical abdomen. The specific management plan must take into consideration:

1. The severity of the symptoms
2. The desire for future children
3. The size of the tumors

Nonpregnant Patients:

Endometrial curettage identifies endometrial abnormalities and rules out the possibility of endometrial malignancy. If the leiomyomas are small, not distorting the endometrial cavity, and if the endometrium indicates anovulatory bleeding, ovarian suppression with estrogen-progestin combination tablets may be considered. These hormones must be used very cautiously, however, since they may provoke growth of preexisting leiomyomas.

Myomectomy may be recommended when the patient wishes to preserve or enhance her childbearing potential. A fibroid polyp that has delivered through a dilated cervix may be removed vaginally by clamping and cutting the pedicle.

Hysterectomy is definitive treatment for persistent symptoms. However, it is recommended primarily for those symptomatic patients who do not desire future children.

Pregnant Patients: During pregnancy, bed rest, analgesia, and observation may be adequate initial therapy. Conservative management is always preferred when the infant is immature. Acute torsion or intra-abdominal hemorrhage, however, requires surgical intervention.

Cesarean section is indicated for delivery when leiomyomas have produced fetal malpresentation, uterine inertia, or mechanical obstruction.

REFERENCES

Birnholz JC: Uterine opacification during excretory urography. Radiology *105*:303-307, 1972; Obstet Gynecol Surv *28*:524-526, 1973

Farrer-Brown G, Beilby JOW, Tarbit MH: Venous changes in the endometrium of myomatous uteri. Obstet Gynecol *38*:743-751, 1971

61 LIVER DISEASE DURING PREGNANCY

GENERAL CONSIDERATIONS

Jaundice, yellow discoloration of the skin or sclerae by bilirubin, is usually apparent when the serum bilirubin concentration exceeds 2 or 3 mg per 100 ml. Hyperbilirubinemia can be caused by one or several mechanisms, including excessive pigment production (hemolysis), reduced hepatic uptake or conjugation of bilirubin, and decreased excretion of conjugated pigment (hepatocellular or biliary tract disease).

Liver diseases unique to pregnancy include cholestatic jaundice of pregnancy (cholestasis of pregnancy), acute fatty liver (very rare), and preeclampsia or eclampsia.

Jaundice during pregnancy may also occur as a result of hepatitis, hemolytic anemia, drug intake, gallstones, or cirrhosis.

Hepatic rupture, although rare, may occur suddenly in late pregnancy and may be associated with preeclampsia or eclampsia.

SUBJECTIVE DATA

Jaundice is usually the first indication of liver disease. Viral hepatitis may appear at any stage of gestation and is usually the most likely diagnosis. Associated symptoms include anorexia, nausea, vomiting, fatigue, fever, abdominal pain, and liver tenderness.

During the last trimester, jaundice preceded by *severe* generalized pruritus suggests cholestasis of pregnancy.

Abdominal pain, severe nausea and vomiting, hematemesis, headache, and impaired states of consciousness developing suddenly in late pregnancy are symptoms of acute fatty liver. Associated hypertension and proteinuria suggest preeclampsia. Shock and acute abdominal pain late in pregnancy can be caused by hepatic rupture with profuse intraabdominal hemorrhage.

OBJECTIVE DATA

General Examination: Icterus, spider angiomas, and palmar erythema are usual signs of liver disease. During uncomplicated pregnancy, spider angiomas and palmar erythema are relatively common, however; thus, they cannot be considered a sign of liver disease.

Abdominal Examination: Liver enlargement usually can be detected easily during early pregnancy; estimation of liver size in late pregnancy can be difficult. Splenomegaly may direct attention to the possibility of long-standing liver disease with secondary portal hypertension.

ASSESSMENT

DIFFERENTIAL DIAGNOSIS

Differential diagnosis of jaundice includes viral hepatitis, cholestatic jaundice of pregnancy, acute fatty liver of pregnancy, gallstones, drug reaction, hemolytic anemia, and cirrhosis (see Table 61-1).

Viral hepatitis, the most common cause of liver disease during pregnancy, follows essentially the same clinical course that it would be expected to follow in a nonpregnant woman of the same age.

Cholestatic jaundice of pregnancy (Table 61-2) is a clinical syndrome consisting of severe pruritus and mild jaundice during the last trimester of pregnancy. Alkaline phosphatase is increased seven- to tenfold, and bilirubin is usually less than 5 mg per 100 ml and virtually never more than 10 mg per 100 ml. Serum transaminases, SGOT and SGPT, may be normal or moderately increased.

Acute fatty liver of pregnancy (Table 61-3) is an extremely rare and highly fatal liver disease that begins abruptly between the thirty-sixth and fortieth weeks of pregnancy. Symptoms include severe and persistent vomiting, followed by abdominal pain, jaundice, and coma. Tachycardia and fever may be associated findings. The bilirubin is usually elevated but less than 10 mg per 100 ml. The level of alkaline phosphatase is higher

TABLE 61-1. Diagnosis of Liver Disease in Third Trimester*

	Histology	Albumin	SGOT†	Bilirubin†	Alkaline Phosphatase†
Normal pregnancy	Normal	↓ 20%	nl	sl ↑	2-fold ↑
Infectious hepatitis	Typical	↓ 20-40%	500-1000	1-5 mg per 100 ml	3-fold ↑
Cholestasis of pregnancy	Cholestasis	↓ 20%	nl	1-5 mg per 100 ml	10-fold ↑
Eclampsia	Sinusoidal fibrin	↓ 20%	100-250	sl ↑	2- to 3-fold ↑
Gallstone	Cholestasis	↓ 20%	nl to sl ↑	↑	3- to 10-fold ↑
Cirrhosis and chronic-active hepatitis	Cirrhosis	↓ 20-40%	50-150	1-5 mg per 100 ml	3-fold ↑
Fatty liver of pregnancy	Steatosis	↓ 40%	300-500	1-10 mg per 100 ml	3-fold ↑
Pyelonephritis	Portal inflammation	↓ 20%	100-300	sl ↑	3-fold ↑

*From Burrow GN, Ferris TF: Medical Complications during Pregnancy. Philadelphia, W.B. Saunders Company, 1975.

†These values indicate the usual range for each disorder.

nl=normal; sl=slight.

than that of normal pregnancy, and the SGOT is most often increased into the range of 300 to 500 units per ml. The prothrombin time is markedly prolonged, and leukocytosis with counts of 20,000 to 30,000 may be expected. Severe hypoglycemia and marked elevation of the level of arterial ammonia contribute to coma.

Hepatic rupture is characterized by the sudden onset of right upper quadrant pain, combined with tenderness upon palpation. Frequently the pain is referred to the right shoulder. Hepatic rupture is most likely to occur during the third trimester in multigravid patients between the ages of 35 and 45 who have associated preeclampsia or eclampsia. Although relatively rare, this possibility should always be considered when a pregnant patient undergoes sudden profound peripheral vascular collapse in association with abdominal symptoms and signs (Portnuff, 1972).

TABLE 61-2. Cholestatic Jaundice of Pregnancy*

Clinical Features	Biochemical Changes	
Pruritus	Alkaline phosphatase	7- to 10-fold ↑
Jaundice	5′-Nucleotidase	2-fold ↑
	Bilirubin (total)	nl to 5 mg per 100 ml
No anorexia or malaise	SGOT	<250 units
	BSP	10-25% retention
Last trimester†	Prothrombin time	nl to 2-fold ↑
Recurrent†	Serum bile acids	10- to 100-fold ↑
Familial†		

*From Burrow GN, Ferris TF: Medical Complications during Pregnancy. Philadelphia, W.B. Saunders Company, 1975.

†These clinical features are not invariably present.

TABLE 61-3. Acute Fatty Liver of Pregnancy*

Clinical Features	Biochemical Changes	
Abrupt onset	Bilirubin	<10 mg per 100 ml
Vomiting	Alkaline phosphatase	sl ↑
Abdominal pain	SGOT	300-500 units
Jaundice	Prothrombin time	2- to 5-fold ↑
Fever,† coma	Leukocytes	20,000-30,000 cells per cu mm
Pre-eclampsia†	Serum glucose	↓
36th-40th weeks	Arterial ammonia	↑

*From Burrow GN, Ferris TF: Medical Complications during Pregnancy. Philadelphia, W.B. Saunders Company, 1975.

†Indicates clinical findings that are most variable.

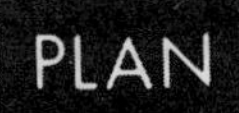

ADDITIONAL DIAGNOSTIC DATA

Liver function tests frequently ordered include total and direct bilirubin, SGOT, SGPT, alkaline phosphatase, prothrombin time, serum protein electrophoresis, and hepatitis B antigen.

TABLE 61-4. Liver Function Tests in Normal Pregnancy*

	Effects	Period of Maximum Change (Trimester)
Albumin	↓ 20%	second
γ-globulin	nl to sl ↓	third
α-globulin	sl ↑	third
β-globulin	sl ↑	third
Fibrinogen	↑ 50%	second
Ceruloplasmin	↑	third
Transferrin	↑	third
Bilirubin	nl to sl ↑	third
BSP	nl to sl ↑	third
Alkaline phosphatase	2- to 4-fold ↑	third
Lactic dehydrogenase	sl ↑	third
SGOT	nl	—
SGPT	nl	—
Cholesterol	2-fold ↑	third

*From Burrow GN, Ferris TF: Medical Complications during Pregnancy. Philadelphia, W.B. Saunders Company, 1975.

Key: nl, normal; sl, slight; ↑, increase; ↓, decrease.

During normal pregnancy, the results of some tests are altered even though the liver is functioning normally (see Table 61-4). Alkaline phosphatase tends to be increased two- to fourfold at term and is apparently derived from the placenta.

In cases of viral hepatitis, hepatitis B antigen can be expected; SGOT and SGPT levels may be two or more times higher than normal.

In cases of cholestasis, serum transaminases tend to be within the normal range or slightly increased. Alkaline phosphatase may be increased seven to ten times.

Liver biopsy, although rarely required, may be the only means of establishing a specific diagnosis in an unusual situation.

Peritoneal tap disclosing blood may indicate hepatic rupture.

MANAGEMENT AND PATIENT EDUCATION

Hepatitis during pregnancy is managed similarly to hepatitis in the nonpregnant patient. A seriously ill patient with severe anorexia must be hospitalized for intravenous fluids, electrolytes, and calories. Supplemental vitamins and iron are often necessary.

Most patients benefit from restrictions of physical activities, although there is no evidence that strict bed rest is essential. Regular activities may be resumed when clinical symptoms have abated and laboratory tests are improved.

Cholestatic jaundice of pregnancy persists until the pregnancy is terminated and the baby delivered. If the pregnancy is far from term and the fetus still immature, therapy may be directed at lowering serum bile acid levels, which may be accomplished with 4 gm of cholestyramine resin three times daily before meals.

Acute fatty liver of pregnancy requires immediate hospitalization. Electrolyte imbalance is corrected, and serum glucose maintained at a normal level. Any impairment of ventilation or circulation must be corrected. Gastrointestinal hemorrhage may necessitate blood transfusion and clotting abnormalities may require the administration of fresh-frozen plasma. As soon as the mother's condition has stabilized, the infant should be delivered, usually by cesarean section.

Hepatic rupture is an emergency necessitating immediate laparotomy with massive fluid and blood replacement. Bleeding vessels are ligated; partial hepatectomy may be required. Pregnancy is usually terminated by cesarean section at the same emergency laparotomy.

REFERENCES

Bis KA, Waxman B: Rupture of the liver associated with pregnancy: a review of the literature and report of 2 cases. Obstet Gynecol Surv *31*:763-773, 1976

Fallon HJ: Liver diseases. *In* Burrow GN, Ferris TF: Medical Complications during Pregnancy. Philadelphia, W.B. Saunders Company, 1975

Hibbard LT: Spontaneous rupture of the liver in pregnancy: a report of eight cases. Am J Obstet Gynecol *126*:334-338, 1976

Portnuff J, Ballon S: Hepatic rupture in pregnancy. Am J Obstet Gynecol *114*:1102-1104, 1972

Utley JR: Spontaneous rupture of the liver during pregnancy. Surg Gynecol Obstet *133*:250-252, 1971; Obstet Gynecol Surv *27*:83-84, 1972

62 MOLAR PREGNANCY

GENERAL CONSIDERATIONS

Hydatidiform mole (Fig. 62-1) is a pathologic condition of the chorion characterized by

1. Cystic degeneration of the villi, with hydropic swelling
2. Avascularity, or absence of fetal blood vessels
3. Proliferation of trophoblastic tissue

The incidence of molar pregnancy in the United States is approximately 1 in 1500 to 1 in 2000 births.

SUBJECTIVE DATA

Vaginal Bleeding: Abnormal uterine bleeding, varying from spotting to profuse hemorrhage, is the most characteristic symptom of molar pregnancy and may be first noted between six and eight weeks following the missed menstrual period. Bloody discharge, continuous or intermittent, may be associated with the passage of grapelike vesicles.

Pregnancy Symptoms: The patient is usually aware of being pregnant. Typical symptoms include two or more missed menstrual periods, abdominal enlargement, and in approximately 14 to 30 per cent of patients, severe nausea and vomiting. Fetal movements are absent. Molar pregnancy is usually diagnosed between the eleventh and twentieth gestational week.

OBJECTIVE DATA

PHYSICAL EXAMINATION

General Examination: The patient may appear dehydrated and emaciated if there is excessive vomiting and weight loss. The blood pressure may be elevated if preeclampsia develops (12 to 20 per cent of patients).

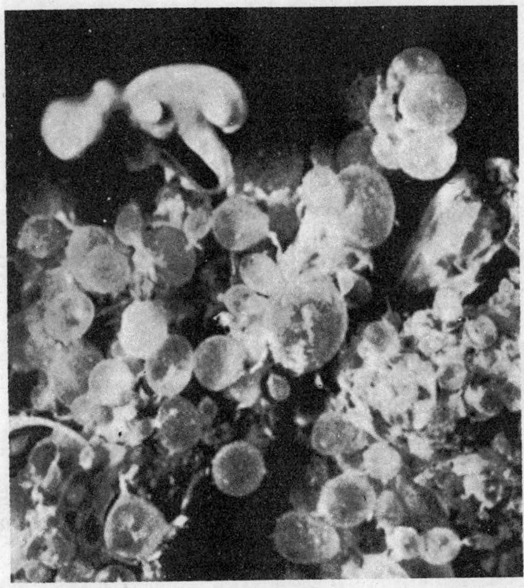

Figure 62-1. Hydatidiform mole with stunted embryo. Magnification ×2. (From Hertig AT: *In* Meigs JV, Sturgis SH (eds): Progress in Gynecology. New York, Grune and Stratton, 1950.)

Less frequently, the thyroid gland may be enlarged, and tachycardia may be associated with hyperthyroidism.

Abdominal Examination: The uterus tends to feel soft and boggy; in 50 per cent of patients, the uterus is larger than expected for the duration of amenorrhea. Uterine size is consistent with gestational dates in approximately 35 per cent of patients and smaller than expected in 10 to 15 per cent. Fetal heart tones are absent.

Pelvic Examination: On speculum examination, blood and possibly grape-like vesicles may be visualized in the vagina or cervical os. Bimanual examination confirms the uterine size. The ovaries may be tender to palpation and enlarged. In approximately 40 per cent of patients, unilateral or bilateral ovarian theca-lutein cysts (up to 10 cm or more in diameter) may result from overstimulation of ovarian lutein elements by the large amounts of chorionic gonadotropin secreted by the proliferating trophoblast.

LABORATORY TESTS

Complete Blood Count with Blood Smear: Iron deficiency anemia is common; megaloblastic erythropoiesis is rare.

Urinalysis is usually normal. Proteinuria suggests associated pre-eclampsia.

ASSESSMENT

DIFFERENTIAL DIAGNOSIS

This includes threatened abortion, missed abortion, multiple pregnancy, erroneous menstrual dates, pregnant uterus enlarged by leiomyomas, and hydramnios.

POTENTIAL COMPLICATIONS

These include hemorrhage (both external and internal), hyperemesis gravidarum (14 to 30 per cent of patients), preeclampsia (12 to 20 per cent of patients), thyrotoxicosis (2 to 10 per cent of patients), torsion or rupture of a theca-lutein cyst, disseminated intravascular coagulation, and trophoblastic invasion or embolization. Acute pulmonary embolization may occur before or following evacuation; the patient develops sudden cyanosis, tachypnea, tachycardia, dyspnea, and in severe cases, signs of right heart failure (see Pulmonary Embolism, p. 585).

PLAN

ADDITIONAL DIAGNOSTIC DATA

One or more of the following tests may be required to establish the diagnosis:

Ultrasound B-Scan (Fig. 62-2): The sonogram characteristic of a molar pregnancy shows multiple diffuse echoes in the enlarged uterus. These

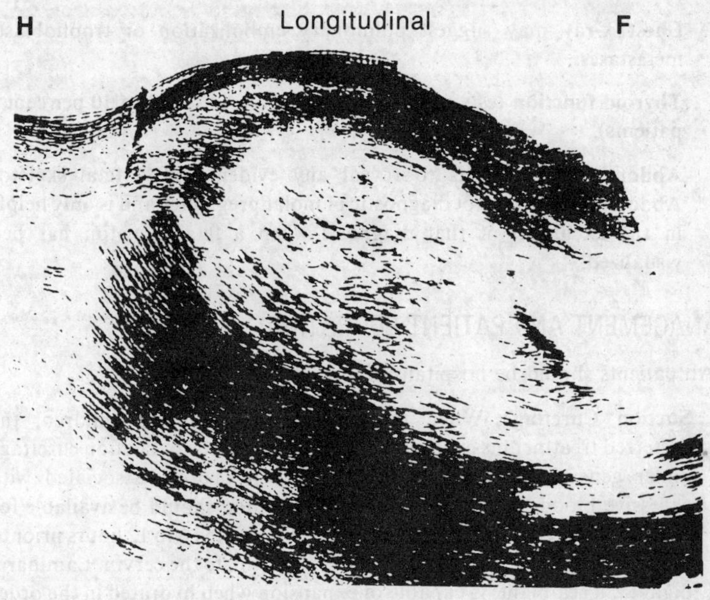

Figure 62-2. Longitudinal ultrasound B scan shows a uterus filled with multiple, fine echoes. No fetal parts are evident. This picture is characteristic of a hydatidiform mole. (From Gosink BB, Squire LF: Exercises in Diagnostic Radiology. Vol. 8. Diagnostic Ultrasound. Philadelphia, W.B. Saunders Company, 1976.)

internal echoes are reflections from multiple interfaces created by molar vesicles. No distinct structures, such as the fetal head, placenta, or fetal body, are visualized. Lutein cysts may be observed in the cul-de-sac or bilateral adnexal areas or above the fundus.

Amniography: Radiopaque contrast material injected transabdominally into the uterine cavity reveals a characteristic "moth-eaten" or "honeycomb" pattern.

Chorionic gonadotropin titers are highly elevated.

Chest x-ray may suggest pulmonary embolization or trophoblastic metastases.

Thyroid function tests may reveal hyperthyroidism (2 to 10 per cent of patients).

Abdominal x-ray fails to reveal any evidence of a fetal skeleton. Abdominal x-ray is not diagnostic of molar pregnancy and is only helpful in the exclusion of that diagnosis when a fetal skeleton has been visualized.

MANAGEMENT AND PATIENT EDUCATION

All patients should be hospitalized for definitive therapy.

Suction Curettage: When the patient desires future children, the preferred treatment is evacuation of the molar tissue by suction curettage under general anesthesia. Since evacuation may be associated with excessive blood loss, two to four units of blood should be available for transfusion as necessary. Laminaria may be inserted 6 to 12 hours prior to the scheduled time of evacuation in order to dilate the cervix. Laminaria digitata, a sea plant, is capable of expansion when hydrated in the order of 1 to 6. This expansion occurs over six to eight hours as the laminaria absorbs moisture from the endocervix. The cervix usually becomes sufficiently dilated to introduce a 10 mm or larger cannula, the size depending on the initial size of the laminaria inserted. For the insertion of the laminaria, the cervix and vaginal vault are cleansed with an antiseptic. The anterior cervical lip is grasped with a tenaculum and the laminaria inserted into the cervical canal just through the internal os. A folded 4×4 gauze sponge is then placed against the cervix to maintain the laminaria in position until sufficient swelling occurs.

Immediately after the patient has been anesthetized in the operating room, intravenous oxytocin (40 units per 1000 ml of lactated Ringer's solution) is initiated. The cervix is then dilated sufficiently to admit a 12 mm suction cannula, and the molar contents are evacuated by suction curettage.

After the uterus shrinks and bleeding diminishes, a sharp curettage is performed. The sharp curettings and the entire molar specimen are sent separately to the laboratory for histologic evaluation.

Abdominal hysterectomy, with the mole *in situ*, may be the preferred treatment for patients who have no desire for future childbearing. Hysterectomy eliminates the possibility of functioning trophoblastic cells' being left in the uterus after suction curettage. Thus, the risk of residual trophoblastic disease is reduced.

Decisions concerning salpingo-oophorectomy are individualized depending, in part, on the patient's age. Since ovarian theca-lutein cysts regress spontaneously after removal of the mole and elimination of the chorionic gonadotropin stimulation, surgical removal is not required unless there is an associated torsion or bleeding.

Follow-Up Program: After evacuation of a molar pregnancy, patients are carefully monitored with weekly quantitative chorionic gonadotropin (HCG) titers in order to select those who risk developing retained, invasive, or metastatic trophoblastic disease.

The most specific indicator of residual trophoblastic disease is the radioimmunoassay of the serum level of the beta subunit of chorionic gonadotropin (HCG) (Goldstein, 1975). The assay is performed at the time of evacuation and weekly thereafter. When the HCG level drops to normal and remains normal for three consecutive weeks, the patient is considered to be in remission. Evaluation of HCG levels is then repeated monthly for six consecutive months. Patients are advised to avoid pregnancy during the entire follow-up period. Usually estrogen-progestin oral contraceptives are prescribed.

Complete disappearance of HCG takes an average of 90 plus or minus 15 days following suction curettage and 55 plus or minus 12 days following abdominal hysterectomy (Goldstein, 1975).

Chest x-ray is also taken at the time of evacuation and may be repeated after four and eight weeks in order to detect any evidence of pulmonary metastases.

The pelvis is examined at two-week intervals to assess the uterus for size, the adnexa for theca-lutein cysts, and the lower genital tract for metastases.

If the serum chorionic gonadotropin level sustains a plateau for more than two consecutive weeks, if the level rises, or if obvious metastases occur, the patient should be treated for residual, proliferative trophoblastic disease. After suction curettage, approximately 15 to 20 per cent of patients may be expected to have a proliferative complication of molar pregnancy. Of this group, approximately 80 per cent acquire nonmetastatic trophoblastic disease while 20 per cent acquire disease that has spread beyond the confines of the uterus, most commonly to the lungs or vagina.

Aside from the persistent chorionic gonadotropin titer, symptoms of residual proliferative trophoblastic disease include vaginal bleeding, intraabdominal hemorrhage, and hemorrhagic lesions in the lung, liver, brain, or other organs.

Proliferative Complications: Whenever proliferative complications are suspected, the patient should be admitted to the hospital for a complete physical and neurologic evaluation. Laboratory tests to be ordered include chest x-ray, complete blood count including differential and platelet counts, blood urea nitrogen, and liver and thyroid function tests. Patients with nonmetastatic trophoblastic disease who desire to retain their childbearing potential are treated with single-agent chemotherapy for five days (usually 0.4 to 0.5 mg/kg/day of methotrexate intramuscularly or 12 mcg/kg/day of actinomycin D intravenously). The response to therapy is monitored with weekly HCG titers; duration of therapy is based on the regression curve of the HCG titer.

For the patient with nonmetastatic trophoblastic disease who has no desire for future childbearing, a five-day course of either methotrexate or actinomycin D is initiated and total abdominal hysterectomy is performed on the third day of chemotherapy. The HCG titer is followed at weekly intervals. As long as the titer regresses, no further therapy is indicated; if the HCG level reaches a plateau or rises, additional courses of chemotherapy are administered.

Patients with metastatic disease of the lungs, vagina, or pelvis are treated with single-agent chemotherapy (methotrexate or actinomycin D). Patients with metastatic disease of the brain, liver, bowel, or kidney are in a high-risk category and are treated with a combination triple chemotherapy.

REFERENCES

Curry SL, Hammond CB, Tyrey L, et al: Hydatidiform mole. Obstet Gynecol *45*:1-8, 1975

Goldstein DP: Endocrine assay in chorionic tumors. Clin Obstet Gynecol *18*:41-60, 1975

Goldstein DP, Pastorfide GB, Osathanondh R, et al: A rapid solid-phase radioimmunoassay specific for human chorionic gonadotropin in gestational trophoblastic disease. Obstet Gynecol *45*:527-530, 1975

Morrow CP, Kletzky OA, DiSaia PJ, et al: Clinical and laboratory correlates of molar pregnancy and trophoblastic disease. Am J Obstet Gynecol *128*:424-430, 1977

Osathanondh R, Goldstein DP, Pastorfide GP: Actinomycin D as the primary agent for gestational trophoblastic disease. Cancer *36*:863-866, 1975

Pastorfide GB, Goldstein DP, Kosasa TS, et al: Serum chorionic gonadotropin activity after molar pregnancy, therapeutic abortion, and term delivery. Am J Obstet Gynecol *118*:293-294, 1974

The management of molar pregnancy. ACOG Technical Bulletin No. 33, August 1975

63 MULTIPLE PREGNANCY

GENERAL CONSIDERATIONS

Multiple pregnancy is the state of being pregnant with two or more fetuses.

Twins occur approximately once in 80 or 90 births. Triplets occur approximately once in 8000 births. Conjoined twins are extremely rare [one in 70,000 in Singapore (Tan, 1971)].

Generally, two kinds of twins are distinguished: those from separate and distinct ova (dizygotic or fraternal) and those arising from one ovum (monozygotic or identical). The frequency of monozygotic twins appears to be relatively constant throughout the world—approximately one set per 250 pregnancies—and is not influenced by race, heredity, parity, or age. Dizygotic twinning results from a double simultaneous ovulation and is influenced by heredity, parity, and age.

SUBJECTIVE AND OBJECTIVE DATA

The uterus may be larger than expected for the gestational dates. Fetal activity may be greater and more noticeable than it is in the case of a single gestation. Frequently, the patient gives a family history of twins. More than one fetal heart beat may be audible.

The maternal hemoglobin and hematocrit are often reduced, since maternal anemia is more common in plural pregnancy.

ASSESSMENT

DIFFERENTIAL DIAGNOSIS

This includes polyhydramnios and uterine leiomyomas. (In early pregnancy rapid uterine growth may be associated with a molar pregnancy. The presence of a fetal heart beat, however, rules out the possibility of molar pregnancy.)

POTENTIAL COMPLICATIONS

These include the following:

1. Premature labor and delivery, which occurs five to ten times more frequently than with single gestation and is the greatest threat to a twin gestation
2. Malpresentation of the first twin, which may be breech, oblique, or transverse, and which may be expected in 25 to 30 per cent of cases
3. Dysfunctional labor, which may be associated with uterine overdistention
4. Fetal malformations
5. Prolapsed cord
6. Hydramnios
7. Maternal iron-deficiency anemia
8. Preeclampsia or eclampsia
9. Antepartum hemorrhage, either placenta previa or placental separation, which may occur in approximately 5 per cent of twin gestations
10. Postpartum hemorrhage

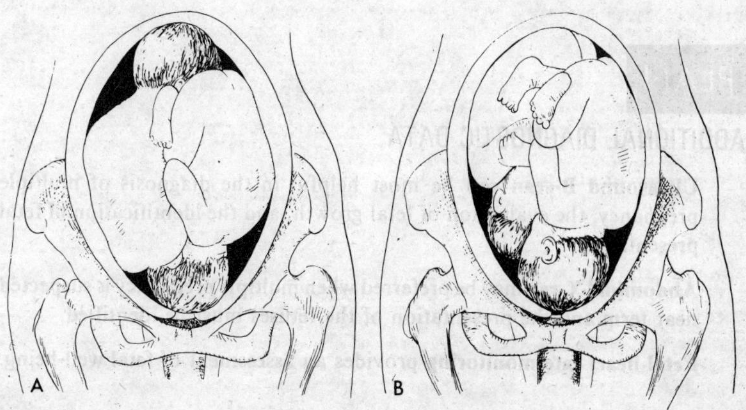

Figure 63-1. *A*, One twin is a cephalic and the other is a breech. *B*, Both twins are cephalic. (From Huffman JW: Gynecology and Obstetrics. Philadelphia, W.B. Saunders Company, 1962.)

Very rare complications include the following:

1. Collision—the contact of any fetal parts of one twin with those of its co-twin that prevents engagement of either
2. Impaction—the indentation of any fetal parts of one twin onto the surface of the other, which thereby permits partial engagement of both twins simultaneously
3. Compaction—the simultaneous full engagement of the leading fetal poles of both twins, which fills the true pelvic cavity and thereby prevents further descent or disengagement of either twin
4. Locked twins—the first twin presents as a breech and the second twin as a vertex. As the first twin descends, its chin impinges on the forelying neck and chin of the second cephalic twin above the pelvic inlet, preventing any further progress.
5. Monoamniotic twins. Mortality rate is extremely high, approximately 50 per cent, owing to tangling and knotting of the cord.
6. Conjoined twins—twins attached to each other. Cases vary widely from those in which two well-developed children have a commonly shared body site, to those in which only a small part of the body is duplicated, or in which amorphous masses of tissue are attached to an otherwise normal child. (Synonym: Siamese twins.)

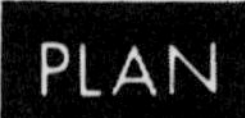

ADDITIONAL DIAGNOSTIC DATA

Ultrasound B-scan can be most helpful in the diagnosis of multiple pregnancy, the evaluation of fetal growth, and the identification of fetal presentation.

Abdominal X-ray may be preferred when multiple pregnancy is suspected near term and the presentation of the fetuses must be identified.

Fetal heart rate monitoring provides an assessment of fetal well-being.

MANAGEMENT

Delivery of First Twin: Usually, the delivery plans for the first baby are similar to those for a single baby in a comparable presentation.

As long as the first baby is in a vertex presentation, spontaneous labor and delivery may be anticipated. Careful fetal monitoring is essential, since the risk of cord prolapse and placental insufficiency is increased. If uterine contractions are ineffective, cesarean section is usually performed, although some obstetricians recommend cautious oxytocin stimulation.

When the first baby presents as a breech, cesarean section appears to offer the optimal perinatal results. (See Breech Presentation, p. 162.)

Cesarean section is indicated for a number of complications, including ruptured membranes without labor, prolapsed cord, fetal distress, placenta previa, premature placental separation, previous cesarean section or uterine surgery, fetal malpresentation, and conjoined twins.

Management of Second Twin after Vaginal Delivery of First Baby: The optimal time interval between the births of the first and second twin appears to be 5 to 20 minutes. When delivery occurs sooner or later, mortality rates are increased. Earlier delivery is associated with trauma as a result of undue haste; delayed delivery may be associated with prolapsed cord or placental separation or both.

As soon as the first twin is born, the position and presentation of the second twin is determined by vaginal examination. If the second twin presents a vertex (approximately 50 per cent do), intravenous dilute oxytocin should be administered in order to activate uterine contractions and encourage fetal descent. Soon thereafter the membranes of the second twin should be ruptured. The patient is encouraged to bear down, and the baby may be delivered either spontaneously or with low forceps.

If the second twin presents as a breech (approximately 38 per cent of cases), the membranes should be ruptured and the breech guided into the pelvis. Intravenous oxytocin may be indicated to reactivate uterine contractions and fetal descent.

If the second twin is in a transverse or oblique lie (approximately 12 per cent of cases), either a cesarean section or an internal version with breech extraction becomes necessary. For version and extraction, an obstetrician skilled in intrauterine fetal manipulation and an anesthesiologist skilled in providing anesthesia for uterine relaxation are essential for a favorable outcome. With the patient asleep and the uterus relaxed, the fetal foot must be distinguished from the fetal hand (Fig. 63-2). Usually, the heel must be identified, since the heel can be clearly distinguished from the wrist. Both feet are secured, if possible, while the membranes are still intact. Then the membranes are ruptured and downward traction is applied to deliver the baby.

Postpartum Management: After the babies have been delivered, the increased risk of postpartum hemorrhage must be anticipated. Twenty to 40 units of oxytocin are added to 1000 ml of 5 per cent dextrose infusion and administered rapidly. In addition, 0.2 mg of ergonovine maleate is given intramuscularly. The uterus should be massaged continuously to prevent atony. (See Postpartum Hemorrhage, p. 537.) Cross-matched blood should be available in the event that transfusion is necessary.

PATIENT EDUCATION

A patient with a multiple pregnancy should be advised of the increased incidence of obstetric complications, including abnormal presentations, cord prolapse, dysfunctional labor, premature labor, preeclampsia, and post-

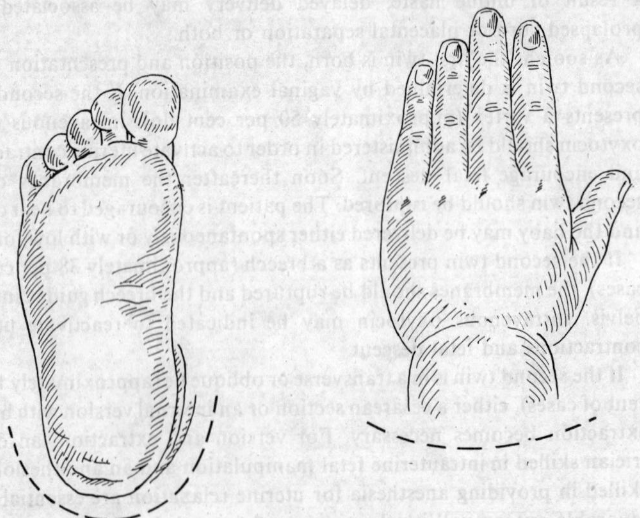

Figure 63-2. Features helpful in distinguishing a fetus' foot from its hand during a vaginal examination. (From Greenhill JP, Friedman EA: Biological principles and modern practice of obstetrics. Philadelphia, W.B. Saunders Company, 1974.)

partum hemorrhage. During the third trimester, bed rest should be encouraged to reduce the risk of premature labor.

When any malformation is suspected and identified, preparation of the parents prior to delivery aids in their acceptance of the situation at the time of birth.

REFERENCES

Farooqui MO, Grossman JH, Shannon RA: A review of twin pregnancy and perinatal mortality. Obstet Gynecol Surv *28*:144-153, 1973

Fox RL, Nathanson HG, Tejani N, et al: Interlocking twins. Obstet Gynecol *46*:53-57, 1975

Powers WF: Twin pregnancy. Obstet Gynecol *42*:795-808, 1973

Sternadel Z, Lysikiewicz: Management of twin labor. Acta Genet Med Gemellol *23*: 70-72, 1974; Obstet Gynecol Surv *30*:432-434, 1975

Tan KL, Goon SM, Salmon Y, Wee JH: Conjoined twins. Acta Obstet Gynecol Scand *50*:373-380, 1971

64 NIPPLE DISCHARGE

GENERAL CONSIDERATIONS

Nipple discharge may be milky, serous, watery, bloody, purulent, or brownish. Serous and bloody breast discharge may be signs of either benign breast disease (fibrocystic disease, intraductal papilloma, ductal ectasia) or malignancy.

Breast milk is ordinarily secreted only after parturition. During pregnancy, prolactin levels rise, reaching a peak at the time of delivery. Estrogen and progesterone levels increase simultaneously and appear to block the action of prolactin on breast tissue. With delivery and the rapid fall in estrogen and progesterone levels, the blockade is lifted and milk production is stimulated. Oxytocin causes contractions of the myoepithelial cells surrounding the milk glands (alveoli and ducts) and breast milk is released.

Suckling induces milk ejection ("letdown") by stimulating oxytocin synthesis and release from the hypothalamus and posterior pituitary. Suckling maintains milk production by suppressing the formation of a hypothalamic substance, prolactin-inhibiting factor (PIF), ensuring adequate prolactin availability. In addition, evidence has accumulated indicating that the hypothalamus contains a prolactin-releasing factor (PRF). It is possible that PRF is released in response to suckling (Reichlin, 1974).

SUBJECTIVE AND OBJECTIVE DATA

Pregnancy, menstrual, and drug history may clarify the possible etiologic factors. Nonpuerperal galactorrhea associated with amenorrhea usually signifies abnormal prolactin secretion. Breast cancer must always be considered when there is a family history of breast malignancy.

Breast palpation is essential. Cysts or masses may be benign or malignant. In the case of a unilateral nipple discharge, methodical, point-by-point palpation circumferentially about the nipple at or just outside the areolar margin usually discloses the lobular duct system containing the responsible abnormality. Any fluid expressed is smeared on a slide and submitted for cytologic examination.

ASSESSMENT

DIFFERENTIAL DIAGNOSIS

The differential diagnosis includes breast manipulation, cancer, drug therapy, ductal ectasia,* fibrocystic disease, hypothalamic-pituitary disorders, infection, inflammation, intraductal papilloma, lactation, Paget's disease, and thyroid disease.

ETIOLOGIC FACTORS

Nonpuerperal galactorrhea (inappropriate lactation) may be caused by hypothalamic-pituitary disorders with elevated prolactin levels, thyroid disease, adrenal disease, drug therapy (phenothiazines, tricyclic tranquilizers, reserpine, methyldopa, sex steroids), breast manipulation, or prolonged irritative lesions of the anterior chest wall, notably after thoracotomy or herpes zoster of the thoracic segments.

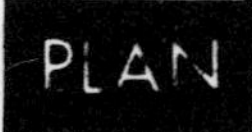

ADDITIONAL DIAGNOSTIC DATA

Cytologic smear of nipple discharge may reveal abnormal cells that give rise to the suspicion of malignancy.

Mammography may aid in breast evaluation when a discrete mass is not palpable.

---

*Mammary duct ectasia is a benign lesion that may appear similar to carcinoma, particularly when nipple retraction, skin adherence, and edema accompany a hard, diffuse mass within the breast. The primary pathologic finding is subacute inflammation of the ductal system, usually beginning in the subareolar area.

Prolactin levels may be helpful when persistent lactation is unrelated to pregnancy. Elevated values may be caused by a prolactin-secreting pituitary tumor or by interference with prolactin-inhibiting factors.

Thyroid function studies are indicated whenever thyroid disease is suspected.

X-ray: Plain skull films or tomograms may demonstrate a pituitary tumor.

MANAGEMENT AND PATIENT EDUCATION

Treatment of nipple discharge depends on the cause. When there is any question of malignancy, surgical biopsy is necessary.

Galactorrhea may respond to estrogen therapy, which directly inhibits the action of prolactin on the breast. Nipple stimulation should be avoided, since breast stimulation tends to prolong lactation.

The patient should be instructed in breast self-examination, and close medical follow-up should be arranged.

(See Breast Masses, p. 158.)

REFERENCES

Reichlin S: Neuroendocrinology. *In* Williams RH (ed): Textbook of Endocrinology. Philadelphia, W.B. Saunders Company, 1974, pp 774-831

Seltzer MH, Perloff LJ, Kelley RI, et al: The significance of age in patients with nipple discharge. Surg Gynecol Obstet *131*:519-522, 1970

65 NIPPLE FISSURE

GENERAL CONSIDERATIONS

Sore nipples are a frequent complication of the first weeks of nursing. Fissures are extremely painful and may inhibit lactation.

SUBJECTIVE AND OBJECTIVE DATA

Pain while nursing and an obvious fissured area adjacent to the nipple establish the diagnosis.

PLAN

MANAGEMENT

Exposure to the air and rest from nursing usually lead to a rapid cure (within 24 to 48 hours). A nipple shield and topical ointments may be helpful. While the fissure persists, the child should not nurse from the affected breast. A breast pump may be used to empty the breast in order to provide milk for the baby and relieve breast distention.

66 OVARIAN ACCIDENTS

Bleeding, Rupture, Torsion

GENERAL CONSIDERATIONS

Ovarian Cycle: During the reproductive years, the ovary undergoes physiologic, cyclic changes at approximately 28-day intervals. Under the influence of pituitary follicle–stimulating hormone (FSH), a primordial follicle, composed of a central ovum encircled by granulosa cells, develops into a mature graafian follicle; granulosa cells proliferate, and fluid spaces between the granulosa cells coalesce to form the fluid-filled cavity or antrum. The granulosa cells lining the antrum and the underlying theca interna are sources of increasing estrogen production.

As the antrum becomes distended by fluid, the follicle protrudes from the ovarian surface and the ovum, surrounded by an investing covering of granulosa cells (cumulus oophorus), is pushed to one side of the follicle. Although ovulation usually follows in the normal course of events, the persistence of a follicle cyst may be associated with acute symptoms of rupture or torsion.

Ovulation involves follicular rupture with discharge of the ovum surrounded by granulosa cells. Usually occurring on day 14 of the average ovarian cycle, ovulation appears to be triggered by a sudden surge of luteinizing hormone (LH). Pain associated with ovulation may be due to slight intraabdominal bleeding or acute antral distention.

Corpus Luteum: Following ovulation, the corpus luteum arises by transformation of the remaining granulosa cells into large, polyhedral lutein cells that secrete estrogen and progesterone. The life cycle of the corpus luteum may be divided into four stages: proliferation, vascularization, maturity, and regression.

Initially, capillary congestion and hemorrhage into the granulosa cell layer are followed by capillary invasion from the theca and luteinization of granulosa cells. Although bleeding into the lumen is usually of a zonal type, more extensive bleeding may distend the entire lumen with blood, forming a corpus luteum hematoma. A recently ruptured follicle filled with sanguinous coagulated material is also called a *corpus hemorrhagicum*. Occasionally, intraperitoneal hemorrhage may occur.

The stage of maturity begins approximately four days after ovulation; the corpus luteum reaches peak functional activity by the eighth day after ovulation.

If pregnancy occurs, corpus luteum development continues under the influence of chorionic gonadotropin. If conception does not occur, the corpus luteum begins to regress approximately nine days after ovulation. Steadily declining estrogen and progesterone production leads to endometrial changes resulting in menstruation.

Normally, the interval from ovulation to menses tends to be consistently close to 14 days. Variability in cycle length is usually due to a variation in the number of days required for follicular growth and maturation during the preovulatory phase. Occasionally, however, the corpus luteum may persist even though conception does not occur. Since estrogen and progesterone production continues, menses fail to appear at the expected time. This syndrome of persistent corpus luteum may be confused with early pregnancy.

Theca-lutein cysts, caused by very high levels of chorionic gonadotropin, usually occur in association with molar pregnancy.

Ovarian accidents—bleeding, rupture, and torsion—may be associated with variations in the normal ovarian cycle (follicle cysts or corpus luteum cysts), inflammatory cysts, endometriomas, and benign or malignant cystic or solid tumors.

Bleeding may occur into the cyst itself, causing acute distention, or into the peritoneal cavity.

Rupture of a cyst may cause peritoneal irritation.

Torsion: When ovarian tumors or cysts twist or rotate around their pedicle, the blood supply becomes compromised; venous congestion leads to hemorrhage within the cyst or to an inflammatory reaction with adhesions to neighboring viscera. With complete torsion, the blood supply becomes thrombosed and the cyst undergoes hemorrhagic necrosis.

In the pregnant patient, torsion of an ovarian cyst is most apt to occur when the uterus is enlarging rapidly (between 8 and 16 weeks) or involuting after delivery.

SUBJECTIVE DATA

Abdominal pain may develop gradually or suddenly, depending on the nature of the accident—gradual bleeding or intermittent torsion; acute hemorrhage, sudden rupture, or torsion.

Pain may be localized to one lower quadrant or generalized over the entire lower abdomen. With peritoneal irritation from fluid or blood, the pain tends to be constant and aggravated by motion. With torsion of an ovarian cyst, the pain may be mild and intermittent if torsion is incomplete, or severe and constant if infarction occurs. Pain associated with a ruptured follicle cyst usually subsides within a few hours.

Nausea or vomiting may occur immediately after sudden excruciating pain or may develop after pain has been present for several hours.

Menstrual History: Timing of symptoms in relation to the menstrual cycle can be variable. Ovarian accidents occur in both pregnant and nonpregnant women. Bleeding from a ruptured corpus luteum, for example, can occur at virtually any time after ovulation, including during early pregnancy. The possibility of a ruptured endometrioma should be considered when the patient gives a history of secondary dysmenorrhea occurring during recent menstrual cycles.

Other Symptoms: Syncope or shock or both suggest profuse intraperitoneal bleeding or acute torsion. Fever and chills are usually absent unless there is a secondary infection. Urinary frequency and the urge to defecate may indicate peritoneal irritation. Shoulder pain suggests diaphragmatic irritation from profuse bleeding or ruptured cystic contents. A history of previous attacks of sharp pain that disappeared spontaneously after a short time is consistent with a diagnosis of ovarian cyst. The possibility of ovarian hemorrhage must be considered whenever a woman is receiving anticoagulant therapy.

OBJECTIVE DATA

PHYSICAL EXAMINATION

General Examination: Temperature is usually normal or slightly elevated. Pulse may be accelerated. Unless profuse intraperitoneal bleeding produces symptoms of hypovolemic shock, blood pressure and respirations are likely to be within the normal range.

Abdominal Examination: Unilateral tenderness in either lower quadrant, with or without rebound tenderness, rigidity, and guarding, suggests a localized process. Bowel sounds are usually normal. More extensive bleeding or rupture of cystic contents causes a more generalized lower abdominal peritonitis, with abdominal rigidity, rebound tenderness, hypoactive or absent bowel sounds, and distention. Only rarely is a tender mass evident on abdominal palpation.

Pelvic Examination: The uterus is usually of normal size unless the patient is pregnant. Cervical motion is often painful. The involved adnexal area tends to be very tender, and with intraperitoneal bleeding, a discrete mass may not be identified. A palpable mass usually represents either hematoma formation around the bleeding site, torsion of a solid or cystic tumor, or bleeding *into* an ovarian cyst. Bleeding into an endometrioma, for example, may cause a previously known cystic mass to enlarge up to 15 cm in diameter. Often the patient is so exquisitely tender that an adequate bimanual examination is impossible unless the patient has been given systemic analgesia or even anesthesia. Bulging in the cul-de-sac suggests extensive intraperitoneal bleeding.

LABORATORY EXAMINATION

Complete Blood Count: Hemoglobin and hematocrit values reflect blood loss. The white count may vary from 5000 to 20,000, and there may be an increased number of immature forms. A declining hematocrit on serial determinations indicates persistent bleeding.

ASSESSMENT

DIFFERENTIAL DIAGNOSIS

This includes ectopic pregnancy, pelvic infection, acute appendicitis, diverticulitis, bowel perforation, and intestinal obstruction.

In acute appendicitis, the initial pain is rarely sudden, severe, sharp, or stabbing.

In the case of pelvic infection, fever and leukocytosis tend to be more marked. Culdocentesis may reveal pus rather than blood.

Ruptured ectopic pregnancy and hemorrhagic corpus luteum may present identical findings.

The patient with colonic diverticulum perforation may give a history of gastrointestinal symptoms (diarrhea, constipation, melena, vomiting).

ETIOLOGIC FACTORS

Ovarian cysts likely to bleed or rupture are the following:

1. Corpus luteum
2. Follicle cyst
3. Endometrioma
4. Theca-lutein cyst
5. Cystic benign teratoma—dermoid cyst
6. Cystadenocarcinoma

Ovarian cysts most likely to undergo torsion are the following:

1. Cystic benign teratoma—dermoid cyst
2. Pseudomucinous cystadenoma
3. Theca-lutein cyst

POTENTIAL COMPLICATIONS

Complications to be anticipated include hemorrhage, infection, intestinal obstruction from adhesions, and necrosis.

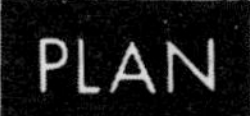

ADDITIONAL DIAGNOSTIC DATA

Culdocentesis may reveal nonclotting blood indicative of intraperitoneal bleeding, or intraperitoneal fluid suggestive of cystic rupture.

Abdominal x-rays (upright, supine, and lateral decubitus views) may reveal free intraperitoneal fluid. Calcified structures or teeth may be found in a dermoid cyst (Fig. 66-1).

Ultrasound B-scan may identify a cystic or solid adnexal mass.

Pregnancy test for chorionic gonadotropin is negative unless pregnancy coexists.

Coagulation tests may disclose coagulation defects associated with anticoagulant therapy or thrombocytopenia.

MANAGEMENT AND PATIENT EDUCATION

Whenever peritoneal bleeding is suspected, the patient should be hospitalized. Observation over 6 to 24 hours frequently clarifies the diagnosis of a self-limited process. Symptoms associated with a ruptured follicle cyst, for example, improve spontaneously.

When symptoms persist or worsen, or an adnexal mass is suspected, examination under anesthesia or laparoscopy may be helpful. Laparoscopy is particularly valuable for direct visualization of the fallopian tubes and ovaries. If a corpus luteum that has ceased to bleed is identified, no additional surgery is required.

Evidence of active intraperitoneal bleeding, an enlarging adnexal mass, torsion, or a ruptured endometrioma are indications for laparotomy. Once the abdomen is opened, the appropriate surgical procedure depends on the extent of the disease process as well as the patient's desire for future childbearing.

Torsion of an ovarian cyst or tumor is generally clockwise. With intense venous stasis, cysts become dark blue or even black. Since the veins in the twisted pedicle are often thrombosed, the cyst and pedicle should be excised without being untwisted lest emboli from the thrombosed vessels be dislodged into the general circulation.

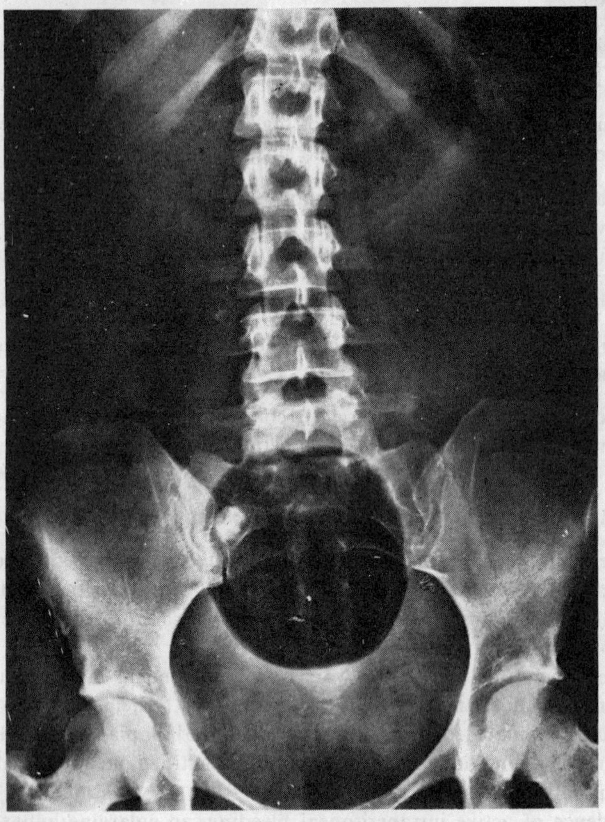

Figure 66-1. History of acute abdominal pain and vomiting over past three hours. Abdominal x-ray shows a round, radiolucent structure overlying the sacrum with a tooth consistent with a dermoid cyst. Emergency surgery confirmed torsion of an ovarian dermoid cyst. (From Squire LF, Colaiace WM, Strutynsky N: Exercises in Diagnostic Radiology. Vol 2. The Abdomen. Philadelphia, W.B. Saunders Company, 1971.)

Ovarian Hyperstimulation Syndrome

GENERAL CONSIDERATIONS

Ovarian hyperstimulation syndrome, characterized by massively enlarged ovaries with multiple follicle cysts, stromal edema, and numerous large cystic corpora lutea, may follow ovulation induction with human menopausal and chorionic gonadotropins. In mild cases, the ovarian enlargement is associated with abdominal distention and weight gain. In severe cases, additional complications include ascites, pleural effusion, hypovolemia, oliguria, and electrolyte disturbances.

SUBJECTIVE DATA

CURRENT SYMPTOMS

Abdominal pain, abdominal distention, nausea, and vomiting are the most consistent symptoms. Weight gain may indicate fluid retention. Dyspnea can be caused by abdominal or pleural fluid.

PRIOR HISTORY

The history of infertility and treatment with fertility hormones (human menopausal gonadotropins or clomiphene followed by chorionic gonadotropin) provides the key diagnostic clue.

OBJECTIVE DATA

PHYSICAL EXAMINATION

General Examination: Hypotension and tachycardia can be caused by the hypovolemia resulting from loss of vascular fluid into the peritoneal cavity.

Abdominal Examination: Distention may be associated with hypoactive or absent bowel sounds, and ascites. Excessive ovarian enlargement may be palpable abdominally.

Pelvic Examination: Ovarian enlargement may exceed 10 cm. Bimanual examination must be done most gently in order to obviate iatrogenic rupture of the hyperstimulated ovaries.

LABORATORY TESTS

Complete Blood Count with Blood Smear: Elevated hematocrit values can be indicative of hemoconcentration due to loss of vascular fluid into the peritoneal or pleural cavity. A decreased hematocrit or falling values on serial determinations may indicate intraperitoneal bleeding.

Urinalysis is usually normal. In cases of hypovolemia, urine output may be reduced.

ASSESSMENT

POTENTIAL COMPLICATIONS

Complications to be anticipated include electrolyte imbalance, coagulation abnormalities, decreased renal perfusion, thromboembolic phenomena, torsion of an ovarian cyst, and intraabdominal hemorrhage.

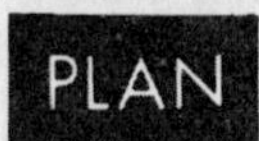

ADDITIONAL DIAGNOSTIC DATA

Chest x-ray may reveal pleural fluid.

Abdominal x-ray (three-way) may reveal abdominal fluid.

Blood Coagulation Studies: Platelet count, fibrinogen, prothrombin time, and partial thromboplastin time may elucidate a coexisting coagulopathy.

Blood Electrolytes; Blood Urea Nitrogen and Creatinine: Severe hypovolemia leads to decreased renal perfusion and, secondarily, to increased water and salt reabsorption in the proximal tubule. With decreased urinary flow, urea reabsorption is increased and blood urea nitrogen rises. Hydrogen and potassium ions accumulate, resulting in hyperkalemia and a tendency to acidosis. Serum electrolyte determinations evaluate the extent of hyperkalemia and hyponatremia.

Electrocardiogram may reveal hyperkalemia.

MANAGEMENT

Hospitalization is usually necessary for careful observation. The patient is placed at complete bed rest, gonadotropin medication is discontinued, and vital signs are monitored frequently.

Intravenous fluids and electrolytes are indicated in order to maintain plasma volume and restore fluid balance. Intake and output are carefully monitored by daily weights, serial hematocrits, serum electrolytes, and central venous pressure, if necessary. Diuretics are avoided, since fluid in the third space is not available for diuresis and if diuresis should occur, additional contraction of the intravascular volume would aggravate the tendency to hypovolemic shock (Engel, 1972).

Exploratory laparotomy is avoided unless there is evidence of torsion or intraabdominal hemorrhage (Schenker, 1975). If surgery is necessary, ovarian tissue should be preserved, if possible.

PATIENT EDUCATION

The patient should be advised of the association of the syndrome with hormonal ovulation induction. Usually self-limited, the syndrome is expected to respond to conservative therapy.

REFERENCES

Engel T, Jewelewicz R, Dyrenfurth I, et al: Ovarian hyperstimulation syndrome. Am J Obstet Gynecol *112*:1052-1060, 1972

McCort JJ: Ruptured corpus luteum with hemoperitoneum. Radiology *116*:65-67, 1975

Pantoja E, Noy MA, Axtmayer RW, et al: Ovarian dermoids and their complications. Obstet Gynecol Surv *30*:1-20, 1975

Pratt JH, Shamblin WR: Spontaneous rupture of endometrial cysts of the ovary presenting as an acute abdominal emergency. Am J Obstet Gynecol *108*:56-62, 1970

Ranney B: Endometriosis: emergency operations due to hemoperitoneum. Obstet Gynecol *36*:437-442, 1970

Schenker JG, Polishuk WZ: Ovarian hyperstimulation syndrome. Obstet Gynecol *46*:23-28, 1975

Shane JM, Naftolin F, Newmark SR: Gynecologic endocrine emergencies. JAMA *231*:393-395, 1975

67 OVULATION AND MITTELSCHMERZ

GENERAL CONSIDERATIONS

Ovulation is the expulsion of a female germ cell (ovum) from a ruptured graafian follicle.

Mittelschmerz is intermenstrual pain in the lower abdomen generally associated with ovulation.

SUBJECTIVE DATA

CURRENT SYMPTOMS

Abdominal pain may be localized to the low back or either lower quadrant. Pain usually develops acutely on the fourteenth day of the average menstrual cycle, or midway between the onset of the menstrual period, and may last a few hours or as long as two days.

Vaginal bleeding: Some patients are not aware of any bleeding; a few report a brownish discharge; others are aware of slight spotting or staining.

PRIOR HISTORY

Frequently, patients have a past history of similar episodes.

OBJECTIVE DATA

PHYSICAL EXAMINATION

General Examination: These findings are normal.

Abdominal Examination: These findings are usually normal. Occasional patients have mild tenderness in one or the other lower quadrant.

Pelvic Examination: These results are usually normal. Slight ovarian tenderness may be present.

LABORATORY TESTS

These are normal.

ASSESSMENT

DIFFERENTIAL DIAGNOSIS

This includes early appendicitis, pelvic infection, ovarian accidents (particularly ruptured corpus luteum with intraabdominal bleeding), and an atypical ectopic pregnancy.

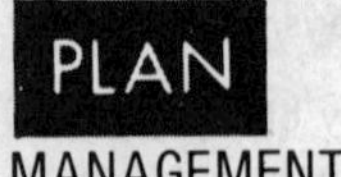

MANAGEMENT

Reassurance and mild analgesics are the only therapy required.

PATIENT EDUCATION

Ovulation pain may be explained by the presence of ovarian follicular distention or peritoneal irritation associated with follicular rupture and is expected to improve within 12 to 24 hours.

The patient should be instructed to report any persistent pain or additional symptoms of weakness, faintness, syncope, or shoulder pain immediately, since a bleeding corpus luteum can cause profuse intraabdominal hemorrhage.

68 PANCREATITIS IN PREGNANCY

GENERAL CONSIDERATIONS

Acute pancreatitis, an acute inflammatory disease of the pancreas, is a relatively rare complication of pregnancy. The incidence is reported to vary from 1 case per 1000 births to 1 in 11,000.

SUBJECTIVE DATA

CURRENT SYMPTOMS

Abdominal pain, usually epigastric, or persistent vomiting are the most typical symptoms of acute pancreatitis. The pain may bore directly through to the back or may be located in the right upper quadrant. Nausea and persistent vomiting are frequently associated symptoms.

PRIOR HISTORY

Some patients report a history of previous attacks of gallbladder disease. An occasional patient reports a history of chronic thiazide therapy.

OBJECTIVE DATA

PHYSICAL EXAMINATION

General Examination: The patient often looks very sick. Shock may be secondary to hypovolemia caused by exudation of plasma into the retroperitoneal space, vasodilatation, sequestration of fluid into the gut, or hemorrhage into the pancreatic bed or the intestine. The temperature elevation, observed in two thirds of the patients, is an indication of tissue injury.

Abdominal examination findings include distention, tenderness with rigidity, and rebound tenderness, particularly in the epigastrium. Bowel sounds are hypoactive or absent.

LABORATORY TESTS

The white cell count tends to be elevated—up to 30,000. Increased hemoglobin and hematocrit values are indicative of hemoconcentration due to exudation of plasma into the retroperitoneal space; decreased values suggest hemorrhage into the pancreatic bed.

ASSESSMENT

DIFFERENTIAL DIAGNOSIS

This includes preeclampsia, perforated peptic ulcer, intestinal obstruction, mesenteric infarction, abdominal trauma, acute cholecystitis, hepatitis, diabetic acidosis, abdominal aortic aneurysm, uremia, acute salpingitis, and ruptured ectopic pregnancy.

PREDISPOSING FACTORS

These include cholecystitis, hyperlipidemia, alcoholism, and the chronic use of thiazide diuretics. A primary bacterial or viral infection elsewhere in the body may cause a secondary pancreatic infection.

POTENTIAL COMPLICATIONS

Complications that may develop include pancreatic abscess, bowel perforation, biliary tract obstruction, pancreatic pseudocyst, intestinal obstruction, pancreatic or gallbladder perforation, thrombophlebitis, bacteremia pulmonary embolism, bronchopneumonia, pleural effusion, hyperglycemia, and diabetic acidosis.

Pancreatic abscesses usually contain enteric organisms, most commonly *Escherichia coli*.

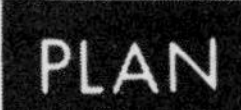

ADDITIONAL DIAGNOSTIC DATA

Serum amylase is usually elevated 2 to 12 hours after the onset of acute pancreatitis. [Eighty per cent of patients have serum amylase above 250 units (Wilkinson, 1973).]

During the latter half of pregnancy, serum amylase values normally may be as high as 200 (Kaiser, 1975). The differential diagnosis of elevated serum amylase includes intestinal obstruction with strangulation, perforated duodenal ulcer with pancreatic involvement, mesenteric vascular occlusion, acute cholecystitis, ruptured aortic aneurysm, mumps, and advanced renal insufficiency.

Serum lipase is usually elevated.

Serum calcium below 7 mg per 100 ml suggests extensive pancreatic damage.

Blood glucose is elevated if the patient has an insulin deficiency.

Serum electrolytes provide a guide to appropriate fluid and electrolyte therapy.

Abdominal x-ray may reveal calcification in the region of the pancreas or nonspecific ileus.

MANAGEMENT

Treatment of acute pancreatitis is fundamentally medical supportive therapy with five major objectives:

1. **Prevention and Correction of Shock:** Intravenous fluids, electrolytes, and blood or albumin are administered to maintain fluid and electrolyte balance. Hypocalcemia is treated by calcium replacement and hyperglycemia with insulin.

2. **Suppression of Pancreatic Secretion:** Nasogastric suction and the elimination of oral intake tend to reduce gastrin stimulation from hydrochloric acid. Sedation and anticholinergic medication (0.4 mg of atropine) appears to be beneficial.

3. **Relief of Pain:** Usually, meperidine (*Demerol*) or codeine are recommended.

4. **Prevention and Treatment of Infection:** Although prophylactic antibiotics are frequently prescribed, there is no conclusive proof that they prevent pancreatic abscess formation. If clinical, radiologic, or bacteriologic evidence of an abscess is present, appropriate antibiotic coverage (usually penicillin and an aminoglycoside, or ampicillin) and surgical drainage are indicated.

5. **Diagnosis and Treatment of Surgical Complications:** These include pancreatic abscess, bowel perforation, biliary tract obstruction, rapidly enlarging pseudocyst, intestinal obstruction, splenic rupture, and gallbladder perforation.

PATIENT EDUCATION

Acute pancreatitis during pregnancy can be life threatening for both mother and baby. Hospital management is essential.

Once the acute phase has subsided, dietary management appears to be an important measure to prevent recurrences. A high-protein, low-fat diet divided into small, frequent meals without alcohol or spicy food is recommended. Following delivery, the patient should have a cholecystogram in order to evaluate gallbladder function.

REFERENCES

Corlett RC, Mishell DR: Pancreatitis in pregnancy. Am J Obstet Gynecol *113*:281-290, 1972

Kaiser R, Berk JE, Fridhandler L: Serum amylase changes during pregnancy. Am J Obstet Gynecol *122*:283-286, 1975

Wilkinson EJ: Acute pancreatitis in pregnancy. Obstet Gynecol Surv *28*:281-303, 1973

69 PEDIATRIC GYNECOLOGY

GENERAL CONSIDERATIONS

Pediatric gynecologic problems most likely to require emergency attention usually result from trauma, infection, or congenital abnormalities. However, virtually every gynecologic disorder that occurs in adults can also happen to children. Although pregnancy is extremely rare under the age of 11, the youngest mother reported was delivered at five years and eight months of age (Huffman, 1968). Genital neoplasia is also extremely rare during childhood. However, since the ovary is the most frequent site of the rare tumors that do occur, this possibility should be considered in the differential diagnosis of any child with abdominal pain and a pelvic mass.

SUBJECTIVE DATA

CURRENT SYMPTOMS

Vaginal Discharge or Bleeding: Children with vaginitis may have a purulent vaginal discharge. Occasionally, the discharge is bloody owing to irritation associated with concomitant pruritus.

The most common cause of bleeding or bloody discharge prior to menarche is a foreign body in the vagina. Bleeding may also result from the ingestion of exogenous hormones, for example, the mother's birth control pills. Precocious puberty as a cause of childhood bleeding is readily recognized by the associated secondary sex characteristics.

Vaginal and ovarian tumors, although extremely rare, should be considered.

Blood-tinged vaginal discharge during the first two weeks after delivery usually signifies withdrawal from maternal estrogen. This bleeding is of short duration, requiring no treatment other than reassurance of the child's parents.

Abdominal Pain: A reproductive tract pathologic condition should be considered whenever sudden abdominal pain develops during childhood.

PRIOR HISTORY

A history of trauma, insertion of a foreign body into the vagina, or hormone ingestion frequently provides the clue to the correct diagnosis.

OBJECTIVE DATA

PHYSICAL EXAMINATION

General Examination: An evaluation of the child's general appearance may detect congenital anomalies, abnormal skeletal growth, or signs of precocious sexual development. Although the average age of menarche is between 12 and 13 years, premature puberty must be considered. Acceleration of growth and weight gain, breast development, and axillary and pubic hair precede the onset of menses.

Abdominal Examination: The presence of an abdominal mass may indicate a reproductive tract pathologic condition (ovarian tumor or mucocolpos in infancy). Other causes of an asymptomatic cystic abdominal mass in a child include mesenteric cyst, urachal cyst, and cyst or tumor of the liver and kidney.

When the patient has an imperforate hymen or a transverse vaginal septum, the vagina may become grossly distended with mucus from the cervical glands. The obstructed mucus balloons out the vagina and may form a lower abdominal mass. (Why some newborns with complete vaginal obstruction collect great quantities of mucus but others do not remains unknown.)

Congenital vaginal abnormalities may not become symptomatic until puberty, at which time the retained menstrual blood can cause painful uterine distention with a lower abdominal mass.

Pelvic Examination: Although genital examination of children tends to be deferred or inhibited for reasons of shyness and modesty, gynecologic examination is *essential* whenever a child has vaginal symptoms or an abdominal mass.

When traumatic injury is suspected, adequate visualization is required to assess the need for surgical repair. In cases of extensive genital trauma, general anesthesia may be necessary for examination and treatment. Straddle injuries can cause large perineal hematomas and lacerations.

Vulvitis, vaginal discharge, or a bulging imperforate hymen distended by mucus or blood can be recognized through genital inspection. For visualization of the vagina and cervix a pediatric vaginoscope (Fig. 69-2), an otoscope, a very narrow long-bladed nasal speculum, or a pediatric laryngoscope may be preferred. The child is usually examined in either the lithotomy position or the knee-chest position.

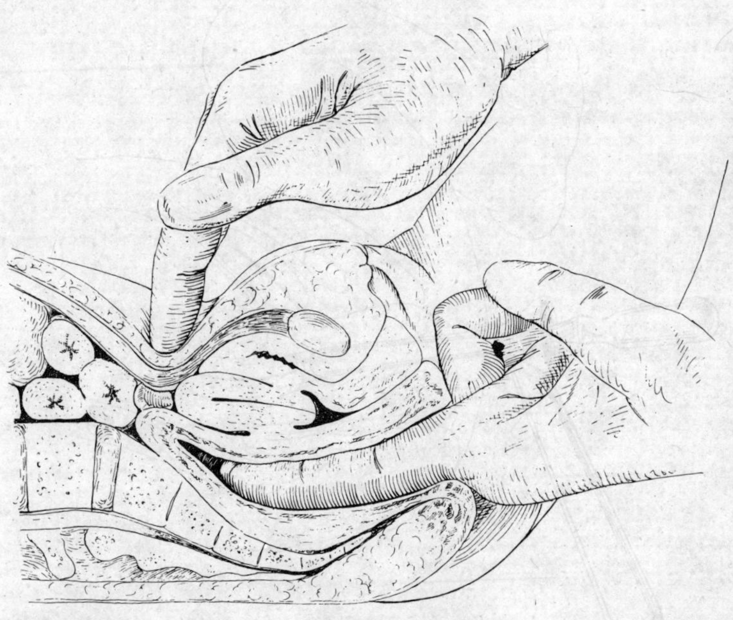

Figure 69-1. Rectoabdominal palpation of the internal genitalia and pelvic cavity in examination of premenarchal child. (From Huffman JW: The Gynecology of Childhood and Adolescence. Philadelphia, W.B. Saunders Company, 1968.)

Rectal Examination: Perianal excoriation may be the first clue to the presence of a pinworm infestation. Prior to puberty, rectal examination is often the best method for evaluation of the internal genital and pelvic cavity. Lower abdominal tumors as well as localized areas of pain are assessed with bimanual rectal abdominal palpation (see Fig. 69-1). In the prepubertal child only a small "button" of cervix is palpated. Any adnexal masses should alert the physician to the possibility of an ovarian cyst or tumor.

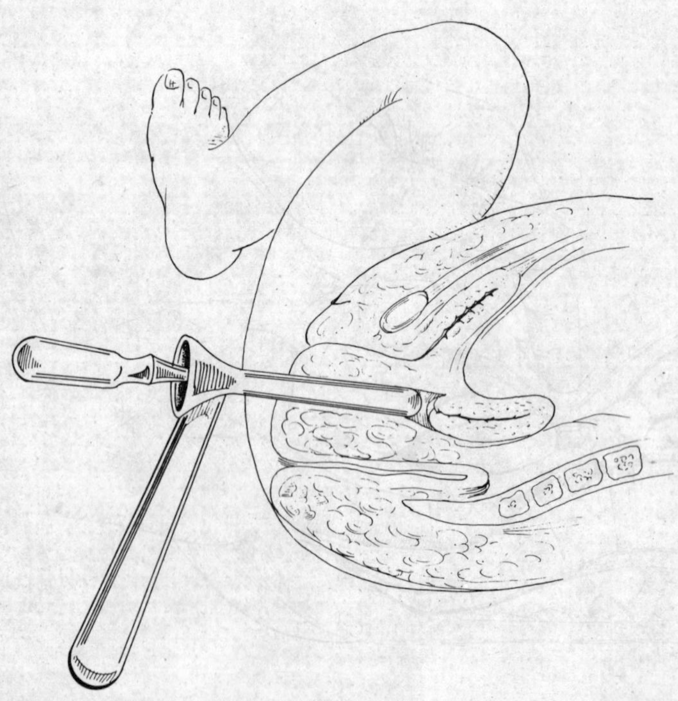

Figure 69-2. Inspection of cervix and vaginal walls by vaginoscopy. (From Huffman JW: The Gynecology of Childhood and Adolescence. Philadelphia, W.B. Saunders Company, 1968.)

LABORATORY TESTS

Complete Blood Count with Blood Smear: Elevated white count suggests a systemic pathologic condition.

Urinalysis: Hematuria or pyuria may indicate an associated urinary tract pathologic condition.

ASSESSMENT

DIFFERENTIAL DIAGNOSIS

Differential diagnosis of pediatric gynecologic problems includes the following:

1. Precocious puberty
2. Trauma
3. Vaginal infections
   a. Foreign body
   b. Bacterial infections
4. Congenital anomalies causing mucocolpos
   a. Imperforate hymen*
   b. Transverse vaginal septum
5. Neoplasia
   a. Benign
   b. Malignant
6. Blood dyscrasias

ETIOLOGIC FACTORS

Etiologic factors in premenarchal vulvovaginitis include specific organisms such as *Neisseria gonorrhoeae*, other organisms of the genus Neisseria, Candida, Trichomonas, *Escherichia coli*, and *Hemophilus vaginalis*. Other causes include soaps, dusting powders, bubble-bath preparations, respiratory infections, pinworms, foreign bodies, and poor perineal hygiene.

---

*Differential diagnosis of imperforate hymen includes vaginal agenesis, vaginal atresia, and testicular feminization.

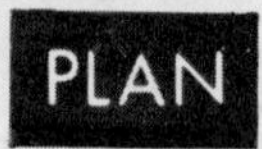

ADDITIONAL DIAGNOSTIC DATA

Microbiology: Samples of vaginal discharge may be obtained for gram-stained smears, cultures, and a wet preparation to identify Candida or Trichomonas.

Vaginal cytologic test or biopsy or both are indicated when neoplasia is suspected.

Cellulose tape examination of the perianal area for pinworm ova may be helpful. This examination should be made first thing in the morning and repeated on consecutive days if necessary.

Pelvic x-ray may aid in identification of a radiopaque foreign body. In the case of a straddle injury, abdominal x-ray may reveal free air and the possibility of visceral injury.

Intravenous Pyelogram: Since congenital abnormalities of the reproductive tract are often associated with congenital anomalies of the urinary tract, an intravenous pyelogram may disclose a urinary tract pathologic condition.

MANAGEMENT AND PATIENT EDUCATION

Therapy depends on the specific diagnosis.

Foreign-Body Vaginitis: Any foreign body in the vagina must be removed. Although extraction, at times, is a simple procedure, sedation or general anesthesia may be required. Usually, the item can be picked out with a long, thin, nasal forceps passed through the vaginoscope. Gentle irrigation may be helpful. Home care consists of sitz baths twice daily and thorough cleansing of the perineum.

Contact or Allergic Vulvovaginitis: Soaps, dusting powders, bubble-bath preparations, or rubberized panties may be responsible for allergic or contact vulvovaginitis. The cornerstone of therapy is removal of the causative factor. Warm sitz baths may be soothing. Topical corticosteroid creams [fluocinolone (0.01 per cent) or the equivalent] usually relieve pruritic symptoms.

Nonspecific Vulvovaginitis: Nonspecific vulvovaginitis usually results from poor perineal hygiene—failure to cleanse the perineum properly following a bowel movement. Warm sitz baths twice daily, as well as thorough cleansing of the perineum with soap and water after defecation, are recommended. The importance of perineal cleanliness (wiping from front to back after bowel movements) and changing soiled underclothes is explained to the child and her parents. The mother is advised to inspect the youngster's genitalia after bathing to be certain that the child is cleansing herself properly.

The patient who has not responded to sitz baths and cleanliness is treated with a local intravaginal antibacterial cream or suppository. One half of a nitrofurazone (Furacin) urethral suppository may be inserted into the child's vagina at bedtime nightly for 14 days. Alternatively, a triple sulfa vaginal cream may be inserted into the vagina with a small plastic applicator. The cream is inserted nightly for two weeks.

Gonorrheal Vaginitis: Uncomplicated gonococcal vulvovaginitis and urethritis may be treated during one visit with aqueous procaine penicillin G (APPG) (75,000 to 100,000 units/kg intramuscularly) and probenecid (25 mg/kg by mouth). Topical and systemic estrogen therapy are of no benefit in vulvovaginitis. All patients should have follow-up cultures, and the source of infection should be identified, examined, and treated.

Infection complicated by peritonitis or arthritis should be treated by hospitalization and administration of aqueous crystalline penicillin G intravenously (75,000 to 100,000 units/kg/day in four doses) or procaine penicillin G intramuscularly (75,000 to 100,000 units/kg/day in two doses for seven days).

Treatment of Patients with Allergy to Penicillin: Patients under six years of age with uncomplicated disease should be treated with erythromycin (40 mg/kg/day in four doses by mouth for seven days). Complicated disease should be treated with cephalothin (60 to 80 mg/kg/day in four doses intravenously for seven days). Patients older than 6 may be treated with an oral regimen of tetracycline (25 mg/kg as an initial dose followed by 40 to 60 mg/kg/day in four doses for seven days or an intravenous regimen of 15 to 20 mg/kg/day of tetracycline in four doses for seven days).

Pinworm Vaginitis: Children with pinworm may be treated with a single oral dose of pyrantel pamoate (Antiminth). The usual dosage is 11 mg/kg of body weight. Alternative agents are piperazine and pyrvinium pamoate. Adjunctive therapy for nonspecific vaginitis is advisable. The entire family may have to be treated.

Imperforate Hymen: An imperforate hymen (see Fig. 69-3) is opened surgically in order to permit drainage of a mucocolpos or hematocolpos or both. In infants and children, the central portion of the membrane is excised. In older girls with retained menstrual blood, a wedge-shaped portion of the thin posterior part of the hymen is removed.

Vulva Trauma: A small vulvar hematoma can usually be controlled by a tight pressure dressing and an ice pack. A large hematoma or one that continues to increase in size should be incised, clotted blood should be removed, and bleeding points should be ligated. If the source of bleeding cannot be found, the cavity is packed with gauze and a firm pressure

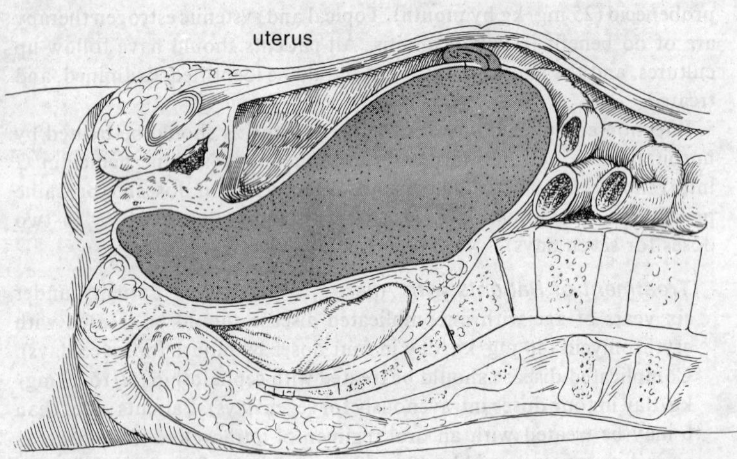

Figure 69-3. During infancy, mucoid material above an imperforate hymen may make a mass simulating a tumor. The tiny uterus sits atop the huge fluid-filled cystlike vagina. (From Huffman JW: The Gynecology of Childhood and Adolescence. Philadelphia, W.B. Saunders Company, 1968.)

dressing is applied. The pack is removed in 24 hours. Blood transfusion may be indicated if there has been excessive blood loss. Antibiotics are given prophylactically when a hematoma is opened.

Vulvar contusions rarely require treatment other than ice packs.

Evidence that a sharp object has penetrated the vagina calls for intravaginal examination under general anesthesia. Although most injuries are superficial and not serious, an extensive vaginal tear or injury of adjacent viscera may be found. In the case of peritoneal perforation, the child's life is in peril unless the condition is quickly diagnosed and promptly treated.

The wound must be carefully inspected to see whether it has extended into the rectum, bladder, or peritoneal cavity. A catheter is gently inserted into the urethra. Difficulty in passing the catheter, or hematuria are indications for urologic study. Bladder rupture and peritoneal perforation must be explored and repaired. If severe trauma to the external genitalia makes primary anatomic reconstruction impossible, additional plastic procedures may be necessary when the girl is older.

A booster dose of tetanus toxoid is given if the child has been previously immunized. Protection against tetanus is essential; antitoxin is indicated if the child has not been previously immunized.

REFERENCES

Altchek A: Symposium on pediatric and adolescent gynecology. Ped Clinics North Am *19*:507-603, 1972

Huffman JW: The Gynecology of Childhood and Adolescence. Philadelphia, W.B. Saunders Company, 1968

70 PELVIC INFECTION

GENERAL CONSIDERATIONS

Pelvic infection is a general term used to describe the state or condition in which the pelvic organs (uterus, fallopian tube, or ovaries) are invaded by pathogenic microorganisms. These organisms, usually bacteria, multiply and produce an inflammatory reaction.

The syndrome of genital infection designated as pelvic inflammatory disease (PID) is frequently a composite one, produced by various degrees of endometrial and tubal involvement, with or without extension to the broad ligament, ovaries, and pelvic peritoneum.

Although bacteria may reach the uterus, tube, and ovary by the blood stream, the usual routes of invasion are either (1) upward migration from the cervix through the endometrial cavity into the endosalpinx (usual route of gonorrheal infection) or (2) the veins and lymphatics of the broad ligaments (see Fig. 70-1).

Endometritis, if not recognized and treated promptly, may be followed by myometritis, parametritis, salpingo-oophoritis with abscess formation, peritonitis, and pelvic thrombophlebitis. The course of the disease depends on the strain and virulence of the invading organisms as well as on the individual host resistance to the microorganisms.

Pelvic infections can be separated into three basic categories: (1) those occurring after curettage and postabortal and postpartum infections; (2) postoperative infections usually developing from organisms that are introduced into the operative site from the skin, vagina, or less frequently, the gastrointestinal tract during surgery; and (3) pelvic infections occurring in nonpregnant patients without preceding surgical entry of the abdominal or endometrial cavity. *Neisseria gonorrhoeae* may be isolated from approximately one third to one half of the last group.

Bacteria usually responsible for pelvic infections are either exogenous organisms (acquired in the community or hospital) or endogenous organisms (normally present in the female genital tract or intestinal

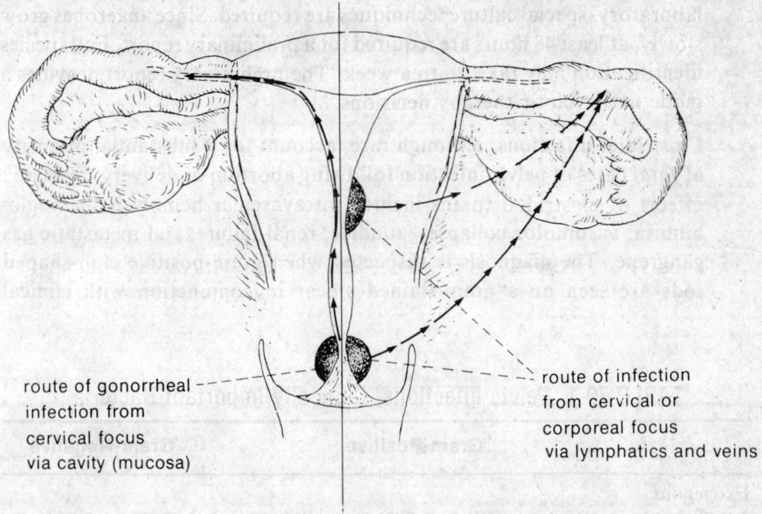

Figure 70-1. The two chief routes of pelvic infection. (From Novak ER, Woodruff JD: Novak's Gynecologic and Obstetric Pathology. 7th ed. Philadelphia, W.B. Saunders Company, 1974.)

tract). Ordinarily nonpathogenic, these endogenous organisms become pathogenic under conditions of altered host resistance. Acute pelvic infections are frequently of polymicrobial cause (Eschenbach, 1975). (See Table 70-1.)

Host resistance to infections seems to be decreased after abortion, delivery, surgery, prolonged rupture of membranes, and trauma. Other predisposing factors to pelvic infection include use of an intrauterine device, retained products of conception, menstruation, and previous gonococcal salpingitis. Gonococcal salpingitis damages the endosalpinx and increases the susceptibility of the fallopian tubes to infection by genital commensal organisms.

Anaerobic Infections: Appropriate specimens for anaerobic cultures include blood, cul-de-sac fluid, and abscess aspirates. It is essential that the specimen be transported to the bacteriology laboratory either in a prereduced transport medium or in an air-free, capped syringe. In the laboratory, special culture techniques are required. Since anaerobes grow slowly, at least 48 hours are required for a preliminary report. Full species identification may take up to a week. The preliminary report provides a guide to antibiotic therapy decisions.

Clostridial infections, although rare, account for a substantial minority of *fatal* cases of pelvic infection following abortion or delivery. Systemic effects of clostridial toxins include intravascular hemolysis, hemoglobinuria, vasomotor collapse, jaundice, renal failure, and metastatic gas gangrene. The diagnosis is suspected when gram-positive club-shaped rods are seen on a gram-stained smear in conjunction with clinical

TABLE 70-1. Pelvic Infections: Clinically Important Bacteria

	Gram-Positive	Gram-Negative
Exogenous		
Cocci	Streptococcus	*Neisseria gonorrhoeae*
	Group A	
	β hemolytic	
	Staphylococcus	
Endogenous		
Aerobes		
Cocci	Streptococcus	
	Group D (Enterococci)	
Bacilli		*Escherichia coli*
		Enterobacter
		Klebsiella
		Proteus
		Pseudomonas
Anaerobes		
Cocci	Peptococcus	Veillonella
	Peptostreptococcus	
Bacilli	Clostridium	Bacteroides
	Eubacterium	Fusobacterium
	Actinomyces*	

*_Actinomyces israelii_ grows as a pleomorphic rod-shaped bacterium and can be cultured from carious teeth, tonsillar crypts, and the region of the cecum. In soft tissue, it can cause a chronic, suppurative, granulomatous lesion. Mycelial clumps in draining pus have been termed sulfur granules.

symptoms of shock, hemolysis, and gas formation. Puerperal clostridial infection is marked by the rapid onset of fever, abdominal pain, uterine tenderness, a foul-sweetish odor of lochia, and marked leukocytosis. [Microbiologic identification of members of the Clostridium genus from sites of infection is of no significance in the absence of clinical findings (Ledger, 1973).]

Mycoplasmas are the smallest free-living organisms, sharing a number of properties with bacteria (growth outside the host cell, susceptibility to antimicrobial drugs, and reproduction by fission). In contrast to bacteria, they do not possess a cell wall.

Mycoplasma hominis and the T mycoplasmas are called genital mycoplasmas and may be recovered from the lower genital tract of asymptomatic women (De Louvois, 1975). Although usually asymptomatic, mycoplasmas may contribute to pelvic infections.

Mycoplasma septicemia is characterized by high temperature, spiking to 103° F, and few localizing signs, in a patient who appears nontoxic. White blood counts range from 6000 to 13,000.

Mycoplasma hominis is sensitive to tetracycline and lincomycin but resistant to erythromycin. T mycoplasmas are sensitive to tetracycline and erythromycin but resistant to lincomycin. Mycoplasmas are also resistant to penicillin, ampicillin, cephalosporins, and aminoglycosides.

Chlamydia are intracellular microorganisms that appear to be responsible for nonspecific urethritis and salpingitis. Usual treatment is oral tetracycline.

DEFINITIONS

Endometritis—inflammation of the endometrium, the inner mucous lining of the uterus, produced by bacterial invasion.

Parametritis—inflammation of the parametrium, the pelvic connective tissue surrounding the uterus. Synonym: *Pelvic cellulitis.*

Salpingitis—inflammation of the fallopian tube.

Oophoritis—inflammation of the ovary.

Tuboovarian abscess—an accumulation of pus involving the fallopian tube and the ovary.

Pyosalpinx—a suppurative inflammation of the fallopian tube resulting from blockage of the tubal lumen at the fimbriated and isthmic ends or obstruction of various segments of the tube. The tube is distended by an accumulation of purulent exudate in the lumen.

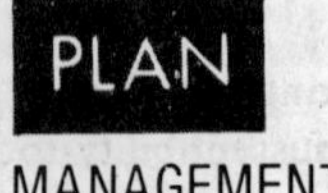

MANAGEMENT

Antibiotic Therapy:

Penicillin G is frequently effective as the primary agent in the treatment of infection produced by Streptococcus, Clostridium, *Neisseria gonorrhoea*, and anaerobic bacteria with the exception of Bacteroides. Enterococcal species (Lancefield group D strepcocci) usually respond to penicillin in combination with an aminoglycoside (streptomycin, gentamicin, or kanamycin).

Gentamicin or one of the other aminoglycosides is the primary agent in the treatment of serious infections caused by the gram-negative bacteria: *Escherichia coli*, Enterobacter, Klebsiella, Proteus, Pseudomonas, and Serratia.

Clindamycin is active against anaerobic gram-negative bacilli, including the Bacteroides species, as well as the gram-positive anaerobic cocci, including peptococci, peptostreptococci, and microaerophilic streptococci. Although clostridia are more resistant than most anaerobes to clindamycin, most strains of *Clostridium perfringens* are susceptible. Susceptibility testing should be done.

When prompt treatment is essential, antibiotic therapy must be initiated prior to the laboratory identification of specific organisms. Antibiotic selection is based on (1) the probable source of infection (community or hospital acquired), (2) the gram-stained smear, (3) previous antibiotic therapy, (4) an estimation of the most likely pathogens from previous experience with similar infections, (5) the current pattern of bacterial resistance in the hospital and community, and (6) the patient's history of allergy or sensitivity. Therapy is continued or modified on the basis of the patient's clinical response as well as the bacteriologic culture and sensitivity data.

TABLE 70-2. Bacterial Susceptibility To Antibiotic Therapy

	Penicillin G	Ampicillin	Carbenicillin	Cephalosporin	Gentamicin	Kanamycin	Clindamycin	Chloramphenicol	Tetracycline *
Actinomyces	S†	S		S			S	S	S§
Bacteroides fragilis			S				S†	S	V
Bacteroides—other	V	V	S				S	S	V
Clostridium perfringens	S†	S	S	V			S	S	S§
Clostridium—other	S†	S	S	V			V	S	S§
Enterobacter			V	V	S†	S		V	V
Escherichia coli	V	S	S	S	S†	S		S	V
Eubacterium	S	S	S				S	S	
Fusobacterium	S	S	S				S	S	S
Klebsiella				S	S	S		S	V
Neisseria gonorrhoeae	S†	S	S						S§
Peptococcus	S	S	S				S	S	V
Proteus	V	S	S	V	S†	S		S	
Pseudomonas			V		S†			V	V
Staphylococcus	V	V	V	S	V	V	S		
Streptococcus—anaerobic	S†	S	S				S	S	V
Streptococcus—Group A β hemolytic	S†	S	S	S			S		V
Streptococcus—Group D Enterococci	‡	S†	V		‡	‡			V

*Although most of the tetracyclines are similar, some have a longer duration of action than others. Doxycycline and minocycline appear to be more active against anaerobic bacteria than the others.

†Usual drug of choice.

‡Most strains of enterococci are sensitive to penicillin and an aminoglycoside (gentamicin or kanamycin) in combination.

§When penicillin is contraindicated, tetracyclines are alternative drugs.

S = Most strains are susceptible.

V = Strains vary in susceptibility. Sensitivity testing is suggested.

Bacterial susceptibility to some of the most commonly prescribed antibiotics is tabulated in Table 70-2.

Multiple-drug regimens are often chosen for severely ill patients or those who have failed to respond to single-agent therapy. The most frequently employed combination regimens are the following:

1. Penicillin G plus gentamicin, which covers virtually all pelvic pathogens with the exception of *Bacteroides fragilis*
2. Clindamycin plus gentamicin, which covers-virtually all pelvic pathogens with the exception of enterococci
3. Penicillin plus chloramphenicol, which covers virtually all pelvic pathogens with the exception of Pseudomonas
4. Cephalosporin plus gentamicin, which covers virtually all pathogens with the exception of *Bacteroides fragilis* and enterococci
5. Penicillin G plus Gentamicin plus Clindamycin, which covers virtually *all* pelvic pathogens

Antibiotics represent only one facet of the treatment of gynecologic and obstetric infections. Failure to respond to a particular antibacterial agent may mean either (1) that the drug or dosage employed or both are inappropriate or (2) that an additional complication coexists. For example, an abscess may require surgical drainage, or a thromboembolism may necessitate anticoagulant therapy.

Intravenous antibiotic dosages for severe pelvic infections are listed in Table 70-3.

TABLE 70-3. Intravenous Antibiotic Dosages for Severe Pelvic Infections

	Initial Dose	**Interval**	**Daily Dose**	
			Total	*Mg/kg/day*
Ampicillin	1-2 gm	q 4 h	6-12 gm	
Carbenicillin	5 gm	q 4 h	30-40 gm	400-500
Cephalosporin				
Cefazolin	0.5-1.0 gm	q 6-8 h	2-4 gm	
Chloramphenicol	1 gm	q 6 h	4 gm (first day)	50
Clindamycin	450-600 mg	q 6-8 h	1.8-2.4 gm	
Gentamicin	60-80 mg	q 8 h	180-240 mg	3-5
Kanamycin	250 mg	q 6-8 h	0.75-1.0 gm	15 max.
Penicillin G	3-5 million units	q 4 h	20-40 million units	
Tetracycline	500 mg	q 6-12 h	1-2 gm	

Treatment of Patients with Impaired Renal Function: Since the kidney is the major route of excretion for most antibiotics, careful consideration must be given to the effect of renal impairment on antimicrobial selection and dosage. When the serum creatinine is elevated, safe but effective blood levels can be attained for most antibiotics through dosage or interval adjustment.

Only moderate dosage reduction is necessary for ampicillin, cephalothin, chloramphenicol, clindamycin, oxacillin, and penicillin G.

Major dosage adjustment is necessary for carbenicillin, gentamicin, kanamycin and streptomycin.

In cases of impaired renal function, cephaloridine and tetracycline should be avoided.

Endometritis

GENERAL CONSIDERATIONS

Endometritis is an inflammation of the endometrium usually due to bacterial infection of the tissue. Endometritis develops most frequently after cesarean section, particularly if the patient has had an immediately preceding chorioamnionitis, prolonged labor, or prolonged rupture of membranes. Other causes of endometritis are retained placental tissue following abortion or delivery.

SUBJECTIVE DATA

Chills, fever, lower abdominal pain with or without vaginal bleeding, a mucopurulent vaginal discharge, and foul-smelling lochia are the most characteristic symptoms.

OBJECTIVE DATA

PHYSICAL EXAMINATION

General Examination: Temperature and pulse rate tend to be elevated. Blood pressure and respiration are usually normal.

A high, spiking temperature with chills within 12 hours of delivery or surgery is suggestive of group A beta-hemolytic streptococcal infection.

Abdominal Examination: Bowel sounds may be hypoactive. The postpartum uterus is often tender to palpation.

Pelvic Examination: The uterus is tender and often boggy (swollen). Foul-smelling lochia suggests anaerobic infection.

LABORATORY TESTS

Complete Blood Count with Blood Smear: Leukocytosis with a shift to the left is the usual finding. (After delivery, however, the white count can be elevated in a normal patient. Hemoglobin and hematocrit determinations may disclose coexisting anemia.

Urinalysis tends to be normal unless there is an associated urinary tract infection.

ASSESSMENT

DIFFERENTIAL DIAGNOSIS

Differential diagnosis of endometritis includes urinary tract infection, respiratory infection, drug fever, septicemia, pelvic thrombophlebitis, and pelvic abscess.

PREDISPOSING FACTORS

Predisposing factors include cesarean section, ruptured membranes, prolonged labor and delivery, anemia, hemorrhage, retained placental tissue, use of an intrauterine device, and systemic diseases that decrease resistance to infection. Women with a poor nutritional status, for example, appear to be more susceptible to bacterial infections.

POTENTIAL COMPLICATIONS

Complications include pelvic cellulitis, pelvic vein thrombophlebitis, peritonitis, pelvic abscess, bacteremia, disseminated intravascular coagulation, and septic shock.

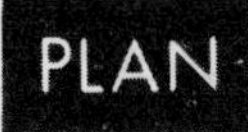

ADDITIONAL DIAGNOSTIC DATA

Bacteriology: Specimens from the endometrial cavity, urine, and blood are sent to the bacteriology laboratory for Gram stain, culture, and antibiotic sensitivity studies. Organisms most frequently isolated include *Escherichia coli*, streptococci, enteric organisms, and Bacteroides (see Table 70-1).

Erythrocyte Sedimentation Rate: The value of this test is very limited, since the sedimentation rate tends to be elevated during pregnancy as well as during times of infection.

MANAGEMENT

Antibiotics and adequate drainage are the cornerstones of therapy. Clinical evaluation and the organisms seen on Gram stain, as well as knowledge of bacteria isolated from previous similar infections, provide a guide to antibiotic therapy.

Intravenous fluids and electrolytes provide replacement therapy for dehydration and maintenance therapy for patients unable to tolerate oral feedings. As soon as feasible, the patient is given an oral diet that will provide essential nutrition.

Blood replacement may be indicated for severe postabortal or postpartum anemia.

Bed rest and analgesia are valuable adjunctive therapy.

Surgical Procedures: Postpartum endometritis is frequently associated with retained placental tissue or cervical obstruction. Adequate lochial drainage is essential. Retained placental tissue is removed by careful, gentle curettage.

Hysterectomy and bilateral salpingo-oophorectomy may be necessary when clostridial infection has extended beyond the endometrium and there is evidence of systemic clostridial sepsis (shock, hemolysis, renal failure).

Salpingitis

DEFINITIONS

Salpingitis—an inflammation of the fallopian tube.

Acute salpingitis—an infection of the fallopian tube that may be gonorrheal or pyogenic.

Subacute salpingitis—a stage of infection intermediate between acute and chronic salpingitis.

Chronic salpingitis—a stage of infection of the fallopian tube following the subacute stage. This type may be manifested in four forms: pyosalpinx, hydrosalpinx, chronic interstitial salpingitis, or salpingitis isthmica nodosa.

SUBJECTIVE DATA

CURRENT HISTORY

Abdominal Pain: Lower abdominal pain is one of the most reliable symptoms of acute pelvic infection. Initially, the pain may be unilateral, bilateral, or suprapubic, and it frequently develops during or shortly after a menstrual period. Gradually increasing in severity over a few hours to a few days, the pain tends to become constant, bilateral in the lower abdomen, and aggravated by motion.

Vaginal Bleeding or Discharge: Intermenstrual bleeding or increased menstrual flow or both may be a direct result of endometritis or an indirect effect of hormonal changes associated with oophoritis. Vaginal discharge may be caused by cervicitis.

Associated Symptoms: Chills and fever are common. Anorexia, nausea, and vomiting are associated with peritoneal irritation. Dysuria and urinary frequency indicate an associated urethritis or cystitis. Shoulder pain or right upper quadrant pain may be symptoms of gonococcal perihepatitis.

Menstrual History: Menses may be increased in amount and duration. Salpingitis may become symptomatic on the fourth or fifth day of the menstrual cycle.

PRIOR HISTORY

Patients with a history of pelvic infections may recognize similar symptoms. Some patients may be using an intrauterine contraceptive device.

OBJECTIVE DATA

PHYSICAL EXAMINATION

General Examination: Temperature is usually elevated, often to 102 or 103° F. Blood pressure is usually normal, although the pulse is frequently rapid. At times, the patient walks into the emergency room with a stooped-over position.

Abdominal Examination: Tenderness is maximal in both lower quadrants. Rebound tenderness, muscular rigidity, guarding, decreased bowel sounds, and distention are signs of peritoneal inflammation. Liver tenderness (perihepatitis) may be noted in up to 30 per cent of patients.

Pelvic examination is often difficult and unsatisfactory because of the patient's severe discomfort and abdominal rigidity. On speculum examination, a purulent discharge may be seen exuding from the cervical os. The cervix is very tender in response to motion. The uterus is of normal size, tender (particularly in response to motion), and often fixed in position. (An enlarged uterus suggests the possibility of septic abortion or ectopic pregnancy.) The adnexa are very tender bilaterally. A definite mass is seldom palpable unless a pyosalpinx or tuboovarian abscess has formed.

LABORATORY TESTS

Complete Blood Count with Blood Smear: The white count tends to be elevated and may be increased to 20,000 with increased polymorphonuclear leukocytes and an increased ratio of band to segmented forms.

Hemoglobin and hematocrit values are usually in the normal range. Elevated values are associated with dehydration.

Urinalysis is usually normal.

ASSESSMENT

DIFFERENTIAL DIAGNOSIS

The most common pelvic conditions that may be mistaken for acute salpingitis are ectopic pregnancy, acute appendicitis, and diverticulitis. (Other diagnoses to be considered include endometriosis, ovarian cysts, regional enteritis, and uterine leiomyomas.) (See Fig. 70-2.)

Ectopic pregnancy must be suspected when there is any history of missed menses, oligomenorrhea, or pregnancy symptoms, particularly if the patient's temperature and white cell count are not significantly elevated. Culdocentesis may disclose nonclotting blood.

Appendicitis should be considered when the pain is localized to the right lower quadrant (particularly McBurney's point). In appendicitis, the classic symptom sequence is initial periumbilical pain, followed by anorexia, nausea or vomiting or both, and a shifting of the pain to the right lower quadrant. Point tenderness over the appendix should be more painful than cervical motion. Mild fever and moderate leukocytosis are associated findings; the white count and temperature are frequently lower than in acute salpingitis. (Note: If a laparotomy is performed for suspected appendicitis and an uncomplicated salpingitis is discovered, the tubes should not be removed or incised.)

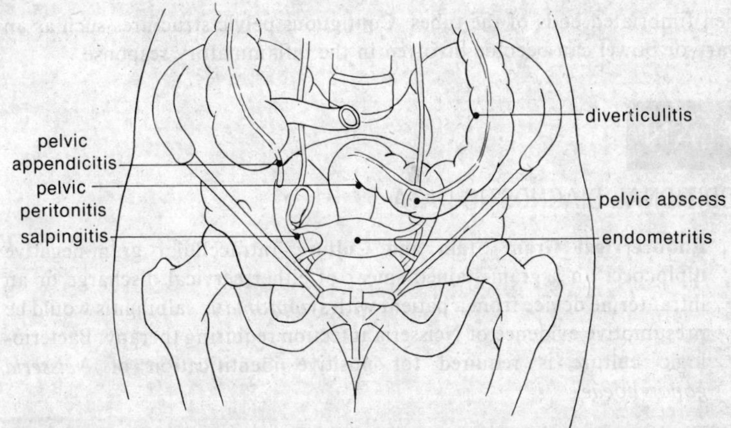

Figure 70-2. Causes and locations of pelvic inflammatory disease. (From Botsford TW, Wilson RE: The Acute Abdomen: An Approach to Diagnosis and Management. Philadelphia, W.B. Saunders Company, 1977.)

Diverticulitis may be difficult to differentiate from left-sided salpingitis. The typical attack of diverticulitis is characterized by left lower quadrant pain, chills, fever, and peritoneal signs. A tender mass over the sigmoid may be palpated. The patient may give a history of attacks of diverticulitis.

ETIOLOGIC ORGANISMS

Neisseria gonorrhoeae accounts for approximately 30 to 50 per cent of the cases of salpingitis. Other pathogenic organisms are aerobic or anaerobic bacteria and Chlamydia. A number of cases appear to have a polymicrobial cause.

POTENTIAL COMPLICATIONS

These include oophoritis, peritonitis, pyosalpinx, tuboovarian abscess, septic thrombophlebitis, lymphangitis, cellulitis, and abscess in the broad ligaments. Peritoneal inflammation occurs either because of serosal inflammation resulting from subepithelial extension of infection of the endosalpinx or because infection spreads directly to the peritoneum via the open fimbriated ends of the tubes. Contiguous pelvic structures such as an ovary or bowel can become involved in the inflammatory response.

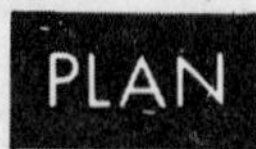

ADDITIONAL DIAGNOSTIC DATA

Endocervical Gram Stain and Culture: Intracellular gram-negative diplococci on a gram-stained smear of either cervical discharge or an intrauterine device from a patient with *symptomatic* salpingitis would be presumptive evidence of Neisseria infection requiring therapy. Bacteriologic culture is required for positive identification of *Neisseria gonorrhoeae.*

Erythrocyte sedimentation rate is frequently elevated. This test can be particularly helpful in the differential diagnosis of appendicitis or unruptured ectopic pregnancy, since the "sed rate" is *rarely* elevated in cases of ectopic pregnancy or within the first 24 hours of acute appendicitis.

Pregnancy test is negative. When the pregnancy test is positive, the possibility of ectopic pregnancy must be excluded.

Culdocentesis rules out hemoperitoneum when nonhemorrhagic fluid is aspirated. Gram stain and cultures (both aerobic and anaerobic) of the peritoneal fluid may provide an accurate bacteriologic diagnosis.

Abdominal x-rays (three-way: supine, upright, and lateral) can be helpful when there is any suspicion of the presence of a foreign body, intraperitoneal fluid, or gas-producing organisms. In acute appendicitis, abdominal x-ray findings are usually nonspecific. Signs that may be suggestive of appendicitis include (1) scoliosis of the lumbosacral spine away from the right lower quadrant due to psoas muscle spasm, (2) air-fluid levels in the cecum (local ileus); (3) a calcified fecalith (appendicolith) in the right lower quadrant, and (4) loss of the psoas shadow and flank stripe on the right side. (See Fig. 70-3.)

In cases of perforation of a hollow viscus, flat and upright films often reveal free air in the peritoneal cavity. Visualization of extraintestinal gas suggests an intraabdominal abscess.

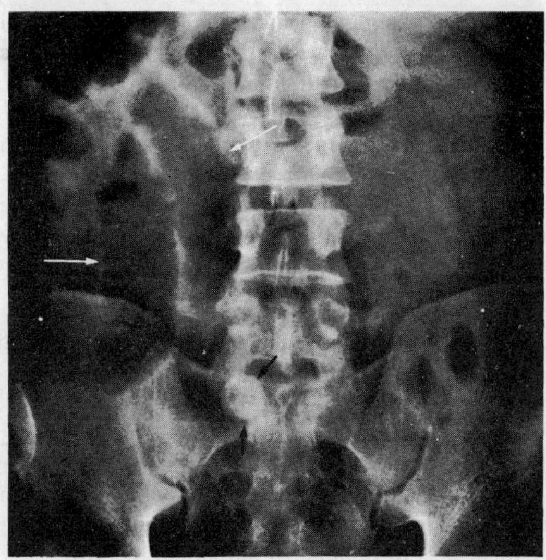

Figure 70-3. Acute appendicitis: sentinel loop and fecalith. In the right lower quadrant, there is a distended loop of ileum (sentinel loop, *white arrows*) that contained fluid levels in erect view. The round density with the calcified rim (*black arrows*) is a fecalith in the appendix. When seen in conjunction with a sentinel loop, it suggests acute appendicitis. A sentinel loop in itself is nonspecific, indicating the presence of a local intra-abdominal inflammatory condition such as appendicitis, cholecystitis, or pancreatitis. (From Teplick JG, Haskin ME: Roentgenologic diagnosis. Philadelphia, W.B. Saunders Company, 1976.)

MANAGEMENT

Outpatient Therapy:

1. Antibiotic therapy: A dosage of 4.8 million units of aqueous procaine penicillin G (APPG) is given intramuscularly, divided into at least two doses and injected at different sites. Alternatively, 3.5 gm of ampicillin may be given orally. One gm of oral probenecid is given along with either the penicillin or the ampicillin. Both are followed by 500 mg of ampicillin given orally four times daily for ten days.

If the patient is allergic to penicillin, alternative therapy is 1.5 gm of tetracycline hydrochloride given as a single oral loading dose, followed by 500 mg given orally four times daily for ten days.

2. An intrauterine device is removed.
3. The patient is given pain medication and advised to remain at bed rest until she is completely asymptomatic.
4. Follow-up cervical culture and pelvic examination are recommended after the termination of therapy. If the culture grows *Neisseria gonorrhoeae*, follow-up examination is essential. (See Gonorrhea, p. 356.)

Hospitalization is recommended in the following circumstances:

1. The diagnosis is uncertain, and surgical emergencies cannot be excluded.
2. Pelvic abscess is suspected.
3. A pregnant patient has salpingitis.
4. The patient is unable to follow an outpatient regimen of oral medication, especially because of nausea and vomiting.
5. The patient fails to respond to outpatient therapy.

Antibiotic Therapy:

1. Aqueous crystalline penicillin G. Twenty million units are given intravenously each day until clear-cut improvement occurs, followed by 500 mg of ampicillin given orally four times daily. Therapy should last a total of ten days.
2. Tetracycline hydrochloride. Five hundred mg are given intravenously four times daily until improvement occurs, followed by 500 mg given orally four times daily. Therapy should last a total of ten days. (This regimen should not be used for pregnant women or for patients with renal failure.)
3. When mixed infections or nongonococcal infections are suspected, an aminoglycoside (usually gentamicin) is administered in addition to the penicillin. If the patient fails to respond within 48 hours, Bacteroides is suspected and clindamycin is recommended.

Adjunctive Therapy: An intrauterine device is removed. Bed rest in Fowler's position is encouraged. Intravenous fluids are initiated. Oral feedings are deferred until any question of surgery has been eliminated and bowel sounds are active.

PATIENT EDUCATION

The patient may be sent home as soon as she is able to comply with oral therapy. Identification of *Neisseria gonorrhoeae* on cervical culture necessitates appropriate follow-up for gonorrhea. (See Gonorrhea, p. 356.)

Pyosalpinx and Tuboovarian (Pelvic) Abscess

GENERAL CONSIDERATIONS

Pyosalpinx is defined as a suppurative inflammation of the fallopian tube subsequent to gonorrheal or postpartum infection. Blockage of the tubal lumen at the fimbriated and isthmic ends results in the accumulation of purulent exudate in the tubal lumen, which causes tubal distention. The distended tube tends to become adherent to the surrounding structures owing to associated perisalpingitis.

Tuboovarian (pelvic) abscess forms when the infected tube becomes adherent to the ovary; tubal and ovarian inflammatory processes become merged. Tuboovarian abscesses can develop as a consequence of puerperal pelvic infection or as a complication of pelvic surgery, as well as from ovarian invasion by pyogenic organisms. Large accumulations of pus result in the formation of an exquisitely tender, nonmobile, poorly defined mass in either of the adnexal regions or in the cul-de-sac.

SUBJECTIVE DATA

CURRENT SYMPTOMS

Abdominal pain is the most typical symptom, tending to be severe, constant, and diffuse over the lower abdomen. As peritonitis spreads, the painful area becomes more extensive; the maximal pain tends to be localized to the abscess site.

Sudden, severe, diffuse abdominal pain associated with shock suggests the possibiity of a ruptured tuboovarian abscess.

Vaginal bleeding, spotting, and discharge are variable symptoms that may indicate ovarian dysfunction, an associated endometritis, or cervicitis.

Associated symptoms include fever, chills, anorexia, nausea, and vomiting. Pain on defecation or diarrhea suggests rectal involvement. Dysuria, frequency, pyuria, or hematuria suggests urinary bladder involvement.

PRIOR HISTORY

A history of recent abortion, obstetric delivery, or pelvic surgery suggests the probable predisposing factor. At times, an adnexal abscess develops late in the postoperative course following cesarean section or pelvic surgery.

Intrauterine devices are associated with an increased incidence of virulent pelvic infection.

Many patients give a history of recent or previous salpingitis or pelvic infection.

OBJECTIVE DATA

PHYSICAL EXAMINATION

General Examination: Temperature tends to be spiking, with elevations up to 103 or 104° F (40° C). The pulse is rapid and the blood pressure normal unless septic shock has caused hypotension, which may be a systemic sign of intraabdominal rupture.

Abdominal Examination: Pelvic tenderness, rebound tenderness, and guarding are characteristic findings of peritoneal inflammation. Bowel sounds are often hypoactive or absent; distention is due to paralytic ileus. A large pelvic abscess may be palpable abdominally.

Generalized muscular rigidity, upper abdominal rebound tenderness, shoulder pain, and absent bowel sounds are signs of generalized peritonitis that may signify intraabdominal rupture of an abscess.

Pelvic Examination: On speculum examination a purulent discharge may be visible in the cervical os. In addition, the string of an intrauterine device may be present.

The uterus is usually of normal size, fixed in position, and possibly deviated to one side. Cervical motion is very painful.

Adnexal masses, either unilateral or bilateral, are palpable. The masses—cystic and exquisitely tender—are irregularly shaped lateral to and behind the uterus. Adhesions often involve the bowel and omentum. Matting together and fixation of tissues add to the apparent size of the tumor masses. The abscess may bulge into the posterior cul-de-sac or point into the vaginal fornix.

Rectovaginal examination may disclose a very tender, fixed abscess dissecting into the rectovaginal septum.

LABORATORY TESTS

Complete Blood Count with Blood Smear: The white count is elevated up to 25,000, with increased polymorphs and band forms. Serial determinations provide an estimate of the patient's response to therapy.

Hemoglobin and hematocrit values are often elevated owing to dehydration. Decreased values indicate anemia, usually due to prior blood loss or hematoma formation.

Urinalysis is normal unless urinary tract infection coexists.

ASSESSMENT

DIFFERENTIAL DIAGNOSIS

Differential diagnosis of tuboovarian abscess includes twisted ovarian cyst, ectopic pregnancy, septic abortion, ruptured ovarian cystadenocarcinoma, degenerating leiomyoma, ruptured urinary bladder, appendiceal abscess, and diverticulitis.

In addition to infection spreading from a pyosalpinx or infected uterus, *general peritonitis* can be caused by disease or rupture of any hollow viscus or ruptured intraabdominal abscess. Diagnoses to be considered are *infection* spreading from pyonephrosis; *intestinal ischemia* following vascular accident or obstruction with strangulation; *ruptured* liver or splenic abscess; and *perforation* of appendix, gastric or duodenal ulcer, intestinal ulcer, diverticulum, gallbladder, or biliary ducts.

The four classic findings in the patient with a pelvic abscess are (1) fever, (2) a tender mass 5 cm or more in diameter, (3) pelvic pain, and (4) signs of pelvic peritonitis.

PREDISPOSING FACTORS

Pelvic abscess may develop as a sequela of salpingitis, puerperal infection, septic abortion, pelvic surgery, appendicitis, or diverticulitis. Other sources of intraabdominal abscess include pancreatitis, urinary tract infection, biliary tract, perforated ulcer (peptic or infectious), inflammatory bowel, ischemic bowel, amebiasis, and actinomycosis.

ETIOLOGIC FACTORS

Etiologic organisms may be either aerobic or anaerobic. Aerobes most commonly isolated include *Escherichia coli*, enterococci, streptococci, staphylococci, Klebsiella, and *Neisseria gonorrhoeae*; anaerobes likely to be identified include Bacteroides, Peptostreptococcus, and Clostridium (Rubenstein, 1976).

Approximately two thirds of the cultures grow multiple organisms.

POTENTIAL COMPLICATIONS

Complications to be anticipated include intraabdominal rupture, bacteremia, septicemia, septic shock, septic thrombophlebitis, and disseminated intravascular coagulation. (Intraperitoneal rupture must always bs suspected when a patient develops acute signs of generalized peritonitis or septic shock and a previously known adnexal mass is no longer palpable.)

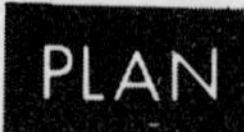

ADDITIONAL DIAGNOSTIC DATA

Bacteriologic studies include

1. Endocervix—gram-stained smear and aerobic cultures
2. Blood—aerobic and anaerobic cultures

3. Abdominal or vaginal wounds—gram-stained smears, aerobic and anaerobic cultures

Erythrocyte sedimentation rate (ESR) tends to be markedly elevated. Values in the range of 60 to 100 mm/hour are indicative of an acute suppurative process.

Serum electrolytes are a useful guide for fluid and electrolyte replacement therapy.

Abdominal x-rays are helpful when there is any suspicion of the presence of a foreign body, intraperitoneal fluid, or gas-producing organisms. A frequent finding is an adynamic ileus.

Intravenous pyelogram may reveal ureteral displacement.

Ultrasound B-scan may aid in the evaluation of the size and location of the abscess cavity. (See Ultrasound, p. 857.)

Culdocentesis may provide purulent fluid to be sent to the bacteriology laboratory for Gram stain, aerobic and anaerobic cultures, and antibiotic sensitivity studies.

MANAGEMENT AND PATIENT EDUCATION

The patient is hospitalized and placed at bed rest in a semi-Fowler's position.

Any intrauterine device is removed.

Nasogastric suction is indicated when vomiting, abdominal distention, and absent bowel sounds are indicative of a paralytic ileus.

An indwelling catheter to record urine output and a central venous pressure line are advisable if septic shock is suspected.

Intravenous fluids and antibiotics are essential. Fluid and electrolyte replacement depends on the patient's hydration as well as on the daily fluid losses. Antibiotics are chosen to cover all suspected aerobic and anaerobic gram-negative and gram-positive organisms. Usually patients are started on a combination of penicillin, gentamicin, and clindamycin, since this combination covers all the most likely organisms. (See Table 70-1.) As soon as a positive bacteriologic culture is obtained, antibiotic therapy is adjusted in accordance with the specific organism(s) identified and the sensitivities known.

The response to therapy is evaluated by the patient's general condition, temperature, and serial white blood counts. Medical therapy is continued as long as the tenderness and size of the mass decline . Sudden deterioration of the clinical situation suggests a ruptured abscess.

If the patient remains febrile after 72 hours of adequate parenteral therapy, there are three possible explanations: (1) The responsible organisms are not susceptible to the antibiotics selected, (2) there is concurrent pelvic thrombophlebitis, or (3) a collection of pus must be drained surgically.

Colpotomy drainage through the posterior vaginal fornix usually benefits patients with a palpable, fluctuant cul-de-sac mass that has dissected into the rectovaginal septum (Rubenstein, 1976). In the operating room, under general anesthesia, the mass is aspirated for Gram stain and culture, then incised and drained with gentle digital exploration of the cavity to break down superficial adhesions (see Fig. 70-4).

Exploratory laparotomy is indicated if the diagnosis is uncertain, the abscess has ruptured intraperitoneally, the patient fails to improve within 72 hours, or the abscess becomes progressively larger. Usually, total abdominal hysterectomy with bilateral salpingo-oophorectomy is necessary. Surgery is difficult because of the extensive inflammatory edema; the risk of bowel and ureteral injury is always present. After the uterus is removed, the vaginal cuff is left open with a drain.

Pyometra

GENERAL CONSIDERATIONS

Pyometra is a condition in which the endometrial cavity becomes filled with pus. This results from an inflammatory process of the endometrium with a concomitant stenosis of the cervix. The uterus is distended and thin-walled. Pyometra may occur with cervical or uterine carcinoma or following cervical amputation, or radiation therapy.

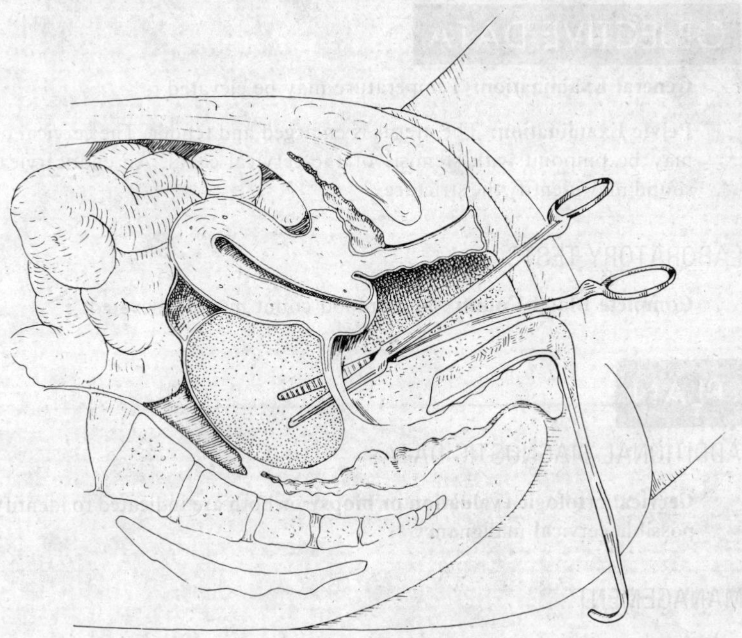

Figure 70-4. Draining the pelvic abscess vaginally. First, the cul-de-sac is aspirated, leaving the needle in place. Then, following alongside the needle with a scalpel or sharp-pointed scissors, the abscess cavity is perforated and the opening is enlarged by spreading the jaws of a clamp, as shown here. (From Greenhill JP, Friedman EA: Biological Principles and Modern Practice of Obstetrics. Philadelphia, W.B. Saunders Company, 1974.)

SUBJECTIVE DATA

Abdominal pain tends to be cramplike. Distention of the uterine cavity causes uterine contractions that attempt to expel the intrauterine material.

Vaginal bleeding may be associated with necrosis and ulceration.

Leukorrhea may be intermittent and purulent.

OBJECTIVE DATA

General Examination: Temperature may be elevated.

Pelvic Examination: The uterus is enlarged and tender. The cervical os may be pinpoint with stenosis of the cervical canal. An endocervical sound may identify the stricture.

LABORATORY TESTS

Complete Blood Count: White blood count may be elevated.

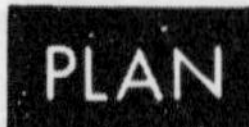

ADDITIONAL DIAGNOSTIC DATA

Cervical cytologic evaluation or biopsy or both are indicated to identify possible cervical malignancy.

MANAGEMENT

The patient should be hospitalized. Initial therapy includes cervical dilatation to release the purulent fluid from the uterus. Uterine contents are cultured and endometrial biopsy obtained to diagnose possible malignancy. Antibiotic therapy is determined by the organisms suspected or identified to be present.

If malignancy is present, appropriate therapy must be arranged.

REFERENCES

Altemeier WA, Culbertson WR, Fullen WD, et al: Intraabdominal abscesses. Am J Surg *125*:70-79, 1973

Charles D: Value of the erythrocyte sedimentation rate in gynecologic infections. Clin Obstet Gynecol *19*:171-193

Chow AW, Malkasian KL, Marshall JR, et al: Bacteriology of acute pelvic inflammatory disease. Am J Obstet Gynecol *122*:876-879, 1975

Chow AW, Marshall JR, Guze LB: Anaerobic infections of the female genital tract: prospects and perspectives. Obstet Gynecol Surv *30*:477-494, 1975

De Louvois J, Stanley VC, Hurley R, et al: Microbial ecology of the female lower genital tract during pregnancy. Postgrad Med J *51*:156-160, 1975; Obstet Gynecol Surv *30*:727-729, 1975

Eschenbach DA: Acute pelvic inflammatory disease: etiology, risk factors and pathogenesis. Clin Obstet Gynecol *19*:147-169, 1976

Eschenbach DA, Buchanan TM, Pollock HM, et al: Polymicrobial etiology of acute pelvic inflammatory disease. N Engl J Med *293*:166-171, 1975

Gibbs RS, Weinstein AJ: Puerperal infection in the antibiotic era. Am J Obstet Gynecol *124*:769-787, 1976

Heaton FC, Ledger WJ: Postmenopausal tuboovarian abscess. Obstet Gynecol *47*: 90-94, 1976

Lamey JR, Foy HM, Kenny GE: Infection with Mycoplasma hominis and T-strains in the female genital tract. Obstet Gynecol *44*:703-708, 1974; Obstet Gynecol Surv *30*: 466-467, 1975

Ledger WJ: Anaerobic infections. Am J Obstet Gynecol *123*:111-118, 1975

Ledger WJ, Hackett KA: Significance of clostridia in the female reproductive tract. Obstet Gynecol *41*:525-530, 1973

Lomax CW, Harbert GM, Thornton WN: Actinomycosis of the female genital tract. Obstet Gynecol *48*:341-346, 1976

McNamar MT, Mead PB: Diagnosis and management of the pelvic abscess. J Reprod Med *17*:299-304, 1976

Mead PB, Beecham JB, Maeck J, Van S: Incidence of infections associated with the intrauterine contraceptive device in an isolated community. Am J Obstet Gynecol *125*:79-82, 1976; Obstet Gynecol Surv *31*:752-754, 1976

Mead PB, Gump DW: Antibiotic therapy in obstetrics and gynecology. Clin Obstet Gynecol *19*:109-129, 1976

Rubenstein PR, Mishell DR, Ledger WJ: Colpotomy drainage of pelvic abscess. Obstet Gynecol *48*:142-145, 1976

Taylor ES, McMillan JH, Greer BE, et al: The intrauterine device and tubo-ovarian abscess. Am J Obstet Gynecol *123*:338-348, 1975; Obstet Gynecol Surv *31*:154-155, 1976

71 PLACENTA ACCRETA

GENERAL CONSIDERATIONS

Placenta accreta is a placenta all or a part of which is inseparable from the uterine wall. It is caused by partial or complete absence of the decidua basalis, especially of the spongy layer.

Placenta increta is a form of placenta accreta in which the chorionic villi invade the myometrium.

Placenta percreta is abnormal penetration of chorionic elements to the serosal layer of the uterus.

The incidence of these abnormalities is rare, ranging from 1 in 2000 to 1 in 14,000 pregnancies.

SUBJECTIVE AND OBJECTIVE DATA

The placenta fails to separate after the birth of the baby. Since a focal placenta accreta is more common than a complete accreta , bleeding tends to be profuse and persistent from partial areas of detachment.

On intrauterine examination, during the course of exploration for manual removal of the retained placenta, no cleavage plane can be identified between the adherent placenta and the uterine wall. In the case of a partial placenta accreta, the cleavage plane may be started, but it cannot be followed completely across the maternal surface of the placenta because dense adhesion is encountered.

Urinalysis may disclose hematuria in the rare case of bladder invasion.

ASSESSMENT

PREDISPOSING FACTORS

These include placenta previa, previous cesarean section, trauma from previous uterine curettage, destruction of endometrium from previous infection, previous manual removal of placenta, and high gravidity.

POTENTIAL COMPLICATIONS

These include profuse hemorrhage, uterine rupture, uterine inversion, and uterine infection (particularly if the placenta is left *in situ*).

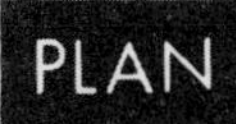

MANAGEMENT AND PATIENT EDUCATION

Intravenous fluids and blood are essential to correct blood-loss hypovolemia.

Abdominal hysterectomy is the preferred treatment for most patients as soon as the diagnosis is made. Since normal placental detachment is impossible, any attempt to remove the adherent placenta manually or with a curette can cause catastrophic hemorrhage or traumatic rupture of the thin uterine muscle.

In the absence of hemorrhage, the placenta may be left *in situ* if the patient strongly desires to have more children and is willing to accept the risk of uterine and pelvic infection. The mortality rate of patients treated without hysterectomy is nearly four times higher than that of patients treated with immediate hysterectomy (Fox, 1972).

REFERENCES

Dick JS, deVilliers VP: Spontaneous rupture of the uterus in the second trimester due to placenta percreta: two case reports. J Obstet Gynaecol Br Commw *79*:187-189, 1972

Fox H: Placenta accreta 1945-1969. Obstet Gynecol Surv *27*:475-490, 1972

Weekes LR, Greig LB: Placenta accreta. Am J Obstet Gynecol *113*:76-82, 1972; Obstet Gynecol Surv *27*:675-677, 1972

72 PREMATURE SEPARATION OF THE PLACENTA

GENERAL CONSIDERATIONS

Premature separation of the placenta is defined as complete or partial detachment of the normally implanted placenta from the uterine wall at 20 weeks or more of gestation. Synonyms are abruptio placentae, accidental hemorrhage, ablatio placentae, and placental apoplexy.

The incidence of premature separation of the placenta ranges between 1 in 55 to 250 deliveries, depending on the diagnostic criteria. All degrees of premature separation of the placenta may occur, from a separation only a few millimeters in diameter to separation of the entire placenta. Placental separation severe enough to cause fetal death may occur in approximately 1 in 400 deliveries.

SUBJECTIVE DATA

CURRENT SYMPTOMS

Vaginal bleeding plus steady uterine pain are characteristic symptoms of premature placental separation. The bleeding may be minimal to profuse, usually occurring suddenly and unexpectedly during the third trimester. Often the bleeding is darker than the bright red blood associated with placenta previa. This dark blood may represent a retroplacental clot dissecting membrane off the uterine wall to drain through the cervix.

Abdominal pain, constant in nature, is usually noted simultaneously with external bleeding. Sudden, severe pain may be a sign of retroplacental bleeding infiltrating the uterine muscle. Abdominal pain may be the only symptom when bleeding is retroplacental and concealed (see Fig. 72-1). Uterine contractions may or may not be evident.

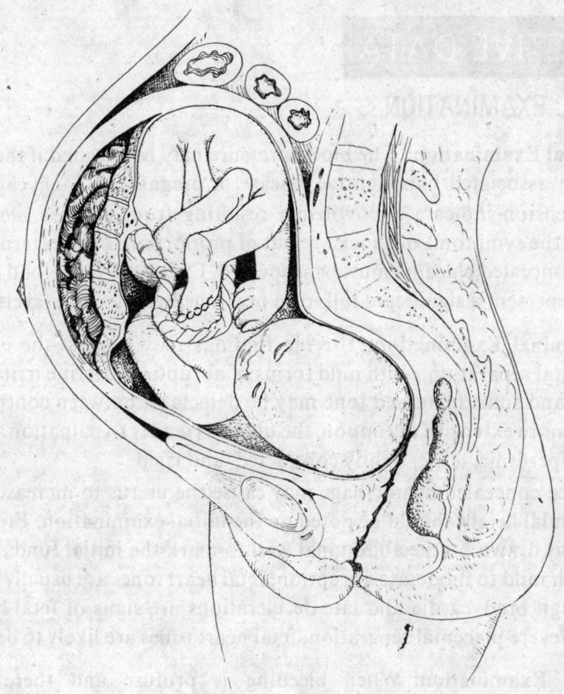

Figure 72-1. Abruptio placentae with concealed hemorrhage. (From Huffman JW: Gynecology and Obstetrics. Philadelphia, W.B. Saunders Company, 1962.)

PRIOR HISTORY

Patients with a history of premature placental separation are more likely to have a recurrent placental abruption. Patients with hypertensive disease of pregnancy have an increased likelihood of premature placental separation.

OBJECTIVE DATA

PHYSICAL EXAMINATION

General Examination: The blood pressure may be elevated if the patient has an associated hypertensive disease of pregnancy. Tachycardia and hypotension indicate hypovolemia resulting from profuse blood loss. When the symptoms of shock are out of proportion to the external blood loss, concealed bleeding must be suspected. Even a normal blood pressure may represent a significant fall from previous hypertensive levels.

Abdominal Examination: Uterine findings may suggest the extent of placental separation. With mild forms of abruption, uterine irritability is slight and some increased tone may be detectable between contractions. With more extensive abruption, the uterus is tender to palpation and may feel hypertonic, tense, tightly contracted, and rigid.

Since concealed hemorrhage may cause the uterus to increase in size, the fundal height should be noted on the initial examination. Frequently a line is drawn on the abdominal wall to mark the initial fundal height.

With mild to moderate abruption, fetal heart tones are usually present, although bradycardia and late decelerations are signs of fetal hypoxia. With severe placental separation, fetal heart tones are likely to be absent.

Pelvic Examination: When bleeding is profuse and there is any possibility of placenta previa, vaginal examination should be deferred until the patient is in an operating room and prepared for an immediate cesarean section, in case this becomes necessary. If ultrasound examination has localized the placenta and has excluded the possibility of placenta previa, a vaginal examination is indicated to assess the status of the cervix (consistency, dilatation, effacement), as well as the station of the presenting part. Placental separation may occur either prior to labor, when the cervix is closed, or during labor, after the cervix has dilated.

LABORATORY TESTS

Complete blood count with blood smear may indicate preexisting anemia and blood loss. Declining hematocrit values on serial determinations may suggest concealed bleeding.

Urinalysis is usually normal. Proteinuria suggests an associated preeclampsia.

Blood Type and Rh: Blood should be cross-matched for transfusion as indicated.

ASSESSMENT

DIFFERENTIAL DIAGNOSIS

Differential diagnosis includes placenta previa, the "bloody show" of labor, ruptured marginal sinus, and vasa previa.

Severe placental abruption must be distinguished from uterine rupture and abdominal pregnancy with intraabdominal hemorrhage. Rare conditions that may simulate premature placental separation include ruptured hemangioma (Dawood, 1972), hepatic rupture, splenic artery rupture (Brass, 1977), and sickle cell crisis.

See Vaginal Bleeding in Late Pregnancy, p. 699.

PREDISPOSING FACTORS

These include hypertension [Forty-seven per cent of patients with a placental abruption severe enough to kill the fetus have associated hypertension (Pritchard, 1970).] multiparity, previous abruption (incidence of recurrence averages 10 per cent), and trauma.

SEVERITY OF PLACENTAL SEPARATION

With mild placental separation, the fetus is alive, with normal heart tones, and there is usually no evidence of distress. Bleeding and abdominal pain are minimal, and there is no evidence of shock or coagulopathy. Uterine contractions are often intermittent, with slightly increased tone between contractions. Maternal vital signs are stable.

Moderate placental separation is characterized by more extensive blood loss and more abdominal pain. The fetus may show fetal heart rate changes suggestive of placental insufficiency.

When severe placental separation occurs, the fetus either dies or is in severe distress. Abdominal pain is persistent, and bleeding may be profuse. Maternal shock and possibly coagulopathy may be evident. Uterine contractions are often tetanic, with no relaxation between contractions.

POTENTIAL COMPLICATIONS

Complications to be anticipated include

1. Disseminated intravascular coagulation (DIC)
2. Renal failure. Hypovolemic shock or DIC may lead to renal ischemia and tubular damage.
3. Couvelaire uterus, the diffuse infiltration of the entire myometrium with blood
4. Postpartum hemorrhage. Postpartum uterine atony may be associated with an increase in fibrin-split products (Basu, 1972).
5. Fetal distress or fetal death. Fetal mortality may be as high as 35 per cent, the main causes being hypoxia and prematurity.

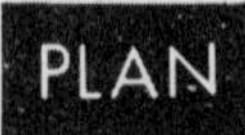

ADDITIONAL DIAGNOSTIC DATA

Coagulation tests may disclose consumption coagulopathy (DIC). Fibrinogen may be depleted, fibrin-split products elevated, platelet count decreased, and prothrombin and partial thromboplastin times prolonged. When fibrinogen levels fall below 100 mg/ml, blood frequently fails to clot.

A clot observation test is easily performed at the bedside. Five ml of the patient's blood is placed in a test tube and observed for clotting. If a clot does not form within 8 to 12 minutes, the patient's fibrinogen concentration is below the critical level. If the blood does clot, the test tube is incubated at 37° C for 30 minutes. Normally the clot remains intact. Disintegration, fragmentation, or dissolution of the clot indicates the presence of fibrinolysins in the blood. (See Coagulation Disorders, p. 210.)

This test should be repeated at 30- to 60-minute intervals, the length of the interval depending on the mother's condition.

Electronic fetal monitoring evaluates fetal well-being and the possibility of placental insufficiency and fetal hypoxia. Fetal heart rate monitoring rules out fetal distress as long as (1) the baseline rate is within a normal range, (2) beat-to-beat variability is normal, (3) accelerations occur with fetal movements, and (4) there are no late decelerations with uterine contractions.

Serum Electrolytes and Blood Chemistries: Determination of these may be helpful in the evaluation of the patient with severe disease.

Ultrasound B-scan may be helpful. The placental site can be localized, and a retroplacental clot may be recognized.

MANAGEMENT AND PATIENT EDUCATION

All patients with third trimester bleeding should be hospitalized immediately. When placental separation is diagnosed, management decisions depend on the maternal blood loss (external and concealed) and fetal maturity, presentation, and well-being.

In cases of moderate and severe placental separation, immediate treatment objectives are to restore blood loss, correct coagulation defects, and effect delivery.

Hemorrhage and hypovolemia are treated by the prompt restoration of an effective circulation. Intravenous fluids are initiated (usually lactated Ringer's solution followed by packed red blood cells or whole blood as necessary). Since blood loss may be concealed behind the placenta, the volume of blood required is often underestimated. Evidence of shock, the patient's response to transfusion, urine output, and central venous pressure serve as guides for blood and fluid replacement. The extent of retroplacental blood loss is not fully known until the placenta is delivered.

In order to recognize continued concealed bleeding, the fundal height is marked on the abdomen when the patient is first seen.

Mild or Moderate Placental Separation: As long as there is no evidence of fetal distress or maternal distress, and the cervix and fetal presentation are favorable for rapid labor and delivery, amniotomy is performed and vaginal delivery anticipated. Oxytocin stimulation appears to provide benefits that override the risks, as long as the fetal heart-rate and uterine contractions are monitored continuously.

Cesarean section is indicated if there is any evidence of fetal distress, if fetal presentation is abnormal, bleeding increases, or labor fails to progress actively.

Severe Placental Separation: When a severe placental separation and intrauterine fetal death occur, vaginal delivery is preferred unless hemorrhage is so brisk that it cannot be managed by vigorous blood replacement or there are obstetric complications that contraindicate vaginal delivery. In order to minimize maternal blood loss, diminish the chances of renal complications, and prevent serious coagulation disorders, the patient should be delivered promptly, usually within six hours of the onset of the abruption.

Membranes are ruptured. Port wine-colored fluid confirms the diagnosis. Uterine contractions are augmented with dilute intravenous oxytocin, if necessary. If labor does not progress rapidly, however, or if there are contraindications to vaginal delivery, cesarean section is necessary.

Hypovolemic shock is corrected with oxygen, intravenous fluids, and blood replacement. Urine output and central venous pressure determinations provide an assessment of volume replacement, helping to guard against over- or under-replacement. Coagulation defects are treated with fresh-frozen plasma or fresh whole blood if available. Cryoprecipitate and platelet packs may also be necessary. (See Blood Transfusion, p. 750.)

Following delivery, hypofibrinogenemia usually corrects itself spontaneously within 24 hours. Repeated coagulation studies (fibrinogen, prothrombin time, partial thromboplastin time, and platelet count) provide the best guide to replacement therapy.

REFERENCES

Basu HK: Some observations on the aetiology and management of coagulation failure complicating abruptio placentae. J Indian Med Assoc *58*:409-416, 1972; Obstet Gynecol Surv *28*:551-553, 1973

Brass P: Splenic artery rupture in pregnancy: a case report. Am J Obstet Gynecol *128*:228-229, 1977

Dawood MY, Teoh EG, Ratnam SS: Ruptured haemangioma of a gravid uterus. J Obstet Gynaecol Br Commw *79*:474-475, 1972

Golditch IM, Boyce NE: Management of abruptio placentae. JAMA *212*:288-293, 1970

Lunan CB: The management of abruptio placentae. J Obstet Gynaecol Br Commw *180*:120-124, 1973; Obstet Gynecol Surv *28*:549-551, 1973

Phillips JM, Evans JA: Acute anesthetic and obstetric management of patients with severe abruptio placentae. Anesth Analg *49*:998-1006, 1970; Obstet Gynecol Surv *26*:435-437, 1971

Pritchard JA, Mason R, Corley M, et al: Genesis of severe placental abruption. Am J Obstet Gynecol *108*:22-27, 1970; Obstet Gynecol Surv *26*:236-237, 1971

Pritchard JA: Haematological problems associated with delivery, placental abruption, retained dead fetus and amniotic fluid embolism. Clin Haematol *2*:563-586, 1973

73 PLACENTA PREVIA

GENERAL CONSIDERATIONS

Placenta previa is the implantation of any part of the placenta in the lower uterine segment. The term expresses the anatomic relationship between the placental site and the lower uterine segment. A placenta previa encroaches on or covers (completely or incompletely) the internal cervical os. (See Fig. 73-1.)

Marginal placenta previa is present when some part of the placenta is attached to the lower uterine segment and extends to, but does not cover, any part of the internal cervical os.

Partial placenta previa is present when any part of the placenta incompletely covers the internal cervical os.

Total placenta previa is present when any part of the placenta completely covers the internal cervical os.

The incidence of placenta previa is approximately 1 in 200 to 400 deliveries.

SUBJECTIVE DATA

Vaginal bleeding is painless, bright red, and apt to occur suddenly during the third trimester. The initial episode is usually slight to moderate and often ceases spontaneously. During active labor, bleeding from a placenta previa may cause profuse hemorrhage. The bleeding results from separation of that portion of the placenta overlying the cervical canal, as a result of cervical effacement and dilatation.

Pregnancy Symptoms: Fetal activity is usually normal. Some patients report previous episodes of bleeding during the first or second trimesters. The dates of the last menstrual period provide the initial estimate of gestational age.

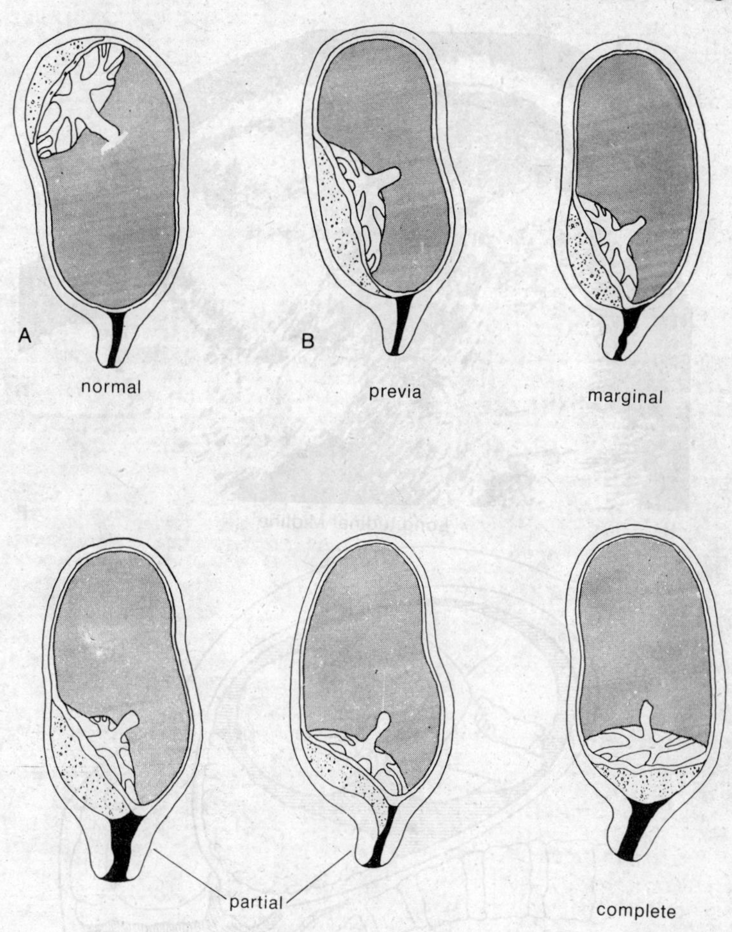

Figure 73-1. The placenta normally implants in the fundus (*A*), but it may implant in the lower corpus, with its lower edge at the margin of the internal os, (*B*) or it may partially or completely cover the internal os. (From Huffman JW: Gynecology and Obstetrics. Philadelphia, W.B.Saunders Company, 1962.)

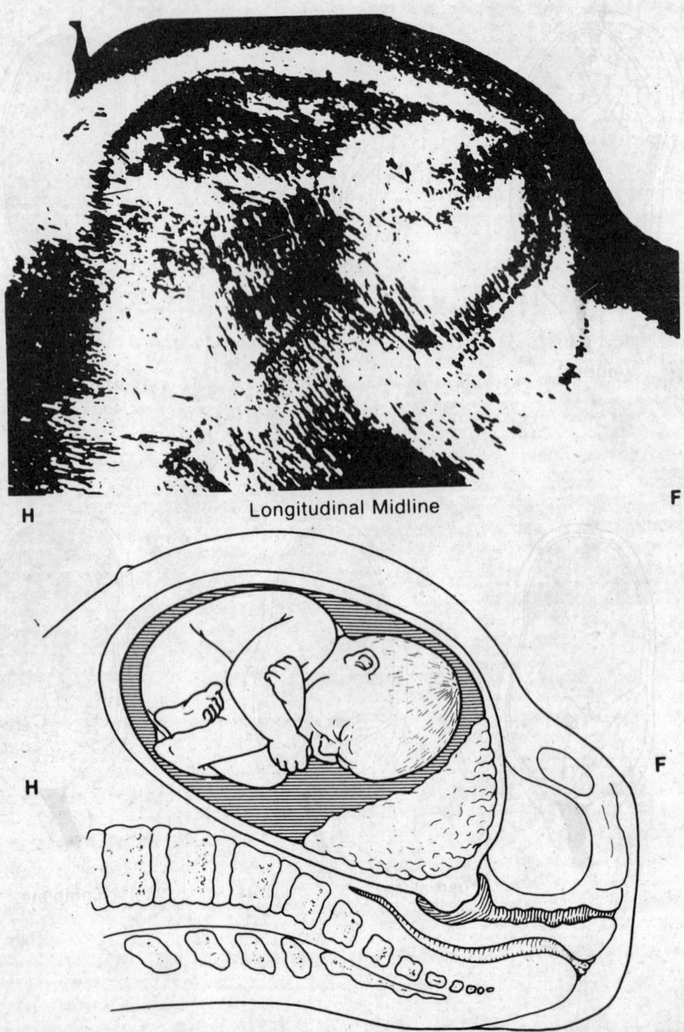

Figure 73-2. Entire fetus displaced superiorly into the uterine fundus in patient with total central placenta previa. (From Gosink BB, Squire LF: Exercises in Diagnostic Radiology 8: Diagnostic Ultrasound. Philadelphia, W.B. Saunders Company, 1976.)

OBJECTIVE DATA

PHYSICAL EXAMINATION

General Examination: Unless the bleeding is profuse (10 to 25 per cent of patients), vital signs are usually normal and the patient appears alert and healthy.

In cases of profuse hemorrhage, hypotension and tachycardia are indicative of maternal hypovolemia.

Abdominal Examination: The uterus is soft and nontender; uterine contractions are usually absent.

Fetal heart tones are usually normal. The presenting part is not engaged in the pelvic inlet. Fetal malpresentation (breech, oblique, or transverse lie) is a frequently associated finding.

Pelvic Examination: The vulva should be carefully examined initially in order to evaluate the quantity of external bleeding and the possibility of urinary tract or rectal bleeding.

Vaginal or rectal examination may stimulate profuse hemorrhage. Consequently, vaginal examination should *never* be done unless the patient is in an operating room prepared for immediate cesarean section.

If bleeding is minimal and placenta previa appears unlikely, a gentle speculum examination may exclude the possibility of vaginal or cervical bleeding (as the result of ruptured varices, cervical erosions, or cervical tumors).

Whenever a fetal source of bleeding is suspected (owing to fetal bradycardia or absent fetal heart tones), the blood should be sent to a laboratory for determination of fetal hemoglobin (See Vasa Previa, p. 706.)

LABORATORY TESTS

Complete blood count should be ordered for every patient in order to assess the degree of anemia.

Urinalysis is usually normal.

Blood Type and Rh: Two to 4 units of blood should be prepared for possible transfusion. The rate and extent of hemorrhage determine the need for blood replacement.

ASSESSMENT

DIFFERENTIAL DIAGNOSIS

The differential diagnosis includes premature separation of the placenta, premature labor, and vasa previa (Table 73-1). (See Vaginal Bleeding, Late Pregnancy, p. 699.)

PREDISPOSING FACTORS

These include multiparity and advanced maternal age.

POTENTIAL COMPLICATIONS

Complications of placenta previa include hypovolemic shock and premature delivery. Rarely, placenta accreta, due to the poorly developed decidua of the lower uterine segment, may be an associated finding.

SEVERITY OF DISEASE PROCESS

The severity of hemorrhage and the rate of blood loss determine the immediate therapeutic plan. Patients in hypovolemic shock with persistent blood loss require termination of pregnancy, usually by immediate cesarean section.

TABLE 73-1. Common Causes of Third Trimester Bleeding

	Placenta Previa	Premature Separation of Placenta	Premature Labor
Vaginal bleeding	Bright red	Darker red	Blood may be mixed with mucus
Blood pressure	Normal	↑ nl ↓	Normal
Uterine pain	Absent	Steady	Intermittent
Uterine tone	Normal	↑	Normal
Fetal heart tones	Normal	Absent, fetal distress	Normal
Coagulation tests	Normal	Abnormal	Normal

↑ nl ↓ = Increased, normal, or decreased
↑ = Increased

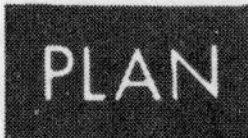

ADDITIONAL DIAGNOSTIC DATA

Ultrasound B-scan may aid in placental localization. In addition, ultrasonic examination clarifies the fetal presentation and the possibility of multiple gestation and provides an estimate of gestational age by measurement of the biparietal diameter.

Amniocentesis: When fetal maturity is questionable, determination of the lecithin-sphingomyelin ratio in the amniotic fluid provides an assessment of fetal lung maturity. (See Amniocentesis, p. 731.)

Coagulation tests (fibrinogen, prothrombin time, partial thromboplastin time, and platelet count) should be ordered whenever there is any possibility of a coagulation disorder.

MANAGEMENT AND PATIENT EDUCATION

Any patient suspected of having a placenta previa should be hospitalized and placed at bed rest. An intravenous infusion is initiated, and blood is drawn for hematocrit, Rh, type, and cross-matching. The patient is carefully observed for any evidence of active bleeding. No oral feedings are permitted. Adequate blood should be available in case transfusion becomes necessary. Immediate questions to be answered include the following:

1. Is the patient in labor?
2. How mature is the fetus?
3. How severe is the hemorrhage?

Specific plans depend on the rate and quantity of bleeding, the presence or absence of uterine contractions, and the gestational age and evidence of fetal maturity. If the fetus is immature and bleeding subsides, the location of the placenta can be determined with ultrasonography. When a placenta previa is visualized, amniocentesis may aid in the evaluation of fetal lung maturity. If the L/S ratio is less than 2.0, the fetus will usually benefit from additional time in the uterus. The patient should be kept under close observation, preferably in the hospital, until fetal maturity permits elective delivery or repeated bleeding endangers the mother and fetus.

If the fetus is mature or if the initial hemorrhage persists or recurs, a double setup examination is performed as soon as blood for replacement is available, in order to determine the optimal route for delivery (vaginal or cesarean section.) A double setup examination is a vaginal examination performed in an operating room, the patient and the medical team being prepared for immediate cesarean section in case this becomes necessary.

Cesarean section is recommended for all cases of partial or total placenta previa, whenever bleeding is profuse, fetal distress is present, fetal presentation is abnormal, or the progress of labor is abnormal.

Opinions differ over the optimal uterine incision. In general, it is best to avoid any incision through the placenta because this would increase maternal and fetal blood loss. As long as the placenta is known to be lying posteriorly, a transverse incision in the lower uterine segment may be selected. In the case of an anterior placenta previa, however, a vertical uterine incision appears to be safer, allowing the physician to find a way around the placental edge, rupture the membranes, and deliver the baby rapidly with minimal fetal blood loss. The cord should be clamped promptly after delivery.

Cesarean hysterectomy is indicated when placenta previa is complicated by placenta accreta.

Vaginal delivery may be elected when the placenta is *marginal* to the cervical os and does not occupy any area of cervical dilatation, bleeding is minimal, the presentation is cephalic, there is no fetal distress, and rapid labor is anticipated. Under these circumstances, amniotomy and intravenous oxcytocin may be administered, as long as the uterine contractions and fetal heart rate can be monitored carefully.

REFERENCES

Crenshaw C, Darnell Jones DE, Parker RT: Placenta previa: A survey of twenty years experience with improved perinatal survival by expectant therapy and cesarean delivery. Obstet Gynecol Surv *28*:461-470, 1973

Scheer K: Ultrasonic diagnosis of placenta previa. Obstet Gynecol *42*:707-710, 1973

74 PLACENTA RETAINED IN UTERUS

GENERAL CONSIDERATIONS

After delivery of the baby, the placenta usually follows spontaneously within ten minutes. While waiting for this to happen, the obstetrician palpates the uterine fundus and observes the perineum for signs of placental separation. These include change in uterine shape from discoid to globular, elongation of the exposed cord, and appearance of increased bleeding.

If at any time bleeding is excessive, the uterus balloons with blood, or the placenta has not separated spontaneously within 10 to 15 minutes, manual removal may be necessary.

SUBJECTIVE AND OBJECTIVE DATA

Either the placenta does not separate spontaneously or active bleeding develops after the baby has been delivered.

On vaginal examination, the placenta is not found in the cervical canal but partially or completely attached within the interior of the uterus.

ASSESSMENT

DIFFERENTIAL DIAGNOSIS

This includes placenta accreta, a placenta abnormally adherent to the myometrium without the physiologic line of cleavage through the spongy layer of decidua.

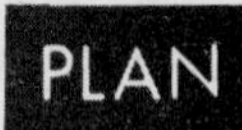

MANAGEMENT

When the placenta is trapped in the cervical canal, it can usually be removed with gentle traction. The uterine fundus must be continually palpated in order to detect the earliest sign of uterine inversion.

If the placenta remains wholly or partially adherent to the uterine wall, manual removal (Fig. 74-1) may be essential in order to control uterine hemorrhage. General anesthesia (usually with halothane) is almost always required for adequate uterine relaxation. Aseptic surgical technique should be employed, making certain that the forearm is covered with a long sterile glove. The uterus is grasped through the abdominal wall with one hand while the other hand is introduced into the vagina and passed into the uterine cavity. When the placental margin is reached, the back of the hand is placed against the uterine wall and the fingers insinuated between the wall and the placenta.

The uterus is supported externally with the abdominal hand while the placenta is separated from its attachment site by blunt digital dissection along the cleavage plane. In the case of a placenta accreta, no cleavage plane can be identified (See Placenta Accreta, p. 500.)

After complete separation, the placenta is grasped with the entire hand and withdrawn. The gloved hand is rinsed and reinserted into the uterine cavity in order to be certain that all placental fragments or cotyledons have been removed. Covering the fingers with a gauze sponge may aid in the removal of adherent membranes.

Anesthesia is discontinued as soon as possible in order to minimize uterine atony and associated hemorrhage. Intravenous oxytocin (20 units/1000 ml of 5 per cent dextrose in lactated Ringer's solution) is administered rapidly to facilitate uterine contractions. Ergonovine (0.2 mg) may be given intramuscularly.

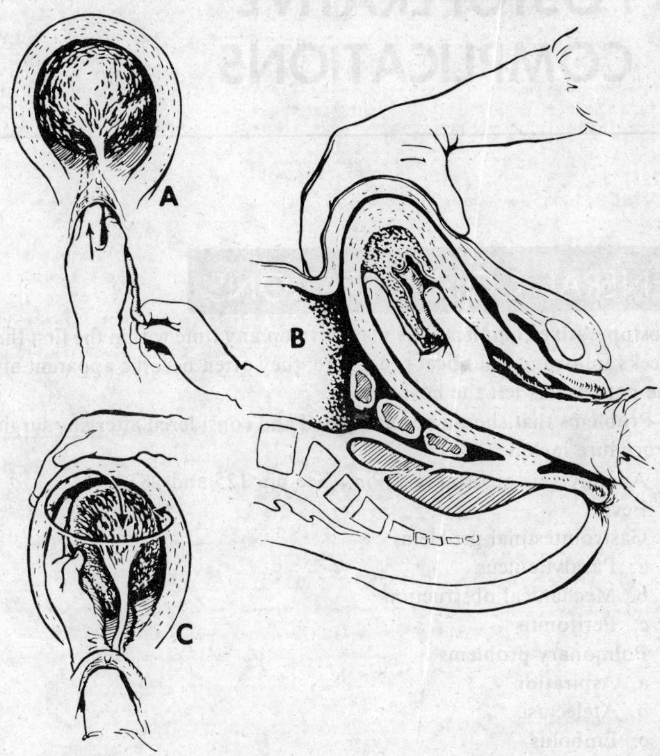

Figure 74-1. Technique for manual removal of the placenta. *A*, The left hand is guided into the uterus along the umbilical cord. *B*, By use of the ulnar side of the hand in a knife motion, the placenta may be carefully separated from the uterus. *C*, After it is certain that the placenta has been completely separated, the hand may cup the placenta from the top and be gently withdrawn. (From Tenney B, Little B: Clinical Obstetrics. Philadelphia, W.B. Saunders Company, 1961.)

75 POSTOPERATIVE COMPLICATIONS

GENERAL CONSIDERATIONS

Postoperative complications may develop any time within the first three weeks following a surgical procedure; they often become apparent after the patient has left the hospital.

Problems that should be anticipated and considered after any surgical procedure include

1. Anaphylaxis or drug reaction. (See pp. 125 and 283.)
2. Fever
3. Gastrointestinal problems
   a. Paralytic ileus
   b. Mechanical obstruction
   c. Peritonitis
4. Pulmonary problems
   a. Aspiration
   b. Atelectasis
   c. Embolus
   d. Pneumonia
5. Shock (see Shock, p. 612)
   a. Cardiogenic
   b. Hypovolemic
   c. Septic
6. Transfusion reactions (see Blood Transfusion, p. 750)
7. Urinary tract
   a. Fistula (see Urinary Incontinence, p. 651)
   b. Infection
   c. Injury
   d. Retention (see Urinary Retention, p. 658)
   e. Suppression (oliguria or anuria) (see Urinary Suppression, p. 660)

8. Venous problems
   a. Bacteremia
   b. Thrombophlebitis (see Thrombophlebitis, p. 644)
9. Wound problems
   a. Bleeding
   b. Dehiscence
   c. Hematoma
   d. Infection (cellulitis or abscess)

Postoperative Fever

GENERAL CONSIDERATIONS

Fever, or elevated body temperature, is one of the most frequent postoperative complications, and it may develop as late as two to three weeks following surgery. (See Table 75-1.)

Infections of the operative site (vaginal cuff, pelvic cellulitis, abdominal wound), urinary tract, lungs, and veins are the most frequent conditions responsible for postoperative febrile morbidity. Other possibilities include drug fever and intraoperative damage to the bowel or urinary tract. When fever resolves only after all medications have been discontinued, a diagnosis of drug fever may be presumed.

SUBJECTIVE DATA

Data such as the time of onset, the type of operative procedure, the known operative complications, the history of bladder catheterization, and the specific localizing symptoms are important clues to the differential diagnosis.

TABLE 75-1. Postoperative Fever

Time of Onset	Possible Diagnosis
Day 1	Contaminated intravenous fluids Aspiration pneumonia Operative wound contaminated with Group A β hemolytic streptococcus Clostridial myonecrosis (gas gangrene)
Days 1-3	Pulmonary atelectasis Pneumonitis
Days 2-4	Ureteral injury Urinary tract infection Endometritis after cesarean section Thrombophlebitis (intravenous infusion) Septicemia—bacteremia
Days 3-5	Vaginal cuff infection after hysterectomy Pelvic cellulitis
Days 5-6	Abdominal wound infection
Days 7-25	Adnexal abscess (frequently anaerobic) Septic pelvic thrombophlebitis

OBJECTIVE DATA

PHSYICAL EXAMINATION

General Examination: The extent of the temperature elevation and the time of onset after surgery may be significant. (See Table 75-1.) Pulmonary atelectasis is suspected if the postoperative patient develops a temperature under 101° F within the first 48 hours. Adnexal abscess or septic pelvic thrombophlebitis is more likely to be associated with high, spiking fevers late in the postoperative period.

Leg Evaluation: Erythema, increased temperature and calf circumference, pain and calf tenderness with dorsiflexion of the foot (Homans' sign) suggest thrombophlebitis.

Chest Examination: Dullness or absent breath sounds suggest atelectasis.

Abdominal Examination: Tender, indurated areas adjacent to the abdominal wound suggest cellulitis or possible abscess. Costovertebral angle tenderness suggests pyelonephritis. Abdominal distention with absent bowel sounds are signs of paralytic ileus.

Pelvic Examination: A tender mass suggests a vaginal cuff abscess or an adnexal abscess.

LABORATORY TESTS

Complete blood count with blood smear may reveal unexpected blood loss, suggesting hematoma formation. The white count and differential count provide an estimate of the patient's response to infection; serial values help evaluate the patient's response to therapy.

Urinalysis may reveal white or red cells, suggesting urinary tract disease.

ASSESSMENT

DIFFERENTIAL DIAGNOSIS

The differential diagnosis must consider the four most likely sources of infection: the lungs, urinary tract, wounds, and thrombophlebitis.

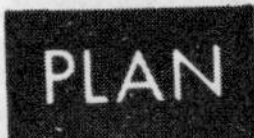

ADDITIONAL DIAGNOSTIC DATA

Bacteriologic studies should include

1. Blood—aerobic and anaerobic cultures
2. Urine—gram-stained smears and aerobic cultures
3. Abdominal and vaginal wounds—gram-stained smears; aerobic and anaerobic cultures.

Chest x-ray may reveal a pulmonary pathologic condition.

Abdominal x-ray may reveal an intraabdominal foreign body.

Ultrasound B-scan may delineate an adnexal abscess.

MANAGEMENT

Specific therapy depends on the specific diagnosis. Appropriate antibiotic therapy and drainage of purulent material are the cornerstones of therapy for infections.

Thrombophlebitis is treated with anticoagulant therapy. (See Thrombophlebitis, p. 644.)

Postoperative Gastrointestinal Problems

Paralytic Ileus: Following abdominal surgery, 12 to 48 hours of gastrointestinal ileus or atony should be expected. Oral feedings are usually withheld until bowel sounds are heard and the patient passes flatus.

Signs and symptoms of persistent paralytic ileus include abdominal distention and discomfort, vomiting, absent bowel sounds, failure to pass flatus, and dehydration.

Therapy consists of the following:

1. Nothing by mouth
2. Intravenous fluids and electrolytes to meet baseline requirements, urinary output and extrarenal losses
3. Nasogastric suction
4. Abdominal x-rays to differentiate ileus from mechanical obstruction

Mechanical obstruction is characterized by vomiting, distention, and intermittent colicky abdominal pain, with associated peristaltic rushes. If a case is seen late, it may be difficult to differentiate between the quiet abdomen of ileus and the relatively quiet abdomen of a neglected small-bowel mechanical obstruction.

X-ray examinations of the abdomen may aid in establishing the diagnosis.

A rise in the white cell count, temperature, and pulse rate is significant. As soon as the diagnosis of mechanical obstruction is established, exploratory laparotomy is indicated. Fluid and electrolyte balance must be corrected.

Postoperative Pulmonary Atelectasis

GENERAL CONSIDERATIONS

Atelectasis and pneumonitis are among the more frequent causes of early postoperative fever. Atelectasis should be suspected in any patient with fever during the first three postoperative days. After obstruction of a portion of the bronchial tree, resorption of alveolar air results in the collapse of a small or massive portion of the lung.

SUBJECTIVE AND OBJECTIVE DATA

The signs and symptoms depend on the area of lung parenchyma involved and the rapidity and completeness of the occlusion. Chest pain, dyspnea, cyanosis, tachycardia, and tachypnea may occur. The temperature tends to be elevated, usually under 101° F, within the first 48 hours after surgery. Chest examination findings include decreased breath sounds, rales, and occasional rhonchi at the lung bases.

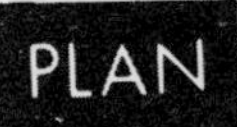

ADDITIONAL DIAGNOSTIC DATA

Chest x-ray may reveal atelectatic streaking of the lungs.

MANAGEMENT

The objective of therapy is increased pulmonary ventilation and the removal of obstructing mucus. Pulmonary parenchyma must be reexpanded before bacterial infection supervenes. Pain medication is prescribed to facilitate adequate chest expansion. Intermittent positive pressure breathing (IPPB), bronchodilators, and humidifiers may be effective. Antibiotics are indicated if there is evidence of pneumonia.

Postoperative Urinary Tract Infection

GENERAL CONSIDERATIONS

Urinary tract infections are among the more common causes of postoperative morbidity. Usually they result from operative manipulation, trauma, or catheterization.

SUBJECTIVE DATA

General Symptoms: Fever and chills are nonspecific signs of infection.

Urinary Symptoms: Dysuria, frequency, urgency, and hematuria point to the urinary tract as the source of infection.

Other Symptoms: Pain, either suprapubic or in the flank, usually is indicative of bladder or renal infection.

OBJECTIVE DATA

PHYSICAL EXAMINATION

General Examination: The temperature is elevated. Pulse and blood pressure tend to be within the normal range.

Abdominal examination findings often include suprapubic or flank tenderness.

LABORATORY TESTS

Complete Blood Count: Leukocytosis is a frequent finding.

Urinalysis may disclose numerous white cells, red cells, and bacteria.

ASSESSMENT

DIFFERENTIAL DIAGNOSIS

Ureteral injuries, with complete or partial ureteral obstruction, may result from accidental ligation, crush injuries, transection, or interference with blood supply. Symptoms include minimal or steadily increasing flank pain, with or without fever; chills; and abdominal distention. In cases of intraperitoneal extravasation of urine, adynamic ileus is associated with abdominal distention and a septic course. In cases of retroperitoneal extravasation, the patient appears critically ill, with an elevated temperature, tachycardia, and leukocytosis. Surgical exploration with deligation or ureteral repair is the treatment usually preferred.

PLAN

ADDITIONAL DIAGNOSTIC DATA

Urine Culture and Sensitivity Studies: A colony count greater than 100,000 per ml of urine in a clean-catch specimen is evidence of bacteriuria. Determination of the organism and antibiotic sensitivity provides a guide to appropriate therapy. Usual etiologic microorganisms are gram-negative enteric bacteria, most commonly *Escherichia coli.*

Intravenous pyelogram is indicated when there is any question of ureteral injury or if the infection fails to respond to antibiotic therapy.

MANAGEMENT

Antibiotic therapy is based on the suspected organism and previously known sensitivity data. Acute febrile urinary tract infections are usually treated with drugs that provide relatively high blood levels as well as urine levels (ampicillin, gentamicin).

Hydration is also beneficial.

Postoperative Venous Bacteremia

GENERAL CONSIDERATIONS

Postoperative venous bacteremia may result from an infection along the course of a vein used for an intravenous infusion. Symptoms and signs include sudden chills, spiking fever, tachycardia, hypotension, oliguria, leukocytosis, and even respiratory distress. Usually, erythema, edema, pain, and tenderness are identified along the course of the vein. Etiologic microorganisms include Bacteroides, Klebsiella, Serratia, and Staphylococcus.

Treatment includes the administration of intravenous antibiotics, the removal of the offending intravenous catheter, and the initiation of intravenous fluids at a new site.

Postoperative Wound Problems

Bleeding

Bleeding from the operative area may not become evident until after surgery has been completed. The cause is usually inadequate control of a severed blood vessel, frequently owing to a slipped ligature. Immediate surgical repair and appropriate blood replacement are essential.

Bleeding from the vaginal vault may appear seven to ten days after hysterectomy. The cause is usually necrosis at the suture site. Arterial bleeding may require a suture ligature. Otherwise, cautery with silver nitrate or vaginal packing may control the bleeding.

Bleeding following cervical biopsy can usually be controlled with Monsel's solution (ferric subsulfate).

Bleeding several days after cervical conization can usually be controlled with vaginal packing. A suture ligature may be required.

The possibility of coagulation disorders must always be considered in the evaluation of postoperative bleeding or wound hematomas. (See Coagulation Disorders, p. 210.)

> **Rectus muscle hematoma** is a rare condition that should be considered when a mass is palpable in the area of the rectus muscle. Characteristic findings are localized exquisite tenderness and spasm, with absence of signs on the opposite side. Treatment includes evacuation of the hematoma combined with identification and ligation of bleeding vessels.

Dehiscence

Dehiscence of an abdominal incision is one of the most serious postoperative complications. Unexpected evisceration (separation of all tissue layers including the peritoneum) is associated with a high mortality rate. Predisposing factors include malignancy, debilitation combined with severe anemia and hypoproteinemia, abdominal wall distention, wound infection, hematomas, and obesity. Evisceration usually occurs between the fifth and twelfth postoperative days. In the usual course of events, a serosanguinous discharge at the incisional site may portend evisceration. Often, there is a low-grade temperature elevation.

Protruding intestinal loops are covered immediately with a sterile, moist dressing, and preparations are made for surgical repair. Intravenous fluids are initiated; pain and anxiety are treated with morphine. Cross-matched blood is ordered in case transfusion becomes necessary. A nasogastric tube is indicated if the abdomen is distended.

The patient is taken to the operating suite as soon as possible in order to replace the bowel and close the abdomen. Through-and-through stainless steel wire, incorporating peritoneum, fascia, and skin, is usually recommended. The sutures are tied over rubber booties and left in place for three weeks.

Infection

Following pelvic surgery, cellulitis or abscess may develop at any wound site: the abdominal incision, adnexal incision, or the vaginal vault. Most wound infections are seen four to ten days postoperatively and should always be suspected in any febrile postoperative patient.

Subjective Data:

Pain over the wound or abdomen tends to increase in severity.

Fever, chills, and malaise are frequently associated symptoms.

Purulent exudate may be observed on a wound dressing.

Objective Data:

Physical Examination

General Examination: Temperature is elevated and frequently spiking. Tachycardia is usually proportional to the temperature elevation. A temperature of less than 102° F three to five days after surgery suggests pelvic cellulitis or vaginal cuff abscess. Temperatures greater than 102° later in the postoperative period may be caused by an ovarian abscess or pelvic thrombophlebitis.

Abdominal Examination: Tender, red, swollen areas usually indicate an abdominal wound infection. A soft, fluctuant area suggests abscess formation. Aspiration of pus confirms the diagnosis of wound abscess.

Pelvic Examination: A tender mass at the vaginal vault suggests vaginal cuff abscess; a tender mass in the adnexal area may represent an adnexal abscess.

Laboratory Tests:

Complete Blood Count with Blood Smear: The white blood count is usually elevated, with increased neutrophils and immature forms.

Assessment: Purulent material with a putrid smell usually indicates an anaerobic infection (Bacteroides, Clostridium, anaerobic Streptococcus). Wound infections without an odor are usually due to *Escherichia coli* or *Staphylococcus aureus.*

Group A beta hemolytic streptococci tend to be very virulent and are likely to produce symptoms on the first postoperative day.

Clostridium perfringens infection may cause shock, tachycardia, fever, and hypotension within the first 24 postoperative hours. In addition, there may be a yellow-brown skin discoloration, crepitation, and a thin, brownish, malodorous discharge.

Plan

Additional Diagnostic Data:

Bacteriology (Gram Stain and Culture): Fluid from fluctuant areas should be aspirated and sent to the laboratory for Gram stain, aerobic and anaerobic cultures, and antibiotic sensitivity studies.

Blood cultures should be drawn whenever there is any suspicion of bacteremia.

Urine cultures are ordered if there is any question of urinary tract infection.

Ultrasound B-scan may reveal an adnexal abscess.

Management and Patient Education: Treatment for any wound infection includes drainage of purulent material and appropriate systemic antibiotic therapy. (See Pelvic Infections, p. 474.)

In cases of severe wound infection and widespread necrosis, the wound should be opened widely and irrigated daily with saline or hydrogen peroxide. Intermittent moist heat may be beneficial.

The infected area closes by granulation from the depths outward.

Postoperative Complications of Laparoscopic Sterilization

Cauterization of fallopian tubes under laparoscopic visualization is one method of permanent sterilization. Often the patient is sent home shortly after the procedure is completed. Potential complications that may require emergency care include intraabdominal bleeding, postoperative infection, and intestinal burn injury.

In the case of an intestinal burn injury, symptoms may not develop until three to seven days after surgery. Usually, the patient complains of nausea and anorexia progressing to crampy, lower abdominal pain. A low-grade fever is an associated finding. Symptoms continue to progress to vomiting combined with ileus and obvious peritonitis.

Findings on abdominal examination include mild distention, lower quadrant pain, and decreased bowel sounds. The temperature may be mildly elevated (99° to 101° F). The white count is usually within the normal range.

The patient should be hospitalized for exploratory laparotomy. The operative procedure depends on the findings at surgery. Antibiotic therapy is initiated to cover a broad spectrum of intestinal microorganisms, both aerobic and anaerobic. Bacterial cultures are taken from the peritoneal cavity at the time of exploratory laparotomy. Postoperative antibiotic therapy is adjusted in accordance with the culture reports and sensitivity studies.

REFERENCES

Altemeier WA, McDonough JJ, Fallen WD: Third day surgical fever. Arch Surg *103*:158-166, 1971

Ledger WJ: OB/GYN infections: changing patterns and management. Hosp Pract *10*:115-121, 1975

Ledger WJ, Headington JT: Group A beta hemolytic streptococcus. Obstet Gynecol *39*:474-482, 1972

Levinson CJ: Hysterectomy complications. Clin Obstet Gynecol *15*:802-826, 1972

Pratt JH: Wound healing—evisceration. Clin Obstet Gynecol *16*:126-134, 1973

Thompson BH, Wheeless CR: Gastrointestinal complications of laparoscopy sterilization. Obstet Gynecol *41*:669-676, 1973

76 POSTPARTUM COMPLICATIONS

DEFINITIONS

In addition to coincidental emergency problems that occur spontaneously during the postpartum period, the Committee on Terminology of the American College of Obstetricians and Gynecologists has defined the following complications of the puerperium.

Puerperium—the period of 42 days following the birth of the fetus and the expulsion or extraction of the placenta and membranes. During this time, the generative organs ordinarily return to normal.

After-pains—painful uterine contractions that occur for one to three days post partum or longer.

Involution of the uterus—the return of the puerperal uterus to its normal nonpregnant state.

Lochia—the vaginal discharge during the puerperium. It usually lasts approximately two weeks and is classified as lochia rubra, lochia serosa, and lochia alba.

Lochia rubra—the bloody discharge occurring during the first one to three postpartum days.

Lochia serosa—a thick, maroon vaginal discharge occurring during the fourth to ninth days post partum. It contains blood, wound exudate, leukocytes, erythrocytes, shreds of decidua in a state of fatty degeneration, mucous from the cervix, and microorganisms.

Lochia alba—a white, creamy vaginal discharge generally occurring from the tenth to the fourteenth postpartum days.

Puerpera—a woman who has given birth to a fetus during the previous 42 days.

Specific Problems

Breast abscess is a late, usually suppurative sequel to acute mastitis. (See Breast Infection, p. 156.)

Breast engorgement is a temporary inflammatory condition caused by increased blood flow preceding the formation of milk. It is characterized by fullness, redness, and hardness of the breast. (See Breast Engorgement, p. 154.)

Postpartum cystitis is infection in the urinary bladder occurring during the puerperium. It is characterized by urgency, dysuria, and a low-grade fever, rarely over 38.3° C (101° F). Diagnosis is made on the demonstration of bacteriuria and pus cells associated with residual urine in the bladder. (See Cystitis, p. 273.)

Puerperal endometritis is infection of the endometrium in association with puerperal infection. (See Postpartum Infection, p. 547, and Pelvic Infection, p. 474.)

Galactocele is a true milk-duct cyst due to an obstruction of a lactiferous duct.

Galactorrhea is the constant leakage of milk from the breast. (See Nipple Discharge, p. 444.)

Hematoma (puerperal) is a collection of blood in the soft tissues of the pelvis. It may occur above or below the levator ani, beneath the vaginal mucosa, or beneath the skin of the external genitalia. (See Vaginal and Vulvar Trauma, p. 679.)

Hemorrhage (postpartum) is excessive bleeding during the puerperium. (See Postpartum Hemorrhage, p. 537.)

Herpes gestationis syndrome is a relatively rare exanthema that occurs as a complication of the latter half of pregnancy or during the early phase of the puerperium. The condition occurs most commonly in women 30 to 35 years old. Symptoms include fever, malaise, dyspnea, burning sensation, neuralgic pain, and an intense pruritus. The cutaneous lesions consist of bullae and vesicles that are present over the chest, abdomen, and extremities. The syndrome may occur with each gestation or during every second or third pregnancy. Exacerbations are likely, even during treatment. Recurrences may occasionally extend into the puerperium as episodes of severe pruritus prior to the first few menstrual periods. These episodes are called *herpes menstrualis recidivans*.

Mastitis (acute) is acute inflammation of the breast, usually associated with a cracked or fissured nipple and occurring in the period of lactation. (See Breast Infection, p. 156.)

Metrophlebitis is inflammation of the uterine veins, usually occurring only in the puerperium. (See Thrombophlebitis, p. 644.)

Milk leg is an extreme edematous swelling of the leg occurring in the puerperium. It is due to thrombosis of the femoral or iliac vein (synonym: phlegmasia alba dolens). (See Thrombophlebitis, p. 644.)

Myometritis (acute) is a severe form of infection of the myometrium resulting from a puerperal streptococcal infection. There is marked edema, muscle hypertrophy, and leukocytic infiltration. (See Postpartum Infection, p. 547, and Pelvic Infection, p. 474.)

Parametritis is a form of puerperal infection that is extended to the pelvic connective tissue surrounding the uterus. Generally, the apex of infection is from the cervix, lower uterine segment, or vagina. (See Postpartum Infection, p. 547, and Pelvic Infection, p. 474.)

Phlebothrombosis is the formation of a thrombus in a vein in the absence of preexisting inflammation. There is a greater danger of pulmonary embolism with this type of thrombosis. The condition may occur in the superficial or deep veins of the legs, or the pelvic veins surrounding the uterus. (See Thrombophlebitis, p. 644, and Pulmonary Embolism, p. 585.)

Polygalactia is the excessive flow of milk from the breast.

Psychoses (postpartum) are characterized by severe degrees of personality disorganization that impair the patient's ability to function responsibly. They are classified as manic-depressive psychosis, puerperal psychosis, schizophrenia, and toxic confusional states. (See Postpartum Psychiatric Problems, p. 550.)

Puerperal infection is any infection of the genital tract occurring during the puerperium. Puerperal infection may be presumed in the presence of a temperature of 38° C (100.4° F) or above on any two successive days, exclusive of the first 24 hours post partum, granted that other causes of fever are not apparent. (See Postpartum Infection, p. 547, and Pelvic Infection, p. 474.)

Thrombophlebitis is the formation of a thrombus after inflammation of the wall of a vein. This condition generally occurs in the leg or pelvic veins during pregnancy or the puerperium. (See Thrombophlebitis, p. 644.)

77 POSTPARTUM HEMORRHAGE

GENERAL CONSIDERATIONS

Postpartum hemorrhage is defined as the loss of 500 ml or more of blood from the reproductive organs after the completion of the third stage of labor (expulsion or extraction of the placenta and membranes). Normally, bleeding from the placental site is controlled primarily by contraction and retraction of the interlacing muscle fibers and secondarily by platelet aggregation and fibrin thrombi in the decidual blood vessels.

Early postpartum hemorrhage is excessive bleeding during the first 24 hours after completion of the third stage of labor.

Late postpartum hemorrhage is excessive bleeding during the puerperium, excluding the first 24 hour period after completion of the third stage of labor.

Early Postpartum Hemorrhage

SUBJECTIVE DATA

CURRENT SYMPTOMS

Vaginal bleeding—copious, profuse, and persistent—is the most characteristic symptom.

PRIOR HISTORY

A history of bleeding disorders may suggest an associated coagulation disorder.

OBJECTIVE DATA

General Examination: Tachycardia and hypotension indicate hypovolemia resulting from excessive blood loss.

Abdominal examination findings depend on the causative factor. Uterine atony is suspected when the uterus is enlarged, soft, and boggy. A firm, contracted uterine fundus suggests genital tract lacerations.

Pelvic examination is essential for the evaluation of uterine contraction, uterine integrity, retained placental tissue, genital tract lacerations, or uterine inversion.

ASSESSMENT

DIFFERENTIAL DIAGNOSIS

Uterine atony is failure of the uterus to maintain normal contractions and retractions. Abnormal relaxation of the uterine fundus accounts for 75 to 90 per cent of cases of postpartum hemorrhage.

Lacerations of the genital tract—cervix, vagina, or perineum—are responsible for 6 to 19 per cent of cases of early postpartum hemorrhage. The uterine fundus is firm and well contracted.

Placenta or Membranes Retained *in Utero:* Bleeding persists because the uterus is unable to contract and retract normally. Diagnosis is suspected when placental inspection reveals incomplete torn or shredded areas.

Placenta Accreta: See Placenta Accreta, p. 500.

Uterine Rupture: See Uterine Rupture, p. 674.

Uterine Inversion: See Uterine Inversion, p. 666.

Coagulation Defect: See Coagulation Disorders, p. 210.

PREDISPOSING FACTORS

Predisposing factors to uterine atony include one or more of the following singly or in combination:

1. General anesthesia
2. Prolonged labor
3. Rapid labor
4. Uterine abnormality—leiomyomata, congenital anomalies
5. Uterine overdistention due to multiple pregnancy, hydramnios, or a very large baby
6. Placenta previa
7. Placental separation (abruptio placenta)
8. Multiparity
9. Preeclampsia or eclampsia

POTENTIAL COMPLICATIONS

Complications of profuse blood loss are hypovolemic shock with inadequate tissue perfusion.

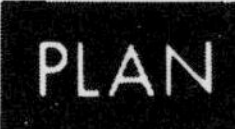

ADDITIONAL DIAGNOSTIC DATA

Since severe postpartum bleeding is more often due to inadequate uterine contractions than to traumatic injury, the uterine fundus is immediately palpated. If the uterus is soft and boggy, particularly if the placenta has not yet been delivered, the placenta should be expressed or manually removed. Intravenous oxytocin (20 to 40 units of oxytocin per 1000 ml 5 per cent dextrose) is infused rapidly.

The integrity of the uterus, cervix, vagina, and perineum are evaluated next. The uterine cavity and lower uterine segment are explored manually in order to detect any evidence of uterine rupture, retained placental tissue, or placenta accreta. Readily detached placental tissue or retained membranes are removed manually.

The cervix and vagina should be carefully visualized in order to identify any possible lacerations. Cervical lacerations can cause severe hemorrhage and are particularly apt to occur when delivery has been very rapid and the baby forced through an incompletely dilated cervix. The most common sites of cervical laceration are three o'clock and nine o'clock.

Profuse bleeding may also result from vaginal tears that extend into the sulci or the fornices. These tears are more likely to be seen in operative forceps deliveries, particularly forceps rotations.

Other possible causes of profuse bleeding are ruptured varices of the vagina or the vulva and lacerations of the clitoris or the bulbocavernosus area of the vestibule.

Coagulation disorders are suspected if there is any evidence of premature placental separation or amniotic fluid embolism. Helpful laboratory tests include platelet count, fibrinogen, fibrin-split products, prothrombin time, and activated partial thromboplastin time.

MANAGEMENT AND PATIENT EDUCATION

General Principles: Intravenous fluids (usually 20 to 40 units of oxytocin in 1000 ml of 5 per cent dextrose in lactated Ringer's solution) are initiated immediately. Two units of blood are cross-matched in case transfusion becomes necessary. A central venous line may be a helpful guide to blood and fluid replacement.

Uterine Atony: Ergonovine maleate or methylergonovine maleate (0.2 mg) is administered intravenously or intramuscularly. The uterine fundus is massaged slowly and evenly through the abdominal wall.

If the fundus remains soft and boggy and uterine atony persists, the uterus is lifted up out of the pelvis and compressed between one hand on the abdomen and the other hand clenched as a fist in the vagina. Elevation and bimanual compression are maintained for two to five minutes.

Laparotomy must be considered when uterine atony persists and bleeding is intractable. Undiagnosed uterine rupture is a possibility, since the lateral walls of the lower uterine segment may be difficult to palpate on vaginal examination. Uterine repair, hysterectomy, or ligation of the hypogastric or uterine arteries may be elected, depending on the patient's age, parity, and general condition, as well as on the extent of trauma.

Uterine packing may be tried as a temporary measure while preparations are made for laparotomy. If the bleeding is coming from a placental site in the lower uterine segment where muscular contractions are inadequate to achieve normal hemostasis, packing may have

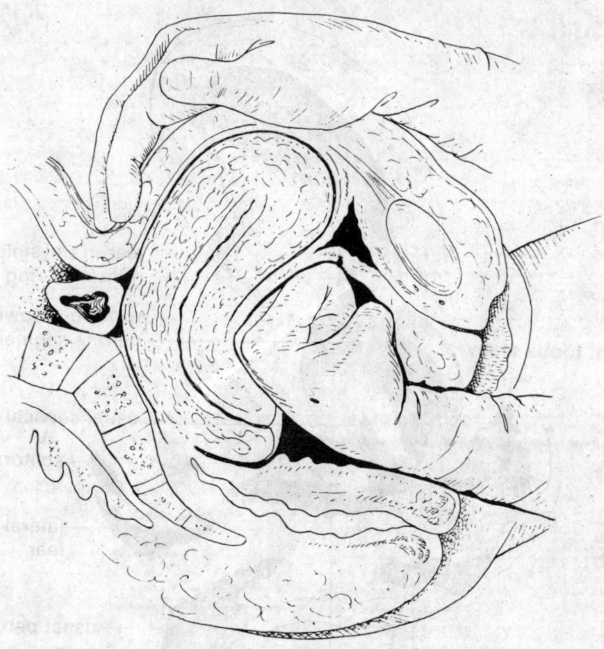

Figure 77-1. Technique for temporarily arresting acute postpartum hemorrhage from uterine atony by compressing the sharply anteflexed uterus between the closed intravaginal fist and the counter-pressure of the suprapubic hand. (From Greenhill JP, Friedman EA: Biological Principles and Modern Practice of Obstetrics. Philadelphia, W.B. Saunders Company, 1974.)

particular value. The uterine packing is placed into the lower uterine segment, with vaginal packing compressing the lower segment between the uterine and vaginal pack. (The material preferred for packing is plain gauze of 4-inch width and six-ply thickness.)

If bleeding is controlled by the packing, surgical intervention may be deferred. However, the patient must be carefully observed and facilities for emergency laparotomy should be immediately available, since packing may do nothing more than mask active bleeding that continues to accumulate behind the pack. (When packing is successful, it is left in place for 12 to 24 hours.)

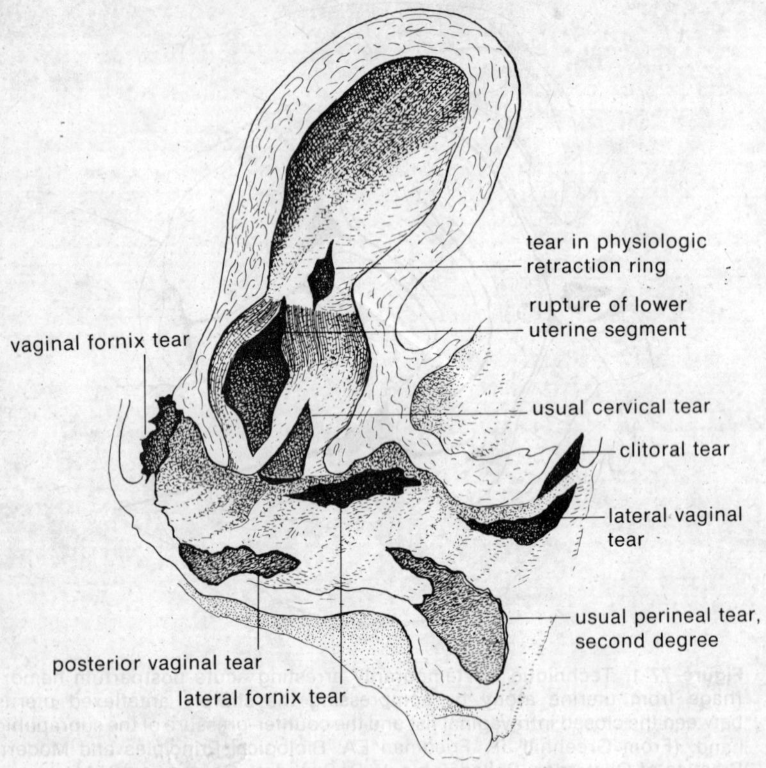

Figure 77-2. Schematic drawing of uterus, vagina, and introitus, illustrating sites of important lacerations occurring in the course of spontaneous or operative delivery. (From Greenhill JP, Friedman EA: Biological Principles and Modern Practice of Obstetrics. Philadelphia, W.B. Saunders Company, 1974.)

Lacerations of the Genital Tract (Fig. 77-2): Bleeding lacerations are repaired with chromic 00 or 000 sutures. Adequate visualization is essential, and an assistant is often required to retract the vaginal walls with right-angle retractors.

Cervical lacerations (Fig. 77-3): are repaired by grasping the cervical lips adjacent to the laceration with ring forceps. Successive stitches of chromic 00 or 000 are passed through the most accessible portion of the cervical tear. Traction on these sutures may be helpful in drawing down the apex of the laceration. Spurting vessels must be ligated in order to prevent retroperitoneal hematomas. The most important suture is the one at the apex of the laceration, which requires careful attention in order to be certain that a retracted vessel does not continue to bleed. Interrupted or continuous sutures may be used, depending on the extent of bleeding, the exposure of the bleeding site, and the operator's preference.

Temporary hemostasis may be achieved by applying ring forceps to the edges of the laceration. When a tear has extended into the lower uterine segment or broad ligament, packing or ring forceps may be of temporary benefit while preparations are made for abdominal surgery.

Vaginal Lacerations: See Vaginal and Vulvar Trauma, p. 679.

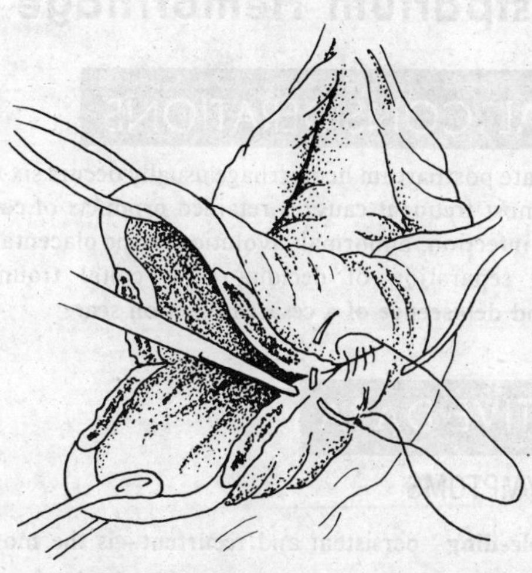

Figure 77-3. The typical cervical tear is sutured with a continuous suture of chromic catgut. It is important that the suturing be started *above* the apex of the wound. (From Greenhill JP, Friedman EA: Biological Principles and Modern Practice of Obstetrics. Philadelphia, W.B. Saunders Company, 1974.)

Varicosities of the vagina or vulva may cause profuse bleeding that is frequently difficult to control with sutures. Under these circumstances, tight vaginal packing may provide essential hemostasis.

Placenta or Membranes Retained in Uterus: Manual removal followed by intravenous oxytocin and ergonovine is usually sufficient therapy. (See Placenta Retained in Uterus, p. 517.)

Placenta Accreta: See Placenta Accreta, p. 500.

Uterine Rupture: See Uterine Rupture, p. 674.

Uterine Inversion: See Uterine Inversion, p. 666.

Coagulation Defect: See Coagulation Disorders, p. 210.

Late Postpartum Hemorrhage

GENERAL CONSIDERATIONS

Delayed or late postpartum hemorrhage usually occurs six to ten days after delivery. The most frequent cause is retained products of conception; other causes include infection, abnormal involution of the placental site, abnormal retention and separation of decidua vera, coital trauma, episiotomy breakdown, and dehiscence of a cesarean section scar.

SUBJECTIVE DATA

CURRENT SYMPTOMS

Vaginal bleeding—persistent and recurrent—is the most characteristic symptom.

Other Symptoms: Chills and fever may indicate an associated genital tract infection.

PRIOR HISTORY

A history of operative delivery, coitus, or trauma may be helpful.

OBJECTIVE DATA

PHYSICAL EXAMINATION

General Examination: Temperature may be elevated if there is an associated infection. Pulse and blood pressure provide an estimate of the severity of blood loss.

Abdominal Examination: Frequently the uterine fundus is palpable abdominally and larger than expected.

Pelvic Examination: The uterus tends to be larger and softer than normally expected. Uterine tenderness may indicate an associated infection. Speculum examination discloses active bleeding from the cervical canal. Often the cervix is sufficiently dilated to admit a 9 or 10 suction cannula.

LABORATORY TESTS

Complete Blood Count: Hemoglobin and hematocrit evaluations determine blood loss and anemia. An elevated white count may be the result of infection, or it may be the normal elevation associated with recent labor and delivery.

Urinalysis is usually normal.

ASSESSMENT

PREDISPOSING FACTORS

Retained products of conception are commonly associated with the following conditions:

1. Primary postpartum hemorrhage of 600 ml or more
2. Suspicion of retained placental tissue after inspection of placenta
3. Morbidity in the first ten days of the puerperium
4. Shock due to severity of secondary postpartum hemorrhage

5. Morbidity (temperature above 38° C) or mild pyrexia (temperature of 37.5 to 38° C) at the time of the secondary hemorrhage
6. Uterine tenderness
7. Bacteriologic evidence of genital tract infection

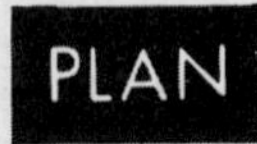

MANAGEMENT AND PATIENT EDUCATION

Minimal Bleeding: Bed rest at home supplemented by oral oxytocic medication (0.2 mg of ergonovine or methylergonovine) is usually adequate therapy. Antibiotics are prescribed if there is any evidence of low-grade endometritis.

Moderate Bleeding: Suction curettage and intravenous oxytocin (20 units per 500 ml of lactated Ringer's solution) remove retained products of conception and aid uterine contractions. As long as there is no evidence of hypovolemia, the patient may return home with a prescription for oral ergonovine (0.2 mg twice daily for three days).

When postpartum bleeding is associated with pelvic infection, hospitalization and intravenous antibiotic therapy are recommended.

Profuse Bleeding: Intravenous fluids, lactated Ringer's solution, blood transfusion, and uterine curettage are the most important therapeutic measures. Hospitalization is necessary for the management of incipient or actual hypovolemic shock. Central venous pressure, urine output, and hematocrit determinations provide valuable guides to fluid replacement therapy. (See Shock, p. 612.)

If bleeding persists after adequate curettage, exploratory laparotomy for arterial ligation or hysterectomy must be considered.

REFERENCES

Hester JD: Postpartum hemorrhage and reevaluation of uterine packing. Obstet Gynecol *45*:501-504, 1975

Kelly JV: Postpartum hemorrhage. Clin Obstet Gynecol *19*:595-606, 1976

MacVicar J, Graham RM: Two unusual cases of secondary postpartum haemorrhage. Br Med J *2*:29, 1973

Rome RR: Secondary postpartum haemorrhage. Br J Obstet Gynaecol *82*:289-292, 1975; Obstet Gynecol Surv *30*:663-664, 1975

78 POSTPARTUM INFECTION

GENERAL CONSIDERATIONS

Postpartum infection is a nonspecific term indicating an infection in any part of the body following childbirth.

Puerperal infection and puerperal sepsis are terms that refer to infection of the genital tract after delivery. (The puerperium is defined as the period of 42 days following the birth of the fetus and expulsion or extraction of the placenta and membranes.) Various manifestations of puerperal infection include endometritis, parametritis, salpingo-oophoritis, pelvic thrombophlebitis, peritonitis, cellulitis of the perineum or vagina, infected hematomas, and wound abscess.

Puerperal morbidity is defined on the basis of oral temperature elevations to 38° C (100.4° F) or more on any two of the first ten postpartum days, exclusive of the first 24 hours. The patient's temperature must be taken at least four times a day to establish the diagnosis.

Since the genital tract is the most common source of postpartum infections, puerperal infection is frequently presumed to be the cause of febrile morbidity, as long as other causes of fever are not apparent.

Puerperal Endometritis and Parametritis

SUBJECTIVE DATA

Chills and fever are usually the first manifestations of puerperal endometritis. The temperature elevation is most likely to occur in the late afternoon or early evening.

OBJECTIVE DATA

PHYSICAL EXAMINATION

Pelvic Examination: The lochia tends to be foul smelling. The uterus may be tender and boggy, with parametrial pain and thickening.

LABORATORY TESTS

The white blood count and differential count are difficult to interpret, since leukocytosis and an increased percentage of immature cells may occur during labor and during the postpartum period although no evidence of infection is present.

ASSESSMENT

DIFFERENTIAL DIAGNOSIS

Differential diagnosis of postpartum fever includes dehydration, atelectasis, drug fevers, and breast engorgement.

Differential diagnosis of postpartum infection includes bacteremia, urinary tract infection, thrombophlebitis (peripheral vein or pelvic vein), respiratory infection, mastitis or breast abscess, and infections at other sites.

Abdominal wound infection may become evident four to seven days after cesarean section (See Postoperative Complications—Wound Infection, p. 530.)

Subgluteal or retropsoal infections, although rare, may follow paracervical or transvaginal pudendal block anesthesia, with spread of infection from the paravaginal or paracervical tissues (Hibbard, 1972). Findings include protracted fever; painful ambulation, with a limp favoring the affected side; and poorly localized hip or pelvic pain. Hip motion may be limited by psoal spasm, and the leg held in a flexed and adducted position. Pelvic x-ray may reveal gas formation in the soft tissues about the hip. Surgical exploration and drainage may be necessary.

POTENTIAL COMPLICATIONS

Complications of postpartum infection include generalized peritonitis, pelvic abscess, septic emboli, and septic shock.

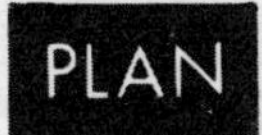

ADDITIONAL DIAGNOSTIC DATA

Bacteriology: Aerobic cultures of the lochia, as well as aerobic and anaerobic blood cultures, may provide information on antibiotic sensitivity.

MANAGEMENT AND PATIENT EDUCATION

After cervical cultures are obtained, adequate drainage from the uterine cavity is established by gently dilating the cervical canal with a sponge forceps and removing any visible membranes.

Antibiotic therapy must be based on the presumptive bacteria. (*Escherichia coli*, streptococci, enterococci, and Bacteroides are most likely.) Usually ampicillin, penicillin, and an aminoglycoside (gentamicin or kanamycin), or clindamycin plus an aminoglycoside will cover the most likely organisms.

(See Pelvic Infections, p. 474.)

Septic shock following term delivery usually results from infection that has extended beyond the endometrial cavity. Although curettage may be performed to rule out necrotic retained placental tissue, abdominal hysterectomy with bilateral salpingo-oophorectomy and drainage may be necessary.

REFERENCES

Gibbs RS, Weinstein AJ: Puerperal infection in the antibiotic era. Am J Obstet Gynecol *124*:769-787, 1976

Hibbard LT, Snyder EN, McVann RM: Subgluteal and retropsoal infection in obstetric practice. Obstet Gynecol *39*:137-150, 1972

Svancarek W, Chirino O, Schaeffer G, et al: Retropsoas and subgluteal abscesses following paracervical and pudendal anesthesia. JAMA *237*:892-894, 1977

79 POSTPARTUM PSYCHIATRIC PROBLEMS

DEFINITIONS

Postpartum depression—an emotional condition characterized by mild, self-limiting crying episodes and sad feelings during the first ten days after delivery. (Synonym: Postpartum blues.)

Postpartum psychoses—severe degrees of personality disorganization that impair the patient's ability to function responsibly. They are classified as manic-depressive psychosis, puerperal psychosis, schizophrenia, and toxic confusional states.

SUBJECTIVE AND OBJECTIVE DATA

CURRENT SYMPTOMS

Depression, crying episodes, and rapid, unpredictable mood changes are relatively common during the first few days following delivery. These symptoms may result from an anticlimactic letdown after the excitement of pregnancy and delivery.

Fatigue, insomnia, irritability, and moodiness are additional symptoms associated with moderate depression.

Anxiety, agitation, delusions, and suicidal and homicidal thoughts are serious symptoms that indicate psychotic decompensation, requiring emergency psychiatric attention.

PRIOR HISTORY

A history of psychiatric and emotional problems or a severely disturbed marital and family relationship may aid in the interpretation of the patient's current symptoms. Postpartum psychosis may represent a latent mental illness that has been uncovered by the stresses of labor and delivery.

ASSESSMENT

DIFFERENTIAL DIAGNOSIS

The differential diagnosis must distinguish the self-limiting emotional disorder of postpartum depression from psychotic decompensation requiring emergency psychiatric therapy. Evaluation takes into consideration the patient's behavior and the potential danger that exists both to the patient and to her child.

ETIOLOGIC FACTORS

These include (1) personality conflicts; (2) environmental stress, and (3) dysfunctional family relationships.

PLAN

MANAGEMENT AND PATIENT EDUCATION

In some instances, reassurance, emotional support, and adequate supervision to minimize the risk of harm to the baby may be adequate. Psychotherapeutic medications, tranquilizing, or mood-elevating drugs or a combination of these may be indicated. Specific therapy depends on the nature of the psychiatric disorder.

Psychiatric consultation is recommended whenever there are serious symptoms of psychotic behavior or depressive symptoms persist or worsen. Short- or long-term psychotherapy may be required.

Hospitalization may be necessary to prevent self-injury or injury to others. Hospitalization may also be necessary if there is incapacitating anxiety or uncontrollable acting-out behavior.

80 PREECLAMPSIA

GENERAL CONSIDERATIONS

Preeclampsia is the development of hypertension with proteinuria, edema, or both due to pregnancy or the influence of a recent pregnancy. It occurs after the twentieth week of gestation but may develop earlier in the presence of trophoblastic disease (molar pregnancy).

Hypertension is a rise in the systolic pressure of at least 30 mm of Hg, or a rise in the diastolic pressure of at least 15 mm of Hg, or the presence of a systolic pressure of at least 140 mm of Hg, or the presence of a diastolic pressure of at least 90 mm of Hg. Hypertension may also be determined by a mean arterial pressure of 105 mm of Hg or more, or by a rise of 20 mm of Hg or more. The levels cited must be manifest on at least two occasions six or more hours apart, and should be based on previously known blood pressure levels.*

Proteinuria is the presence of urinary protein in concentrations greater than 0.3 gm per liter in a 24-hour urine collection, or in concentrations greater than 1 gm per liter (1+ to 2+ by standard turbidometric methods) in at least two random urine collections six hours apart. The specimens must be clean, voided midstream or obtained by catheterization.*

Vasospasm, especially arteriolar spasm, is basic to the disease process of preeclampsia and eclampsia. Increased vascular sensitivity to angiotensin appears to precede clinically apparent hypertension. Vascular constriction imposes resistance to blood flow and accounts for the arterial hypertension. Blood volume is contracted. The net effect is decreased perfusion of various organs—the uterus, kidney, liver, and brain.

Glomerular capillary endotheliosis is the most typical renal lesion of preeclampsia and eclampsia. The glomerular endothelial cells are swollen

*Hughes EC (ed): Obstetric-Gynecologic Terminology. Philadelphia, FA Davis Company, 1972

to such an extent that the capillary lumina are almost obstructed. There is hyperplasia and hypertrophy of the intercapillary cells. Electron-microscopic examination of the cytoplasm of the glomerular endothelial cell shows vacuolation, droplet formation, and deposition of an amorphous material against the basement membrane. This material has been identified as a fibrinogen derivative.

These changes in the glomerular capillaries appear responsible for the proteinuria, the reduced renal blood flow, and the reduced glomerular filtration rate.

Once preeclampsia is established, there appears to occur some type of "vicious circle," which is interrupted completely only after delivery of the placenta (See Fig. 80-1). The pathologic physiologic condition may begin at any point, and the various predisposing factors that favor the development of preeclampsia may operate at different segments of this circle (Page, 1976).

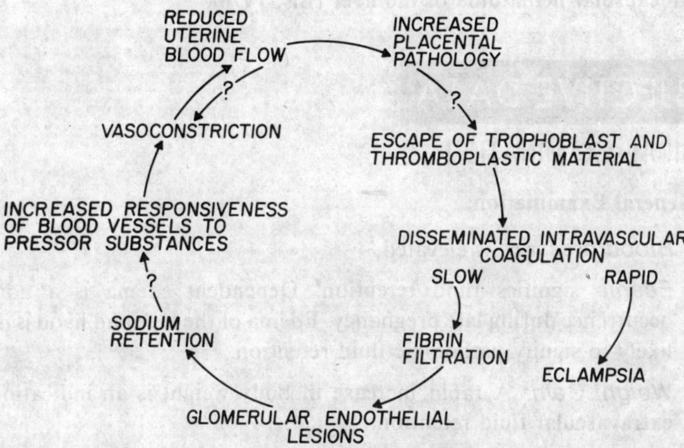

Figure 80-1. A concept of the sequence of events that may constitute a "vicious circle" in the pathogenesis of preeclampsia and eclampsia. (From Page EW, Villee CA, Villee DB: Human Reproduction. Philadelphia, W.B.Saunders Company, 1976.)

SUBJECTIVE DATA

Weight gain occurring rapidly over a short period of time signifies fluid retention and may be the earliest symptom of preeclampsia. The patient may be aware of generalized edema, particularly puffiness of her face and hands. A common complaint is tightness of rings on the fingers. In order to distinguish gestational edema, a benign process, from preeclampsia, the patient's blood pressure must be known.

Headache: Although headache is a relatively common symptom during pregnancy, headache can also be the initial symptom of cerebral edema. Consequently, any patient complaining of headache must have a blood pressure examination. (See Headache during Pregnancy, p. 367.)

Visual disturbances are symptoms of severe preeclampsia and may indicate retinal edema.

Epigastric pain is a potentially ominous symptom of hepatic swelling associated with severe preeclampsia. Rarely, it may portend rupture of a subcapsular hematoma of the liver (Bis, 1976).

OBJECTIVE DATA

PHYSICAL EXAMINATION

General Examination:

Blood pressure is elevated.

Edema signifies fluid retention. Dependent edema is a normal occurrence during late pregnancy. Edema of the face and hand is more likely to signify pathologic fluid retention.

Weight Gain: A rapid increase in body weight is an indication of extravascular fluid retention.

Retinal Examination: Arteriolar spasm and a retinal sheen may be observed.

Chest Examination: Since pulmonary edema is one of the most serious complications of severe preeclampsia, the lungs must be carefully examined.

Deep Tendon Reflexes (Knee and Ankle): Hyperreflexia and clonus are indications of increased irritability of the central nervous system and may portend an eclamptic convulsion.

Abdominal Examination: Liver tenderness is a potentially ominous sign of severe preeclampsia and may portend liver rupture.

Uterine examination is essential to assess gestational age, the presence of uterine contractions, and the fetal presentation.

Pelvic Examination: The status of the cervix and the station of the presenting part are important considerations in plans for vaginal or abdominal delivery.

LABORATORY TESTS

Complete Blood Count with Blood Smear: Elevation of the hematocrit from previously known values suggests hemoconcentration, or decreased plasma volume. If the hematocrit is lower than expected, the possibility of intravascular hemolysis resulting from a microangiopathic hemolytic process should be considered. Careful analysis of the peripheral blood smear may disclose severely distorted red blood cells and schistocytes.

Urinalysis: Proteinuria is a typical finding in patients with preeclampsia. If the random urine specimen contains 3+ or 4+ protein or the 24-hour urine contains 5 gm or more, preeclampsia is considered "severe."

ASSESSMENT

DIFFERENTIAL DIAGNOSIS

The differential diagnosis of preeclampsia includes chronic hypertensive disease, renal disease, gestational edema,* and gestational proteinuria.†

---

*Gestational edema is the occurrence of a general and excessive accumulation of fluid in the tissues of greater than 1+ pitting edema after 12 hours' rest in bed, or a weight gain of five pounds or more in one week due to the influence of pregnancy.

†Gestational proteinuria is the presence of proteinuria during or under the influence of pregnancy in the absence of hypertension, edema, renal infection, and known intrinsic renovascular disease.

Preeclampsia symptoms may imitate many disorders, including hepatitis, cholelithiasis, pancreatitis, appendicitis, retinal hemorrhage, gastrointestinal bleeding, idiopathic thrombocytopenia, cardiac failure, renal disease, and central nervous system disease (Goodlin, 1976).

SEVERITY OF DISEASE PROCESS

Preeclampsia generally is classified as "severe" if any one of the following signs or symptoms occurs:

1. Blood pressure of 160 mm Hg or more systolic or 110 or more diastolic, on at least two occasions at least six hours apart, with the patient at bed rest.
2. Proteinuria of 5 gm or more in 24 hours (3+ or 4+ on qualitative examination)
3. Oliguria (500 ml or less in 24 hours)
4. Cerebral or visual disturbances
5. Epigastric pain
6. Pulmonary edema or cyanosis

PREDISPOSING FACTORS

These include

1. Being a teen-aged nullipara
2. Being an indigent patient with little or no prenatal care and poor nutrition, especially with a protein-deficient diet
3. Having a family history of preeclampsia or eclampsia
4. Having a preexisting hypertensive vascular disease
5. Pregnancies with a superabundance of trophoblast plus chorionic villi
   a. Multiple pregnancy
   b. Hydatidaform mole
   c. Diabetes mellitus
   d. Rh isoimmunization (Fetal Hydrops)

POTENTIAL COMPLICATIONS

Maternal complications include eclampsia, premature placental separation, renal failure, liver necrosis, liver rupture, disseminated intravascular coagulation, hemolysis, cerebral hemorrhage, pulmonary edema, and retinal detachment.

Fetal complications include prematurity, uteroplacental insufficiency, and intrauterine fetal death.

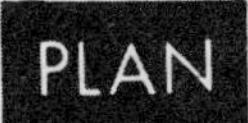

ADDITIONAL DIAGNOSTIC DATA

Evaluate the severity of the maternal disease. The patient should be hospitalized for evaluation and definitive therapy as indicated.

Blood Chemistry Tests: Blood urea nitrogen, creatinine, creatinine clearance, and uric acid determinations assess renal function. Usually creatinine and urea concentrations are not elevated; uric acid is more likely to be elevated, as a result of decreased renal clearance of uric acid, a decrease that exceeds the reduction in glomerular filtration and the creatinine clearance. (Elevations of creatinine or blood urea nitrogen suggest associated renal disease.)

Liver function tests [bilirubin, lactic dehydrogenase (LDH), and serum glutamic oxalacetic transaminase (SGOT)] assess liver disease. Elevations in these are indicative of serious disease.

Blood Electrolytes: Dehydration and abnormalities of intravascular and extravascular volume may cause electrolyte disturbances.

Coagulation Studies: Coagulation abnormalities may be caused by a disseminated intravascular coagulation. Decreased platelet counts may be the first manifestation of a serious coagulopathy.

Urine output measurements are an important indicator of the severity of the disease process. Oliguria is a perilous sign of impaired renal function.

Evaluate fetal well-being:

Amniocentesis: Determination of the lecithin-sphingomyelin (L/S) ratio provides an assessment of fetal lung maturity.

Ultrasound B-Scan: Serial sonography may identify fetal growth retardation.

Oxytocin Challenge Test: A positive test suggests fetal jeopardy.

Estriol determinations provide an assessment of fetal-placental function. Low or declining values suggest fetoplacental insufficiency.

Human placental lactogen (HPL) values less than 4 mcg/ml suggest abnormal placental function and fetal danger.

Fetal heart rate monitoring rules out fetal distress as long as the (1) baseline heart rate is within a normal range, (2) beat-to-beat variability is normal, (3) accelerations occur with fetal movements, and (4) there are no decelerations with uterine contractions.

MANAGEMENT AND PATIENT EDUCATION

General Principles: Preeclampsia persists pathophysiologically until the pregnancy terminates. Consequently, delivery of the fetus and placenta is the only true cure. Objectives of management are

1. Prevention of convulsions and other complications
2. Delivery of a surviving child, if possible
3. Delivery with minimal trauma to mother and child
4. Prevention of a residual pathologic condition

Delivery is recommended when the fetus is mature, the fetus shows evidence of intrauterine distress, or preeclampsia is severe. The choice between induction of labor and cesarean section depends on the fetal presentation and the status of the cervix.

Every patient with a blood pressure elevated above 140/90 should be hospitalized.

Mild Preeclampsia and Mature Fetus: Sedation with 100 mg of phenobarbital may be administered initially. If evidence of mild preeclampsia persists, labor is induced with intravenous oxytocin, as long as the fetus is in a vertex presentation, the cervix is soft and partially effaced, and there are no contraindications to oxytocin.

Mild Preeclampsia and Immature Fetus: When the fetus is immature, the risks of allowing pregnancy to continue, with the hazards of severe preeclampsia and possible intrauterine death, must be weighed against the risks associated with cesarean section and the possibility of neonatal morbidity and mortality from prematurity.

Initially, fetoplacental function is assess with estriol determinations and an oxytocin challenge test. If both these tests indicate fetal distress, termination of pregnancy is recommended. As long as there is no evidence of fetal jeopardy and preeclampsia remains mild, there is often a tendency to postpone delivery in the hope that additional intrauterine stay will give the infant a better chance for survival. The patient is advised to remain under constant surveillance in the hospital. Blood pressure is checked four times daily. Weight, urine protein, and urine output are recorded daily. In addition, serial platelet counts, estriol determinations, oxytocin challenge tests, and serial sonography aid in the evaluation of maternal and fetal well-being.

Diuretic therapy is not recommended, since there is no proof that diuretic agents are beneficial in the management of preeclampsia or eclampsia (except for the treatment of pulmonary edema).

Maternal risks from thiazide diuretics include pancreatitis, volume contraction, alkalosis, decreased carbohydrate tolerance, severe hypokalemia, hyponatremia, and hyperuricemia. Fetal risks include bleeding diatheses and hyponatremia (Lindheimer, 1973).

Severe Preeclampsia and Mature or Immature Fetus: The patient is hospitalized and treated with sedation and bed rest initially. No oral feedings are permitted, since general anesthesia may be required for delivery.

The blood pressure, weight, urinalysis, urine output, and fluid intake are monitored.

Intravenous fluids are administered—initially 5 per cent dextrose in water at a rate of 100 ml per hour. Electrolyte replacement depends on the serum electrolyte values. If oliguria exists, overhydration must be avoided.

Magnesium sulfate is administered to prevent convulsions. The initial dose is 4 gm diluted in 100 ml of 5 per cent dextrose in water administered intravenously over a period of 30 minutes. This is followed by 1 gm per hour administered in a dilute intravenous infusion (10 gm in 1000 ml of 5 per cent dextrose infused at the rate of 100 ml per hour.)

Alternatively, 10 gm of magnesium sulfate may be administered intramuscularly—10 ml of a 50 per cent solution injected deeply in the upper outer quadrant of both buttocks through a 3-inch long needle.

Whenever magnesium sulfate is administered, the following precautions must be observed: the patellar reflex must be present, urinary output must be at least 30 ml per hour, and respirations must not be depressed. If respiratory depression develops, 10 ml of a 10 per cent solution of calcium gluconate is given intravenously over a period of three minutes.

Antihypertensive Therapy: If the blood pressure is acutely elevated above 170 to 180 mm Hg systolic or 110 to 120 mm Hg diastolic, hydralazine is recommended to reduce the risk of cerebral hemorrhage and possibly improve renal blood flow. An initial dose of 5 mg is administered intravenously and the blood pressure monitored every five minutes. If the diastolic pressure is not lowered to 90 to 100 mg Hg in 20 minutes, a 10 mg dose is administered, and the blood pressure is monitored as described above. This dose is repeated at 20-minute intervals until the diastolic pressure is lowered to 100 mg Hg.

Delivery: After the patient is well stabilized, plans should be made for delivery. If the fetal presentation and cervix are favorable, labor may be induced with oxytocin and amniotomy. The fetal heart rate and uterine

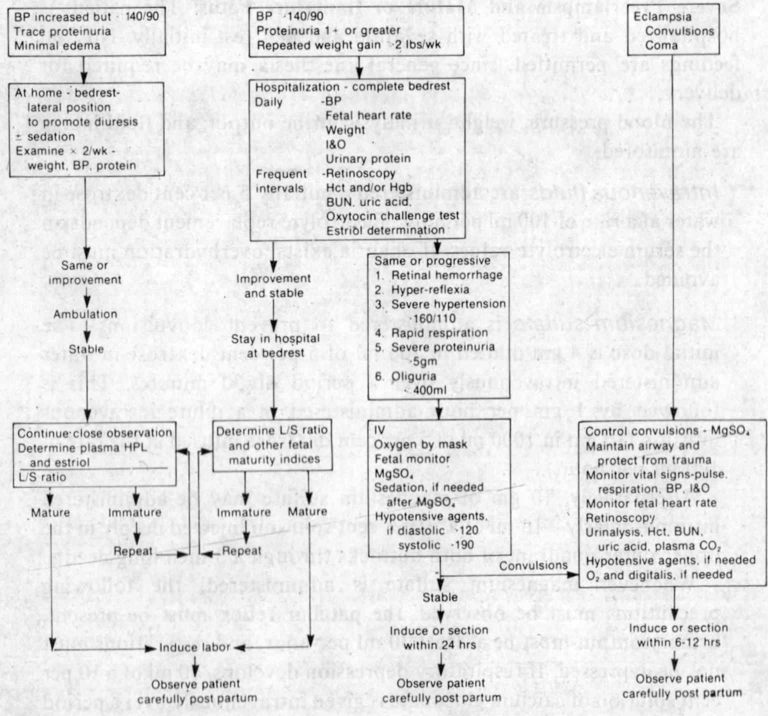

Figure 80-2. Schematic flow diagram illustrating management of patients with preeclampsia and eclampsia.

contractions are monitored continuously. In cases of fetal malpresentation or unsuccessful induction, cesarean section is necessary.

(Additional therapy indicated for specific complications includes digitalization for congestive heart failure and furosemide for pulmonary edema.) A flow chart showing the sequence of management for preeclampsia is presented in Figure 80-2.

(See Eclampsia, p. 303.)

REFERENCES

Baskett TF, Bradford CR: Active management of severe preeclampsia. Can Med Assoc J *109*:1209-1211, 1973; Obstet Gynecol Surv *29*: 458-460, 1974

Beecham JB, Watson WJ, Clapp JF: Eclampsia, preeclampsia, and disseminated intravascular coagulation. Obstet Gynecol *43*:576-585, 1974

Birmingham Eclampsia Study Group: Intravascular coagulation and abnormal lung scans in preeclampsia and eclampsia. Lancet *2*:889-891, 1971; Obstet Gynecol Surv *27*:244-246, 1972

Bis KA, Waxman B: Rupture of the liver associated with pregnancy: a review of the literature and report of 2 cases. Obstet Gynecol Surv *31*:763-773, 1976

Goodlin RC: Severe pre-eclampsia: another great imitator. Am J Obstet Gynecol *125*: 747-753, 1976

Koch-Weser J: Hydralazine. N Engl J Med *295*:320-323, 1976

Lindheimer MD, Katz AI: Sodium and diuretics in pregnancy. N Engl J Med *288*: 891-894, 1973; Obstet Gynecol Surv *28*:708-710, 1973

Newcombe DS: Hyperuricemia of pre-eclampsia and eclampsia. Obstet Gynecol Surv *27*:543-551, 1972

Page EW: On the pathogenesis of preeclampsia and eclampsia. J Obstet Gynecol Br Commonw *79*:883-894, 1972

Speroff L: Toxemia of pregnancy. Am J Cardiol *32*:582-591, 1973

81 PREMATURE RUPTURE OF MEMBRANES

GENERAL CONSIDERATIONS

Premature rupture of membranes, that is, rupture of the amniotic sac at least one hour before the onset of uterine contractions, occurs in approximately 7 to 12 per cent of pregnancies. Most often, membranes rupture at or near term; labor spontaneously ensues within a few hours. When premature rupture of the membranes is associated with a premature gestation, there is an increased risk of perinatal morbidity and mortality due to fetal immaturity; if delivery does not occur within 24 hours, there is also an increased risk of intrauterine infection.

SUBJECTIVE DATA

Involuntary gushing or leakage of clear fluid from the vagina is the characteristic symptom. Neither pain nor uterine contractions are evident.

Menstrual History: The gestational age is estimated by the date of the last menstrual period.

OBJECTIVE DATA

PHYSICAL EXAMINATION

General Examination: Temperature is normal unless there is an associated infection.

Abdominal Examination: The uterus is soft and nontender. The fundal height should be measured and compared with the height expected according to the date of the last menstrual period. Abdominal palpation provides an estimate of fetal size and presentation as well as engagement of the presenting part. Fetal heart tones should be normal.

Pelvic Examination:

Sterile speculum examination is performed initially in order to verify the presence of amniotic fluid in the vagina. Since the alkaline amniotic fluid alters the normal acid pH of the vagina, nitrazine paper can be used to measure the vaginal pH. The nitrazine paper turns blue in the presence of the alkaline amniotic fluid. If there is any suspicion of infection, a swab is taken from the cervical canal for culture and sensitivity. If the pregnancy is preterm, amniotic fluid in the vagina may be sent to the laboratory for a determination of the lecithin-sphingomyelin ratio in order to evaluate fetal lung maturity. (See Amniocentesis, p. 731.)

Sterile vaginal examination determines cervical effacement and dilatation. Vaginal examination also identifies the presenting part and the station of the presenting part and excludes the possibility of a prolapsed cord.

LABORATORY TESTS

Complete Blood Count with Blood Smear: Leukocytosis combined with increased band forms on the peripheral smear suggests intrauterine infection.

ASSESSMENT

DIFFERENTIAL DIAGNOSIS

The differential diagnosis must include the possibility of urinary incontinence. Since urine is usually acid, a comparison of the pH of the urine and the pH of the vagina is helpful in the differentiation.

PREDISPOSING FACTORS

These include chorioamnionitis, cervical incompetence, multiple pregnancy, hydramnios, and fetal malpresentation.

POTENTIAL COMPLICATIONS

Complications that must be anticipated include prolapsed cord, intrauterine infection, and fetal malpresentation.

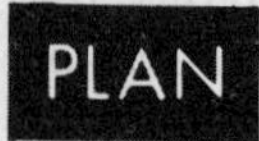

ADDITIONAL DIAGNOSTIC DATA

Diagnostic procedures are concerned with evaluation of fetal maturity and the possibility of intrauterine infection.

Ultrasound B-scan provides an estimate of gestational age through measurement of the biparietal diameter. In addition, sonography can localize the placenta, as well as a pocket of amniotic fluid for amniocentesis.

Amniocentesis: Amniotic fluid may be sent to the laboratory for determinations of the lecithin-sphingomyelin (L/S) ratio. In addition, amniotic fluid may be sent to the bacteriology laboratory for Gram stain, bacterial culture, and smear for polymorphonuclear leukocytes in order to determine the possibility of bacterial infection.

Fetal monitoring aids in fetal evaluation. With intrauterine infection and elevated maternal temperature, fetal tachycardia would be expected.

MANAGEMENT

Recommendations concerning the optimal management of pregnancies complicated by premature rupture of the membranes depend on the gestational age of the fetus, the evidence for intrauterine infection, and the patient population. In general, it appears most reasonable to admit all patients with ruptured membranes to the hospital and to deliver all babies older than 34 to 36 weeks, as well as all babies with a mature lecithin-sphingomyelin ratio within 24 hours of definite rupture of the membranes in order to minimize the risk of intrauterine infection. Labor is induced with oxytocin as long as the fetal presentation is cephalic. If induction fails, cesarean section is performed. Cesarean section is also recommended for breech presentation, transverse lie, or fetal distress, unless the fetus is so immature that hope of salvage is minimal.

In the case of the smaller fetuses, the risk of infection must be weighed against the risks stemming from premature birth—mainly, respiratory distress syndrome (RDS)—in order to determine the best course of management.

If the risk of intrauterine infection is low, continuous observation without vaginal examination is most likely to benefit the premature fetus. Observation in the hospital allows for treatment at the earliest sign of infection and for continuous assessment of fetal welfare.

In those institutions in which puerperal febrile morbidity is common, the mother and even the premature fetus may be more likely to benefit from delivery within 24 hours.

If the patient has had a cervical suture for an incompetent cervix and presents with ruptured membranes, the suture should be removed, unless cesarean section is planned, to obviate the hazard of infection and serious trauma to the cervix.

Respiratory Distress Syndrome: The effect of premature rupture of the membranes on the incidence of respiratory distress syndrome (RDS) in premature infants is controversial.

Richardson and co-workers reported that the lecithin-sphingomyelin ratio in the amniotic fluid may mature at an accelerated rate after premature rupture of the membranes. Others have reported a lower incidence of respiratory distress syndrome in fetuses of 28 to 33 weeks' gestation when membranes were ruptured longer than 24 hours (Sell, 1977; Berkowitz, 1976). On the other hand, Jones and co-workers concluded that prolonged rupture of the membranes does *not* provide protection against the development of respiratory distress syndrome.

Betamethasone and dexamethasone have been reported to accelerate fetal lung maturation and to prevent respiratory distress syndrome in the premature newborn (Liggins, 1972; Caspi, 1975, 1976; Ballard, 1976). Neither the ultimate risks and benefits nor the optimal regimen have been established. Dosages under evaluation vary from 12 mg per day given intramuscularly in three divided doses until delivery to 12 mg initially given intramuscularly followed by a second dose of 12 mg after 12 to 24 hours.

When intrauterine infection is present, appropriate antibiotics—usually ampicillin or cephalosporin—are administered in high dosages intravenously. Labor is induced with intravenous oxytocin, as long as the fetal presentation is cephalic. If induction fails, cesarean section is performed. Cesarean section is usually indicated for breech presentation, transverse lie, or fetal distress, unless the fetus is so immature that there is no hope for fetal survival.

Cesarean hysterectomy should be considered when abdominal delivery is indicated and the uterus is grossly infected.

See Chorioamnionitis, p. 205, and Premature Labor, p. 413.

PATIENT EDUCATION

The risks of prematurity and intrauterine infection are discussed with the patient in order to formulate the optimal management plan. At times, a patient who had planned for months on a natural childbirth at term may be severely upset and disappointed by the premature rupture of the membranes and the prospect of premature delivery.

Most patients have not completed their preparation for childbirth when membranes rupture a number of weeks before term. Appropriate emotional support is essential.

If the fetus is premature and a nonintervention course is chosen, the patient is advised neither to douche nor to have sexual intercourse.

REFERENCES

Ballard RA, Ballard PL: Use of prenatal glucocorticoid therapy to prevent respiratory distress syndrome. Am J Dis Child *130*:982-987, 1976

Berkowitz RL, Bonta BW, Warshaw JE: The relationship between premature rupture of the membranes and the respiratory distress syndrome. Am J Obstet Gynecol *124*: 712-718, 1976

Caspi E, Schreyer P, Weinraub Z, Bukovsky I, Tamir I: Changes in amniotic fluid lecithin-sphingomyelin ratio following maternal dexamethasone administration. Am J Obstet Gynecol *122*:327-331, 1975

Caspi E, Schreyer P, Weinraub Z, et al: Prevention of the respiratory distress syndrome in premature infants by antepartum glucocorticoid therapy. Br J Obstet Gynecol *83*:187-193, 1976

Gunn GC, Mishell DR, Morton DG: Premature rupture of the fetal membranes. Am J Obstet Gynecol *106*:469-483, 1970

Jones MD Jr, Burd LI, Bowes WA Jr, et al: Failure of association of premature rupture of membranes with respiratory distress syndrome. N Engl J Med *292*:1253-1257, 1975; Obstet Gynecol Surv *31*:8-9, 1976

Larson JW, Goldkrand JW, Hanson TM, Miller CR: Intrauterine infection on an obstetric service. Obstet Gynecol *43*:838-843, 1974

Liggins GC, Howie RN: A controlled trial of antepartum glucocorticoid treatment for prevention of the respiratory distress syndrome in premature infants. Pediatrics *50*:515-525, 1972

MacVicar J: Chorioamnionitis. *In* Charles D, Finland M: Obstetric and Perinatal Infections. Philadelphia, Lea & Febiger, 1973

Martin JE: Management of premature rupture of the membranes. Clin Obstet Gynecol *16*:213-225, 1973

Richardson CJ, Pomerance JJ, Cunningham MD, Gluck L: Acceleration of fetal lung maturation following prolonged rupture of the membranes. Am J Obstet Gynecol *118*:1115-1118, 1974

Sell EJ, Harris TR: Association of premature rupture of membranes with idiopathic respiratory distress syndrome. Obstet Gynecol *49*:167-169, 1977

82 PROLAPSED UMBILICAL CORD

GENERAL CONSIDERATIONS

Prolapse of the umbilical cord occurs approximately once in 200 deliveries. Three degrees of prolapse may be distinguished (Fig. 82-1): (1) *Occult* prolapse is the condition in which the cord is located at or near the pelvis but not within reach of the fingers on vaginal examination. (2) The cord may be *forelying*, that is, palpable through the cervical os, but within the intact amniotic sac. (3) The cord may be *prolapsed* into the vagina or even outside the vulva after the membranes have ruptured.

SUBJECTIVE AND OBJECTIVE DATA

Aside from when the cord can be palpated on vaginal examination, cord prolapse should be suspected when fetal heart tones become irregular in combination with sudden periodic episodes of bradycardia of variable duration.

ASSESSMENT

PREDISPOSING FACTORS

These include anything that causes maladaptation of the presenting part to the lower uterine segment or that prevents engagement of the head: a contracted pelvis with a high head when the membranes rupture, fetal malpresentation (breech, oblique, or transverse lie), premature labor, multiparity, premature rupture of the membranes, and hydramnios.

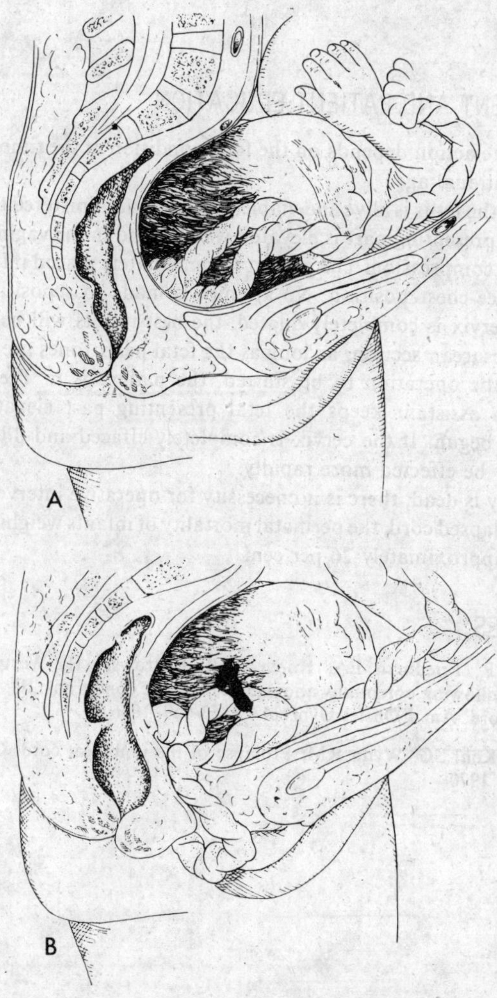

Figure 82-1. *A*, Cord presentation. *B*, Prolapse of cord. (From Huffman JW: Gynecology and Obstetrics. Philadelphia, W.B.Saunders Company, 1962.)

PLAN

MANAGEMENT AND PATIENT EDUCATION

Appropriate action depends on the fetal condition at the time of diagnosis and the gestational age.

As long as the fetus is alive and viable, oxygen is administered to the mother and the fetal presenting part is elevated with a hand in the vagina in order to prevent cord compression. The patient is immediately placed into Trendelenburg's or knee-chest position. No attempt is made to reposition the cord. Unless the cervix is completely dilated, the best results will be obtained by immediate cesarean section, as long as the fetal heart tones are good. While waiting for the operation to be started, the patient is in Trendelenburg's position. An assistant keeps the fetal presenting part elevated until the operation is begun. If the cervix is completely effaced and dilated, vaginal delivery may be effected more rapidly.

If the baby is dead, there is no necessity for operative intervention. In the case of a prolapsed cord, the perinatal mortality of infants weighing more than 1000 gm is approximately 26 per cent.

REFERENCES

Niswander KR, Friedman EA, Hoover DB, Pietrowski H, Westphal M: Fetal morbidity following potentially anoxigenic obstetric conditions. III. Prolapse of the umbilical cord. Am J Obstet Gynecol *95*:853-859, 1966

Savage EW, Kohl SG, Wynn RM: Prolapse of the umbilical cord. Obstet Gynecol *36*:502-509, 1970

83 PRURITUS VULVAE

GENERAL CONSIDERATIONS

Pruritus vulvae (vulvar itching) can be caused by a wide variety of local and systemic disorders. Although usually a chronic problem and more frequent in older women, intense genital itching may affect females of any age, who may request emergency care.

SUBJECTIVE DATA

Vulvar Itching: Details of onset, duration, and associated symptoms (vaginal discharge, incontinence, and so forth) aid in the diagnostic evaluation. Pruritus in other areas of the body suggests the probability of a generalized systemic or dermatologic disorder.

OBJECTIVE DATA

Vulvar skin is examined carefully for redness, excoriation, maceration, lichenification, scaling, fissuring, and visible lesions. Nits and lice may be visualized with a magnifying lens. Examination of other skin surfaces may disclose characteristic dermatologic lesions (psoriasis, contact dermatitis, and so forth).

Vaginal examination may reveal an irritating discharge.

ASSESSMENT

ETIOLOGIC FACTORS

1. Vaginal discharge
   a. Candida
   b. Trichomonas
2. Atrophy or dystrophy
   a. Estrogen deficiency
   b. Hyperplastic dystrophy
3. Infestations or infections
   a. Pediculosis pubis (pubic lice)
   b. Scabies
   c. Insect bites
4. Dermatologic disorders
   a. Contact dermatitis
   b. Allergic dermatitis
   c. Psoriasis
   d. Apocrine miliaria (Fox-Fordyce disease)*
5. Psychogenic factors
6. Systemic disease
   a. Diabetes
   b. Jaundice
   c. Allergy

---

*Fox-Fordyce disease is a chronic itching papular eruption of apocrine gland-bearing areas, particularly the axillae and pubes. It results from obstruction and rupture of the intraepidermal portion of the ducts of affected apocrine sweat glands. The onset of the disease is usually between 13 and 35 years of age.

The lesions of Fox-Fordyce disease are small papules, usually rounded and smooth because of scratching. On close examination, the lesions are principally follicular in location. The limitation of the papular changes to apocrine gland-bearing areas, the follicular or parafollicular orientation of the individual papules, the decrease or absence of apocrine sweat at affected follicular orifices, and the oft-noted diminished axillary odor are characteristic features of this disease. Skin biopsy confirms the diagnosis.

There is no method of management that offers a permanent cure. Local measures, including antibiotics and steroid lotions and creams, have only limited value. Usually the disease regresses during pregnancy. Some patients have benefited from oral contraceptive medication.

7. Rectal disease
   a. Fissures
   b. Hemorrhoids
   c. Pinworms

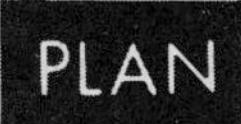

ADDITIONAL DIAGNOSTIC DATA

Wet smear of vaginal discharge may disclose Candida or Trichomonas.

Urinalysis may disclose glucose.

Vaginal cytologic test may show estrogen deficiency.

Biopsy of the vulva is indicated when chronic epithelial changes, dystrophy, or malignancy are suspected. The area to be biopsied is cleansed with an antiseptic solution and then infiltrated with 1 per cent lidocaine. A 4- or 6-mm dermal punch is twisted into the recently made wheal and the base of the tissue plug severed with small scissors. The local application of Monsel's solution followed by pressure is usually adequate to control bleeding. If necessary, a suture can be used to close the skin edges.

Toluidine blue dye is a valuable diagnostic aid that delineates suspicious skin areas for biopsy. In a normal keratin layer there are no surface nuclei; the toluidine blue stain is decolorized and washed away with dilute acetic acid. If nuclear material is present at the skin surface, the dye becomes fixed to cell nuclei and is retained. The stained areas are biopsied for microscopic evaluation.

MANAGEMENT

The specific cause is identified, if possible, and specific therapy is initiated. (See Vulvovaginitis, p. 709.)

Local irritants (deodorants, douches, perfumes, and other cosmetics) are eliminated.

Warm sitz baths or wet dressings with Burow's solution (aluminum acetate) or both often provide symptomatic relief and aid in cleansing the perineal area. Between treatments, the skin should be clean and dry. Shake lotions (calamine) or dusting powders (talc or cornstarch) may be useful.

Topical corticosteroids [fluocinolone acetonide (Synalar) cream or solution (0.01 per cent) or an equivalent] are effective antipruritic, anti-inflammatory preparations. (Anesthetic or other ointments are avoided, since they may irritate or macerate vulvar skin, rendering it more susceptible to injury.)

Trimeprazine tartrate (Temaril), a phenothiazine with antipruritic and antihistaminic properties, may benefit the nonpregnant patient. The usual dosage is 2.5-mg tablets four times daily or 5-mg capsules every 12 hours.

PATIENT EDUCATION

The patient is advised to avoid underclothes made of synthetic fabrics and tight, constricting garments, since they prevent adequate evaporation of moisture. Either no underpants or cotton underpants are recommended.

84 PUBIC SYMPHYSIS SEPARATION

GENERAL CONSIDERATIONS

Pregnancy may be associated with relaxation of the pubic symphysis, evidenced by a separation of the pubic bones. Beginning during the first half of pregnancy, antepartum softening and separation of the symphysis pubis appear to be due to the hormones of pregnancy, although the exact mechanisms by which these changes arise are unknown. The amount of separation varies considerably; possibly, congenital or acquired weakness of the pubic joint may predispose to symptomatic separation. The incidence of this complication varies from 1 in 1000 to 1 in 2000 deliveries.

SUBJECTIVE AND OBJECTIVE DATA

Pain on walking or during exertion may occur for the first time during the sixth or seventh month of pregnancy. Some patients complain only of symphysis pain or tenderness radiating down the inner aspects of the thighs; others walk with a painful broad-based, side-to-side waddle.

Pain may occur suddenly shortly after delivery, at which time the patient is unable to get out of bed, since any motion causes severe discomfort. If she does get out of bed and attempts to walk, she may find that she cannot flex her thighs and walks with eversion of her lower extremities (duck waddle).

Tenderness: On palpation, the pubic symphysis is very tender.

PLAN

ADDITIONAL DIAGNOSTIC DATA

Pelvic X-ray examination shows a separation of the symphysis pubis greater than 1 or 2 cm (see Fig. 84-1).

MANAGEMENT

Bed rest is usually adequate therapy for most patients. Prior to delivery, a snug maternity corset may be helpful. After delivery, the patient is usually able to ambulate within a week and gradually recovers within four weeks.

In the most serious cases, patients are confined to bed and require the use of pelvic slings similar to those used for the treatment of pelvic fractures.

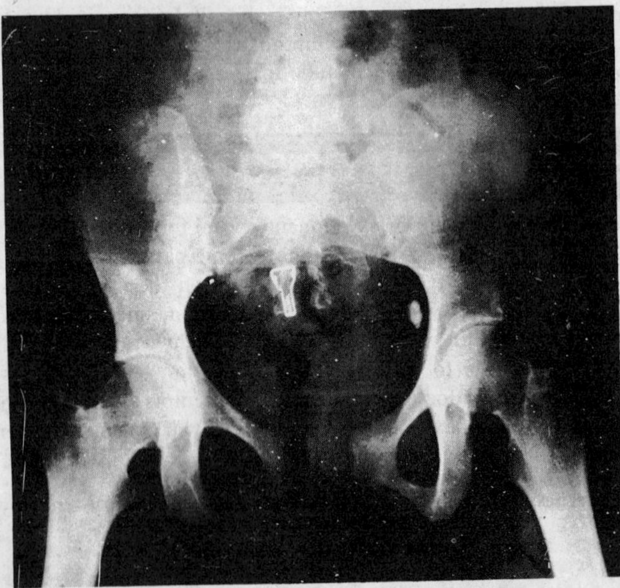

Figure 84-1. Anteroposterior x-ray view of a patient taken after a spontaneous delivery showing abnormally wide separation of the symphysis pubis. (From Greenhill JP, Friedman EA: Biological Principles and Modern Practice of Obstetrics. Philadelphia, W.B.Saunders Compa. y, 1974.)

85 PULMONARY ASPIRATION

GENERAL CONSIDERATIONS

Pulmonary aspiration (Table 85-1) of gastric contents, a leading cause of maternal anesthetic mortality, may occur whenever regurgitation or vomiting coincides with the impairment of normal pharyngeal reflexes and the protective mechanisms of glottic closure. Larger pieces of particulate matter can cause sudden tracheal obstruction or bilateral obstruction of the major bronchi, resulting in acute asphyxia and death. Particulate matter of smaller size may obstruct bronchi to various lung segments, resulting in atelectasis and pulmonary abscess.

Aspiration of acid gastric juice (pH of less than 2.5) can produce a diffuse chemical bronchiolitis and pneumonitis (Mendelson's syndrome). In order to reduce this risk, gastric contents may be neutralized by the

TABLE 85-1. Pulmonary Aspiration

Material Aspirated	Pulmonary Reaction	Therapy
Gastric acid	Chemical pneumonitis	Oxygen Clear airway Intravenous fluids Bronchodilators Corticosteroids
Oropharyngeal Bacterial	Infiltrate in dependent pulmonary segment	Antibiotics
Particulate matter	Airway obstruction	Tracheal suction Extraction of offending material Bronchoscopy for larger particles

administration of 15 ml of a liquid antacid every three hours during labor or prior to anesthesia (Roberts and Shirley, 1976).

SUBJECTIVE AND OBJECTIVE DATA

Regurgitation or Vomiting: During the induction of general anesthesia, silent regurgitation of acid vomitus may occur. At other times, vomiting occurs, which is usually followed by coughing and respiratory distress (dyspnea, expiratory wheezing).

General Appearance: Cyanosis, tachypnea, tachycardia, and hypotension indicate the severity of respiratory obstruction. Fever may indicate pulmonary infection.

Pulmonary findings may include bronchospasm, atelectasis, wheezes, rhonchi, and rales.

ASSESSMENT

DIFFERENTIAL DIAGNOSIS

This includes congestive heart failure, asthma, pulmonary emboli, pulmonary edema, adult respiratory distress syndrome, and amniotic fluid emboli.

ETIOLOGIC FACTORS

General anesthesia with its associated loss of protective upper airway reflexes is the usual precipitating factor. Oversedation with narcotics, tranquilizers, and hypnotics may also obtund both consciousness and the protective upper airway reflex. Hypotension associated with conduction anesthesia can result in the loss of upper airway reflexes.

Overdosage of local anesthetic drugs may cause convulsions that predispose to pulmonary aspiration.

Women during labor are particularly vulnerable to aspiration for various reasons. First, compression of the abdominal contents by the gravid uterus results in an elevated intragastric pressure. Second, gastric-emptying time is appreciably delayed during labor, and women have often eaten shortly before the onset of labor. Since vomiting occurs commonly during labor, antiemetic medications, such as promethazine hydrochloride (Phenergan) (25 to 50 mg), may be useful.

When general anesthesia is necessary in a patient with a full stomach, a crash induction is usually advisable. The patient is rapidly anesthetized with intravenous pentothal and then given succinylcholine intravenously to produce muscular relaxation for endotracheal intubation. During the time from loss of consciousness to the placement and inflation of the cuffed endotracheal tube, the patient's vulnerability to pulmonary aspiration of stomach contents is minimized by cricoid pressure, which obstructs the esophagus between the trachea and the bodies of the cervical vertebrae. As soon as the cuffed endotracheal tube is passed, the cuff is immediately inflated to occlude the trachea.

SEVERITY OF DISEASE PROCESS

Pulmonary aspiration produces a syndrome that may rapidly progress from subtle respiratory distress to respiratory failure, pulmonary edema, and circulatory collapse.

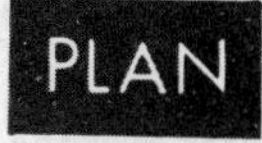

ADDITIONAL DIAGNOSTIC DATA

Chest X-ray: Aspiration of particulate matter may produce a pulmonary, lobar, or segmental collapse. The chest x-ray may show atelectasis, with areas of increased density usually in a dependent segment. Aspiration of gastric acid produces diffuse, mottled, irregular densities. Aspiration of bacteria may produce an infiltrate in a dependent pulmonary segment.

Arterial Blood Gases: Decreased pO_2 indicates hypoxemia.

MANAGEMENT

As soon as aspiration is suspected, the patient should be placed on her right side, with her head tilted down to allow dependent drainage of vomitus from the pharynx. The airway is immediately cleared with pharyngeal suction, and oxygen is administered continually. Intubation with a cuffed endotracheal tube prevents further aspiration and provides an airway for positive pressure ventilation and the removal of aspirated material. Repeated suctioning with intermittent oxygenation is continued until no more solid material is recovered. Bronchoscopy may be necessary to remove large food particles.

At the time of initial tracheal suction, the pH of the pulmonary aspirate is determined. If the pH is less than 2.5, therapy for acid aspiration is initiated. If the pH is greater than 2.5, a gastric tube is passed after tracheal intubation in order to determine the pH of the gastric contents. Whenever the pH is 2.5 or less therapy for acid aspiration is initiated.

The objectives of therapy are correction of hypoxia, oxygenation, adequate ventilation, and treatment of bronchospasm.

Oxygen is administered, and arterial blood gases are determined. The therapeutic objective is an arterial oxygen tension in the range of 70 to 90 mm Hg. Prolonged mechanical positive pressure ventilation may be required to maintain adequate pulmonary exchange and to prevent pulmonary edema. A clear airway is essential.

Bronchospasm is treated with aminophylline (500 mg in 500 ml of 5 per cent dextrose in water) or isoproterenol [0.01 to 0.02 mg (0.5 to 1 ml of a 1:50,000 diluted solution)]. Intravenous corticosteroids may be beneficial. An initial dose of 250 mg to 1000 mg of hydrocortisone is administered. Baggish and Hooper recommend 1 gm of hydrocortisone every six hours followed by 1 gm daily for one or two days.

Antibiotics are usually prescribed to prevent secondary bacterial invasion when pathogenic organisms are aspirated, although opinions differ over the benefits of prophylactic antibiotic therapy. Antibiotics are mandatory after infection has developed.

Repeated arterial blood gas and pH determinations provide guidelines for management.

REFERENCES

Baggish MS, Hooper S: Aspiration as a cause of maternal death. Obstet Gynecol *43*: 327-336, 1974

Cameron JL, Mitchell WH, Zuidema GD: Aspiration pneumonia: clinical outcome following documented aspiration. Arch Surg *106*:49-52, 1973

Gutsche BB: Anesthetic emergencies in obstetrics. Clin Obstet Gynecol *19*:519-531, 1976

Roberts RB, Shirley MA: The obstetrician's role in reducing the risk of aspiration pneumonitis. Am J Obstet Gynecol *124*:611-617, 1976

Ruggera G, Taylor G: Pulmonary aspiration in anesthesia. West J Med *125*:411-414, 1976

Tinstman TC, Dines DE, Arms RA: Postoperative aspiration pneumonia. Surg Clin North Am *53*:859-862, 1973

86 PULMONARY EDEMA

GENERAL CONSIDERATIONS

Pulmonary edema is one of the most serious emergency problems resulting from increased pulmonary capillary pressure or permeability associated with cardiac, pulmonary, or renal disease.

SUBJECTIVE AND OBJECTIVE DATA

Dyspnea; orthopnea; rapid, shallow breathing; wheezing; tachycardia; frothy sputum; cough; and moist rales are typical symptoms and signs. The onset may be acute or gradual.

ASSESSMENT

DIFFERENTIAL DIAGNOSIS

See Dyspnea during Pregnancy, p. 298.

ETIOLOGIC FACTORS

These include increased blood volume, fluid overloading, cardiac failure, increased intracranial pressure, preeclampsia and eclampsia, and abnormal permeability of pulmonary capillaries resulting from shock, sepsis, the inhalation of hot or irritant fumes or chemicals, and burns.

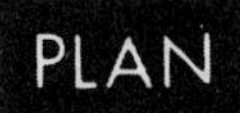

ADDITIONAL DIAGNOSTIC DATA

Chest X-rays: Loss of definition of pulmonary vascular markings, haziness of hilar shadows, and thickening of the interlobular septa (Kerley's B lines) may be seen in cases of interstitial edema. Diffuse, confluent shadows of uniform density randomly scattered throughout the lung fields or bilateral perihilar homogeneous alveolar densities (butterfly or batwing configuration) with air bronchograms may be seen with alveolar edema.

Arterial Blood Gases: Decreased oxygen tension, increased carbon dioxide tension, and decreased arterial pH are associated with severe pulmonary edema.

Electrocardiogram may reveal cardiac arrhythmias.

MANAGEMENT

Oxygenation: Oxygen is provided by mask, nasal catheter, or intermittent positive pressure. Positive pressure breathing increases intrathoracic pressure, retards venous return, and inhibits the movement of fluid into the alveoli. With abnormal pulmonary capillary permeability, respirator therapy via a tracheostomy or endotracheal tube may be required.

Sedation:

Morphine (7 to 15 mg given intravenously or subcutaneously) helps allay anxiety and decrease tachypnea; it is particularly beneficial for attacks of acute pulmonary edema resulting from failure of the left ventricle. Morphine should be avoided, however, in chronic obstructive lung disease and during the late stages of pulmonary edema, when respiration is depressed because of severe hypoxia.

Reduction of Pulmonary Blood Volume:

Diuretics: Furosemide (Lasix) (10 to 40 mg intravenously) or ethacrynic acid (Edecrin) (25 to 50 mg) usually produces a prompt diuresis.

Rotating tourniquets on three extremities every 15 minutes may also be beneficial. The tourniquet should occlude venous return but not arterial inflow.

Treatment of Underlying Cause: See Cardiac Failure During Pregnancy, p. 176, Eclampsia, p. 303, and Preeclampsia, p. 552.

87 PULMONARY EMBOLISM

GENERAL CONSIDERATIONS

Pulmonary embolism is an obstruction of the pulmonary artery or one of its branches by a previously detached thrombus, amniotic fluid, or air. The most common source for pulmonary embolus is a venous thrombus arising in the deep veins of the lower extremities or in the pelvic veins.

Emboli lodging in the pulmonary arterial tree acutely reduce the circulation distal to the site of obstruction. Potential effects are fourfold: (1) Less blood proceeds through the pulmonary circuit to the left side of the heart and systemic circulation, (2) blood is dammed back behind the mechanical obstruction (pulmonary hypertension), (3) hemorrhagic necrosis of the ischemic area (infarction) occurs, and (4) pulmonary function is impaired. The clinical picture depends on the size of the obstructed vessel. When embolism occludes more than 60 per cent of the pulmonary vasculature, the resultant pressure load can cause acute dilatation of the right ventricle combined with venous engorgement and an elevated central venous pressure. Consequences of impaired pulmonary venous return are a sharp reduction in left ventricular filling, diminished cardiac output, and acute circulatory failure resulting from shock or cardiac arrest.

Although pulmonary embolism can affect women of all ages and occur at any time, acute episodes are most apt to occur following surgery or delivery.

SUBJECTIVE DATA

CURRENT SYMPTOMS

Dyspnea and chest pain (substernal or pleuritic) are the most common symptoms. Other symptoms, depending on the degree of vascular obstruction, include anxiety, apprehension, syncope, cough, hemoptysis, an urgent desire to defecate, and cardiovascular collapse. Abdominal pain (midepigastric or right upper quadrant), although uncommon, may be due to hepatic congestion from right ventricular failure or referred pain from diaphragmatic pleural irritation (Potts, 1976).

PRIOR HISTORY

A history of thromboembolism may be elicited from approximately 25 per cent of patients.

OBJECTIVE DATA

PHYSICAL EXAMINATION

General examination may disclose acute circulatory failure due to shock or cardiac arrest. Tachypnea, a respiratory rate greater than 16 per minute, is the most common abnormality encountered (Bell, 1977). Tachycardia, hypotension, syncope, cyanosis, and distended neck veins are suggestive of massive pulmonary embolism. Low-grade fever (100° F) and an increased pulse rate can be manifestations of pulmonary infarction. Peripheral venous thrombosis may be apparent.

Chest examination may disclose absent breath sounds, a pleural friction rub, rales, or reduced expansion of the affected side. Other possible findings include accentuation of the pulmonic second sound, systolic or diastolic murmurs in the second left interspace, and S_3 or S_4 gallop rhythm.

Abdominal examination may disclose a tender, enlarged liver.

LABORATORY TESTS

Complete Blood Count with Blood Smear: Leukocytosis may be associated with pulmonary infarction.

ASSESSMENT

DIFFERENTIAL DIAGNOSIS

This includes pulmonary aspiration, pneumonia, atelectasis, asthma, pleuritis, pleural effusion, myocardial infarction, congestive heart failure, pulmonary edema, cerebral vascular accident, pneumothorax, sickle cell disease, and emotional reactions.

PREDISPOSING FACTORS

Risk factors for thromboembolism during pregnancy and the puerperium include

1. Increasing age
2. Multiparity
3. A prior episode of thrombosis or embolism
4. Operative delivery
5. Obesity
6. Prolonged bed rest or immobilization
7. Vascular injury
8. Dehydration

(See Thrombophlebitis, p. 644.)

The role of estrogen in the pathogenesis of thromboembolic problems remains controversial, since numerous studies have reached different conclusions (Goldzieher, 1975). Nonetheless, various studies estimate that users of oral contraceptives are 4 to 11 times more likely than nonusers to acquire idiopathic thromboembolic disease. (See Contraceptive Emergencies, p. 249.)

Some patients with fatal pulmonary embolism following delivery had received estrogens for lactation suppression. Since many of these patients also had other predisposing factors to thromboembolism, it is not possible to conclude that there is a positive association between the embolism and estrogenic medications (Report on Confidential Enquiries into Maternal Deaths in England and Wales, 1967-1969).

SEVERITY OF DISEASE PROCESS

The clinical syndrome depends on the degree of obstruction in the pulmonary circulation, which varies from cardiovascular collapse to acute cor pulmonale, pulmonary infarction, or symptoms mimicking bronchopneumonia or postoperative atelectasis.

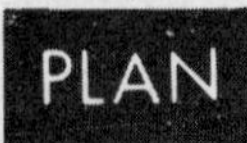

ADDITIONAL DIAGNOSTIC DATA

Arterial Blood Gases: Arterial oxygen tension (pO_2) aids in screening patients suspected of having pulmonary embolism. With an embolus, both pO_2 and pCO_2 are usually decreased. Although the absence of arterial hypoxemia does not exclude the diagnosis, pulmonary embolus is very unlikely if the arterial pO_2 is greater than 90 mm Hg.

Chest x-ray findings are often nonspecific (normal films, pulmonary infiltrates, pleural effusion, atelectasis). Findings suggestive of pulmonary emboli are prominent pulmonary arteries and segmental decreased pulmonary vasculature. Enlargement of the right ventricle and pulmonary conus are signs of acute cor pulmonale. A peripheral wedge-shaped density, caused by segmental infarction, is seen in less than one third of the cases.

Electrocardiogram often shows only sinus tachycardia and nonspecific ST- and T-wave abnormalities. ECG patterns highly suggestive of pulmonary emboli are the following (Humphries, 1976):

1. Inverted T (V_1 to V_4)
2. Right bundle-branch block (especially if transient)
3. S_1, O_3, or S_1, S_2, S_3 (especially if transient)
4. Right axis deviation
5. Right-ventricle hypertrophy
6. Tall and peaked P-waves in leads II, III, and a V_F

Pulmonary perfusion scans can be helpful when pulmonary emboli are suspected. A completely normal scan virtually excludes the diagnosis of embolization.

Since the perfusion scan is extremely sensitive, defects can be due not only to pulmonary emboli but also to pleural effusion, pneumonitis, atelectasis, pulmonary congestion, or chronic lung disease. When the chest X-ray shows changes of parenchymal or pleural disease, the interpretation of defects on the perfusion scan is more difficult. A ventilation scan may be helpful.

If the scan and the clinical picture are highly suggestive of pulmonary emboli, treatment may be initiated. If the perfusion scan is abnormal, pulmonary angiography is recommended to confirm the diagnosis.

Pulmonary angiography is the most specific diagnostic criterion currently available. A normal angiogram excludes the diagnosis of pulmonary embolism.

MANAGEMENT AND PATIENT EDUCATION

Objectives of therapy are twofold:

1. To provide general supportive measures
2. To prevent recurrent embolism

Supportive Measures:

The patient is hospitalized at bed rest.

Respiratory Support:

Oxygen is administered by nasal catheter, mask, or positive pressure, as indicated.

Circulatory Support:

Intravenous fluids (1000 ml of 5 per cent dextrose in water) are initiated slowly.

In the management of shock, dopamine or *isoproterenol* may be a useful adjunct. Isoproterenol tends to increase cardiac output and relax bronchial smooth muscle. One mg of a 1:5000 solution is added to 500 ml of dextrose injection and infused at a rate of 1 to 5 mcg per minute (0.5 to 2.5 ml of a 1:500,000 solution diluted). The infusion rate is adjusted on the basis of heart rate, central venous pressure, systemic blood pressure and urine flow. If the heart rate exceeds 110 beats per minute, it may be advisable to decrease the infusion rate or temporarily discontinue the infusion.

Sedation to Allay Pain and Apprehension: Morphine (5 to 15 mg) or meperidine (25 to 100 mg) is given.

Other Measures: Stool softeners are recommended to prevent constipation.

Prevention of Recurrent Embolism:

Intravenous heparin is initiated as soon as the diagnosis is established. Since most initial episodes of pulmonary embolism are not massive or fatal but additional episodes could be, prevention of recurrent emboli is one of the most important aspects of treatment.

The heparin may be administered by continuous intravenous infusion (an initial loading dose of 5000 units followed by 1000 units per hour) via infusion pump. The activated partial thromboplastin time (APTT) is determined approximately every four hours during the early stages of treatment. The heparin infusion is adjusted to keep the APTT between one and one half and two and one half times the control level. The average daily dose is 20,000 to 40,000 units.

Oral anticoagulation therapy with coumarin compounds is initiated several days before discontinuation of heparin, except during pregnancy when coumarin compounds are avoided if at all possible because of fetal risks (hemorrhage, intrauterine death, and congenital malformations). During pregnancy, subcutaneous heparin is preferable for long-range therapy.

Surgical ligation of the inferior vena cava and ovarian veins may be necessary if emboli recur despite anticoagulant therapy.

After having a pulmonary embolism, the patient is advised never to take oral contraceptive medications since she has a greater risk of recurrent embolism.

Air Embolism

GENERAL CONSIDERATIONS

Air embolism is a very rare event that may occur following delivery if air enters the large venous sinuses at the placental site. Three hundred ml of air or more in the vascular system can be lethal, since the air collects in the right ventricular outflow tract and creates an acute cor pulmonale.

SUBJECTIVE AND OBJECTIVE DATA

Acute symptoms include cyanosis, hypotension, shock, and cardiovascular collapse. Gasping respiration or focal seizures may also occur.

A millwheel heart murmur, a loud churning sound audible over the entire precordium, is a characteristic finding.

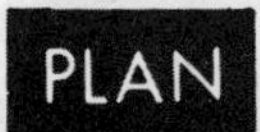

MANAGEMENT

The patient is immediately placed in a left lateral decubitus position to allow the air bubble in the right ventricular outflow tract to rise toward the apex of the heart and permit resumption of right ventricular output. A needle or catheter inserted into the right ventricle may release the trapped air.

Respiratory and circulatory support are essential.

Amniotic Fluid Embolism

GENERAL CONSIDERATIONS

Amniotic fluid embolism is a very rare and frequently fatal complication of labor and delivery. Particulate matter from the amniotic fluid causes a mechanical obstruction in the distal pulmonary tree.

Sudden pulmonary hypertension leads to a vagus-mediated vasoconstriction of both pulmonary and coronary arteries. Blood flow to the left heart decreases and cardiac output falls, leading to peripheral vascular collapse. Acute cor pulmonale and right heart failure lead to pulmonary edema.

Hemorrhage associated with amniotic fluid embolism is a result of a disseminated intravascular coagulation (DIC) as well as of a coincident diminution in uterine tone.

The route by which amniotic fluid enters the maternal circulation is not clear; lacerations in the endocervical veins during cervical dilatation, subplacental venous sinuses, and lacerations in the lower uterine segment are all possibilities.

SUBJECTIVE DATA

Sudden, acute dyspnea immediately after a precipitous delivery or during a precipitate labor is the most characteristic symptom.

If the patient has delivered enroute to the hospital, she may enter the emergency room in shock with profuse vaginal bleeding.

Other possible symptoms include chest pain, convulsions, restlessness, anxiety, coughing, and vomiting.

OBJECTIVE DATA

PHYSICAL EXAMINATION

General Examination: Cyanosis and shock are usually profound. Hypotension and tachycardia are indications of the extent of cardiovascular collapse. Other possible findings include convulsions, coma, pulmonary edema with pink, frothy sputum, and even cardiac arrest.

Pelvic Examination: Persistent vaginal bleeding is usually due to uterine atony, with or without disseminated intravascular coagulation.

LABORATORY TESTS

Complete blood count and blood smear provide an indication of blood loss and preexisting anemia.

Urinalysis is usually normal.

Blood Type and Rh: Blood is sent to the blood bank for type and Rh determination. Four units are cross-matched for transfusion as indicated. (A coagulation defect is immediately suspected if the blood in the tube fails to clot.)

ASSESSMENT

DIFFERENTIAL DIAGNOSIS

The triad of *dyspnea*, *cyanosis*, and *sudden shock* occurring during strong labor or immediately post partum, particularly if associated with profuse vaginal bleeding and a coagulopathy, favors the diagnosis of amniotic fluid embolism. Other possibilities to be considered include uterine rupture, uterine inversion, placental abruption, eclampsia, myocardial infarction, cerebrovascular accident, and congestive heart failure.

POTENTIAL COMPLICATIONS

Complications to be expected include disseminated intravascular coagulation and uterine atony. The maternal mortality rate is in the range of 80 per cent.

PREDISPOSING FACTORS

These include rapid, tumultuous labor with hypertonic uterine contraction, precipitous delivery, multiparity, intrauterine fetal death, meconium in the amniotic fluid, operative delivery, and placenta previa.

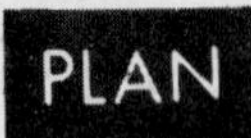

ADDITIONAL DIAGNOSTIC DATA

Arterial Blood Gases: The pO_2 is usually decreased.

Central Venous Pressure may be elevated, normal, or subnormal, depending on the quantity of blood lost. Central venous blood may contain amniotic-fluid cellular debris.

Coagulation profile (fibrinogen, platelet count, prothrombin time, and partial thromboplastin time) is usually abnormal, indicating disseminated intravascular coagulation.

Electrocardiogram may show acute right heart strain.

Urine output may be decreased, indicating inadequate renal perfusion.

Chest x-ray is usually nondiagnostic but may show infiltrates. A lung scan may show perfusion defects consistent with a pulmonary embolic process.

MANAGEMENT AND PATIENT EDUCATION

Crucial therapy includes immediate *resuscitation, ventilation*, and *circulatory support* and the correction of specific defects: uterine atony, coagulation defects, and pulmonary arteriolar spasm.

Oxygen is always indicated and should be administered under positive pressure through an endotracheal tube, if necessary.

Intravenous fluids and blood replacement are necesasry to correct hypovolemia and blood loss. Fluid therapy may be monitored by determinations of the central venous pressure or pulmonary artery diastolic or wedge pressure. Fresh-frozen plasma and platelet packs may be required for correction of coagulation defects.

Oxytocin added to the intravenous infusion aids in the management of uterine atony. Bimanual uterine compression may also be necessary. (See Postpartum Hemorrhage, p. 537.)

Morphine (10 mg) may aid in the relief of dyspnea and apprehension.

Aminophylline (250 to 500 mg) by slow intravenous infusion may be beneficial if bronchospasm is present.

Isoproterenol (1 to 2 mg diluted in 500 ml of 5 per cent dextrose in water) tends to produce peripheral vasodilatation, relax bronchial smooth muscle, and increase the rate and force of the heart. It is administered slowly intravenously to sustain the systolic blood pressure at approximately 100 mm Hg.

Heparin has been advocated to impede intravascular defibrination by inhibiting the clotting process. Efficacy and dosage remain controversial. A typical course of therapy is an initial dose of 2500 to 3000 units intravenously followed by 500 units per hour administered with a constant infusion pump.

Digitalization may be indicated if there is evidence of cardiac failure.

Amniotic fluid embolism is highly fatal; survival depends in part on the extent of pulmonary obstruction. Support of the cardiovascular system and control of coagulation defects are essential therapeutic measures.

REFERENCES

Aaro LA, Juergens JL: Thrombophlebitis and pulmonary embolism as complications of pregnancy. Med Clin North Am *58*:829-834, 1974

Artz DP, Hardy JD (eds): Management of Surgical Complication. 3rd ed. Philadelphia, W.B. Saunders Company, 1975

Bell WR, Simon TL, DeMets DL: The clinical features of submassive and massive pulmonary emboli. Am J Med *62*:355-360, 1977

Chung AF, Merkatz IR: Survival following amniotic fluid embolism with early heparinization. Obstet Gynecol *42*:809-814, 1973; Obstet Gynecol Surv *29*:394-397, 1974

Courtney LD: Amniotic fluid embolism. Obstet Gynecol Surv *29*:169-177, 1974

Goldzieher JW, Dozier TS: Oral contraceptives and thromboembolism: a reassessment. Am J Obstet Gynecol *123*:878-914, 1975

Gottlieb JD, Ericsson JA, Sweet RB: Venous air embolism. Anesth Analg *44*:773-779, 1965

Gregory MG, Clayton EM: Amniotic fluid embolism. Obstet Gynecol *42*:236-244, 1973

Henry M: Pulmonary embolism and maternal mortality 1966-1973. J Irish Med Assoc *68*:175-177, 1975

Humphries JO, Bell WR, White RI: Criteria for the recognition of pulmonary emboli. JAMA *235*:2011-2012, 1976

Moser KM: Pulmonary Embolism. Am Rev Respir Dis *115*:829-852, 1977

Peterson EP, Taylor HB: Amniotic fluid embolism: an analysis of 40 cases. Obstet Gynecol *35*:787-793, 1970

Potts DE, Sahn SA: Abdominal manifestations of pulmonary embolism. JAMA *235*: 2835-2837, 1976

Report on confidential enquiries into maternal deaths in England and Wales, 1967-1969, London, HMSO, 1972

Resnik R, Swartz WH, Plumer MH, et al: Amniotic fluid embolism with survival. Obstet Gynecol *47*:295-298, 1976

Salzman EW, Deykin D, Shapiro RM, et al: Management of heparin therapy. N Engl J Med *292*:1046-1050, 1975

Sasahara AA: Therapy for pulmonary embolism. JAMA *229*:1795-1798, 1974

Szucs MM, Brooks HL, Grossman W, et al: Diagnostic sensitivity of laboratory findings in acute pulmonary embolism. Ann Intern Med *74*:161-166, 1971

Turnbull AC, Daniel DG, McGarry JM: Antenatal and postnatal thromboembolism. Practitioner *206*:727-735, 1971

88 PYELONEPHRITIS

GENERAL CONSIDERATIONS

Pyelonephritis is usually caused by ascending infection from the bladder, that involves the ureter, renal pelvis, and parenchyma. The kidney may also become infected by the hematogenous route.

During pregnancy, acute pyelonephritis is a serious complication, occurring in approximately 2 per cent of pregnancies. The disease may be bilateral or unilateral; if unilateral the right side is more frequently involved. Acute pyelonephritis is most likely to develop during the latter half of pregnancy or post partum.

SUBJECTIVE DATA

Lumbar pain in the costovertebral area is the most characteristic symptom. The pain is usually unilateral but may be bilateral if both kidneys are involved.

Urinary symptoms include dysuria, burning, frequency, urgency, and hematuria. Often there is a past history of urinary tract infections.

Fever and chills are common symptoms associated with acute pyelonephritis.

Anorexia, nausea and vomiting may be associated symptoms.

OBJECTIVE DATA

PHYSICAL EXAMINATION

Temperature is usually elevated above 100.4° F (38° C).

Tenderness over the kidney in the costovertebral area is a characteristic finding.

LABORATORY TESTS

Complete Blood Count with Blood Smear: The white count is usually elevated, with increased polymorphonuclear leukocytes and immature forms.

Urinalysis: The urine specimen tends to be loaded with white blood cells and bacteria. The sediment often shows white cells in clumps or casts and numerous bacteria. On Gram stain, the bacteria are usually determined to be gram-negative bacilli.

ASSESSMENT

DIFFERENTIAL DIAGNOSIS

The differential diagnosis of acute flank pain includes ureteral calculus, labor, premature placental separation, leiomyoma with infarction, and uterine infection. In addition, with right-sided pain, appendicitis and biliary colic should be considered.

PREDISPOSING FACTORS

Predisposing factors during pregnancy include ureteral obstruction and bacteriuria.

Ureteral obstruction may be caused by the mechanical effects of the enlarged uterus or by dilated ovarian veins. The latter are more likely to occur on the right side and have been proposed as the explanation for the more frequent occurrence of right-sided pyelonephritis (Bellina, 1970). Stasis induced by ureteral dilatation and decreased persistalsis contributes to a partial obstruction of urinary flow, increasing the susceptibility to renal infection.

Ovarian vein syndrome is a urologic disorder in which an aberrant right ovarian vein compresses the ureter, predisposing the patient to either pyelonephritis or hydronephrosis.

Bacteriuria (a colony count of 100,000 or more) is persistent and asymptomatic in approximately 3 to 8 per cent of pregnant women. The incidence varies with age, parity, and socioeconomic factors. Unless patients with asymptomatic bacteriuria are treated, approximately 20 to 25 per cent subsequently acquire an acute symptomatic urinary tract infection during the course of pregnancy. Bladder catheterization may be a source of bacteriuria.

Postpartum predisposing factors include trauma to the bladder and urethra during delivery. In addition, anesthesia may remove the sensation of bladder filling, thereby leading to bladder overdistention. During the early puerperium, the bladder has a greater capacity and less sensitivity to intravesical fluid tension than it has in the nonpregnant state. This contributes to overdistention, with incomplete emptying and residual urine. If bacteria have been introduced by catheterization, the residual urine in a traumatized bladder provides an excellent environment for bacterial multiplication.

POTENTIAL COMPLICATIONS

These include premature labor, septicemia, septic shock, and chronic pyelonephritis.

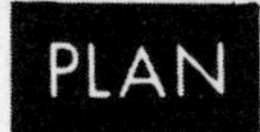

ADDITIONAL DIAGNOSTIC DATA

Bacteriologic Evaluation: Urine culture and antibiotic sensitivities are essential to determine the specific bacteria and the appropriate therapy. *Escherichia coli* is the organism grown on culture most frequently. The next most likely bacteria are Klebsiella, Enterobacter, and Proteus.

Blood cultures should also be taken to evaluate the possibility of bacteremia.

Blood Chemistries: Blood urea nitrogen and blood creatinine are usually normal, unless chronic renal disease is present.

Serum electrolytes are usually normal, unless persistent nausea and vomiting have caused severe dehydration.

X-ray: Abdominal x-ray (KUB) may be helpful if a ureteral calculus is suspected and the stone is opaque. An intravenous pyelogram may be indicated if renal calculi or other renal diseases are suspected. X-radiation is avoided during pregnancy, if at all possible.

MANAGEMENT

During pregnancy, the patient should be hospitalized until clinical improvement occurs. Close observation is essential in order to detect the earliest evidence of bacterial shock. Urine output, pulse, and blood pressure are evaluated at frequent intervals.

Intravenous fluids are recommended for hydration, since elevated temperatures tend to be associated with excessive fluid loss.

Antibiotic therapy is initiated immediately, based on a Gram stain of the urine specimen and knowledge of the most likely infecting organisms. Ampicillin is often preferred, unless the patient is sensitive to penicillin, since high blood levels are effective against potential bacteremia. The initial dosage is 1 gm intravenously every six hours, followed by oral therapy after the patient has responded. Total duration of therapy is ten days.

When sensitivity data are not available and infection is severe and life threatening, gentamicin sulfate provides the most reliable coverage against gram-negative rods. If gram-positive cocci are present in addition to gram-negative rods, ampicillin and gentamicin in combination are preferred for initial therapy. When infecting organisms are identified and sensitivities known, therapy may be altered according to the clinical and bacteriologic responses.

Clinical response is usually apparent within 48 hours. A urine culture should be repeated after 72 hours in order to verify the absence of bacteriuria.

PATIENT EDUCATION

During pregnancy, physiologic changes in the urinary tract that may predispose to infection are not altered by treatment. Consequently, reinfection is always possible. Repeated follow-up cultures are essential in order to be certain that the urine remains sterile.

Pyelonephritis resistant to treatment may be due to underlying renal disease, ureterolithiasis, or stasis with impaired drainage. Thorough urologic investigation may be necessary to elucidate the diagnosis and plan appropriate therapy.

REFERENCES

Bellina JH, Dougherty CM, Mickal A: Pyeloureteral dilatation and pregnancy. Am J Obstet Gynecol *108*:356-363, 1970

Cunningham FG, Morris GB, Mickal A: Acute pyelonephritis of pregnancy: a clinical review. Obstet Gynecol *42*:112-117, 1973

Fass RJ, Klainer AS, Perkins RL: Urinary tract infection. JAMA *225*:1509-1513, 1973

89 SEXUAL ASSAULT — ALLEGED RAPE

GENERAL CONSIDERATIONS

Rape is unlawful carnal knowledge (sexual intercourse) through force or deception and without consent. This definition may be extended to "any orifice" in order to allow for forced penetration of the mouth or anus. The rape victim is traumatized by both a sexual and a violent crime.

The act of rape is one of the most psychologically devastating encounters a person can experience. It is a brutal, violent act that robs its victims of self-identity and carries ramifications of guilt and fear that can persist long after the patient receives emergency medical care. The rape victim has undergone a dehumanizing, emotionally shattering experience, which creates intense psychologic stress. Gentle, sympathetic care is essential for the recovery of self-identity and emotional health.

Whether rape occurred is a *legal* matter for court decision and *not* a medical diagnosis. Unlawfulness, carnal knowledge, and lack of consent must be shown individually in every case.

An act's unlawfulness depends in part on marital status and age. Sexual activity by a married couple is not unlawful. Therefore, although there can be sexual assault in marriage, there cannot, according to present laws, be rape. In addition, there is a statutory age of consent that varies from state to state and below which consent is invalid. Intercourse in such a situation constitutes statutory rape, unless the couple is married.

Medical evidence may be necessary to establish carnal knowledge and help to show lack of consent.

When a woman who is allegedly the victim of rape is seen in an emergency department or requests medical care, she has special emergency needs:

Medical Needs: These are immediate treatment of any physical injuries, evaluation for pregnancy and venereal disease, and appropriate referral for follow-up evaluations.

Psychologic needs include minimization of psychologic stress and appropriate referral for follow-up.

Legal needs are collection of medicolegal evidence, maintenance of a legal record, and protection of the chain of evidence for police.

Informed Consent: The patient should give a written, witnessed, informed consent for physical examination, collection of laboratory specimens, photographs, release of information to proper authorities, and medical treatment. The patient should always be advised of the benefits and risks of medical examination and treatments.

Since the results of the medical examination may be used as evidence in a courtroom, the patient has the right to request medical treatment only and to refuse examination for the collection of legal evidence. The patient should be informed, however, if the hospital is required to report cases of suspected assault and battery to the local authorities.

Implied consent applies to situations when the patient presents herself for treatment or is brought to a medical facility by the local police.

SUBJECTIVE DATA

The patient's history should be recorded by quoting the patient's own words concerning time, place, circumstances and degree of penetration. Information concerning the ejaculation site may aid the physician in the search for semen staining. The occurrence of fellatio or anal intercourse is indication for examination of oral or anal areas.

The patient should be asked if she has bathed, douched, changed clothing, or taken any medications since the alleged assault.

The date of the last menstrual period and details of contraceptive usage aid in the evaluation of pregnancy risk. If the patient is known to be pregnant, this should be recorded. Preexisting pregnancy affects the discussion of treatment as well as medical and psychologic follow-up.

Questioning and examination should always be done in the presence of a witness.

OBJECTIVE DATA

PHYSICAL EXAMINATION (See Table 89-1)

General Examination: The patient's general appearance, emotional state, behavior (hysterical, stoical, intoxicated, and so forth) and the appearance of her clothing are noted. The skin is inspected for evidence of trauma: abrasions, contusions, lacerations, and scratches, especially about the mouth, throat, wrists, arms, breasts, and thighs. If dried seminal stains are found on the skin, they should be removed with saline-moistened swabs, which are then preserved for evidence in glassine envelopes or stoppered test tubes.

The oral cavity is inspected for signs of trauma, especially if fellatio occurred. A gonorrhea culture is taken from the pharynx.

Photographs are taken if they are required.

Pelvic Examination: The external genitalia are inspected for evidence of trauma. The pubic hair is combed for foreign material; hairs containing seminal stains are trimmed out and preserved as evidence.

The condition of the hymen is described (for example, the hymen is present and intact without evidence of trauma; the hymen is bleeding; the hymen is absent).

For examination of the cervix and vagina, a nonlubricated, water-moistened speculum is used. A vaginoscope or nasal speculum may be preferred prior to puberty.

Any lacerations are noted. The following specimens should be obtained:

1. Secretions in the vagina fornix for evidence of semen
2. Cervical culture for gonorrhea
3. Cytologic smear from the cervix for sperm
4. Saline vaginal washing (4 ml) for evidence of semen

Bimanual examination is performed to check for preexisting pregnancy, infection, or other signs of trauma.

Rectal Examination: If the patient has reported anal intercourse, a gonorrhea culture is taken and the rectal vault washed with saline.

TABLE 89-1. Sexual Assault: An Outline of Medical Examination

Procedure	Material Needed	Comment
History	Sexual assault forms	
Photography of clothing or wounds or both	Camera, film	Photograph patient in the clothes in which she allegedly was attacked. Photograph any signs of trauma
Clothing collection	Paper bags	Handle clothing as little as possible. Place each item in a separate, labeled paper bag.
Physical examination	Sexual assault forms	
Urine for pregnancy test and drug screen	Urine containers	
Removal of dried seminal stains from skin	Saline, cotton-tipped swabs, test tubes and stopper	Moisten swab with saline and gently rub stain from skin. Place swab in a test tube, seal, and label.
Fingernail scrapings	Fingernail file, glassine envelope	Scrape beneath fingernails and place debris in the envelope.
Pubic hair trimming	Forceps, scissors, glassine envelope	Trim any hair thought to be matted with semen, place in the envelope, and affix a label.
Pubic hair combing	Plastic comb, envelope	Comb the mons pubis and place hairs in the envelope.
Aspiration of vaginal contents	Vaginal speculum, gloves, aspiration pipette, test tube and stopper	Insert a water-lubricated speculum into the vagina and check for signs of trauma. If secretions are present, aspirate them, place in a test tube, seal and label.
Swab of posterior fornix of vagina	Saline, cotton-tipped swab, test tube and stopper, glass slides	Moisten swab with saline and wipe the posterior fornix. Smear glass slides and air dry. Place slides in a container, seal, and label. Place swab in the test tube, seal, and label.

TABLE 89-1. Sexual Assault: An Outline of Medical Examination (Continued)

Procedure	Material Needed	Comment
Vaginal washing	Saline, aspiration pipette, test tube and stopper	Irrigate vaginal vault with 4 ml saline, aspirate fluid, place in the test tube, seal, and label.
Pap smear	Clean slides, cervical scraper, pap fixative	
Cervical gonorrhea culture	Thayer-Martin plate or Transgrow medium, cotton-tipped swab	
Bimanual pelvic examination	Gloves, lubricant	
Perianal examination		Look for signs of trauma and lubrication.
Rectal gonorrhea culture	Thayer-Martin plate or Transgrow medium, cotton-tipped swab	
Pharyngeal gonorrhea culture	Thayer-Martin plate or Transgrow medium, cotton-tipped swab	
Blood samples for syphilis serologic test	Blood tube	

LABORATORY TESTS (See Table 89-1)

All specimens should be obtained by the physician in the presence of an attendant who acts as a witness and handed personally to the pathologist, technician, or investigating police officer. The police officer's badge number is recorded on the chart. Unless specimens are positively identified, they cannot be used as evidence.

Tests include

1. Cervical culture for gonorrhea
2. Vaginal washing for semen
3. Pubic hairs

Examination of
Allegedly Sexually Assaulted Patient

HISTORY: (May be obtained by nurse or physician)

If female, was vaginal penetration attempted or accomplished? ____________

Did assailant attempt anal intercourse or any other act? If yes, explanation ________
____

When did patient last have intercourse? ______________________________

If female, when was her last period? ________________________________

If female, is she currently taking birth control pills, or does she have an I.U.D.? ____
____

Is patient under the care of a physician? If yes, explanation ______________
____

PHYSICAL EXAMINATION: (Nurse will record physical appearance of all clothing, and have victim in hospital gown to facilitate exam.)

Appearance of clothing ______________________________________

Emotional state of victim ____________________________________

Evidence of trauma – record on the other side of this form location of abrasions, contusions, lacerations, burns, fractures, or rope burns. Also please note any evidence of dirt, vegetation or other foreign material.

Examination of Genitalia – note evidence of trauma and appearance of:

- Perineum ____
- Hymen ____
- Vagina ____
- Cervix ____
- Anus ____
- Uterus, Adnexa ____

LABORATORY TESTS:

Saline suspension for sperm ☐ positive ☐ negative? ☐ motile ☐ non-motile

Cervical culture for gonorrhea to bacteriology ☐ yes ☐ no?

Saline vaginal washing obtained for investigating officer ☐ yes ☐ no?
(USE MAXIMUM of 4cc.)

Loose pubic hair obtained for investigating officer ☐ yes ☐ no?

If indicated, culture of rectum ☐ of mouth ☐ to bacteriology.

TREATMENT: (Include prophylactic medication given for gonorrhea and pregnancy, if any suturing was necessary, if x-rays were taken and results, if hospitalization was required, and if psychiatric consultation was obtained.)
____
____
____

______________________ R.N. ______________________ M.D.
(Nurse) (Emergency Resident, Gynecology resident, or attending)

____
(Officer requesting report) (Agency) (Badge number)

Figure 89-A.

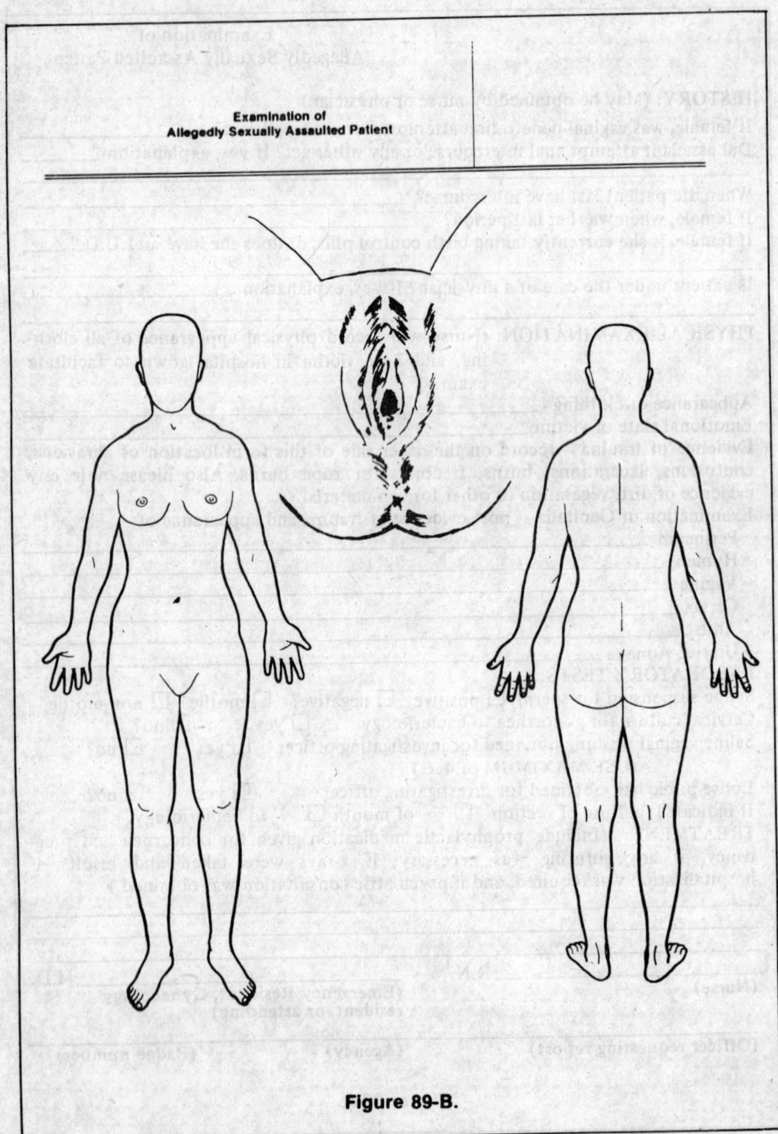

Figure 89-B.

4. Rectal or pharyngeal gonorrhea culture or both, as indicated by the patient's history
5. Pregnancy test
6. Serologic test for syphilis

RECORDS

Written, accurate records are essential, since each instance of sexual assault is a potential court case. The examining physician should expect either to give a legal deposition or to make a statement of his findings in court.

The record should contain the patient's statements, the physician's findings, and the procedures carried out. In addition, the record should show the names of the witnesses and the person to whom the laboratory specimens, clothing, or photographs were delivered.

The physician should not express any conclusions or opinions or make any diagnosis (either orally or in writing) concerning whether the victim has been raped. Only the phrases "suspected rape" or "alleged rape" should be used. However, any specific diagnosis of traumatic injury or preexisting pregnancy should be recorded.

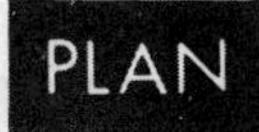

MANAGEMENT

Psychologic Trauma: Having undergone a crisis that has threatened her life and safety, a woman needs to feel that the medical environment is nonthreatening. With emotional support, the medical staff helps establish this feeling of safety.

Details of the examination and reasons for the procedures are explained calmly. The patient should be reassured that psychologic distress is a normal response to a crisis situation. Medications for anxiety [diazepam (Valium) or an equivalent] may be indicated.

Physical Trauma: Lacerations or physical injuries may require surgical repair under local or general anesthesia. The patient's tetanus immunization status should be reviewed and tetanus toxoid offered if it is needed.

Prevention of Venereal Disease: Since the assailant may have gonorrhea or syphilis, the patient should be offered prophylactic antibiotic therapy. For prophylaxis of gonorrhea, 1 gm of probenecid followed by 4.8 million units of procaine penicillin is usually recommended, unless the patient gives a history of penicillin allergy. (See Gonorrhea, p. 356, for alternative treatments.)

Pregnancy Prevention: If the patient is not pregnant and not using contraceptive methods, the possibility of pregnancy resulting from the sexual assault, as well as the benefits and risks of antipregnancy measures, should be considered. A pregnancy test is recommended whenever there is any possibility of preexisting pregnancy.

Diethylstilbesterol, 25 mg twice daily for five days, appears to be an effective postcoital (postovulatory) contraceptive. The major side effects are nausea and vomiting, which may be treated with promethazine (Phenergan) rectal suppositories (25 mg every six hours).

(Diethylstilbesterol is not recommended when a woman has thrombophlebitis, breast or genital cancer, or a history of these disorders. Side effects associated with diethylstilbesterol include nausea, vomiting, headache, menstrual irregularities, and breast tenderness. Since recent reports have shown that diethylstilbesterol during pregnancy may be associated with an increased incidence of vaginal tumors in female offspring, abortion should be strongly considered if the woman is found to have been pregnant or becomes pregnant despite the stilbesterol treatment.)

PATIENT EDUCATION

The importance of follow-up medical and psychologic care must be emphasized. The patient should have a reexamination at six weeks to be certain that serologic tests and gonorrhea cultures remain negative, that she has not become pregnant, and that she has received appropriate psychologic support.

Referral to a psychologic counselor or to a counseling organization such as Women Organized Against Rape may be helpful. The patient may be offered a prescription for chlordiazepoxide hydrochloride (Librium), diazepam (Valium), or an equivalent medication to help her cope with the acute fear and anxiety.

REFERENCES

Glover D, Gerety M, Bromberg S, et al: Diethylstilbesterol in the treatment of rape victims. West J Med *125*:331-334, 1976

Guidelines for the interview and examination of alleged rape victims. West J Med *123*: 420-422, 1975

90 SHOCK

GENERAL CONSIDERATIONS

Shock is a generalized state of severe circulatory failure. Inadequate organ blood flow fails to provide the tissue oxygen perfusion necessary for normal cellular metabolism. Cellular hypoxia leads to cellular anoxia, anaerobic metabolism, and cellular death.

Clinical manifestations of hypoperfusion are pallor and decreased skin temperature caused by cutaneous vasoconstriction; oliguria indicates diminished renal blood flow.

Although hypotension is a frequent clinical finding, shock and hypotension are not necessarily synonymous. Severe shock may exist in the presence of a normal systemic pressure, and conversely, adequate perfusion may be present despite hypotension. Reduced blood flow rather than reduced blood pressure is the critical pathologic physiologic condition.

Reduced blood flow stems from reduced cardiac output—either inadequate venous return or intrinsic cardiac defect. Inadequate venous return is the most common cause and results from diminished circulatory volume (hypovolemia), peripheral vasodilatation, or mechanical obstruction.

SUBJECTIVE DATA

Anxiety, apprehension, mental confusion, disorientation, and agitation, followed by apathy or even stupor, are symptoms of cerebral ischemia. Weakness, paleness, restlessness, and intense thirst are additional symptoms of inadequate perfusion.

The history of onset helps distinguish the various types of shock.

OBJECTIVE DATA

PHYSICAL EXAMINATION

General Examination: Hypotension and tachycardia are typical findings. The pulse tends to be rapid, feeble, and of small volume. Respiratory rate is frequently increased. (Bradycardia may be a sign of vagal stimulation or a cardiac pathologic condition.)

The skin is usually cold, moist, clammy, and cyanotic or pale. Sweating and peripheral vasoconstriction are manifestations of the body's adrenergic response to a suddenly reduced blood volume.

Urine output is scant or absent.

Neck veins tend to be flat in cases of hypovolemic shock and engorged in cases of cardiogenic shock. Peripheral or pulmonary edema suggests cardiogenic shock.

See Table 90-1 for methods for rapid clinical monitoring of cellular metabolism and organ perfusion and Tables 90-2 and 90-3 for normal hemodynamic and respiratory measurements.

Abdominal Examination: Diffuse peritoneal irritation suggests intraabdominal hemorrhage, a ruptured tuboovarian abscess, or a ruptured viscus.

Pelvic Examination: Findings may elucidate the reasons for external hemorrhage or suggest peritoneal irritation from blood or pus. A bulging cul-de-sac may be found in cases of profuse intraabdominal hemorrhage.

LABORATORY TESTS

Complete Blood Count with Blood Smear: Hemoglobin and hematocrit determinations are indirect measures of the circulating oxygen-carrying capacity (see Table 90-2). Decreased or declining values are an indication of acute blood loss. Elevated values may indicate hemoconcentration associated with the loss of vascular fluid into a "third space". An elevated white count with increased neutrophils and immature forms is evidence of infection.

TABLE 90-1. Methods for Rapid Clinical Monitoring of Cellular Metabolism and Organ Perfusion*

Parameter	Primary Organ or System
Respiratory rate, tidal volume (estimated and measured), skin color, temperature, capillary blanching and filling	Pulmonary and ventilatory system Peripheral cellular metabolism and perfusion
Pupillary size: sensorium	Central nervous system
Pulse and heart rate: stethoscope; oscilloscope with electrocardiograph (cardiac rate and rhythm; ventricular depolarization and repolarization)	Heart
Urinary output determined by indwelling bladder catheter	Kidney
Tilt test, jugular vein filling, capillary blanching test, venous and pulse pressure	Extracellular and intravascular fluid volume

Other periodic measurements: cardiac output, blood pH, expired air and arterial blood gas determinations and blood volume may be necessary in some cases but are not as simple or immediately available as those listed above.

*From Flint T, Cain HD: Emergency Treatment and Management. Philadelphia, W.B. Saunders Company, 1975.

TABLE 90-2. Guidelines for Normal Hemodynamic Measurements in Patients*

Determinations	Normal Adult Range
Central venous pressure	5-10 cm H_2O
Pulmonary arterial pressure	25-30/8-10 mm Hg
Pulmonary wedge pressure	8-10 mm Hg
Systemic arterial pressure	120/80 mm Hg
Cardiac index	3.0-4.5 l/min/M^2
Heart rate	70-80/min
Hematocrit	37-45%
Urine flow	30-50 ml/hr

*Modified from Artz CP, Hardy JD: Management of Surgical Complications. 3rd ed. Philadelphia, W.B. Saunders Company, 1975.

TABLE 90-3. Guidelines for Normal Respiratory Function Measurements in Patients

Determination	Normal Adult Range
Arterial Po_2 (on room air)	80-100 mm Hg
Arterial Pco_2	37-45 mm Hg
Arterial pH	7.35-7.45
Venous Po_2	35-50 mm Hg
Venous Pco_2	42-51 mm Hg
Venous pH	7.30-7.40
Alveolar-arterial oxygen difference (A-aDo_2)	
Room air	5-10 mm Hg
100% O_2	10-60 mm Hg
Dead space-tidal volume ratio (V_D/V_T)	0.3-0.35
Vital capacity	3-4.8 l
Respiratory rate	12-15/min
Compliance	10-30 ml/cm H_2O

*From Artz CP, Hardy JD: Management of Surgical Complications. 3rd ed. Philadelphia, W.B. Saunders Company, 1975.

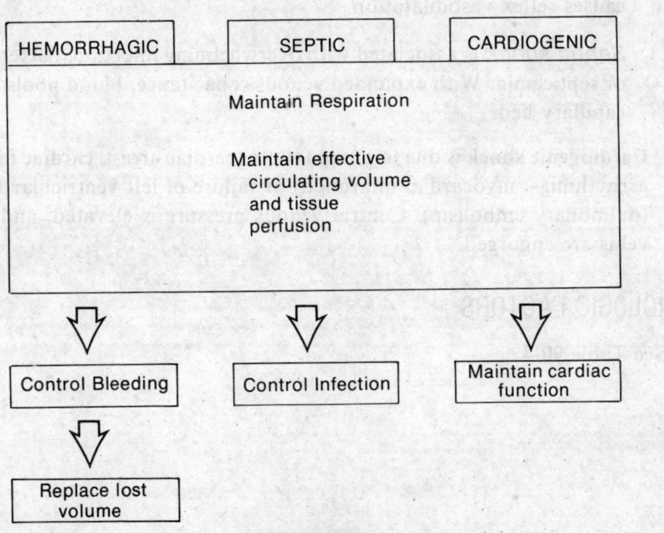

Figure 90-1.
Therapy of Shock Syndrome

ASSESSMENT

DIFFERENTIAL DIAGNOSIS

Hypovolemic shock is due to inadequate circulatory volume. Blood, plasma, or water may be lost externally or into an inaccessible third compartment (peritoneum, soft tissues). Examples include hemorrhage, hematomas, intestinal obstruction, peritonitis, tissue injury, and diabetic acidosis.

The central venous pressure is low and neck veins are flat.

Vasogenic shock is due to peripheral vasodilation or expanded venous capacitance. Blood becomes pooled in the peripheral circulation; venous return is inadequate and circulation becomes ineffective.

Anaphylactic shock is associated with the release of allergic mediators. (See Anaphylaxis, p. 125.)

Neurogenic shock, a central form of vasogenic shock, is usually associated with spinal or epidural anesthesia. Autonomic blockade causes reflex vasodilatation.

Septic shock is associated with overwhelming infection, bacteremia, or septicemia. With expanded venous capacitance, blood pools in the capillary bed.

Cardiogenic shock is due to pump failure (cardiac arrest, cardiac failure, arrhythmias, myocardial infarction) or failure of left ventricular filling (pulmonary embolism). Central venous pressure is elevated, and neck veins are engorged.

ETIOLOGIC FACTORS

See Table 90-4.

TABLE 90-4. Etiologic Factors of Intrapartum or Postpartum Shock

Hemorrhage	Uterine atony Lacerations of vagina or cervix Uterine rupture Uterine inversion Placental abnormalities: premature separation, Placenta accreta, retained fragments Coagulation defects
Sepsis	Endometritis Pelvic thrombophlebitis Peritonitis Pyelonephritis
Pulmonary embolism	Thrombotic Amniotic fluid Air
Cerebral vascular accident	Intracranial hemorrhage Subarachnoid hemorrhage

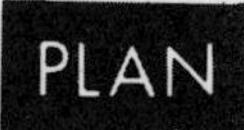

ADDITIONAL DIAGNOSTIC DATA

Blood Tests:

1. Complete blood count with blood smear. Initial values may not reflect acute blood loss.
2. Blood type, Rh and antibody screen. Blood is cross-matched for transfusion if necessary.
3. Blood chemistries—glucose, blood urea nitrogen, creatinine
4. Blood electrolytes—sodium, potassium, chloride, carbon dioxide
5. Coagulation tests if there is any question of a coagulopathy
6. Arterial blood gases— pO_2, pCO_2, pH (see Table 90-3)

Urine: A Foley catheter is inserted into the bladder to obtain a urine specimen and monitor urine output.

1. Urinalysis—protein, sugar, acetone, specific gravity, culture, and sensitivities if infection is suspected
2. Urine output

Electrocardiogram should be done if cardiogenic shock is suspected.

Central venous pressure: (see Table 90-2).

Central venous pressure (CVP) provides an approximation of the efficacy of venous return. The normal range is 2 to 10 cm of water. When the central venous pressure is low (0 to 5 cm of water), hypovolemia is suspected and intravenous fluids administered. Elevation of the central venous pressure with an acute volume infusion suggests impairment of the cardiac pumping mechanism or overloading of the right heart.

The pulmonary artery pressure (see Table 90-2) may be measured directly by a Swan-Ganz catheter (Swan, 1970). Monitoring pulmonary wedge pressure or pulmonary arterial end-diastolic pressure (Table 90-2) provides a more accurate measure of the filling pressure in the left ventricle and is more sensitive to fluid overloading than monitoring the central venous pressure.

MANAGEMENT

General Principles: Primary goal is restoration of an effective blood flow through the microcirculation in order to maintain tissue oxygen perfusion.

General therapeutic principles include

1. Cardiorespiratory support*
2. Effective circulating blood volume
3. Normal acid-base and electrolyte balance
4. Definitive therapy directed toward underlying disease

*Respiratory support with an adequate airway is essential, since the most frequent cause of death in a shock unit is failure of respiratory gas exchange. All patients with dyspnea and tachypnea are given oxygen. Respiratory rate and arterial blood gas measurements assess the respiratory exchange. Depressed pO_2, elevated pCO_2 and decreased pH are evidence of hypoxia and respiratory acidosis, indicating the need for mechanical ventilatory assistance. The response to therapy is monitored through serial blood gas determinations.

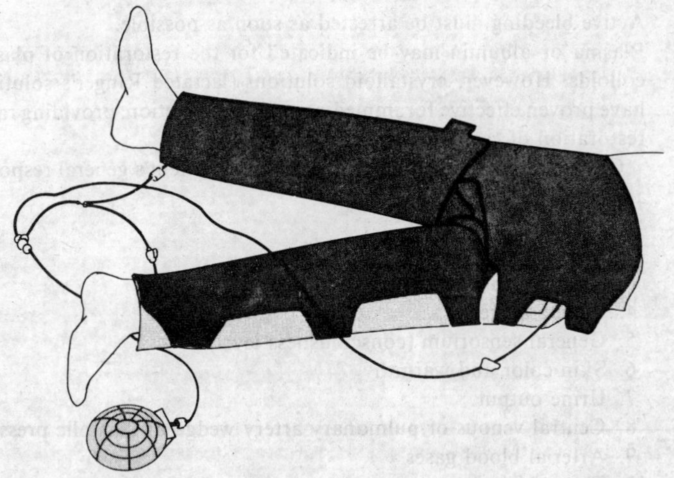

Figure 90-2. Pneumatic pants.

Specific Measures for Management of Hemorrhagic Shock

Respiratory Support: Oxygen and an adequate airway are essential.

Vascular Volume Replacement: Intravenous fluids are essential for the restoration of circulatory volume. Lactated Ringer's solution or normal saline is initiated immediately at a rapid rate. This must be followed by blood (whole blood or packed cells) if shock is due to hemorrhage.

A sample of blood is sent to the blood bank immediately for determination of type and Rh, and antibody screen. Two to four units of blood are cross-matched for transfusion. If blood loss is extreme, type-specific red cells are administered. In cases of exsanguinating hemorrhage, when the blood type cannot be determined, O Rh-negative red cells are administered.

Patients in hemorrhagic shock have usually lost at least one third of their normal blood volume; consequently, they may require 2 to 4 units of blood acutely, and additional transfusions to keep up with progressive losses.

Active bleeding must be arrested as soon as possible.
Plasma or albumin may be indicated for the restoration of plasma colloids. However, crystalloid solutions (lactated Ringer's solution) have proven effective for immediate volume repletion, providing rapid restoration of cardiac output.

Circulatory volume replacement and the patient's general response are monitored by

1. Blood pressure
2. Heart rate
3. Respiration
4. Temperature
5. General sensorium (consciousness level)
6. Skin color and warmth
7. Urine output
8. Central venous or pulmonary artery wedge or diastolic pressure
9. Arterial blood gases
10. Electrolytes
11. Hematocrit

Body heat should be conserved.

Pain and apprehension are controlled as soon as the respiratory and circulatory systems are stable.

Vasoactive drugs are *not* recommended for the management of hemorrhagic shock. Endogenous sympathetic overactivity accounts for many of the patient's symptoms; additional alpha adrenergic activity could only produce additional vasoconstriction, impeding tissue perfusion and increasing ischemic injury to the viscera.

G-suit (antigravity suit) may diminish or control intraabdominal hemorrhage either as an interim measure while the patient is being prepared for surgery, or when multiple surgical procedures have failed to arrest bleeding. The G-suit, wrapped around both legs and the lower abdomen, is inflated to 20 mm Hg. Its effectiveness in improving systemic circulation while diminishing intraabdominal bleeding stems from the circumferential compression or hoop stress applied to the vascular tree. This encircling force overcomes tangential tension in the blood vessel wall, which, in large part, is responsible for the bleeding (Gardner, 1966). (See Fig. 90-2.)

Acidosis and electrolyte imbalance are corrected by improving tissue perfusion with intravenous fluids.

Appropriate obstetric and surgical procedures are directed toward definitive control of bleeding.

Septic Shock

GENERAL CONSIDERATIONS

Septic shock is a state of circulatory collapse associated with the intravascular dissemination of bacteria or their products. Although bacteremia with both gram-positive and gram-negative pathogens can elicit circulatory collapse, the gram-negative organisms are responsible for the majority of cases. These bacteria (*Escherichia coli*, Klebsiella, Enterobacter, Pseudomonas, Proteus, Bacteroides) contain a complex lipopolysaccharide (endotoxin) in their cell walls. When bacterial death occurs, the endotoxin is released into the bloodstream, deranging circulatory control.

During the early pyrogenic phase of acute circulatory failure, arterial vasodilatation predominates, with an increased pulse pressure and cardiac output. Endotoxin causes intense arteriolar and venous spasm, leading to pooling of blood in the venous capacitance bed. (A primary cellular defect may be responsible for reduced oxygen uptake.)

With impaired tissue perfusion, stagnant anoxia occurs and anaerobic metabolism leads to increased blood lactate. The local acidosis promotes relaxation of the arteriolar sphincters while the venules remain constricted. Blood pools in the capillary bed and the increased hydrostatic pressure leads to plasma leakage into the interstitial spaces. This, in turn, results in a sharp decrease in the effective circulating blood volume, lowered cardiac output, and systemic arterial hypotension. If perfusion of the vital organs is ineffective, metabolic acidosis and severe parenchymal damage ensue.

Septic shock may also have a cardiogenic or a hypovolemic component or both.

SUBJECTIVE DATA

CURRENT SYMPTOMS

A shaking chill followed by fever is the most typical symptom of gram-negative bacteremia. Mental confusion and disorientation may indicate reduced cerebral blood flow. Syncope and coma are associated with advanced circulatory collapse.

PRIOR HISTORY

Frequently, there is a history of prior surgery, abortion, delivery, or severe infection.

OBJECTIVE DATA

PHYSICAL EXAMINATION (Table 90-5)

General Examination: Hypotension and tachycardia are the usual findings. Temperature tends to be variable: It is usually elevated initially and then becomes subnormal, since endotoxins often cause hypothermia.

The skin is warm and dry initially; peripheral cyanosis may be noted. Later, the skin becomes cold, pale, and moist.

Tachypnea, or hyperventilation, may be caused by acidosis.

TABLE 90-5. Septic Shock: Clinical Findings

	Early Phase	Late Phase
Temperature	101°-105°	Subnormal
Pulse	Rapid	Rapid
Blood pressure	Decreased	Decreased
Mental status	Alert, apprehensive	Mental confusion
Skin	Flushed, warm	Pale, cold, clammy
Urine output	Normal or increased	Decreased
Blood lactate	Increased	Increased
Blood pH	Decreased	Decreased
Cardiac output	Normal or increased	Decreased
Respiratory rate	Increased	Increased

Abdominal and pelvic examinations may aid in the elucidation of the underlying disease process.

LABORATORY TESTS

Complete Blood Count with Blood Smear: The white blood count is usually elevated (15,000 to 30,000), with an increased number of immature band forms. Hematocrit values may indicate anemia or hemoconcentration. The blood smear may reveal evidence of hemolysis, suggesting clostridial sepsis.

Urinalysis: In cases of pyelonephritis, the urine contains a large number of bacteria and pus cells. Urine output tends to be variable, often increased during the early phase of septic shock and then decreased during the later phase.

Blood Type and Rh: Blood is cross-matched in case transfusion becomes necessary.

ASSESSMENT

PREDISPOSING FACTORS

Predisposing obstetric and gynecologic problems include

1. Adnexal (tuboovarian) abscess, leaking or ruptured, with pelvic peritonitis
2. Chorioamnionitis, which is often associated with prolonged rupture of membranes
3. Postpartum infection
4. Pyelonephritis during pregnancy
5. Septic abortion

ASSOCIATED PROBLEMS

Previous blood loss or current hemorrhage may contribute to the shock syndrome.

POTENTIAL COMPLICATIONS

Complications to be anticipated include disseminated intravascular coagulation, respiratory failure (shock lung), and renal failure.

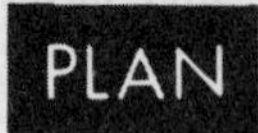

ADDITIONAL DIAGNOSTIC DATA

Bacteriology (Aerobic and Anaerobic): Specimens of blood, urine, and abscess cavities are sent to the bacteriology laboratory for Gram stain, culture, and sensitivity studies. When uterine infection is suspected, a cervical specimen is evaluated for the presence of *Neisseria gonorrhoeae* and Clostridium. (See Pelvic Infection, p. 474.)

Arterial blood gas measurements assess the adequacy of tissue perfusion and the extent of pulmonary involvement. A base deficit of 5 or greater is an indication of metabolic acidosis; less than 70 mm Hg of pO_2 is an indication of anoxemia.

Monitoring of urine output and urinalysis help determine the extent of renal perfusion. If the urinary osmolality is greater than 400 mOsm and the ratio of urine to plasma osmolality is greater than 1.5, renal function is normal, and oliguria is usually due to volume depletion. A urine osmolality of less than 400 mOsm and a urine-plasma ratio of less than 1.5 are indications of renal failure.

Blood electrolytes (sodium, potassium, chloride, and carbon dioxide) and blood chemistry (blood urea nitrogen, creatinine, glucose, lactate) determinations aid in the evaluation of fluid replacement therapy and renal function. When creatinine values are elevated, antibiotic dosages may have to be adjusted.

Determination of central venous pressure or pulmonary artery diastolic or wedge pressure can be a very helpful guide for fluid replacement therapy.

Coagulation studies may provide evidence of a coagulation disorder, necessitating appropriate replacement therapy. (See Coagulation Disorders, p. 210.)

Electrocardiograms aid in the evaluation of cardiac rhythm and electrolyte imbalances.

X-rays of the chest or abdomen may disclose free air in the peritoneal cavity (uterine perforation, intestinal perforation), a foreign body in the peritoneal cavity, or a pulmonary pathologic condition.

MANAGEMENT

General Principles:

1. Infection must be eradicated with antibiotic therapy, plus surgery when indicated.
2. Cardiovascular and respiratory homeostasis must be maintained.
   a. Intravascular volume deficit must be corrected.
   b. Oxygenation must be adequate.
   c. Tissue perfusion must be restored.

Specific Measures:

Respiratory Support: Oxygen and an adequate airway are essential. Repeated measurements of arterial blood gases assess the oxygen requirements and the need for endotracheal intubation and mechanical ventilation.

Circulatory Support: When sepsis is present, large volumes of fluid may be sequestered at the sites of inflammation. In addition, substantial fluid deficits stem from fever, vomiting, diarrhea, and hemorrhage. Intravenous fluids, usually lactated Ringer's solution or normal saline, are essential to expand plasma volume.

Central venous pressure measurements provide a guide to fluid replacement. In the patient whose basic defect is peripheral vasoconstriction, the central venous pressure may be high at the outset and volume must be replaced very cautiously.

Packed red cells or whole blood transfusions are indicated for patients with reduced red cell mass, usually when the hematocrit is less than 30.

Acidosis is due to a failure of tissue perfusion, which results in the accumulation of acid metabolites. This is treated by augmentation of intravascular volume, improving tissue perfusion, rather than by the administration of sodium bicarbonate (Shubin and Weil, 1976).

Antibiotics Intravenously: Before one has knowledge of the specific organisms, the antibiotic choice is based on the site of the infection, whether it was acquired in the hospital, previous antibiotic therapy, the underlying host disease, previous cultures and sensitivities, and the individual hospital's antibiogram. Microorganisms usually responsible for serious pelvic infections include gram-negative bacilli, anaerobic streptococci, Bacteroides, and clostridia.

Gentamicin (60 to 80 mg every eight hours) is usually selected, since it is bactericidal and effective against more than 95 per cent of the common strains of gram-negative enteric organisms, except the Proteus species, for which the sensitivity approximates 75 per cent (Shubin and Weil, 1976). If there is any evidence of renal failure, these dosages must be reduced.

Penicillin (3 to 5 million units every four hours) is prescribed to cover the gram-positive organisms. Alternatively, ampicillin (2 gm every six hours) may be preferred.

Clindamycin (600 mg every eight hours) is usually recommended whenever Bacteroides is suspected.

Corticosteroids may suppress systemic reactions to endotoxin and tend to prevent nonspecific cellular injury by stabilizing lysosomal membranes. In addition, these drugs may improve tissue perfusion, increase cardiac output, and decrease peripheral arterial resistance. The early administration of steroids, in addition to other therapeutic measures (antibiotics, fluid replacement, reparation of acid-base balance), appears to decrease the overall mortality rate (Schumer, 1976). (Dosages evaluated by Schumer were 3 mg/kg of dexamethasone in 100 ml of saline and 30 mg/kg of methylprednisolone in 100 ml of saline. Treatment was administered at the time of diagnosis as a single bolus infusion through a central venous catheter over a period of 10 to 20 minutes. The initial dose was repeated, when necessary, after four hours.)

Alternative regimens are methylprednisolone (Solu-Medrol) (15 to 30 mg/kg given intravenously initially, followed by 200 to 1000 mg given at six-hour intervals for 24 hours) or dexamethasone (Decadron) (3 to 5 mg/kg given intravenously initially, followed by 30 to 100 mg given at six-hour intervals for 24 hours).

Vasoactive Drugs are *not* recommended unless the patient has failed to respond to augmentation of the intravascular volume. Under these circumstances, treatment with the $\alpha\beta$ adrenergic agonist dopamine or the β adrenergic isoproterenol may be considered (Shubin, 1976).

Dopamine (Intropin) tends to increase myocardial contractility as well as visceral blood flow. Two hundred mg are diluted into 250 to 500 ml of 5 per cent dextrose or lactated Ringer's solution.) Two to

5 mcg per kg per minute may evoke a satisfactory response. Once an effective dose is established, the lowest infusion rate consistent with adequate renal perfusion is maintained. Dopamine is discontinued or decreased if an established urine flow rate decreases, tachycardia increases, or arrhythmias develop.

Isoproterenol is a potent myocardial stimulant that also decreases venous pooling. It has the potential risk of inducing tachycardia and cardiac arrhythmias, however. Isoproterenol should be used only after the plasma volume has been fully repleted. Doses usually range from 0.5 mcg to 5.0 mcg per minute (Shubin and Weil, 1976).

Surgery is frequently required to eradicate a focus of infection responsible for septic shock in obstetric and gynecologic patients. Infected products of conception must be removed from the uterus. Abscess cavities must be drained or eradicated.

Laparotomy may be necessary if there is evidence of a ruptured tuboovarian abscess, the patient fails to improve after curettage, or there is evidence of a perforated viscus or foreign body in the peritoneal cavity. Hysterectomy with bilateral salpingo-oophorectomy may be necessary for eradication of uterine infections complicated by parametritis and tuboovarian abscesses or postpartum fulminating infections that fail to respond to curettage.

Other Measures:

Morphine tends to allay pain and anxiety.

Digitalis and diuretics are indicated for the management of cardiac failure.

Heparin may be indicated for the management of disseminated intravascular coagulation or infected venous thrombosis.

REFERENCES

Gardner WJ, Storer J: The use of the G suit in control of intra-abdominal bleeding. Surg Gynecol Obstet *123*:792-798, 1966

Gibbs RS, Weinstein AJ: Puerperal infection in the antibiotic era. Am J Obstet Gynecol *124*:769-787, 1976

Goldberg LI: Dopamine—clinical use of an endogenous catecholamine. N Engl J Med *291*:707-710, 1974

Kitzmiller JL: Septic shock: an eclectic view. Obstet Gynecol Surv *26*:105-132, 1971

MacLean LD: The patient in shock. *In* Committee on Pre- and Postoperative Care, American College of Surgeons: Manual of Preoperative and Postoperative Care. Philadelphia, W.B. Saunders Company, 1971

Pelligra R, Trueblood HW, Mason R, et al: Anti-G suit as a therapeutic device. Aerospace Med *41*:943-945, 1970

Rosenbaum RW, Hayes MF, Matsumoto T: Efficacy of steroids in the treatment of septic and cardiogenic shock. Surg Gynecol Obstet *136*:914-918, 1973

Schumer W: Steroids in the treatment of clinical septic shock. Ann Surg *184*:333-341, 1976

Shires GT, Canizaro PC: Fluid resuscitation in the severely injured. Surg Clin North Am *53*:1341-1366, 1973

Shubin H, Weil MH: Bacterial shock. JAMA *235*:421-424, 1976

Swan HJ, Ganz W, Forrester J, et al: Catheterization of the heart in man with use of a flow-directed balloon-tipped catheter. N Engl J Med *283*:447-451, 1970

Weil MH, Shubin H. Carlson R: Treatment of circulatory shock. JAMA *231:1280-1286, 1975*

91 SHOULDER PRESENTATION

GENERAL CONSIDERATIONS

Shoulder presentation (transverse lie, transverse presentation, acromion presentation) means that the long axis of the fetus is perpendicular to the long axis of the mother. The shoulder (acromion process of the scapula) is the presenting part (Fig. 91-1).

Although uncommon, shoulder presentation occurs about once in 300 to 400 deliveries and in 10 to 12 per cent of deliveries of second twins.

SUBJECTIVE AND OBJECTIVE DATA

Usually, the patient is unaware of the fetal malpresentation.

The abdomen tends to be unusually wide from side to side; prior to labor, there is no presenting part in the pelvic inlet. If the patient is seen in advanced labor after the membranes have ruptured, the shoulder may be tightly wedged in the upper part of the pelvis with a hand and arm prolapsed into the vagina.

Vaginal bleeding may be an associated symptom if a placenta previa is preventing normal fetal presentation.

ASSESSMENT

PREDISPOSING FACTORS

These include placenta previa, multiple pregnancy, uterine malformations (bicornuate uterus, leiomyoma), pelvic tumors, fetal anomaly, hydramnios, prematurity, pelvic contracture, and multiparity (abnormal relaxation of the abdominal wall, with a pendulous abdomen).

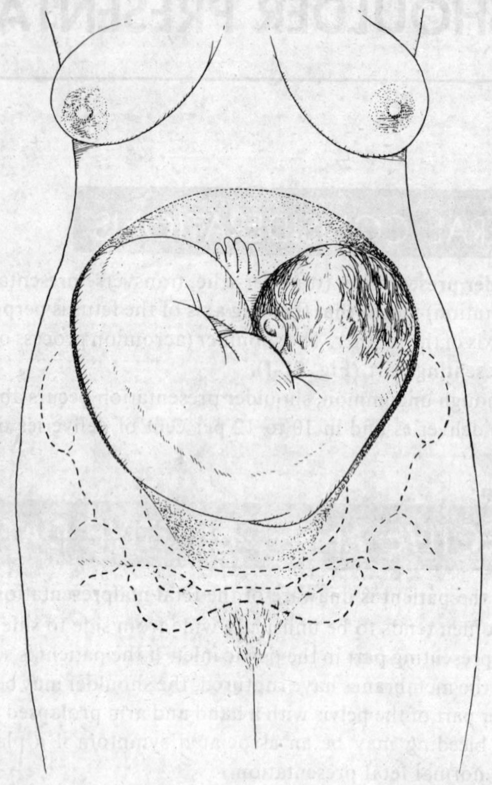

Figure 91-1. Transverse lie. (From Huffman JW: Gynecology and Obstetrics. Philadelphia, W.B. Saunders Company, 1962.)

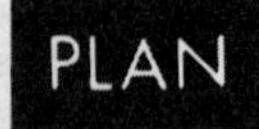

ADDITIONAL DIAGNOSTIC DATA

Abdominal x-ray or ultrasound B-scan (Fig. 91-2) can provide diagnostic confirmation when fetal malpresentation is suspected.

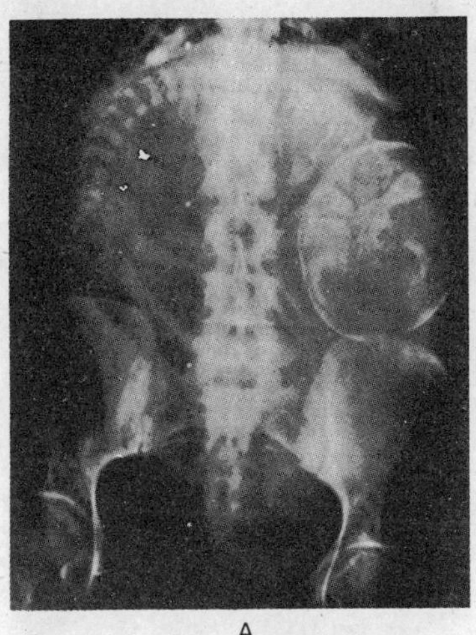

A

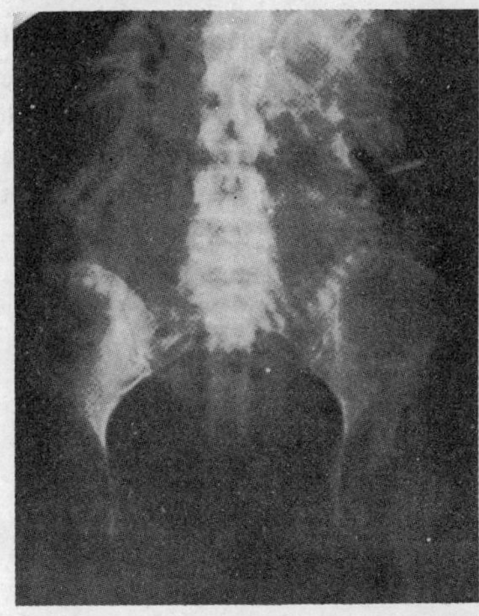

B

Figure 91-2. X-ray findings in transverse presentation. *A*, Fetal small parts are over the inlet. *B*, Fetal back is over the inlet. (From Reid DE, Ryan KJ, Benirschke K: Principles and Management of Human Reproduction. Philadelphia, W.B. Saunders Company, 1972.)

MANAGEMENT

Cesarean section is always recommended when the fetus is alive and viable. A vertical uterine incision facilitates delivery of the baby. The only exception to this policy would be in the management of shoulder presentation in the delivery of a second twin (see Multiple Pregnancy, p. 438).

Even with a neglected transverse lie and a dead baby, cesarean section is usually preferred, since the uterus is tightly contracted around the baby and spontaneous delivery is impossible, unless the fetus is very small or macerated. Cesarean hysterectomy may be indicated if the uterus is infected and the patient does not desire additional children.

Decapitation and other destructive procedures can cause extensive maternal trauma, including uterine rupture; in most instances, these procedures are *more* hazardous than cesarean section or cesarean hysterectomy.

Antibiotic Therapy: Patients with a neglected shoulder presentation and prolonged rupture of membranes almost invariably have an associated intrauterine infection. Bacteriologic culture and sensitivity studies are obtained from the uterine cavity. Antibiotic therapy is initiated immediately, with broad spectrum coverage. (See Pelvic Infection, p. 474.)

92 SYNCOPE DURING PREGNANCY

GENERAL CONSIDERATIONS

Syncope, or fainting—transient loss of consciousness—is usually due to a hypotensive reduction of cerebral blood flow. Some patients use the term "fainting" to mean faintness, that is, a feeling of unsteadiness or lightheadedness combined with a sensation of *impending* loss of consciousness.

Syncope must be distinguished from other disturbances of cerebral function, particularly epilepsy. Although epilepsy resembles syncope in that it also involves loss of consciousness, the epileptic attack is characteristically more sudden in onset, since the arrest in mental function is a consequence of an electrical discharge that causes paroxysmal activity in certain cerebral neurons. Syncope, on the other hand, is not as sudden, since there is a more gradual failure of the cerebral circulation.

Epileptic attacks tend to be stereotyped in their nature and often occur without warning. Even when there is an aura, it bears little resemblance to the prodromal symptoms of syncope.

Injury from falling is also more likely to occur with epilepsy, since the protective reflexes are instantaneously abolished. Tonic-convulsive movements with upturning eyes are a feature of epilepsy but not of syncope. In epilepsy, the period of unconsciousness tends to be longer, urinary incontinence may occur, and cyanosis can be caused by apnea. After an epileptic attack, consciousness returns slowly. Disorientation, mental confusion, headache, and drowsiness are common sequelae. The blood pressure may be slightly elevated.

The electroencephalogram may establish the diagnosis.

Classification of Causes of Syncope or Faintness:

1. Inadequate vasoconstrictor mechanisms
   a. Vasovagal
   b. Postural hypotension
2. Hypovolemia—acute blood loss
3. Mechanical reduction of venous return
   a. Supine hypotensive syndrome
4. Cardiac lesions with reduced cardiac output
   a. Bradyarrhythmias—atrioventricular block with Stokes-Adams attacks; ventricular asystole; sinus bradycardia
   b. Tachyarrhythmias—episodic ventricular fibrillation; ventricular tachycardia
   c. Myocardial infarction with pump failure
   d. Obstruction of left ventricular outflow—aortic stenosis
   e. Obstruction of pulmonary flow: pulmonic stenosis; primary pulmonary hypertension, pulmonary embolism
   f. Pericardial—cardiac tamponade
5. Hyperventilation syndrome
6. Hypoglycemia
7. Anemia—hypoxia
8. Cerebrovascular disturbances—cerebral ischemia
9. Emotional disturbances—anxiety attacks

Vasovagal syncope is the most frequent cause of loss of consciousness during pregnancy. Predisposing factors include emotional stress, pain or the anticipation of pain, fatigue, being in a warm crowded room, prolonged standing, and prolonged dining, during which time alcohol may add to a tendency to peripheral vasodilatation.

Autonomic manifestations preceding unconsciousness include cold sweating, pallor, nausea, slow pulse, yawning, and overbreathing. As the blood pressure falls, there may be a blurring of vision and weakness.

Physiologically, the attack is characterized by peripheral vasodilatation that is not compensated by an increased cardiac output. Vagal activity leads to marked bradycardia, resulting in further lowering of arterial pressure and reduction of cerebral perfusion.

Vasovagal syncope is transient, lasting only a few seconds to several minutes. Once the patient is in a horizontal position, cerebral blood flow improves and consciousness is regained rapidly.

Therapy: The patient should be encouraged to remain recumbent on her side until the episode passes. Inhalation of spirits of ammonia is customary.

Hypovolemia causes syncope as a direct result of the fall in central venous pressure. When external bleeding is present, there is no diagnostic difficulty. In the case of occult internal bleeding, syncope may be the initial symptom. The pulse is rapid, pallor is striking, and the neck veins are collapsed.

Supine Hypotensive Syndrome: The pressure of the enlarged uterus on the inferior vena cava impedes venous return. Prodromal symptoms include a feeling of weakness, nausea, sweating, and epigastric discomfort. Typically, the patient is lying on her back in bed or on an examining table when the acute hypotensive episode occurs. As soon as the patient is turned to her side, her blood pressure returns to normal.

Cardiac syncope results from a sudden reduction of cardiac output. The most common cause is cardiac arrhythmia. Upright posture, cerebrovascular disease, anemia, and coronary, myocardial, or valvular disease all reduce the tolerance to alterations in heart rate.

Complete atrioventricular block causes syncopal episodes known as the Stokes-Adams syndrome. Ventricular tachycardia or fibrillation may also be responsible for cardiac syncope.

Other causes of reduced cardiac output include acute massive myocardial infarction, aortic stenosis, primary pulmonary hypertension, pulmonary embolism, and pericardial tamponade.

When syncope results from a disorder of cardiac function, there is likely to be a combination of pallor, cyanosis, pronounced dyspnea, and distended neck veins.

The electrocardiogram usually clarifies the responsible cardiac pathologic condition.

Hyperventilation impairs consciousness, producing a feeling of lightheadedness that may be described as faintness even though syncope seldom occurs. Symptoms tend to develop gradually. First, the patient may complain of tightness of the chest and a feeling of suffocation. Excessive deep sighing may be observed. Other symptoms include palpitations, fullness in the throat, epigastric discomfort, and numbness and tingling of the hands and feet. In a prolonged attack, carpopedal spasm or jerky muscular movements may occur.

Hyperventilation is almost always a manifestation of acute anxiety. The symptoms can be reproduced readily by having the patient breathe rapidly and deeply for two or three minutes. This test is often of therapeutic value because the underlying anxiety tends to be lessened when the patient learns that she can produce and alleviate her symptoms at will simply by controlling her breathing.

Treatment includes reassurance and conscious breath holding and rebreathing into a paper bag. A mild sedative such as hydroxyzine (Vistaril, Atarax) may be given during late pregnancy.

Hypoglycemia: The clinical picture can vary from confusion to weakness, syncope, or coma. Symptoms tend to develop gradually. The diagnosis depends largely upon the patient's history (for example, insulin therapy, fasting) and documentation of reduced blood sugar during the attack.

Treatment is specific: the administration of glucose orally or intravenously.

See Diabetic Emergencies, p. 276.

Anemia: See Anemia during Pregnancy, p. 130.

Cerebrovascular Disturbances: See Cerebrovascular Accident during Pregnancy, p. 185.)

Emotional disturbances, including anxiety, may be considered if the physical examination, including a neurologic examination, is normal and there is no evidence of any specific pathologic condition. Appropriate psychiatric consultation may be helpful.

REFERENCE

Noble RJ: The patient with syncope, JAMA *237*:1372-1376, 1977

93 SYPHILIS

GENERAL CONSIDERATIONS

Syphilis is a chronic infectious disease caused by the spirochete *Treponema pallidum.* The initial lesion, or *primary chancre* (Fig. 93-1) usually appears within two to six weeks at the site of the infectious contact and may be seen on the labia, vagina, or cervix. The typical chancre of primary syphilis is a 1.0- to 1.5-cm solitary, punched-out, indurated, *painless* ulcer with a smooth base (Fig. 93-1). Bilateral lymphadenopathy may be palpated. The nodes are firm, freely movable, and painless. The chancre tends to heal spontaneously over two to six weeks.

Secondary manifestations of syphilis may appear at about the sixth week of infection and include skin lesions (usually macular, papular, or papulosquamous), mucous membrane lesions, and lymphadenopathy.

Macular lesions—pale red, roundish patches 5 to 10 mm in diameter, neither infiltrated, pruritic, nor scaling—are usually bilateral and distributed over the trunk and proximal parts of the extremities. Papular lesions—coppery red round infiltrates 3 to 10 mm in diameter—may be distributed anywhere, including on the scalp, soles, and palms, and sometimes leave pigmented patches on healing.

Large hypertrophic papules—condylomata lata—may be localized to skin folds, for example, on the vulva, on the axillae, and under pendulous breasts, and are often moist and eroded.

Superficial lymph nodes are frequently palpable, firm, freely movable, and painless.

ASSESSMENT

DIFFERENTIAL DIAGNOSIS

The differential diagnosis of a syphilitic chancre includes herpes genitalis and chancroid.

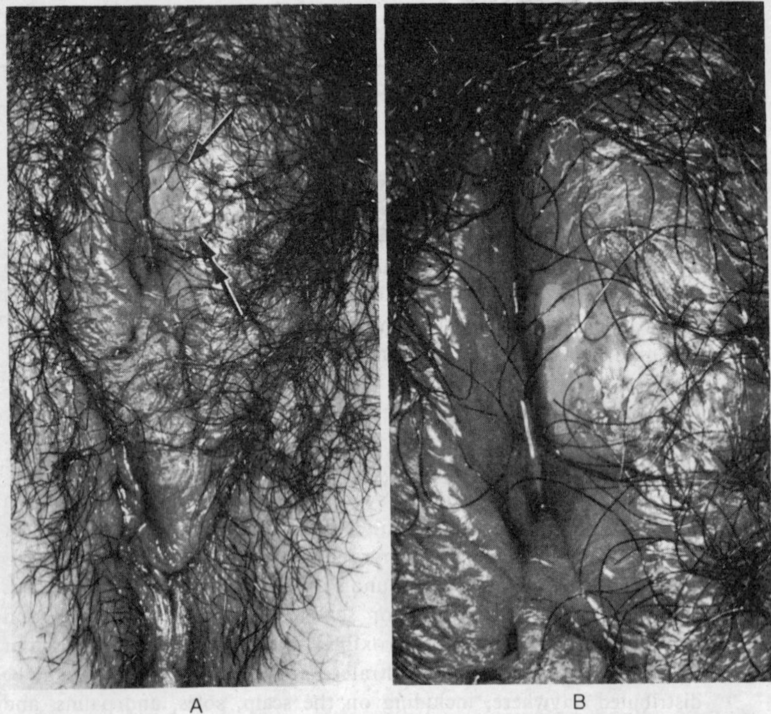

Figure 93-1. Primary chancres. (From Burrow GN, Ferris TE: Medical Complications During Pregnancy. Philadelphia, W.B. Saunders Company, 1975.)

Herpes genitalis begins with grouped vesicles accompanied by burning, pricking pain. After the vesicles rupture, shallow, irregular, painful ulcerations appear. Pelvic and inguinal lymph nodes may be painful.

Chancroid ulcer is acutely inflamed and extremely painful, with a large surrounding inflammatory zone. The ulcer edge is undermined. Lymphadenopathy tends to be unilateral, with severe inflammation and possibly ulceration. The diagnosis is confirmed by identification of Ducrey's bacillus.

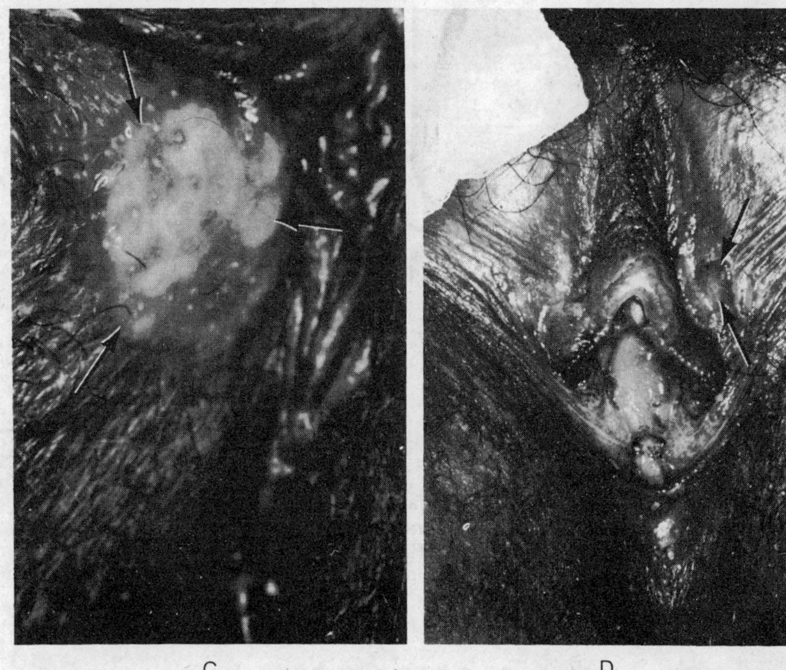

C D

Figure 93-1. Primary chancres. (Continued)

PLAN

ADDITIONAL DIAGNOSTIC DATA

Dark-field examination of a smear from the chancre or condyloma may reveal *Treponema pallidum* and confirm the diagnosis of syphilis. To obtain material for examination, the purulent matter, scab, or epithelium is cleaned from the surface of the lesion, and the serous exudate from the base of the lesion is placed on a glass slide.

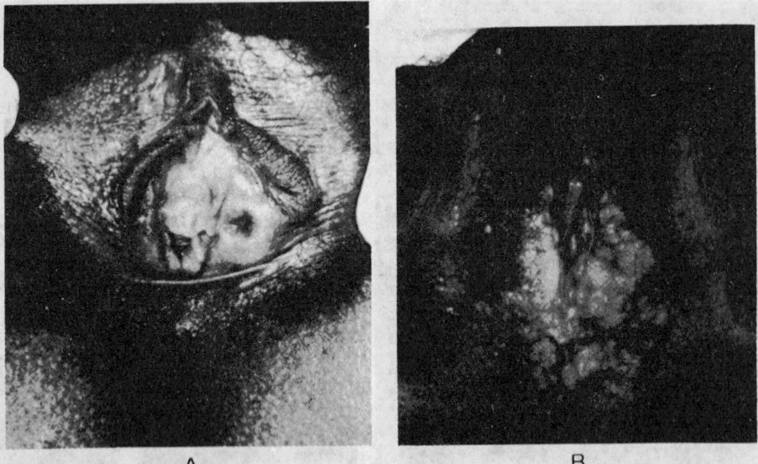

Figure 93-2. *A*, Chancre on inner surface of left labium minus. *B*, Condylomata lata confluent in central area, with individual ulcerative lesions on perineum and inguinal adenitis. (From Novak ER, Woodruff JD: Novak's Gynecologic and Obstetric Pathology. 7th ed. Philadelphia, W.B. Saunders Company, 1974.)

Serologic Tests:

Reagin tests [such as Venereal Disease Research Laboratories (VDRL)] are recommended for screening purposes because of their high reliability and low cost. The reagin titer should be determined when the test is reactive and a second specimen obtained to verify the reaction. After treatment, the patient is followed-up with the same quantitative reagin test, since different reagin tests may have different titers. After effective treatment of early syphilis, reagin tests usually revert to nonreactive within two years. (Serologic tests are not likely to become reactive until 10 to 14 days after the primary lesion appears.)

Treponemal tests (such as FTA-ABS) utilize treponemal antigens to detect specific treponemal antibody. If the VDRL test is reactive, a diagnosis of syphilis is confirmed by the fluorescent antibody technique (FTA-ABS test). FTA tests remain positive despite treatment, however. (To establish a new diagnosis of syphilis in patients previously treated for syphilis, there must be a fourfold increase in the quantitative reagin titer or the dark-field examination must be positive.)

Indications for Spinal Fluid Examination (Lumbar Puncture):

1. Not indicated in examination or treatment of early syphilis except in treated cases with
   a. Persistent high titer one year or more after treatment
   b. Increase in the titer of two or more dilutions after treatment
2. In late symptomatic syphilis (patients with positive serologic tests and any symptoms or signs suggestive of central nervous system lues)
   a. Performed before treatment. If negative, there is no need to repeat it.
   b. If it is positive, repeat it every three to six months until protein and cell count are normal. Repeat in two years.
   c. Indicated to rule out central nervous system syphilis in patients with suggestive signs or symptoms and negative VDRL but reactive FTA
3. In late latent or late congenital syphilis
   a. May be performed before treatment at the physician's discretion (high titer or suggestive signs).
   b. Usually, it is preferable to treat patients with 7.2 million units of benzathine penicillin and not perform lumbar puncture.
4. All late syphilis patients treated with alternate drugs should have lumbar puncture as part of their follow-up.

MANAGEMENT

Early Syphilis [primary, secondary, or latent syphilis of less than one year's duration as determined by clinical or serologic evidence (Fig. 93-3)]: The treatment of choice is 2.4 million units of benzathine penicillin G given by intramuscular injection in one dose.

An alternative treatment schedule is 600,000 units of aqueous procaine penicillin G given by intramuscular injection daily for eight days. The total dosage is 4.8 million units.

Patients allergic to penicillin may be given tetracycline hydrochloride—500 mg orally four times daily for 15 days. The total dosage is 30 gm. Another alternative for allergic patients is erythromycin (stearate, ethylsuccinate)—500 mg given orally four times daily for 15 days.

For follow-up, quantitative nontreponemal tests are performed 3, 6 and 12 months after treatment.

Syphilis of More Than One Year's Duration: The treatment of choice is 7.2 million units of benzathine penicillin G (2.4 million units given by intramuscular injection weekly for three successive weeks).

An alternative treatment schedule is 9.0 million units of aqueous procaine penicillin G given by intramuscular injection in doses of 600,000 units daily for 15 days.

Patients allergic to penicillin may be given tetracycline hydrochloride—500 mg orally four times daily for 30 days—*or* erythromycin—500 mg orally four times daily for 30 days.

For follow-up, quantitative nontreponemal tets are performed 3, 6, 12, and 24 months after treatment.

Syphilis in Pregnancy: The treatment of choice, for patients not allergic to penicillin, is penicillin in the same dosage schedules appropriate for the particular stage of syphilis as those recommended for nonpregnant patients.

Patients allergic to penicillin are given erythromycin (stearate, ethylsuccinate) in the same dosage schedules appropriate for the particular stage of syphilis as those recommended for the treatment of nonpregnant patients. (Erythromycin estolate and tetracycline are not recommended for syphilitic infections in pregnant women because of the potentially adverse effects they may have on mother and fetus.)

For follow-up, quantitative nontreponemal serologic tests are performed monthly for the remainder of the current pregnancy. Women who show a fourfold rise in titer should be retreated. After delivery, follow-up is the same as that outlined for nonpregnant patients.

Epidemiologic Treatment: Patients who have been exposed to infectious syphilis within the preceding three months and other patients who, on epidemiologic grounds, are at high risk for syphilis should be treated as for early syphilis. Every effort should be made to establish a diagnosis in each case.

PATIENT EDUCATION

Every patient must be made aware of the importance of follow-up evaluations. After treatment for early syphilis, the patient is advised to have a quantitative nontreponemal test after 3, 6, and 12 months.

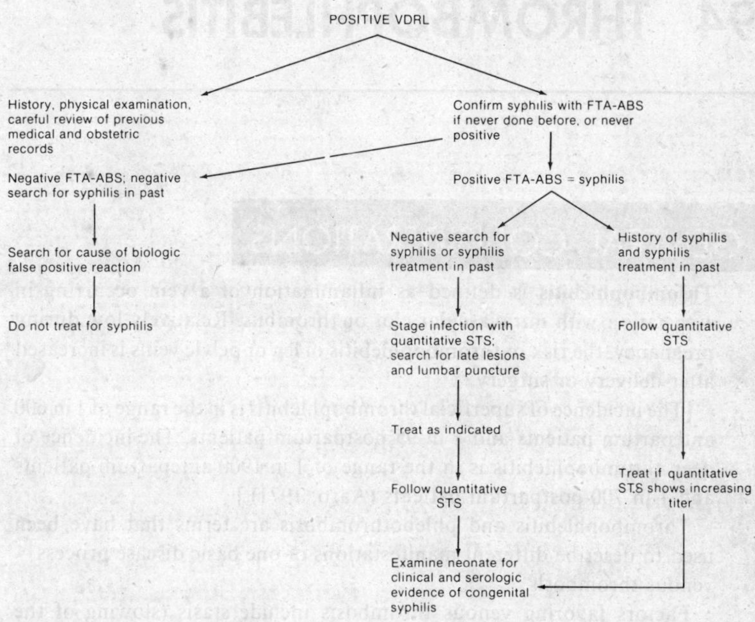

Figure 93-3. Steps in the management of a pregnant patient with a positive serologic test for syphilis. (From Burrow GN, Ferris TF: Medical Complications during Pregnancy. Philadelphia, W.B. Saunders Company, 1975.)

All sexual partners of patients with syphilis should have serologic and clinical evaluations.

REFERENCES

Barrett-Connor E: Current status of the treatment of syphilis. West J Med *122*:7-11, 1975

Center for Disease Control: Syphilis—CDC recommended treatment schedules, 1976. U.S. Dept of HEW. Publ No 76-8017. Morbidity and Mortality Weekly Report *25*:101-107, 1976; Obstet Gynecol *48*:727-729, 1976

94 THROMBOPHLEBITIS

GENERAL CONSIDERATIONS

Thrombophlebitis is defined as inflammation of a vein occurring in association with intravascular clot or thrombus. Relatively low during pregnancy, the risk of thrombophlebitis of leg or pelvic veins is increased after delivery or surgery.

[The incidence of superficial thrombophlebitis is in the range of 1 in 600 antepartum patients and 1 in 95 postpartum patients. The incidence of deep thrombophlebitis is in the range of 1 in 1900 antepartum patients and 1 in 700 postpartum patients (Aaro, 1971).]

Thrombophlebitis and phlebothrombosis are terms that have been used to describe different manifestations of one basic disease process—venous thrombosis.

Factors favoring venous thrombosis include stasis (slowing of the blood stream), injury to the blood vessel lining (local irritation, infection), and physical or chemical alterations in blood constituents.

The manifestation of symptoms depends on

1. The degree of impairment to blood flow with tissue engorgement or ischemia
2. The inflammatory response around the involved veins
3. Associated bacterial infections

Venous Thrombosis of the Peripheral Veins

GENERAL CONSIDERATIONS

Venous thrombosis occurs most commonly in the superficial and deep veins of the lower extremities. Deep leg vein thrombi are most likely to develop in the soleal arcade of the calf muscles, where they may resolve, organize, extend, or trigger additional thrombi at independent sites. Less frequently, thrombi may arise in the pelvic venous network, the right cardiac chambers, and veins of the upper extremities.

SUBJECTIVE DATA

Unilateral leg pain, swelling, and redness may be symptoms of venous thrombosis. Approximately 50 per cent of patients with x-ray evidence of venous thrombosis are asymptomatic, however.

OBJECTIVE DATA

General Examination: An elevated pulse rate and a slight temperature elevation may be the only systemic signs.

Leg Examination: Pain in the calf or popliteal space produced by dorsiflexion of the foot (Homans' sign) may be the only evidence of deep venous thrombosis. Other signs of thrombosis are swelling of the limb, resulting in increased circumference, tenderness, and redness along the course of the involved vessel.

ASSESSMENT

DIFFERENTIAL DIAGNOSIS

This includes cellulitis, varicose veins, trauma with subfascial hematoma, lymphangitis, and arthritis.

PREDISPOSING FACTORS

Risk factors for thrombophlebitis include increasing age, prior episodes of thromboembolism, surgery, delivery, obesity, immobilization, vascular injury, and dehydration.

The role of *estrogen* in the pathogenesis of thromboembolic problems remains controversial, since numerous studies have reached different conclusions (Goldzieher, 1975). Nonetheless, various studies estimate that users of oral contraceptives are 4 to 11 times more likely than nonusers to acquire idiopathic thromboembolic disease. (See Contraceptive Emergencies, p. 249.)

Some patients who acquired fatal pulmonary embolism following delivery had received estrogens for lactation suppression. Since many of these patients also had other predisposing factors to thromboembolism, it is not possible to conclude that there is a positive association between the embolism and estrogenic medications (Report on Confidential Enquiries into Maternal Deaths in England and Wales, 1967-1969).

POTENTIAL COMPLICATIONS

The most serious complication to be avoided is pulmonary embolism (see Pulmonary Embolism, p. 585). Other complications include circulatory obstruction and venous valve damage.

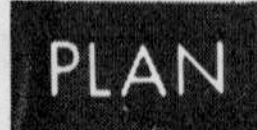

ADDITIONAL DIAGNOSTIC DATA

Phlebography may be helpful when the diagnosis is questionable.

MANAGEMENT

Bed rest, analgesics, moist heat, and elevation of the affected limb are traditional treatment for local thrombophlebitis (superficial and deep).

Anticoagulant therapy with heparin is recommended as soon as a diagnosis of deep venous thrombosis is established, in order to prevent further propagation of the thrombus. The initial dose is 5000 units given intravenously, followed by a continuous infusion of approximately 1000 units per hour.

The continuous intravenous infusion may be prepared by adding 20,000 to 40,000 units of heparin to 1000 ml of 5 per cent dextrose solution. A continuous infusion pump is desirable. Levels of heparin activity are monitored by measuring the activated partial thromboplastin time approximately every four hours during the early stages of treatment. The heparin dosage is adjusted to keep the activated partial thromboplastin time between one and one half and two and one half times the control level. The usual dosage is 20,000 to 40,000 units given over a period of 24 hours.

Hemorrhagic complications of anticoagulant therapy may require termination of the treatment. (In cases of heparin overdosage, 1 per cent protamine sulfate solution given by slow infusion neutralizes heparin. Each mg of protamine sulfate neutralizes approximately 100 units of heparin. Thirty minutes after a dose of heparin, approximately 0.5 mg of protamine is sufficient to neutralize each 100 units of administered heparin. No more than 50 mg of protamine should be administered, very slowly, in any ten-minute period.)

During pregnancy, heparin is the preferred anticoagulant, since it does not cross the placenta.

PATIENT EDUCATION

The patient should be warned of the risk of embolization and told of the necessity for anticoagulant therapy. After symptoms of thrombophlebitis have subsided, the patient may begin walking, her leg supported by an elastic stocking.

Patients receiving anticoagulant treatment should be cautioned to avoid aspirin, since it may exacerbate any bleeding tendency.

Oral contraceptive medications should also be avoided in the future because of the increased risk of recurrent thromboembolism.

Septic Pelvic Thrombophlebitis

GENERAL CONSIDERATIONS

Septic pelvic thrombophlebitis—thrombus formation in an infected pelvic vein—is an uncommon but potentially serious complication of pyogenic pelvic infection. Veins that may be affected include the ovarian, uterine, iliac, hypogastric, and inferior vena cava. Bacteria usually associated with septic thrombophlebitis include anaerobic streptococci and bacteroides.

SUBJECTIVE DATA

Fever and chills are the most consistent symptoms. Some patients acquire abdominal pain and an elevated temperature within 2 to 21 days following delivery, abortion, or pelvic surgery. Often the patient appears well, with minimal, poorly localized pain, despite a recurrent spiking temperature.

Chest pain or dyspnea or both suggest pulmonary emboli.

OBJECTIVE DATA

PHYSICAL EXAMINATION

General Examination: The temperature is elevated, persistent, and spiking, despite antibiotic therapy. Tachycardia and, occasionally, tachypnea may be associated findings.

Abdominal examination is variable. Some patients have manifestations of an acute abdomen—tenderness, guarding, rebound tenderness, distention—whereas others have minimal abdominal tenderness. A palpable mass is an inconsistent finding.

Pelvic examination is often normal or vague. Rarely, a tender thrombosed vein is palpable. Frequently, only vague parametrial tenderness is evident.

LABORATORY TESTS

White blood count varies from normal to 25,000.

Urinalysis is normal.

ASSESSMENT

DIFFERENTIAL DIAGNOSIS

This includes acute appendicitis, twisted ovarian cyst, broad ligament hematoma, pelvic abscess, urinary tract infections, and wound infections.

Septic pelvic thrombophlebitis is suspected in postabortal, postpartum, and postoperative patients who continue to run a septic febrile course despite appropriate antibiotics when other causes of fever have been excluded. A presumptive diagnosis of septic pelvic thrombophlebitis may be based on the rapid reduction of fever (within 48 to 72 hours) after the initiation of intravenous heparin therapy.

PREDISPOSING FACTORS

These include pelvic surgery and obstetric complications (puerperal sepsis, prolonged rupture of membranes, abortion, pelvic infection).

POTENTIAL COMPLICATIONS

These include septic pulmonary emboli, septicemia, and empyema.

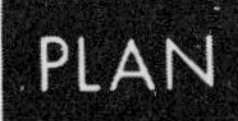

ADDITIONAL DIAGNOSTIC DATA

Blood cultures, both aerobic and anaerobic, may be helpful. Organisms to be anticipated include aerobic and anaerobic streptococci, *Staphylococcus aureus, Escherichia coli,* and Bacteroides.

Endometrial cultures may be helpful if there is an associated endometritis.

Chest x-ray is often nonspecific, since septic pulmonary emboli tend to be small and multiple.

MANAGEMENT AND PATIENT EDUCATION

The patient should be hospitalized and kept at bed rest.

Antibiotic therapy depends on the suspected organisms. (See Pelvic Infections, p. 474.)

Heparin anticoagulant therapy in conjunction with antibiotics may effect a dramatic clinical response. Since certain species of Bacteroides produce enzymes capable of degrading heparin, the dosage may have to be increased above the usual range in order to achieve a therapeutic prolongation of the partial thromboplastin time or clotting time.

Surgery may be necessary if the patient fails to respond to heparin therapy within 48 hours, if her general condition worsens, or if pulmonary emboli occur or recur despite adequate anticoagulation therapy. Surgical procedures include ligation of the inferior vena cava and ovarian veins. If a pelvic abscess is found, the infected pelvic organs are excised.

If the abdomen is opened after a preoperative diagnosis of appendicitis, twisted ovarian cyst, or pelvic abscess and ovarian vein thrombophlebitis is discovered, the ovarian veins should be ligated bilaterally. Heparin and antibiotics are prescribed postoperatively.

REFERENCES

Aaro LA, Juergens JL: Thrombophlebitis associated with pregnancy. *109*:1128-1136, 1971

Chow AW, Marshall JR, Guze LB: Anaerobic infections of the female genital tract. Obstet Gynecol Surv *30*:477-494, 1975

Goldzieher JW, Dozier TS: Oral contraceptives and thromboembolism. Am J Obstet Gynecol *123*:878-914, 1975

Josey WE, Staggers SR: Heparin therapy in septic pelvic thrombophlebitis. Am J Obstet Gynecol *120*:228-233, 1974

Ledger WJ, Peterson EP: Use of heparin in the management of pelvic thrombophlebitis. Surg Gynecol Obstet *131*:1115-1121, 1970; Obstet Gynecol Surv *26*:403-405, 1971

Perry MO: Detection and management of deep vein thrombosis. West J Med *125*:195-202, 1976

95 URINARY INCONTINENCE

GENERAL CONSIDERATIONS

Urinary incontinence, or involuntary loss of urine, may be continuous or intermittent.

Classification:

1. Continuous incontinence
   a. Congenital defects
   b. Fistula formation following operative procedures, delivery, pelvic malignancy, or radiation therapy.
2. Intermittent incontinence
   a. Stress incontinence
   b. Detrusor dyssynergia—unstable bladder
   c. Urge incontinence
   d. Overflow incontinence
      (1) Hypotonic bladder
      (2) Neurogenic bladder
   e. Urethral deformity

SUBJECTIVE DATA

A detailed history of the onset and nature of the urinary symptoms is the first prerequisite for accurate diagnosis.

Involuntary voiding associated with coughing, sneezing, straining, laughing, or lifting, and without any sensation of bladder fullness, is characteristic of stress incontinence. Involuntary voiding immediately after a sensation of bladder fullness unassociated with any stress is usually due to vesical irritation (urge incontinence). Symptoms of an associated urinary tract infection include frequency, burning, dysuria, and possibly fever.

If voiding occurs spontaneously without any sensation or any specific action, the possibility of a neurogenic bladder or overflow incontinence must be considered.

Continuous urinary leakage is suggestive of a fistula—ureterovaginal or vesicovaginal. A history of pelvic surgery, obstetric delivery, radiation, or accidental injury involving a pelvic fracture or urinary tract laceration provides the key diagnostic clue.

OBJECTIVE DATA

Vulvar Examination: Diffuse erythema, moistness, and maceration may be associated with a vaginal fistula or an ectopic ureter.

Vaginal Examination: The site of a vesicovaginal or ureterovaginal fistula may be visualized.

Cystocele and urethrocele are likely to be associated with stress incontinence. If urine is lost when the patient is asked to bear down or strain, stress incontinence is evident (Fig. 95-1 *A*).

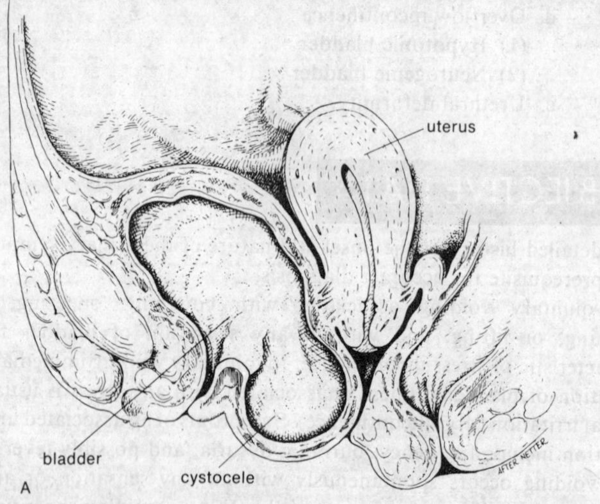

Figure 95-1. *A*, Cystocele associated with stress incontinence.

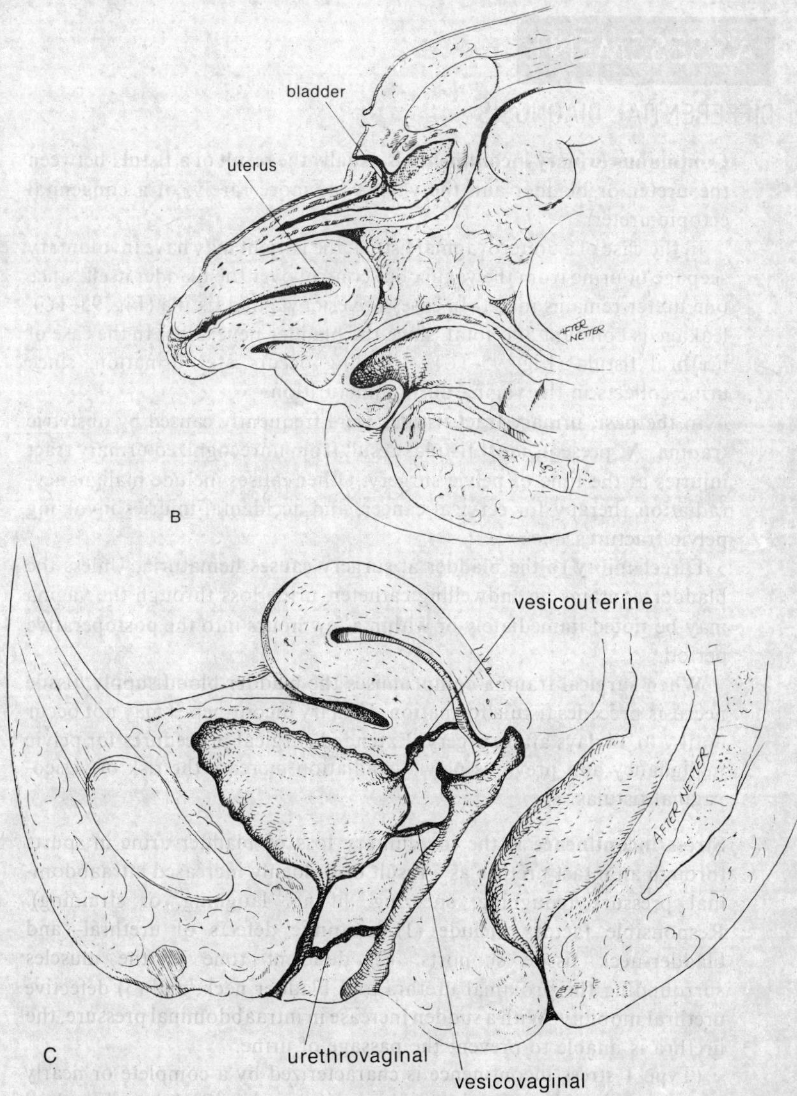

Figure 95-1 Continued. *B*, Uterine prolapse. *C*, Various sites of urinary tract fistulas.

ASSESSMENT

DIFFERENTIAL DIAGNOSIS

Continuous urinary incontinence is usually the result of a fistula between the ureter or bladder and the vagina or, more rarely, of a congenital ectopic ureter.

In the case of a ureterovaginal fistula, the patient may have involuntary seepage of urine from the vagina but control over the bladder itself, since one ureter remains intact. In cases of vesicovaginal fistula (Fig. 95-1*C*), leakage is constant and total, since the bladder never fills. In the case of urethral fistula (Fig. 95-1*C*), dribbling occurs afer urination, since urine collects in the vagina during micturition.

In the past, urinary tract fistulas were frequently caused by obstetric trauma. At present, most fistulas result from unrecognized urinary tract injuries at the time of pelvic surgery. Other causes include malignancy, radiation therapy for cervical cancer, and accidental injuries involving pelvic fractures.

Direct injury to the bladder at surgery causes hematuria. Unless the bladder contains an indwelling catheter, urine loss through the vagina may be noted immediately or within a few hours into the postoperative period.

When surgical trauma compromises the bladder blood supply, tissue necrosis precedes fistula formation. Urinary incontinence may not occur until 7 to 14 days after surgery. Extended surgical procedures for pelvic malignancy and previous pelvic irradiation increase the risk of vesicovaginal fistulas.

Stress incontinence is the involuntary loss of bladder urine in spurts through an intact urethra as a result of suddenly increased intraabdominal pressure (coughing, sneezing, lifting, laughing, or straining). Responsible factors include (1) anatomic defects of urethral- and bladder-neck tissue supports, (2) deficient tone in the muscles surrounding the proximal urethra and bladder neck, and (3) defective urethral mobility. With a sudden increase in intraabdominal pressure, the urethra is unable to prevent the passage of urine.

(Type 1 stress incontinence is characterized by a complete or nearly complete loss of the posterior urethrovesical angle with a normal urethral angle of inclination. Type 2 stress incontinence is characterized by increase and reversal of the normal axis of urethral inclination due to urethral descent, as well as by loss of the posterior urethrovesical angle.)

Detrusor dyssynergia (unstable bladder) is characterized by *spontaneous* detrusor contractions with involuntary urine loss. The detrusor appears to be overresponsive to sudden motion, thoughts, temperature changes, sounds of running water, and so forth. If coughing or jumping cause detrusor contraction, urine loss does not occur simultaneously with the stress but a few seconds later.

Urge Incontinence: The bladder tends to be hyperirritable, usually as a result of trauma or inflammatory conditions (trigonitis, cystitis). Often the bladder is contracted. Urine is lost shortly after the patient recognizes the urge to void.

Overflow Incontinence:

Hypotonic Bladder: With overdistention due to urethral obstruction or the inhibition of vesical smooth muscle by drugs or anesthetics, constant or intermittent dribbling of urine occurs.

Neurogenic Bladder: Lower neurologic lesions produce an atonic bladder with increased capacity and large quantities of residual urine. Etiologic factors include radical surgery, spinal cord injuries, spinal tumors, diabetes, tabes dorsalis, multiple sclerosis, and paralytic poliomyelitis.

Urethral Deformity: The patient with urethral stenosis or a diverticulum often continues to dribble moderate amounts of urine after emptying her bladder.

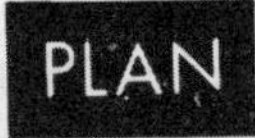

ADDITIONAL DIAGNOSTIC DATA

Urinalysis is essential in order to evaluate urinary tract disease. Bacteriuria and pyuria indicate infection.

Residual urine should be measured after voiding in order to identify overflow incontinence.

Urine culture and sensitivity studies identify urinary tract pathogens.

Cystoscopy is indicated whenever an intrinsic bladder pathologic condition is suspected. The exact site and extent of a vesicovaginal fistula may be visualized.

X-ray cystourethrograms depict the anatomic relationship of the posterior urethrovesical angle, as well as the urethral angle of inclination. Metallic bead chain cystourethrograms are often useful.

Elevation of the urethrovesical junction (Bonney test) may relieve symptoms of stress incontinence.

Intravenous pyelogram may disclose ureteral obstruction or uretero-vaginal fistulas.

Urodynamic studies may be helpful in the evaluation of detrusor dyssynergia. As the bladder becomes distended, a desire to void can normally be suppressed until the bladder contains approximately 500 ml of fluid.

Fistula Identification: For differentiation between a vesicovaginal and ureterovaginal fistula, a dry sponge or tampon may be placed in the vagina. Methylene blue or indigo carmine is then instilled into the bladder. If the dye stains the sponge, the fistula involves the bladder and the vagina. If the sponge remains dry, indigo carmine is injected intravenously. Discoloration of the sponge indicates a communication between the ureter and the vagina.

MANAGEMENT AND PATIENT EDUCATION

Stress incontinence may be managed initially with exercises designed to strengthen the pubococcygeus musculature. Surgical repair is usually required when urine loss results in social embarrasment, the necessity to wear protective pads or garments, or chronic vulvar maceration.

Detrusor Dyssynergia: Fifteen mg of propantheline bromide (Pro-Banthine) or 5 mg of oxybutynin chloride (Ditropan) three to four times daily may be helpful.

Urge Incontinence: An intrinsic bladder pathologic condition requires appropriate therapy. Urinary tract infections are treated with antibiotics, the specific antibiotic depending on the pathogen isolated.

Overflow incontinence is treated by the use of an indwelling catheter to prevent the accumulation of residual urine.

Urinary tract damage recognized at surgery or resulting from acute trauma is repaired immediately.

Fistulas are not repaired surgically until the tissues have had an adequate chance to heal completely.

Occasionally, a vesicovaginal fistula may heal spontaneously, particularly if bladder drainage prevents vaginal leakage. The principle of treatment is the prevention of bladder distention until the fistula edges have firmly healed. Prolonged drainage for four to eight weeks may be necessary. Antimicrobial therapy is prescribed to prevent urinary tract infection. If catheter drainage does not prevent seepage of vaginal urine, a complete urologic evaluation is essential.

REFERENCES

Beck RP, Arnusch D, King C: Results in treating 210 patients with detrusor overactivity incontinence of urine. Am J Obstet Gynecol *125*:593-596, 1976; Obstet Gynecol Surv *31*:824-826, 1976

Graber EA: Stress incontinence in women: a review—1977. Obstet Gynecol Surv *32*:565-577, 1977

Green TH Jr: Urinary stress incontinence: differential diagnosis, pathophysiology and management. Am J Obstet Gynecol *122*:368-400, 1975

Moolgaoker AS, Ardran GM, Smith JC et al: The diagnosis and management of urinary incontinence in the female. J Obstet Gynaecol Br Commonw *79*:481-497, 1972; Obstet Gynecol Surv *28*:350-354, 1973

Urinary incontinence in the female. ACOG Technical Bulletin, No 36, February 1976

Williams TJ: Urinary incontinence in the female. Med Clin North Am *58*:729-741, 1974

96 URINARY RETENTION

GENERAL CONSIDERATIONS

Acute urinary retention in females is most likely to occur post partum or following pelvic surgery. Other causes include urethral obstruction by an incarcerated pregnant uterus and herpes genitalis.

Postpartum urinary retention may occur in a patient who had a normal delivery, as a result of stretching and trauma of the bladder base with edema of the trigone. Other factors predisposing to urinary retention include anesthesia, with temporarily disturbed neural control of the bladder, and trauma to the genital tract, especially large hematomas.

When the bladder becomes overdistended, the patient is either unable to void or can void only small quantities of urine. On abdominal examination, the uterine fundus is higher than expected, since it is displaced upward by the distended bladder.

Once the bladder has become overdistended, catheterization is required. A Foley catheter is left in the bladder for 24 to 48 hours in order to keep the bladder completely empty and allow the bladder muscle to recover normal tone and sensation.

When the catheter is removed, the patient should be able to void spontaneously in approximately four hours. Five mg of bethanechol chloride (Urecholine) may be helpful. After spontaneous voiding, the bladder should be catheterized again in order to be certain that residual urine is minimal. If the bladder contains more than 100 ml of urine, continuous bladder drainage is reinstituted.

Postoperative urinary retention is usually caused by trauma to the bladder, pain, or temporary interference with bladder innervation. Often, postoperative pain discourages the voluntary effort necessary to initiate urination. In addition, large amounts of intravenous fluids may have been administered while the patient was depressed from the anesthetic. Under these circumstances, the bladder becomes overdistended at a time when the desire and ability to void are at a low ebb. Although small quantities of urine may be voided, the bladder contains a large residual. Catheterization is essential.

Frequently, a suprapubic catheter is preferred, since it allows a patient to void spontaneously as soon as her bladder tone has returned to normal. Furthermore, a suprapubic catheter permits assessment of residual urine after spontaneous voiding without the necessity for additional catheterization.

Bethanechol Chloride (Urecholine): Postpartum or postoperative bladder atony may respond to 5 mg of bethanechol given subcutaneously or 10 mg given orally. Bethanechol increases the tone of the detrusor urinae muscle, usually producing a contraction sufficiently strong to initiate micturition and empty the bladder.

Bethanechol should not be used, however, whenever there is any question of the strength or integrity of the gastrointestinal or bladder wall, or in the presence of mechanical obstruction. Other contraindications include hyperthyroidism, pregnancy, peptic ulcer, latent or active bronchial asthma, pronounced bradycardia or hypotension, vasomotor instability, coronary artery disease, epilepsy, and parkinsonism. With hypersensitivity or overdosage, violent symptoms of cholinergic overstimulation include circulatory collapse, hypotension, abdominal cramps, bloody diarrhea, and sudden cardiac arrest. Atropine (0.6 mg) given subcutaneously, or in an emergency, intravenously, is a specific antidote for toxic reactions.

Incarcerated Pregnant Uterus: Near the end of the fourth gestational month, a retroverted uterus may become incarcerated in the hollow of the sacrum. As the uterus enlarges, the cervix is pushed forward behind the symphysis pubis, impinging on the bladder neck. The patient complains of abdominal discomfort and inability to void. With increased bladder pressure, overflow incontinence occurs. The patient gives a history of increasing difficulty in voiding; even with straining, she releases only a dribble of urine.

Treatment includes bladder catheterization and repositioning of the uterus outside the pelvis with the patient in the knee-chest position. A retention catheter may be required until normal bladder tone returns.

97 URINARY SUPPRESSION — OLIGURIA AND ANURIA

GENERAL CONSIDERATIONS

Urinary suppression —anuria or oliguria—is a life-threatening crisis, demanding immediate medical attention.

Anuria is the absence of urine excretion, that is, complete urinary suppression.

Oliguria indicates diminished urine volume, usually less than 400 to 500 ml over a period of 24 hours. A sustained urinary output less than 20 ml per hour in a patient with previously normal renal function is evidence of significant oliguria. The minimal volume of urine necessary for adequate solute excretion under basal conditions is approximately 450 ml per day.

CLASSIFICATION

Prerenal suppression of urine formation results from inadequate perfusion of an anatomically and physiologically normal kidney and collection system. Usual causes include hypotension and hypovolemia from any condition that depletes vascular volume (hemorrhage, dehydration, diarrhea, vomiting, and so forth.) Prolonged impairment of renal perfusion leads to renal ischemia, necrosis, and intrinsic renal failure.

Renal disease with structural damage can be caused by ischemia or nephrotoxic agents. Acute tubular necrosis is the major cause of acute renal failure associated with pregnancy complications. (Oxytocin has a temporary antidiuretic effect, primarily by direct action on the distal tubules causing reabsorption of free water.)

Postrenal obstructive lesions of the ureter, bladder, or urethra include surgical trauma (ureteral ligation), urethral obstruction from vaginal packing, and urethral spasm. Urinary retention in the bladder must be distinguished from anatomic obstruction.

SUBJECTIVE AND OBJECTIVE DATA

The history of the preceding events may provide a key diagnostic clue. Anuria following surgery or delivery suggests postrenal obstruction or bladder atony. Oliguria occurring a number of days after surgery or delivery is more likely to be associated with an intrinsic renal lesion.

Suprapubic pain suggests bladder distention. The patient is unable to void even though she feels the desire. The distended bladder may be palpable above the symphysis pubis.

Unilateral lumbar pain may be symptomatic of an acute ureteral obstruction.

Anorexia, nausea, vomiting, convulsive muscular twitchings, dyspnea, headache, lethargy, and mental confusion are symptoms of advanced renal failure (uremia).

Weight gain is a sign of fluid retention.

Complete blood count with blood smear is usually normal unless there is an associated infection or hemolytic process.

Urinalysis: A catheterized specimen is essential in order to measure the quantity of urine in the bladder and the output per hour. White cells suggest urinary tract infection. Hematuria is associated with bladder or ureteral trauma.

ASSESSMENT

DIFFERENTIAL DIAGNOSIS OF OLIGURIA

See Table 97-1 for the differential diagnosis of oliguria.

ETIOLOGIC FACTORS OF ACUTE RENAL FAILURE

1. Disseminated intravascular coagulation
2. Intravascular hemolysis
   a. Clostridial sepsis
   b. Mismatched blood transfusion
3. Nephrotoxins—bacteria, drugs, heavy metals
4. Operative trauma
5. Postpartum hemolytic uremic syndrome*
6. Preeclampsia or eclampsia
7. Premature separation of the placenta
8. Septic Abortion or intrauterine sepsis
   a. Clostridial sepsis with hemolysis
   b. Toxic compounds to induce abortion [soap, disinfectant (Lysol)]
9. Septicemia
10. Shock—hypovolemic and septic

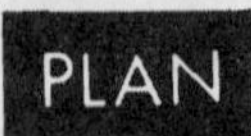

DIAGNOSTIC TESTS AND PROCEDURES

Catheterization of the bladder or ureter or both differentiates bladder retention or ureteral obstruction from intrinsic renal disease or prerenal oliguria.

Urinalysis (specific gravity, albumin, hemoglobin, sodium, osmolality, and urea) provides important diagnostic information.

---

*Postpartum hemolytic uremic syndrome may occur two weeks to six months after delivery and is characterized by renal failure and microangiopathic hemolytic anemia. Intravascular thrombosis in the kidney leads to tissue necrosis. Laboratory findings are anemia, thrombocytopenia, microangiopathic red blood cell changes, elevated fibrin-split products, blood urea nitrogen greater than 20, hematuria, proteinuria, and urine casts. Hypertension and left ventricle failure are usually associated findings. Heparin therapy may improve chances for survival (Strauss, 1976).

Prerenal oliguria is associated with high urine osmolality (greater than 600 mOsm/l), very low urine sodium concentration (less than 10 mEq/l), and high urine urea concentration (greater than 1000 mg/100 ml). The urine-plasma urea ratio is greater than 10, and the urine-plasma osmolality ratio is greater than 1.5. The specific gravity is greater than 1.020.

Acute tubular necrosis is associated with iso-osmolar urine (300 mosm/l), low urine urea concentration, and high urine sodium concentration (greater than 40 mEq/l). The urine-plasma urea ratio is less than 10, and the urine-plasma osmolality ratio is less than 1.5. The

TABLE 97-1. Differential Diagnosis of Oliguria*†

	Hypoperfusion (Hypovolemic Kidney)	**Hyperperfusion ("Conduit" Syndrome; Diffuse Nephron Disease)**
Examples:	Shock	"Shock kidney"
	Congestive heart failure	Acute renal failure
	Hepatorenal syndrome	Acute tubular necrosis
	Nephrotic syndrome (especially with hypotension)	Chronic renal insufficiency (end stage)
	Acute glomerulonephritis	Severe transfusion reaction
	Acute urinary tract obstruction	Chronic urinary tract obstruction
FINDINGS		
Urine sp. gr.	> 1.020	< 1.015
U/P ratio: Creatinine	> 40	< 15
Urea	> 20	< 5
Osmolal	> 1.2	< 1.1
Urine [Na] mEq/l.	< 20	> 30

*From Davidsohn IS, Henry JB: Todd-Sanford Clinical Diagnosis. Philadelphia, W.B. Saunders Company, 1974. (Modified from Weisberg HF: Osmolality. ASCP Commission on Continuing Education Council on Clinical Chemistry, Check Sample CC-71, 1971.)

†Most useful in absence of azotemia or urinary tract obstruction.

specific gravity is 1.010. Examination of the urine sediment discloses large numbers of tubular epithelial cellular casts and granular casts.

Blood Studies: Serum electrolytes, osmolality, blood urea nitrogen, and creatinine determinations provide important diagnostic information concerning the status of renal function. Hyperkalemia may be caused by intravascular hemolysis or tissue necrosis.

Radiographic Studies: A plain film (kidney, ureter, bladder) may reveal radiopaque calculi. An intravenous pyelogram or retrograde pyelogram may be helpful in the elucidation of surgical ureteral obstruction.

Coagulation tests (fibrinogen, fibrin-split products, platelets) and a blood smear may reveal evidence of a coagulation disorder with or without hemolysis.

MANAGEMENT AND PATIENT EDUCATION

Prerenal Oliguria: Shock must be adequately treated by restoration of blood and extracellular volume. Large volumes of intravenous fluid may be required and should be monitored by pulmonary wedge pressure or, at least, central venous pressure.

Mannitol may be indicated if volume replacement does not restore urinary output and dehydration must be differentiated from acute renal failure. A test dose of approximately 0.2 gm/kg body weight (100 ml of a 15 per cent solution) is infused intravenously over a period of five minutes. If the urine flow increases to 40 ml/hour, further doses of mannitol may be given. Lack of a diuretic response to mannitol usually means renal failure; in this case, further mannitol administration is futile and dangerous.

Acute Renal Failure: The primary goal of therapy is maintenance of fluid balance and prevention of uremia while the damaged kidneys regenerate.

Strict control of fluid and electrolyte intake is essential. Intravenous fluids are administered only to replace vascular deficits, insensibly lost water, and observed extrarenal and urinary output. The diet should minimize protein catabolism, potassium accumulation, and sodium overload.

Body weight and plasma electrolytes are guides to fluid balance. Weight gain indicates overhydration.

Infection must be treated. Antibiotic dosages may have to be adjusted for renal failure. Usually, full loading doses are used, with subsequent doses determined by creatinine values or serum antibiotic levels.

Dialysis may be necessary and should be initiated before serious metabolic derangements develop. Indications for dialysis include uremic toxicity, fluid overload, hyperkalemia, and acidosis.

Postrenal Obstruction: The early recognition of urinary tract obstruction is vital to prevent renal failure with nephron destruction. Whenever obstruction is suspected, bladder catheterization or ureteral catheterization or both are essential.

Appropriate therapy, surgical repair, nephrostomy, and so forth depend on the underlying pathologic condition.

REFERENCES

Harkins JL, Wilson DR, Muggah HF: Acute renal failure in obstetrics. Am J Obstet Gynecol *118*:331-336, 1974

Strauss RG, Alexander RW: Postpartum hemolytic uremic syndrome. Obstet Gynecol *47*:169-173, 1976

98 UTERINE INVERSION

DEFINITIONS

Uterine inversion—abnormal turning of the uterus inside out, with the internal surface of the corpus lying in or outside of the vagina. This is a rare obstetric emergency (1 per 2000 to 12,000 deliveries) occurring during or immediately following the third stage of labor.

Incomplete inversion—the uterine fundus does not invert beyond the cervix.

Complete inversion—the entire uterus, turned inside out, extends through the cervical ring.

Forced inversion—uterine inversion created by pulling on the cord or by forceful manual expression of the placenta when the uterus is atonic.

Spontaneous inversion—uterine inversion following a spontaneous action of the patient such as bearing down, sudden abdominal muscle contraction, coughing, or increased intraabdominal pressure.

SUBJECTIVE DATA

Vaginal bleeding is frequently profuse, occurring immediately after the baby has been delivered.

Uterine pain may be suddenly severe.

Labor and delivery are often uncomplicated. The patient is frequently young and para 1 or 2.

OBJECTIVE DATA

General Examination: Shock tachycardia and hypotension may be both hypovolemic and neurogenic in origin.

Abdominal Examination: The uterine fundus is not palpable, and a craterlike depression may be noted.

Pelvic Examination: The uterine fundus may protrude through the vaginal orifice or may be found in the vagina or cervical canal. Blood loss is usually profuse. Frequently, the placenta is partially attached to the uterine wall.

ASSESSMENT

DIFFERENTIAL DIAGNOSIS

This includes other causes of postpartum shock (see Shock, p. 612). With uterine inversion, however, the findings are usually distinctive.

PREDISPOSING FACTORS

These include fundal pressure, cord traction, fundal insertion of the placenta, a markedly lax or thin uterine wall, and suddenly increased intraabdominal pressure associated with uterine atony.

POTENTIAL COMPLICATIONS

Complications to be anticipated include hypovolemic shock, placenta accreta, and uterine rupture.

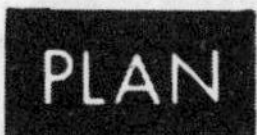

MANAGEMENT

Supportive therapy for shock and blood loss must be initiated immediately: Oxygen and intravenous fluids with lactated Ringer's solution are given, as well as plasma and blood to restore intravascular fluid volume. Oxytocic agents are withheld.

The uterus is repositioned immediately, if possible. The placenta, if attached, is not removed until the inversion has been corrected, in order to prevent additional hemorrhage. It may be preferable, however, to remove the placenta if all but a small portion is already separated, or if it appears necessary to reduce the bulk of the inverted mass in order to replace the uterus through a narrowed cervical ring.

Initially, a prolapsed uterus is replaced within the vagina. General anesthesia, usually halothane, is frequently required for uterine relaxation.

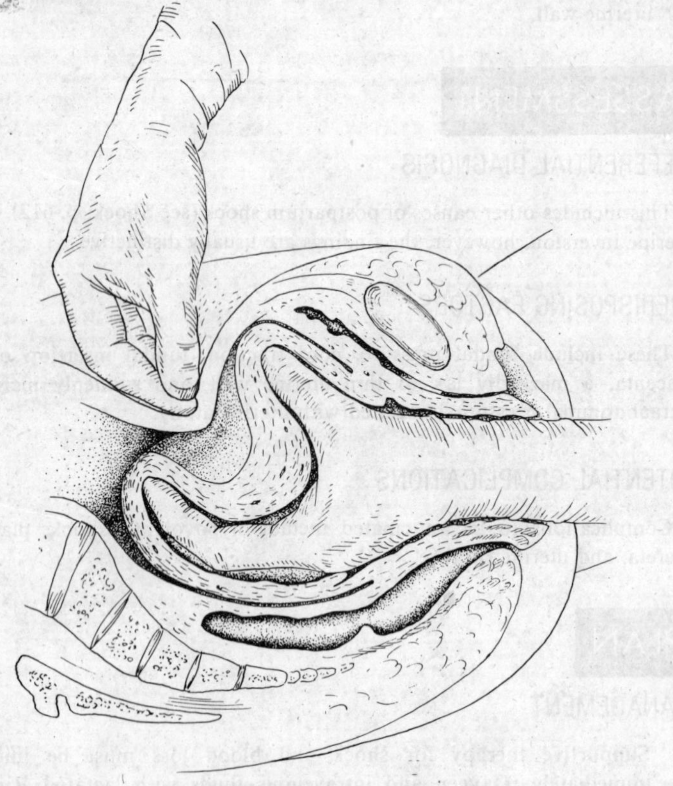

Figure 98-1. Replacement of inverted uterus. (From Greenhill JP, Friedman EA: Biological Principles and Modern Practice of Obstetrics. Philadelphia, W.B. Saunders Co., 1974.)

The entire hand is placed in the vagina with the palm on the center of the fundus. Pressure is applied with the fingertips at the junction of the cervix and corpus to push the fundus upward through the cervical canal (see Fig. 98-1). As soon as the inversion has been corrected, the anesthetic agent that provided uterine relaxation is stopped. The entire uterus is lifted out of the pelvis and held up for three to five minutes while uterine contractions are stimulated with intravenous oxytocin (40 units per 1000 ml of lactated Ringer's solution) and 0.2 mg of ergonovine. Bimanual compression helps control further hemorrhage until uterine tone is restored.

Surgery may be necessary if attempts at vaginal repositioning fail. Laparotomy is usually preferred. After the abdomen is opened and the inverted uterus identified, the fundus may be simultaneously pushed upward from below and pulled upward from above. A constriction ring, preventing repositioning may have to be incised through the posterior wall of the uterus. After the uterus has been reinverted with gentle traction, the posterior defect in the uterine wall is repaired.

PATIENT EDUCATION

Without prompt treatment, uterine inversion can be fatal. After successful treatment the likelihood of recurrence in subsequent pregnancy is difficult to predict.

In former years, high recurrence rates were recorded. Nonetheless, there are numerous reports of uncomplicated deliveries in subsequent pregnancies (Kitchin, 1975).

REFERENCE

Kitchin JD, Thiagarajah S, May HV Jr, et al: Puerperal inversion of the uterus. Am J Obstet Gynecol *123*:51-58, 1975

99 UTERINE PERFORATION

GENERAL CONSIDERATIONS

Uterine perforation may occur any time an instrument is introduced into the uterine cavity. Insertion of intrauterine devices and abortion procedures are the most common causes of uterine perforation.

SUBJECTIVE DATA

CURRENT SYMPTOMS

Lower abdominal pain can be caused by peritoneal irritation, intraperitoneal bleeding, or bleeding into the broad ligament.

Syncope and shock are manifestations of acute blood loss.

PRIOR HISTORY

A history of instrumentation (intrauterine device insertion or abortion) is the key diagnostic clue.

OBJECTIVE DATA

PHYSICAL EXAMINATION

General Examination: Tachycardia and hypotension are signs of hypovolemia, usually acute blood loss.

Abdominal Examination: Tenderness and rigidity are signs of intraperitoneal or retroperitoneal bleeding.

Pelvic Examination: The uterus is likely to be acutely anteflexed or retroflexed. A mass lateral to the uterus suggests a broad ligament hematoma; an enlarging mass is characteristic of an expanding hematoma.

LABORATORY TESTS

Complete Blood Count with Blood Smear: Initial hemoglobin and hematocrit values do not reflect the true extent of acute hemorrhage. Declining serial values are more accurate indications of blood loss. White blood count is usually normal initially; an elevated white count is a sign of infection.

Urinalysis: Hematuria suggests associated trauma to the urinary tract.

ASSESSMENT

ETIOLOGIC FACTORS

These are uterine instrumentation: intrauterine device insertion and uterine curettage.

POTENTIAL COMPLICATIONS

Complications to be anticipated include bacterial peritonitis, broad ligament hematoma, and intestinal laceration.

SEVERITY OF DISEASE PROCESS

Often the injury is minimal, particularly if the perforation is caused by a small, blunt instrument such as a uterine sound. When the perforation is caused by a sharp curette, there may be associated intestinal trauma or active bleeding. The most serious instances of uterine perforation are encountered in women who have had illegal abortions. Under these circumstances, infection is often present and the extent of perforation is unknown.

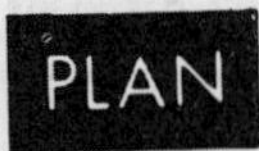

ADDITIONAL DIAGNOSTIC DATA

Abdominal X-ray Examination: Three-way films (supine, upright, and lateral decubitus) may reveal free air or free fluid in the peritoneal cavity. An intrauterine device may be visualized.

Serial hematocrit determinations may suggest continuing occult bleeding.

Laparoscopy may aid in the visualization of the perforation site and in the determination of the extent of the bleeding.

MANAGEMENT AND PATIENT EDUCATION

The patient is hospitalized for observation. Intravenous fluids are initiated; *nulle per os* is permitted in the event that surgical exploration becomes necessary. Blood is prepared for transfusion in case this becomes necessary. Antibiotics may be prescribed to prevent infection.

A single, small uterine perforation incidental to a diagnostic or therapeutic curettage usually heals spontaneously and rarely requires surgical repair, unless there are signs of continued intraperitoneal or retroperitoneal bleeding.

Exploratory abdominal surgery is indicated when there is evidence of intestinal tract injury or persistent intraperitoneal or retroperitoneal bleeding. At times, the uterine laceration can be repaired. Hysterectomy may be necessary if a lateral perforation into the broad ligament involves the uterine vessels.

Hysterectomy may be preferred when extensive uterine trauma is accompanied by pelvic infection.

A periuterine hematoma should be opened and the bleeder sought. If the bleeding is arterial, a pumping vessel is isolated. With venous bleeding, there is a welling up of blood from a plexus of damaged veins. The main danger is ureteral damage.

If a bleeding artery cannot be isolated and ligated, hypogastric artery ligation may arrest the bleeding. In addition, the uterine vessels as well as the ovarian vessels may have to be dissected out and ligated individually.

At times, Avitene or a hemovac catheter placed into the retroperitoneal space may be necessary to control bleeding or prevent the reaccumulation of blood and serum.

REFERENCES

Lauersen NH, Birnbaum S: Laparoscopy as a diagnostic and therapeutic technique in uterine perforations during first-trimester abortions. Am J Obstet Gynecol *117*: 522-526, 1973

100 UTERINE RUPTURE

GENERAL CONSIDERATIONS

Uterine rupture, disruption of the uterine wall, is one of the most serious obstetric emergencies and may occur in the antepartum or intrapartum period. Maternal mortality ranges from 3 to 15 per cent; fetal mortality is approximately 50 per cent.

Uterine rupture during the second trimester is usually due to a cornual implantation.

Uterine rupture during the third trimester may be classified as incidental rupture, traumatic rupture, or spontaneous rupture.

Incidental rupture is an asymptomatic variety of spontaneous rupture of the gravid uterus. Such a rupture may involve all or a small part of a previous scar (synonyms—silent rupture, occult rupture).

Traumatic rupture includes ruptured uteri associated with pharmacologic agents (oxytocics), intrauterine manipulations, external pressure, or instrumental procedures. Traumatic rupture may occur in a scarred or unscarred uterus, and usually occurs during labor, *with* the rupture site being in the lower uterine segment.

Spontaneous rupture occurs in the absence of iatrogenic trauma. Ruptured uteri associated with an unstimulated obstructed labor fall into this category. Spontaneous rupture may occur in a scarred or unscarred uterus.

The incidence of uterine rupture varies greatly from hospital to hospital. At the Charity Hospital in New Orleans, Louisiana, an incidence of 1 per 2500 deliveries has been reported (**Beacham,** 1970).

SUBJECTIVE DATA

CURRENT SYMPTOMS

Abdominal pain may be sudden, sharp, and knifelike, particularly when the rupture occurs suddenly during labor.

Vaginal bleeding may be symptomatic of active bleeding from torn blood vessels.

Other Symptoms: Shock tends to be out of proportion to external blood loss because of the occult hemorrhage. Shoulder pain may be associated with intraperitoneal bleeding.

PRIOR HISTORY

Uterine rupture should always be anticipated if the patient gives a history of previous uterine surgery, cesarean section, myomectomy or cornual resection.

OBJECTIVE DATA

PHYSICAL EXAMINATION

General Examination: Tachycardia and hypotension are indications of acute blood loss, usually external bleeding and intraabdominal hemorrhage.

Abdominal Examination: During labor, a sudden change in uterine contour may indicate extrusion of the fetus into the peritoneal cavity. The uterine fundus feels contracted and firm, with fetal parts palpable close to the abdominal wall above the contracted fundus. Uterine contractions cease abruptly and fetal heart tones suddenly disappear.

If the rupture occurs during or immediately after delivery, the abdomen is frequently extremely tender, with rebound tenderness indicating intraperitoneal bleeding.

Pelvic Examination: Prior to delivery, the presenting part regresses and is no longer palpable vaginally after the fetus has been extruded into the peritoneal cavity. Vaginal bleeding may be profuse.

Uterine rupture after delivery is recognized by manual exploration of the lower uterine segment and uterine cavity. The lower uterine segment is the most common site of rupture. When the tear is complete, the obstetrician's fingers pass through the rupture site directly into the peritoneal cavity, which may be recognized by (1) the smooth, slippery surface of the uterine serosa, (2) the presence of intestines and omentum, and (3) the great freedom of motion for the fingers and hand.

LABORATORY TESTS

Complete Blood Count with Blood Smear: Base-line hemoglobin and hematocrit values may not reveal the extent of blood loss.

Urinalysis: Hematuria frequently indicates associated bladder injury.

Blood Type and Rh: Four to six units of blood are prepared for transfusion as necessary.

ASSESSMENT

ETIOLOGIC FACTORS

1. Uterine scar (cesarean section, myomectomy, cornual resection, prior abortion)
2. Trauma
   a. Operative delivery (version, breech extraction, forceps)
   b. Oxytocin stimulation [particularly when women have had five or more babies (Awais, 1970)]
   c. Automobile accidents
3. Spontaneous rupture of the unscarred uterus (persistent uterine contractions in the face of pelvic obstruction)
   a. Cephalopelvic disproportion
   b. Fetal malpresentation
   c. Fetal anomaly (hydrocephalus)
   d. Multiparity without other cause
   e. Uterine leiomyomas

4. Other factors
   a. Placenta accreta or percreta
   b. Cornual pregnancy
   c. Invasive trophoblastic disease

SEVERITY OF RUPTURE

Rupture of a previous cesarean section scar may be complete or incomplete. The former are characterized by a tear through all layers of the uterus, the latter by an incomplete tear,. usually dehiscence of the uterine wall with minimal bleeding. The complete tears are the most dangerous, particularly if they occur in the uterine fundus. Whenever the tear involves major blood vessels, bleeding is profuse and hemorrhagic shock quickly ensues.

POTENTIAL COMPLICATIONS

Complications to be anticipated include injury to adjacent organs. Bladder injury has been reported in association with 22 per cent of uterine rupture cases (Raghavaiah, 1975). The diagnosis is suggested by finding hematuria or meconium-stained urine.

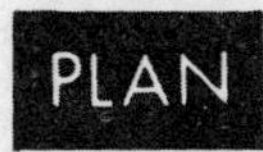

MANAGEMENT AND PATIENT EDUCATION

Supportive Therapy: Correct shock and blood loss. This includes the administration of oxygen, intravenous fluids, blood for replacement, and antibiotics for infection.

Immediate Laparotomy: As soon as the diagnosis is made, preparations are made for surgery. In the meantime, blood volume is restored with intravenous fluids and blood.

After the extent of injury has been determined, the surgeon may have to choose between repairing the uterine defect and performing a hysterectomy. The decision is based on the rupture site, the nature of the tear, the extent of bleeding, the cause of rupture, the presence of a uterine scar, the stage of gestation, the patient's general condition, and her desires concerning future childbearing.

If the tear is smooth, regular, and not excessively friable, repair may be not only feasible but also preferable. Patients in poor condition may tolerate repair of the tear better than they would hysterectomy (Sheth, 1969).

If the tear is irregular, zigzag, edematous, and friable, repair is usually impossible and the only choice is hysterectomy. If the rupture extends into the lower uterine segment, cervix, and vagina, total hysterectomy is virtually always required for control of bleeding. The vagina must be carefully inspected lest hemorrhage persist from an undiscovered vaginal laceration.

When hematuria suggests an associated bladder injury, the latter must also be repaired. Since devitalization of the bladder wall adjoining the uterine tear occurs even more frequently than bladder injury, postoperative bladder drainage with an indwelling catheter for 10 to 14 days is an important aid to healing of the contused, devitalized bladder (Raghavaiah, 1975).

REFERENCES

Awais GM, Lebherz TB: Ruptured uterus. A complication of oxytocin induction and high parity. Obstet Gynecol *36*:465-472, 1970

Beacham WD, Beacham DW, Webster HD, Fielding SL: Rupture of the uterus at New Orleans' Charity Hospital. Am J Obstet Gynecol *106*:1083-1097, 1970

Borenstein R, Katz Z, Lancet M: External rupture of the uterus. Obstet Gynecol *40* 211-213, 1972

Dick JS, de Villiers VP: Spontaneous rupture of the uterus in the second trimester due to placenta percreta: Two case reports. J Obstet Gynaecol Br Commonw *79*:187-189, 1972

Groen GP: Uterine rupture in rural nigeria. Obstet Gynecol *44*:682-687, 1974; Obstet Gynecol Surv *30*:372-373, 1975

Raghavaiah NV, Indira Devi A: Bladder injury associated with rupture of the uterus. Obstet Gynecol *46*:573-576, 1975

Sheth SS: Suturing of the tear as treatment in uterine rupture. Am J Obstet Gynecol *105*:440-443, 1969

Yussman MA, Haynes DM: Rupture of the gravid uterus. Obstet Gynecol *36*:115-120, 1970

101 VAGINAL AND VULVAR TRAUMA

GENERAL CONSIDERATIONS

Vaginal and vulvar trauma may be caused by obstetric lacerations, blows to the perineum, straddling injuries, forcible intercourse (sexual assault), foreign bodies inserted into the vagina, or abortion attempts.

The most frequent sites of injury from coitus are the lateral vaginal wall, posterior fornix, and vaginal vault (after a hysterectomy). Labial hematomas are more likely to result when the perineum absorbs the brunt of the impact from straddle accidents involving the edges of chairs, bathtubs, toilet seats, or the central bar of a bicycle.

SUBJECTIVE DATA

CURRENT SYMPTOMS

Vulvar and vaginal pain, bleeding, and swelling are the most characteristic symptoms. Difficulty in urination and ambulation are other possible symptoms.

PRIOR HISTORY

A history of spontaneous or operative delivery, trauma, or forcible intercourse explains the nature of the injury.

OBJECTIVE DATA

PHYSICAL EXAMINATION

Vulvar examination reveals the severity and extent of contusions, lacerations, or hematoma formations. Vulvar swelling and edema are often associated findings.

Vaginal or rectal examination is necessary to identify vaginal or rectal lacerations or hematomas. Rectovaginal examination may disclose retroperitoneal hematomas. Speculum examination reveals deep vaginal lacerations.

Abdominal Examination: These findings are normal unless there is associated intraperitoneal trauma.

LABORATORY TESTS

Complete blood count assesses blood loss. Serial values are particularly helpful in the identification of persistent concealed bleeding.

Urinalysis, usually a catheter specimen, reveals hematuria when there is associated bladder or urethral trauma.

Blood type and Rh are determined in order to prepare blood in the event that transfusion becomes necessary.

ASSESSMENT

CLASSIFICATION

Obstetric lacerations may be classified as

1. First degree (Fig. 101-1*A*)—tears involving the fourchette, perineal skin, and vaginal mucous membrane without involving underlying muscles.
2. Second degree—tears involving, in addition to perineal skin and vaginal mucous membrane, the muscles of the perineal body but not the sphincter ani.
3. Third degree—tears extending completely through the perineal skin, vaginal mucous membrane, perineal body, and sphincter ani.

4. Fourth degree (Figs. 101-1*B–D*)—tears extending completely through the perineal skin, vaginal mucous membrane, perineal body, sphincter ani, and rectal mucosa.

POTENTIAL COMPLICATIONS

Complications to be anticipated include vesicovaginal or rectovaginal fistulas with incontinence, secondary infections with abscess formation or septicemia or both, and associated injuries to the bony pelvis, bowel, bladder, and peritoneal cavity.

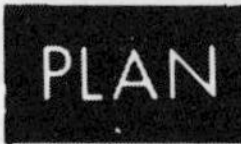

ADDITIONAL DIAGNOSTIC DATA

Pelvic or abdominal x-rays or both may disclose associated bone injuries or free air in the peritoneal cavity.

MANAGEMENT

Lacerations: As long as bleeding is minimal, superficial wounds with simple splitting of the skin and mucous membrane seldom require suturing, since the edges become apposed when the legs are brought together. Deeper lacerations and actively bleeding lacerations require thorough cleansing and surgical repair in order to achieve hemostasis and anatomic reapproximation of the perineum. Careful repair is always essential when injuries involve adjacent structures—urethra, bladder, and rectum—in order to prevent fistula formation.

When blood loss is profuse, intravenous fluids and blood transfusions are indicated.

Hymeneal tears and small vaginal lacerations may be repaired with chromic 000 sutures under local anesthesia. Subsequent cold compresses reduce swelling and pain. More extensive vaginal lacerations may require general anesthesia for adequate repair. Young, frightened patients may also require general anesthesia for adequate repair.

At times, vaginal trauma is so extensive that primary surgical repair is not feasible; under these circumstances, a tight vaginal packing may be

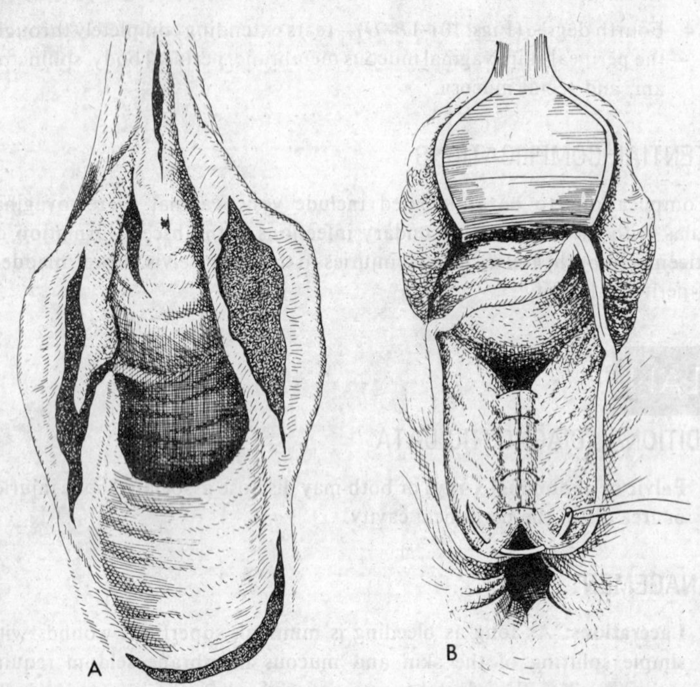

Figure 101-1. *A*, The vulvar structures showing the different varieties of lacerations that can be sustained during delivery. *B*, The first step in repair of fourth degree laceration, showing suturing of rectal mucosa with interrupted atraumatic 000 or 0000 chromic catgut introduced submucosally. A second reinforcing layer of sutures may be placed if the tear is extensive. *C*, Second step in repair, illustrating method for reaching into sphincter pit with Allis or tissue

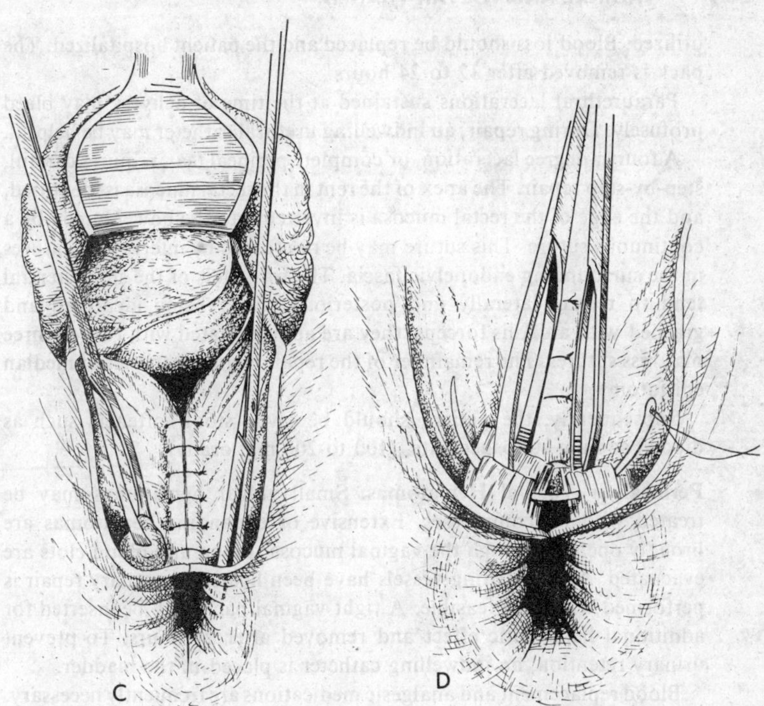

Figure 101-1 *(Continued)*
forceps to grasp and draw up the retracted ends of the sphincter ani muscle. *D*, Third step in the repair, uniting the cut ends of the sphincter ani with figure-eight sutures of 0 chromic catgut. The remainder of the repair is the same as for second degree laceration or episiotomy. (From Greenhill JP, Friedman EA: Biological Principles and Modern Practice of Obstetrics. Philadelphia, W. B. Saunders Co., 1974.)

utilized. Blood loss should be replaced and the patient hospitalized. The pack is removed after 12 to 24 hours.

Paraurethral lacerations sustained at the time of delivery may bleed profusely. During repair, an indwelling urethral catheter may be helpful.

A fourth-degree laceration, or complete perineal tear, requires careful, step-by-step repair. The apex of the rent in the rectal mucosa is identified, and the edge of the rectal mucosa is inverted into the bowel lumen by a continuous suture. This suture may be reinforced by interrupted sutures in the surrounding endopelvic fascia. The torn ends of the sphincter ani tend to retract laterally and posteriorly. After being identified and grasped with an Allis forceps, they are approximated with two or three mattress sutures. The remainder of the repair is similar to that of median episiotomy.

Subsequently, the patient should be given stool softeners such as dioctyl sodium sulfosuccinate, (100 to 200 mg, orally).

Perineal or Vaginal Hematomas: Small vulvar hematomas may be treated with ice compresses. Extensive or expanding hematomas are broadly opened through the vaginal mucosa. Blood and blood clots are evacuated. After bleeding vessels have been ligated, a primary repair is performed whenever feasible. A tight vaginal pack may be inserted for additional hemostatic effect and removed after 24 hours. To prevent urinary retention, an indwelling catheter is placed in the bladder.

Blood replacement and analgesic medications are frequently necessary. Prophylactic antibiotics are usually recommended. Tetanus immunization is also recommended if the hematoma has resulted from external trauma.

Infected hematomas are evacuated and drained. After cultures are obtained, antibiotics are prescribed.

Enlarging broad ligament hematomas require laparotomy for definitive management.

Foreign bodies in the vagina are most commonly encountered in young children. Occasionally, adult females may forget a tampon or sponge in the vagina. Elderly, senile patients are particularly prone to forget a pessary, which can become calcified.

Foreign bodies produce a vaginitis with an unpleasant, malodorous discharge. Sharp objects may cause vaginal lacerations. Most foreign bodies are easily identified and removed in the examining room. Lacerations are repaired and vaginitis treated with an antibacterial cream.

Ruptured vaginal or vulvar varix is treated with compression, initially. Actively bleeding vessels should be ligated.

Penetration of the cul-de-sac warrants exploratory laparotomy in order to rule out injury to intraabdominal viscera.

REFERENCE

Sheikh GN: Perinatal genital hematomas. Obstet Gynecol *38*:571-575, 1971; Obstet Gynecol Surv *27*:247-249, 1972

102 VAGINAL BLEEDING

GENERAL CONSIDERATIONS

Vaginal bleeding at periodic intervals is a normal occurrence from the second to the fifth decades of a woman's life.

Menstruation is the cyclic physiologic discharge of blood, mucus, and cellular debris from the endometrial mucosa that results from hormonal changes produced by the interaction of the ovaries and the anterior pituitary gland. The usual menstrual flow lasts three to seven days, with an average blood loss of 30 to 100 milliliters.

Menarche is the appearance of the first menstrual period, generally between ages 11 and 16. The average age of onset is 12.

Menopause is the transitional phase in a woman's life during which menstrual function ceases. Synonyms include *climacteric* and *change of life*. Age 50 is the median age for the last menstrual period.

Menstrual cycle is the period extending from the onset of one normal menstrual period to the onset of the next normal period; generally, it lasts from 21 to 37 days. Histologic and biochemical events occurring in the endometrium, characterized by endometrial proliferation, secretion, and regression, are produced by the cyclic stimulation of estrogen and progesterone.

Proliferative phase of the menstrual cycle begins at the end of menstruation and ends at the time of ovulation. During the early proliferative phase, the superficial epithelium is thin, glands are sparse and nontortuous, and the lumina are narrow. As proliferation continues, under the stimulus of estrogen from the ovarian follicle, endometrial glands become more tortuous and mitoses are seen in both the glands and stroma. Variations of menstrual cycle length reflect a longer or shorter proliferative phase.

Secretory Phase: Immediately after ovulation (36 to 48 hours), subnuclear glycogen-containing vacuoles develop between the nuclei of the glandular cells and the basement membrane. Under the influence of estrogen and progesterone, endometrial glands increase in tortuosity and have pseudostratified nuclei. From the sixth postovulatory day to the time of menstruation, the glands show marked tortuosity and maximal secretion into the lumina. The secretory or luteal phase generally lasts 14 plus or minus 2 days, and specific endometrial changes during this time permit relatively exact endometrial dating.

The blood supply to the endometrium increases progressively during the menstrual cycle. The *straight* arteries, arising from arcuate vessels of the myometrium, supply the basal portion of the endometrium and are not greatly affected by estrogen and progesterone. The *spiral* arteries of the endometrium grow rapidly following estrogen stimulation during the proliferative phase. During the secretory phase, the spiral arteries become coiled as they outgrow the thickness of the endometrium.

Menstruation is the normal endometrial response to the withdrawal of estrogen and progesterone hormones. Modest shrinking of tissue height, diminished blood flow within the spiral vessels, decreased venous drainage, and vasodilatation are the initial, immediate effects of hormone withdrawal. Thereafter, the spiral arterioles undergo rhythmic vasoconstriction and relaxation. Each successive spasm is more prolonged and profound, leading to endometrial blanching, ischemia, and stasis. Interstitial hemorrhage results from breaks in superficial arterioles and capillaries. With progressive disorganization, the endometrium shrinks further, and coiled arterioles are buckled.

Ischemic breakdown causes stromal degeneration and desquamation.

Important characteristics of normal estrogen-progesterone withdrawal bleeding, contributing to its self-limiting nature, are the following:

1. Menstrual changes tend to be initiated simultaneously in all segments of the uterine endometrium.
2. The endometrial tissue that has responded to estrogen and progesterone is structurally stable. The events leading to ischemic

disintegration are orderly and progressive, being related to increasing waves of vasoconstriction.

3. The vasomotor rhythmicity inherent in the initiation of menstruation is also responsible for its termination. Just as waves of vasoconstriction initiate the ischemic events provoking menses, so does prolonged vasoconstriction, abetted by the stasis associated with endometrial collapse, account for the cessation of menstrual flow. Resumed estrogen secretion effectuates endometrial reconstruction and growth.

During normal menstrual flow, platelets adhere to blood vessel walls; platelet aggregation, plus serum glycoproteins, forms a temporary vascular plug. A permanent fibrin clot is never formed, as is evidenced by the absence of fibrin-split products in the menstrual flow. Consequently, factors associated with fibrin formation from fibrinogen are *not* required for cessation of menstrual flow. Abnormalities of platelets and platelet aggregation, however, are associated with abnormalities of menstrual bleeding.

Abnormal Vaginal Bleeding: Vaginal bleeding is considered abnormal if the woman has never established a regular pattern, if the bleeding pattern changes, or if bleeding occurs during the interval between menstrual periods. Abnormal bleeding can occur at any age, lasts a few hours to several weeks, varies from spotting to profuse, life-threatening hemorrhage, and may be associated with the passage of clots or tissues (Table 102-1). Abnormal vaginal bleeding may be classified into three major categories:

1. *Anatomic factors*—pregnancy complications or organic pelvic disease (see Table 102-2)
2. *Systemic problems* reflected in pelvic symptoms—blood dyscrasias,* hypertension, exogenous medications
3. *Dysfunctional uterine bleeding*—abnormal bleeding unassociated with tumor, inflammation, or pregnancy (usually endocrine dysfunction.) (see Dysfunctional Uterine Bleeding, p. 286)

*Associated with abnormalities of platelets or platelet aggregation.

TABLE 102-1. Causes of Abnormal Uterine Bleeding By Age Groups

Age	Cause
Newborn	Maternal estrogen Bleeding tendencies
3 to 7 years	Foreign body in vagina Trauma Sarcoma botryoides Granulosa cell tumors
Menarche	Precocious puberty Blood dyscrasias Emotional states Anovulation

Reproductive age	Organic causes
	  Pelvic inflammation
	  Chronic cervicitis
	  Polyps
	  Fibroids
	  Cancer of cervix or uterus
	  Hormones
	  Blood dyscrasias
	  Granulosa cell tumors
	Pregnancy
	  Abortion
	  Ectopic pregnancy
	  Hydatid mole
	Endocrine causes
	  Thyroid disturbances
	  Emotional states
	  Excess estrogen
	  Anovulation
	  Irregular shedding

Menopause	Cancer of cervix or endometrium Anovulation
Postmenopausal	Cancer of uterus or cervix Exogenous hormones Granulosa cell tumor Senile vaginitis Retained pessaries Benign polyps

TABLE 102-2. Anatomical Factors of Abnormal Vaginal Bleeding

Site	Diagnosis
Vulva and Vagina	Infection—vulvitis, vaginitis Trauma—coitus, obstetric trauma, accidents Tumor Foreign body—most common cause of bleeding in children
Cervix	Cervicitis—erosion, ectropion, eversion Polyp Carcinoma Postconization or cauterization Cervical pregnancy Endometriosis
Uterus	Pregnancy complications Endometritis Endometrial hyperplasia Tumors—benign, malignant Cirsoid aneurysm—arteriovenous fistula Adenomyosis Exogenous estrogens or oral contraceptives Intrauterine device
Adnexa	Ectopic Pregnancy Salpingo-oophoritis Ovarian cysts and tumors Endometriosis Fallopian tube tumor

DEFINITIONS (Abnormal Vaginal Bleeding)

Menorrhagia or **hypermenorrhea**—excessive or prolonged menstrual bleeding.

Metrorrhagia—uterine bleeding independent of the menstrual period.

Menometrorrhagia—irregular or excessive bleeding during menstruation and between menstrual periods.

Polymenorrhea—increased frequency of menstrual bleeding.

SUBJECTIVE DATA

CURRENT SYMPTOMS

Vaginal Bleeding: Attention is paid to its quantity, duration, and color and to the interval between this episode and previous bleeding.

Quantity:

Gushing vaginal bleeding usually suggests a pregnancy complication, malignancy, fibroid polyp, or dysfunctional uterine bleeding.

Spotting or staining following a missed period may represent a threatened abortion or ectopic pregnancy. Oral contraceptives may be associated with intermenstrual spotting, particularly during the initial cycles.

Duration of bleeding often helps distinguish normal menses from reproductive tract abnormalities. Once menses have become established, the patient is usually aware of the normal duration of menstrual flow; any deviation from normal tends to be a cause for concern.

The presence of an intrauterine device may be associated with profuse and prolonged menstrual periods. The necessity for removal of the device depends on the extent of the patient's discomfort.

Repeated episodes of hypermenorrhea (menorrhagia) may imply an ovulatory cycle complicated by leiomyomas or adenomyosis. Heavier than usual bleeding may be caused by endometrial polyps, although intermenstrual bleeding or spotting, postmenstrual staining, and postmenopausal bleeding are also symptoms of endometrial polyps.

Systemic diseases of nonreproductive organs can cause abnormal cyclic bleeding manifested by hypermenorrhea. Menorrhagia is seen more frequently with hypothyroidism than with hyperthyroidism, although it can be present with either condition.

Blood dyscrasias associated with platelet abnormalities and the use of anticoagulant drugs are also possible explanations for excessive menstrual bleeding.

Endometrial hyperplasia, polyps, or *cancer* may be responsible for profuse hemorrhage or persistent endometrial bleeding. Endometrial hyperplasia results from persistent estrogenic stimulation, secondary to either anovulation or exogenous hormone therapy.

Color of the blood helps distinguish current active bleeding from a more chronic process. Bright red bleeding is active bleeding that may be caused by a pregnancy complication, acute laceration, and so forth. Brown staining is an indication that blood in the vagina has been altered by cervical or vaginal secretions.

Interval between the onset of the current bleeding episode and the previous menses must be interpreted in relation to the patient's menstrual history. *Cyclic* bleeding, occurring at regular, predictable intervals, usually implies ovulation. *Noncyclic* bleeding, unpredictable bleeding episodes without a regular rhythm, may be due to irregular ovulation, anovulation, or a specific pelvic pathologic condition. Bleeding after an interval of amenorrhea is usually due to a pregnancy complication. Persistent bleeding of less-than-normal volume at the time of an expected period may be symptomatic of ectopic pregnancy or threatened abortion. (Implantation bleeding may produce bleeding for one day similar to or less than that of the first day of a normal cycle.)

Intermenstrual bleeding may be caused by adenomyosis, leiomyomata, polyps, hyperplasia, and uterine carcinoma. Endometrial hyperplasia is generally associated with lack of ovulation and persistent estrogenic stimulation of the endometrium. Although patients with endometrial hyperplasia may have regular periods combined with intermenstrual bleeding, they are most likely to have noncyclic bleeding and episodes of prolonged, profuse uterine hemorrhage (see Dysfunctional Uterine Bleeding, p. 286).

Intermenstrual bleeding following intercourse or douching may be caused by cervical eversion, ectropion, erosion, polyps, or malignancy.

Midcycle bleeding is attributed to the decrease of estrogen levels prior to ovulation. Although gross bleeding or spotting is uncommon, many women are aware of slight staining associated with lower abdominal pain due to stretching of the ovarian capsule at the time of ovulation.

Associated Symptoms:
Fever and pain tend to suggest pelvic infection. Uterine cramps and pregnancy symptoms suggest a gestational abnormality.

The patient's age may provide a clue to the likely pathologic condition. Anovulatory, dysfunctional bleeding is most common during the perimenarchal and perimenopausal years. After the menopause, bleeding may be caused by cancer, polyps, or estrogen-induced hyperplasia.

Generalized petechiae or ecchymoses or both, epistaxis, or bleeding from other sites suggests a coagulation disorder.

PRIOR HISTORY

Contraceptive history is helpful. The patient taking oral contraceptives is not likely to be pregnant, although she may have breakthrough bleeding or even an ectopic pregnancy. On the other hand, the patient with an intrauterine device is more likely to have a heavy period, pelvic infection, or ectopic pregnancy.

A history of easy bruising, bleeding tendencies, recent surgery or trauma, exogenous hormonal therapy, or anticoagulant therapy must be considered in the diagnostic evaluation.

OBJECTIVE DATA

PHYSICAL EXAMINATION

General Examination: Temperature elevation suggests pelvic infection. Tachycardia and hypotension may signify hypovolemia (profuse blood loss or sepsis). When external blood loss is not sufficient to account for the patient's symptoms, intraperitoneal bleeding must be suspected.

Generalized petechiae or ecchymoses may be the first clue to a coagulation disorder.

Abdominal Examination: Inspection and palpation may reveal an obvious pregnancy or evidence of peritoneal irritation.

Pelvic examination is essential to determine the exact site and cause of vaginal bleeding. During the latter half of pregnancy, however, special precautions are necessary since vaginal bleeding may be due to placenta previa. (See Vaginal Bleeding—Late Pregnancy, p. 699.)

Initially, speculum examination discloses the quantity of blood in the vagina as well as the source of bleeding. Visualization of the vagina and cervix identifies vaginal lacerations, cervical lesions, and bleeding from the cervical os.

Severe vaginitis or a foreign body in the vagina may cause sufficient mucosal irritation to produce a bloody discharge. Foreign bodies are more likely to be found in young children or mentally defective adults. However, a forgotten tampon or a pessary may cause severe vaginitis with bleeding and a fetid odor.

Malignant cervical and vaginal lesions tend to be friable and bleed readily.

Scant, dark blood in the vagina indicates older bleeding, whereas bright red blood, particularly with clots, suggests an active bleeding process. Bleeding associated with a foul-smelling vaginal discharge implies pelvic infection.

The diagnosis of incomplete or complete abortion becomes obvious when the cervical os is dilated and products of conception are visualized in the cervical canal or vagina.

Bimanual examination frequently identifies the pelvic pathologic condition responsible for bleeding. Symmetrical uterine enlargement during the childbearing years is usually the result of pregnancy; asymmetrical, irregular uterine enlargement is more characteristic of multiple leiomyomata. Correlating the depth of the uterine cavity, measured with a uterine sound, with the bimanual examination may be helpful. Adenomyosis and uterine malignancy are other possible explanations for uterine enlargement. Particularly after the menopause, malignancy must always be considered.

If the uterus is smaller than expected from the menstrual history, a diagnosis of ectopic pregnancy, missed abortion, or complete abortion should be considered. A uterus larger than the expected gestational size may result from a molar pregnancy, multiple pregnancy, or pregnancy in a fibroid uterus.

Palpation of the adnexa is essential in order to assess the possibility of ovarian cysts, tumors, pelvic infection, or ectopic pregnancy. Adnexal tenderness combined with vaginal bleeding is a frequent finding in cases of pelvic infection or ectopic pregnancy. The triad of missed menses, vaginal bleeding, and unilateral adnexal pain and tenderness is always highly suspicious of ectopic pregnancy.

An adnexal mass associated with postmenopausal bleeding may be caused by a carcinoma of the fallopian tube.

LABORATORY TESTS

Complete Blood Count with Blood Smear: Hemoglobin and hematocrit determinations provide an indirect measurement of blood loss. With dehydration, these values tend to be elevated. During acute hemorrhage, the hematocrit remains normal until compensatory mechanisms come into play. (Time is required for the fluid shift from the extravascular compartment to replenish the circulating blood volume and cause a dilutional decrease in the hematocrit.) Allowing for mixing time, each 500 ml of blood lost causes approximately a 3 per cent fall in hematocrit.

Evaluation of red cell indices and the cells on blood smear helps distinguish acute hemorrhage from chronic blood loss. With chronic bleeding, the red cells are usually hypochromic and microcytic, whereas with acute hemorrhage, the red cells are normochromic and normocytic unless the patient has a preexisting anemia.

Leukocytosis with a shift to the left in the differential count, increased bands, and increased polymorphonuclear leukocytes usually signifies infection.

ASSESSMENT

ETIOLOGIC FACTORS

1. Pregnancy complications
   a. Implantation bleeding
   b. Abortion
   c. Ectopic pregnancy
   d. Molar pregnancy, trophoblastic disease
   e. Placental complications
   f. Vasa previa
   g. Retained products of conception
   h. Subinvolution of uterus after pregnancy
2. Infection and inflammation
   a. Vulvitis with excoriation
   b. Vaginitis
   c. Cervicitis

d. Endometritis
e. Salpingo-oophoritis

3. Hyperplasia and neoplasia—benign and malignant
   a. Vagina—carcinoma, metastatic trophoblastic disease, sarcoma botryoides
   b. Cervix—polyp, papilloma, carcinoma
   c. Endometrium—hyperplasia, polyp, carcinoma, sarcoma, trophoblastic disease
   d. Myometrium—Leiomyoma, leiomyosarcoma, endolymphatic stromal myosis (hemangiopericytoma)
   e. Ovary—Granulosa theca-cell tumors produce estrogen; other tumors or cysts may stimulate ovarian stromal hormones.
   f. Fallopian tube—Carcinoma
4. Hormonal abnormalities
   a. Hypothalamic-pituitary-ovarian dysfunction
      (1) Anovulatory bleeding—see Dysfunctional Uterine Bleeding, p. 286
      (2) Ovulatory bleeding (irregular shedding or irregular secretory development)
   b. Ovarian functional cysts producing hormones
      (1) Follicle cysts producing estrogen
      (2) Corpus luteum or luteal cysts producing estrogen and progesterone
   c. Exogenous hormones
      (1) Estrogens
      (2) Estrogen-progestin oral contraceptives
   d. Thyroid dysfunction—hypothyroidism is more likely than hyperthyroidism to cause irregular vaginal bleeding
   e. Psychogenic disturbances
5. Trauma
   a. Postoperative bleeding
   b. Obstetric lacerations
   c. Foreign body in vagina
   d. Intrauterine device
6. Endometriosis
7. Adenomyosis
8. Cirsoid aneurysm—arteriovenous fistula
9. Hematologic or systemic disorders
   a. Thrombocytopenia
   b. Von Willebrand's disease

c. Anticoagulant therapy
d. Disseminated intravascular coagulation
e. Hypertension
f. Hypothyroidism (or hyperthyroidism)
g. Leukemia
h. Hepatic disease

DIFFERENTIAL DIAGNOSIS

The differential diagnosis of bleeding following missed menses includes the following:

1. Bleeding within six to eight weeks of the last menstrual period
   a. Early pregnancy: implantation bleeding, abortion, ectopic pregnancy
   b. Anovulatory bleeding
   c. Delayed ovulation or persistent corpus luteum with subsequent withdrawal bleeding
2. Bleeding within 8 to 20 weeks following last menstrual period
   a. Pregnancy complication: abortion, ectopic pregnancy, molar pregnancy
   b. Anovulatory bleeding

SEVERITY OF BLEEDING

The quantity of bleeding must be evaluated. Severe anemia, hypovolemia, and shock demand immediate measures to stop the bleeding as well as appropriate fluid and blood replacement.

Any bleeding, even spotting, after the menopause is abnormal. The possibility of cancer must be ruled out by a cervical cytologic test and endometrial curettage.

PLAN

ADDITIONAL DIAGNOSTIC DATA

Endometrial biopsy or curettage provides a specific histologic diagnosis. Curettage has the added advantage of controlling excessive bleeding and is often both diagnostic and therapeutic.

Endometrial polyps may be discovered and removed in the course of uterine curettage for the diagnosis of unexplained endometrial bleeding.

Bleeding after the menopause may be due to exogenous estrogenic stimulation, endogenous estrogens, endometrial cancer, or atrophic changes. A tissue diagnosis is mandatory.

Endometrial carcinoma is predominantly a disease of postmenopausal women, most prevalent in women 60 to 70 years old. Associated diseases may include obesity, hypertension, and diabetes. Associated genital disease may include leiomyomas and polycystic ovaries. When an early lesion is present, the uterus is frequently of normal size or only slightly enlarged or softened. Treatment depends on uterine size, tumor differentiation, myometrial invasion and endocervical involvement. Usually, surgery, with or without radiotherapy, is indicated.

Biopsy of Vulva, Vagina, or Cervix: Actively bleeding lesions of the vulva, vagina, or cervix should be biopsied, with the exception of a dark, hemorrhagic vaginal nodule resembling a thrombosed varix that appears subsequent to a molar pregnancy. Such a lesion is typical of metastatic trophoblastic disease and could bleed profusely if biopsied. (See Molar Pregnancy, p. 430.)

Cervical discharge should be sent to the bacteriology laboratory for Gram stain and culture, particularly if pelvic infection is suspected.

Pregnancy test for chorionic gonadotropin is often very helpful. A positive test strongly suggests functioning trophoblastic tissue, either intrauterine or extrauterine. A negative test, however, does not rule out an extrauterine pregnancy.

Serial Hematocrit Determinations: During and immediately after a major hemorrhage, the hematocrit remains unchanged, since whole blood is lost from the circulation and time is required for the fluid shift from the extravascular compartment to replenish the circulating blood volume and cause a dilutional decrease in the hematocrit. Serial determinations, however, are of great value in the assessment of blood loss.

Coagulation tests (platelet count, prothrombin time, partial thromboplastin time, fibrinogen, and fibrin-split products) can be very helpful whenever a coagulation disorder is suspected.

Thyroid function tests are rarely required under emergency situations. They may be indicated during follow-up evaluations, however.

MANAGEMENT AND PATIENT EDUCATION

The necessity for emergency hospitalization depends on the quantity of blood lost and evidence of anemia or hypovolemia. When vaginal bleeding is profuse, emergency management includes intravenous fluids, blood transfusion, and an immediate etiologic diagnosis. Therapy must be based on the specific diagnosis; arrangements for follow-up care are essential.

Specific measures that may be indicated include

1. Endometrial curettage for retained products of conception (see Abortion, p. 84.)
2. Antibiotics for pelvic infection (see p. 474)
3. Hormonal therapy for dysfunctional uterine bleeding (see p. 286)
4. Vaginal or cervical packing for malignant cervical lesions (see p. 189)
5. Laparotomy for ectopic pregnancy (see p. 311)
6. Suturing for vaginal lacerations (see p. 679)
7. Radiation for malignant lesions
8. Removal of an intrauterine device
9. Hysterectomy for leiomyomata

Vaginal Bleeding During Late Pregnancy (After 20 Weeks)

GENERAL CONSIDERATIONS

The dividing line between abortion and premature labor is the twentieth gestational week. A fetus with a gestational age of 20 weeks weighs approximately 400 gm and is considered legally viable. Vaginal bleeding during the latter half of pregnancy, after the twentieth week, occurs in approximately 3 per cent of all pregnancies. Not only is this abnormal symptom associated with an increased maternal risk, but also there is a high rate of perinatal loss.

Although vaginal bleeding may be either maternal or fetal in origin, most bleeding results from a placental abnormality or a lesion in the reproductive tract. In general, any patient with painless, bright red bleeding during the latter half of pregnancy, must be suspected to have a placenta previa, until it is proved that she does not.

SUBJECTIVE DATA

CURRENT SYMPTOMS

Vaginal bleeding associated with placenta previa is usually bright red. Bleeding associated with premature placental separation tends to be darker in color, since this type of bleeding is often initially concealed.

Abdominal pain is usually absent in cases of placenta previa, unless there are associated uterine contractions. Continuous, persistent abdominal pain is frequently associated with premature placental separation and may signify blood distending or infiltrating the myometrium.

Intermittent abdominal pain associated with vaginal bleeding with bloody mucous suggests the bloody show of labor.

Severe lower abdominal pain with systemic evidence of shock may signify uterine rupture.

PRIOR HISTORY

A history of previous abruption, hypertensive disease, or renal disease suggests premature placental separation.

OBJECTIVE DATA

PHYSICAL EXAMINATION

General Examination: With placenta previa, all blood loss is external. Therefore, blood pressure and pulse reflect the external blood loss.

Bleeding in cases of premature separation of the placenta may be both external and concealed. Consequently, tachycardia and hypotension may be out of proportion to the external blood loss. Patients with hypertension must always be suspected of having premature placental separation.

Abdominal Examination: The uterine size is compared with gestational age; when it is larger than expected, concealed bleeding should be suspected.

In cases of placenta previa, the uterine tone tends to be normal, without any evidence of uterine tenderness. In cases of premature placental separation, the uterus tends to be hypertonic, firm, and rigid, with generalized or localized tenderness.

Uterine contractions coincident with vaginal bleeding suggest cervical dilatation and bleeding from the cervix or placental margin.

Fetal presentation may aid in the differential diagnosis. When placenta previa occurs, the fetal presenting part is palpable above the pelvic brim, since the placenta occupies the lower uterine segment; the fetus may be in a breech, oblique, or transverse lie.

When premature placental separation occurs, the fetal presenting part is more likely to be well engaged in the pelvis.

Fetal heart tones are usually normal in cases of placenta previa, whereas with a severe placental separation, fetal demise or fetal distress may be expected.

Vaginal examination is *never* performed in the emergency room when there is any question of placenta previa, since vaginal or rectal examination could produce a torrential, fatal hemorrhage. Until placenta previa has been ruled out, vaginal examination should be performed only under "double set-up" conditions, that is, in an operating room or delivery suite prepared for immediate cesarean section in the event this becomes necessary.

LABORATORY TESTS

Urinalysis is usually normal unless there is an associated preeclampsia. Hematuria may, on occasion, be mistaken for vaginal bleeding.

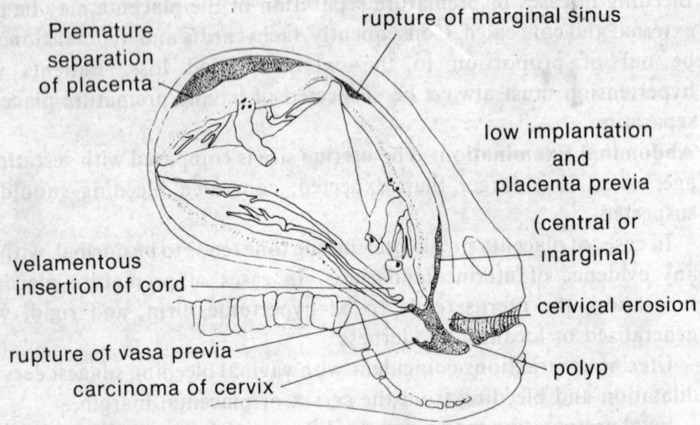

Figure 102-1. Causes of bleeding in late pregnancy. (From Douglas RG, Buchman MI, Macdonald FA: Premature separation of the normally implanted placenta. J Obstet Gynaecol Br Empire 62:710, 1955.)

ASSESSMENT

DIFFERENTIAL DIAGNOSIS

This includes *placental*, *fetal*, and *maternal* sources of bleeding. (See Table 102-3.)

Placenta previa and placental separation are the most frequent serious causes of bleeding in late pregnancy.

Ruptured marginal sinus or circumvallate placenta are diagnoses that can be made only in retrospect after delivery. Bleeding is usually minimal and not accompanied by abdominal pain. Rarely is there any danger to the mother or fetus.

Vasa previa is a rare but serious cause of painless vaginal bleeding caused by a velamentous insertion of the umbilical cord, which allows placental vessels to traverse the membranes. The umbilical vessels may be ruptured by pressure from the fetal head or as a result of spontaneous or artificial rupture of the membranes. The blood loss is fetal. Absent or abnormal

TABLE 102-3. Bleeding in Late Pregnancy

Source	Diagnosis	Clinical Features
Placental	Placenta previa	Painless, bright red bleeding—sudden onset
	Placenta, premature separation	Bleeding associated with painful, tender, irritable uterus
	Marginal sinus rupture	Painless bleeding—diagnosis only made after delivery when an organized thrombus is identified at placental margin.
	Placenta, circumvallate	Painless, intermittent bleeding. Diagnosis made after delivery by recognition of placenta with peripheral portion of chorion turned inward forming a cufflike ring.
Fetal	Vasa previa	Fetal blood identified
Maternal	Bloody show	Blood mixed with mucus, uterine contractions
	Cervical dilatation	Cervical dilatation
	Cervicitis, erosion polyp, malignancy	Identification by speculum examination
	Laceration of genital tract	Identification by speculum examination or history
	Uterine rupture	Sudden severe pain and shock
	Varicose vein rupture, vaginal or vulvar	Visual identification
	Vaginal infections	Speculum examination
	Coagulation disorders	Other systemic evidence of bleeding
	Hemorrhoids	Rectal bleeding
	Cystitis	Hematuria

fetal heart sounds associated with painless vaginal bleeding suggest the diagnosis. (See Vasa Previa, p. 706.)

Uterine rupture is very rare and characterized by sudden severe pain. (See Uterine Rupture, p. 674.)

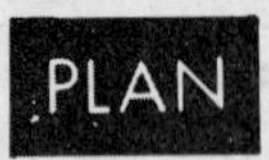

MANAGEMENT

Any patient with active vaginal bleeding during the latter half of pregnancy is admitted to the hospital for evaluation. Whenever there is any question of placenta previa, vaginal or rectal examination is *not* done until or unless the patient is in an operating room prepared for immediate cesarean section which may become necessary. (See Placenta Previa, p. 510.)

Initial emergency management depends on the extent of blood loss and the stage of gestation.

Vital signs (blood pressure, pulse, and respiration) are closely monitored.

Ventilation and oxygen exchange (clearing of the airway and giving of oxygen, if necessary) are essential.

Intravenous fluids, usually 1000 ml of 5 per cent dextrose in lactated Ringer's solution, are initiated.

Blood is prepared for transfusion in case this becomes necessary.

Abdominal examination provides an evaluation of the approximate duration of pregnancy; fetal size, presentation, and heart rate; and uterine contractions, resting tone, and tenderness.

Fetal monitoring provides an evaluation of the base-line fetal heart rate, variability, and reactivity, as well as evidence of intermittent uterine contractions.

Urine output is closely monitored if there is any suggestion of hypovolemia. Proteinuria suggests premature placental separation associated with preeclampsia.

Serial hemoglobin and hematocrit determinations are particularly helpful when there is any question of occult bleeding.

Coagulation tests may disclose a coagulopathy associated with severe placental separation. (See Premature Separation of the Placenta, p. 502.)

Kleihauer test on the vaginal blood may detect fetal bleeding. Although rare, vasa previa should be considered as a possible cause of painless vaginal bleeding associated with fetal distress. (See Vasa Previa, p. 706.)

Ultrasound B-scan is the preferred method for placental localization when bleeding is minimal and the fetus is premature. (See Placenta Previa, p. 510.)

Double Set-up Precautions: When bleeding is life threatening or the pregnancy is near term, the patient is examined in an operating room prepared for immediate vaginal or abdominal delivery.

Speculum examination of the vagina and cervix can rule out local traumatic or neoplastic causes of bleeding. The time and place for such an examination depends on the strength of the suspicion of placenta previa versus that of a vaginal or cervical pathologic condition.

103 VASA PREVIA

GENERAL CONSIDERATIONS

Vasa previa is a rare anomaly of the umbilical cord resulting from a velamentous insertion, a condition in which the umbilical vessels separate in the membranes some distance from the edge of the placenta. The fetal blood vessels cross the internal cervical os and present ahead of the fetal presenting part. Vasa previa is associated with a high rate of fetal mortality, which results from exsanguination from torn vessels or vascular occlusion by the presenting part. The fetal vessels may be torn when the membranes rupture or by pressure from the fetal head.

SUBJECTIVE AND OBJECTIVE DATA

Vaginal bleeding, bright red and painless, is the most characteristic symptom.

Fetal heart tones may be slow and irregular, indicating fetal distress. Absent fetal heart tones indicate fetal exsanguination.

Fetal vessels may be palpated on vaginal examination. There is no evidence of maternal blood loss.

ASSESSMENT

DIFFERENTIAL DIAGNOSIS

This includes maternal causes of third trimester bleeding (placenta previa, premature placental separation, bloody show, and so forth.) See Vaginal Bleeding, Late Pregnancy, p. 699.)

PLAN

ADDITIONAL DIAGNOSTIC DATA

A sample of the vaginal blood is sent to the laboratory for determination of fetal hemoglobin.

Kleihauer test is very sensitive to small amounts of fetal blood. The blood film is examined after incubation at an acid pH (Fig. 103-1); maternal cells lyse, and fetal blood cells are counted.

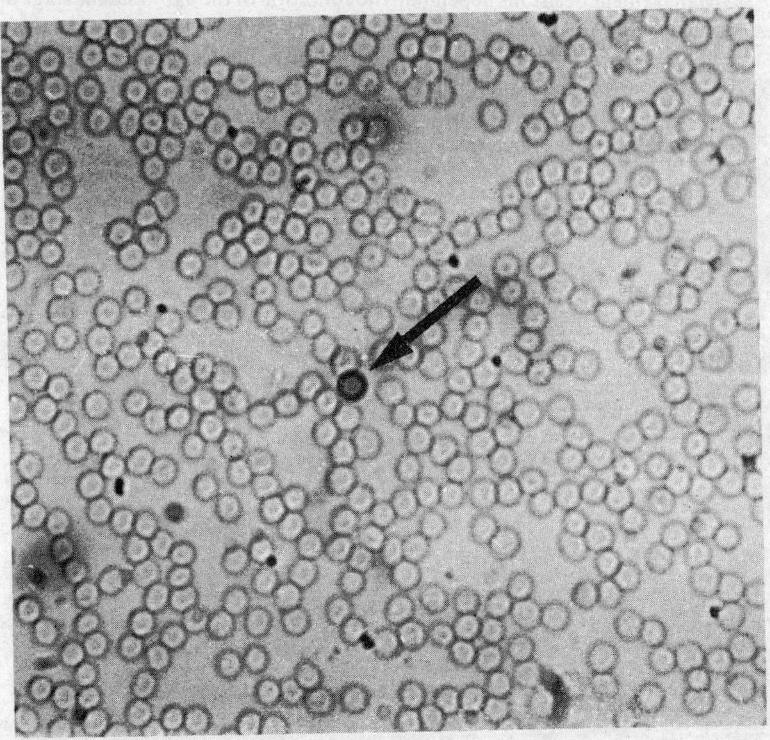

Figure 103-1. Kleihauer-Betke smear of maternal blood showing a fetal erythrocyte (arrow). (From Barber HBK, Graber EA: Surgical Disease in Pregnancy. Philadelphia, W. B. Saunders Co., 1974.)

Apt test is based on the resistance of fetal hemoglobin to alkali. Fetal hemoglobin remains pink, whereas maternal hemoglobin turns yellow.

Blood smear may reveal fetal nucleated red cells.

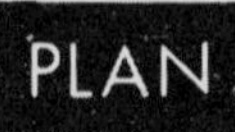

MANAGEMENT AND PATIENT EDUCATION

Management decisions depend on the condition of the baby and the stage of maturity. If the baby is alive and viable, prompt delivery, usually by cesarean section, is essential for fetal survival. Often the infant is anemic and may require blood transfusion after birth.

If the heart tones are absent and the baby is dead, there is no urgency for immediate delivery, since vasa previa does not create any maternal danger.

104 VULVOVAGINITIS

GENERAL CONSIDERATIONS

Vulvovaginitis—inflammation of the vulva and vagina—may be caused by a number of different irritants, most commonly, *Candida albicans, Trichomonas vaginalis, Hemophilus vaginalis,* and herpes simplex virus. Other causative factors include estrogen deficiency (atrophic vaginitis), chemical irritants, allergic reactions, and foreign bodies.

SUBJECTIVE DATA

Age of Patient: Prior to puberty, a foreign body in the vagina is a common cause of foul-smelling vaginal discharge. After the menopause, atrophic vaginitis is a common cause of vulvar irritation and pruritus.

Vaginal Discharge: The color, odor, and consistency of the vaginal discharge provide the first clue to diagnosis. Candidiasis is characterized by a white, curdlike discharge. Trichomoniasis tends to cause a greenish-gray, frothy, fetid discharge. *Hemophilus vaginalis* produces a grayish, thin, malodorous discharge.

Normal vaginal discharge is clear and acid (pH 3.5 to 4.5), tending to be maximal at the midportion of the menstrual cycle. During pregnancy, there is an increased physiologic discharge, possibly due to estrogenic stimulation and increased vascularity.

Vaginal bleeding or spotting may be caused by atrophic vaginitis in postmenopausal patients.

Pruritus may be caused by candidiasis or trichomoniasis.

Irritation: Swelling, redness, and burning are nonspecific symptoms usually associated with vulvar and vaginal inflammations.

Associated Symptoms: Fever and malaise suggest the possibility of a disseminated viral or bacterial infection. Skin lesions on other parts of the body suggest the possibility of a generalized dermatologic disorder with vulvar manifestations (psoriasis, seborrheic dermatitis, lichen planus). Dysuria, or urinary retention, may be associated with herpes genitalis.

PRIOR HISTORY

Use of vulvar sprays or douches, cosmetics, or contraceptive jellies or creams may cause a chemical irritation. A history of diabetes, antibiotic therapy, or pregnancy suggests the possibility of candidiasis.

OBJECTIVE DATA

Vulvar Examination (skin color, ulceration, induration):

Erythema is most commonly observed with candidiasis, contact vulvitis, allergic vulvitis, and urinary incontinence.

Ulcerations (see Figs. 104-1 to 104-6): Multiple vesicles or superficial ulcers or both are usually due to herpes simplex virus, Type II. A single, painless, indurated ulcer may be a syphilitic chancre. A tender, painful, suppurative ulcer, irregular in shape and softer than the syphilitic chancre, may represent chancroid.

Papillary warts are usually condylomata acuminata. The lesions are flesh-colored, cauliflower-like papules occurring singly or in groups.

Bartholin's and Skene's Glands: Acute inflammation of these glands can be caused by *Neisseria gonorrhoeae.* The gland duct is surrounded by erythema and exudes a purulent discharge.

Inguinal lymphadenopathy may be associated with herpes genitalis, chancroid, lymphogranuloma venereum, or syphilis.

Speculum Examination of Vagina and Cervix:

Vaginal Discharge: Thick white, curdlike ("cottage cheese") exudate adherent in patches to the vaginal mucosa is suggestive of candidiasis. A greenish-gray, frothy, fetid fluid discharge pooled in the vaginal fornix close to the cervix and associated with numerous red points

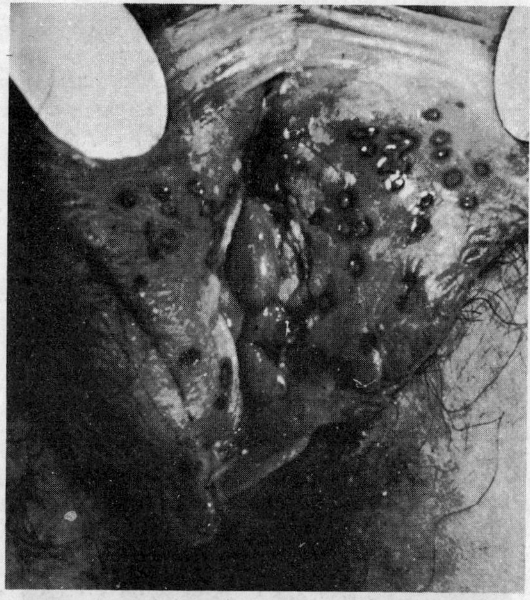

Figure 104-1. Herpes genitalis on labia. (From Domonkos AN: Andrews' Diseases of the Skin. 6th ed. Philadelphia, W.B. Saunders Co., 1971.)

("strawberry patches") scattered over the vaginal surface and cervix is indicative of trichomoniasis. A homogeneous, gray, malodorous discharge adherent to the vaginal wall in a thin film suggests *Hemophilus vaginalis* infection.

A foreign body in the vagina, including a forgotten tampon or diaphragm, may produce a foul-smelling discharge.

Vaginal Mucosa: Hyperemia and petechiae are seen in cases of trichomoniasis. Pale, flat, dry, fissured vaginal mucosa with capillary petechiae and small areas of superficial hemorrhage are characteristic of atrophic vaginitis associated with estrogen deficiency, particularly in the postmenopausal patient.

Purulent cervical discharge may be caused by *Neisseria gonorrhoeae.*

(Text continued on p. 715)

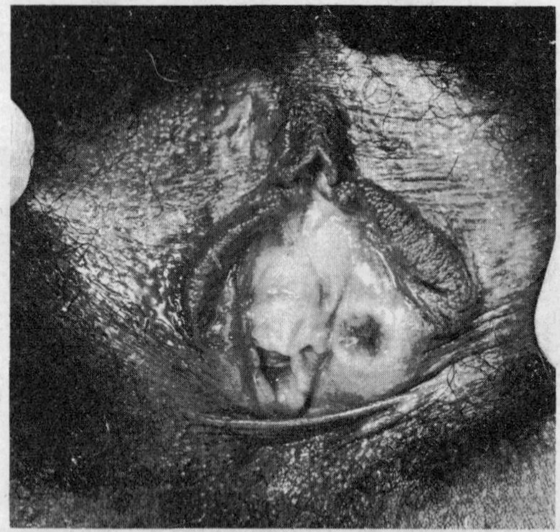

Figure 104-2. Chancre on inner surface of left labium minus. (From Novak ER, Woodruff JD: Novak's Gynecologic and Obstetric Pathology. 7th ed. Philadelphia, W.B. Saunders Co., 1974.)

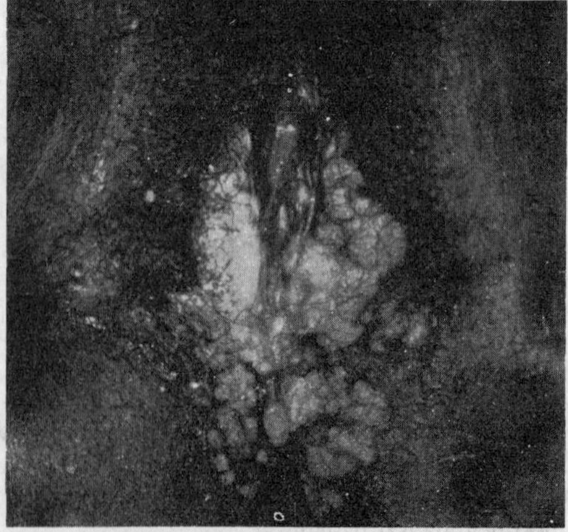

Figure 104-3. Condylomata lata confluent in central area, with individual ulcerative lesions on perineum and inguinal adenitis. (From Novak ER, Woodruff JD: Novak's Gynecologic and Obstetric Pathology. 7th ed. Philadelphia, W.B. Saunders Co., 1974.)

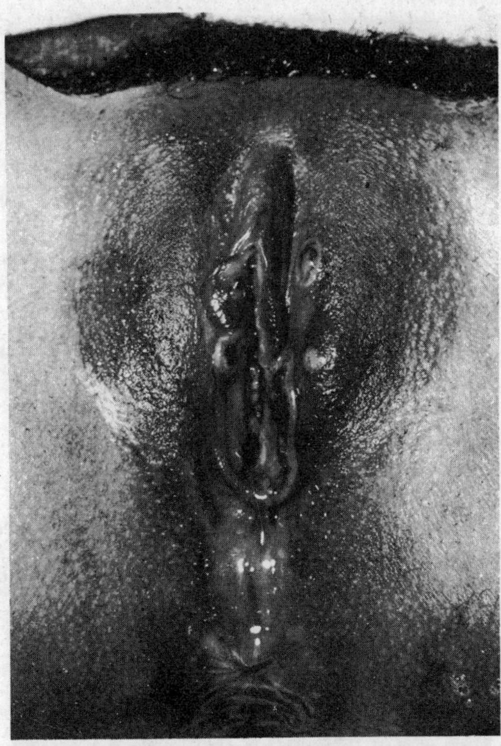

Figure 104-4. Granuloma inguinale. Large ulcerative area at outlet on left, with satellite lesions above and on right labium minus. (From Novak ER, Woodruff JD: Novak's Gynecologic and Obstetric Pathology. 7th ed. Philadelphia, W.B. Saunders Co., 1974.)

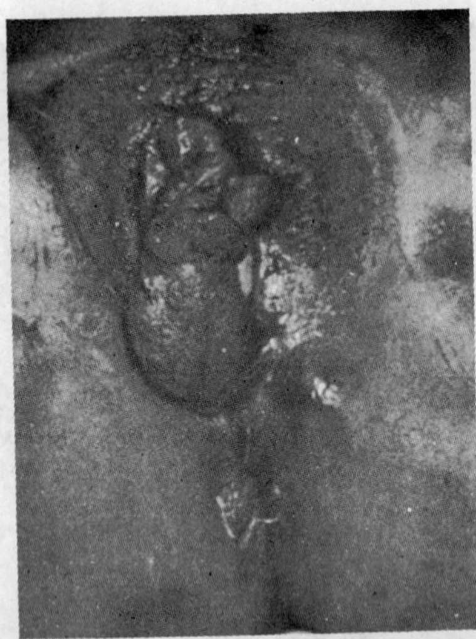

Figure 104-5. Lymphopathia venereum (L.G.V.) showing lymphedema of right labium and draining sinuses in perineum on left. (From Novak ER, Woodruff JD: Novak's Gynecologic and Obstetric Pathology. 7th ed. Philadelphia, W.B. Saunders Co., 1974.)

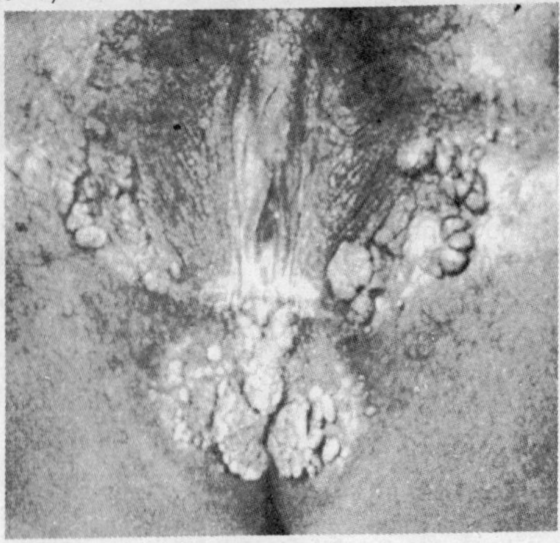

Figure 104-6. Multiple condylomata acuminata of vulva and perineum. Note similar positions on opposite sides. (From Novak ER, Woodruff JD: Novak's Gynecologic and Obstetric Pathology. 7th ed. Philadelphia, W.B. Saunders Co., 1974.)

ASSESSMENT

DIFFERENTIAL DIAGNOSIS

Atrophic vulvovaginitis is usually due to estrogen deficiency. The skin and mucous membrane of the postmenopausal patient appear thin, red, atrophic, and excoriated. The condition may also occur following radiation therapy.

Bartholin's abscess is an infection of a Bartholin's duct cyst characterized by varying degrees of pain and tenderness over the infected gland. Objective signs include unilateral swelling over the site of the infected gland, redness of the overlying skin, and edema of the labia. The abscess is palpable as an extremely tender, fluctuant mass. (See Bartholin's Abscess, p. 152.)

Candidiasis (moniliasis) (see Fig. 104-7 and Table 104-1) is caused by organisms belonging to the genus Candida, usually *Candida albicans*. The major symptom is vaginal or vulvar burning and itching, with or without vaginal discharge. Burning may be aggravated by urination. The labia may be reddened and edematous. Frequently, there is a history of antibiotic therapy; diabetes and pregnancy are additional predisposing factors. The typical vaginal discharge is thick, white, and curdlike. The diagnosis is made by spreading a small amount of discharge on a glass slide, adding a drop of 10 to 20 per cent potassium hydroxide, and visualizing the spores and hyphae.

Carcinoma of the vulva usually appears after age 50 as an ulcerated or exophytic lesion. The surface may be fungating, infected, polypoid or a shallow ulcer with indurated rolled edges.

Chancroid, a venereal infection caused by *Hemophilus ducreyi,* is characterized by one or more shallow, soft, painful, ragged ulcers with erythematous haloes and little induration. Unilateral, painful inguinal adenitis with marked redness of the overlying skin occurs in 25 to 60 per cent of cases.

Condylomata acuminata are wartlike papillomata of the genitalia caused by a virus. Usually they produce few symptoms, although they may be a source of chronic annoyance to the patient. Located on the vulva,

(Text continued on p. 719)

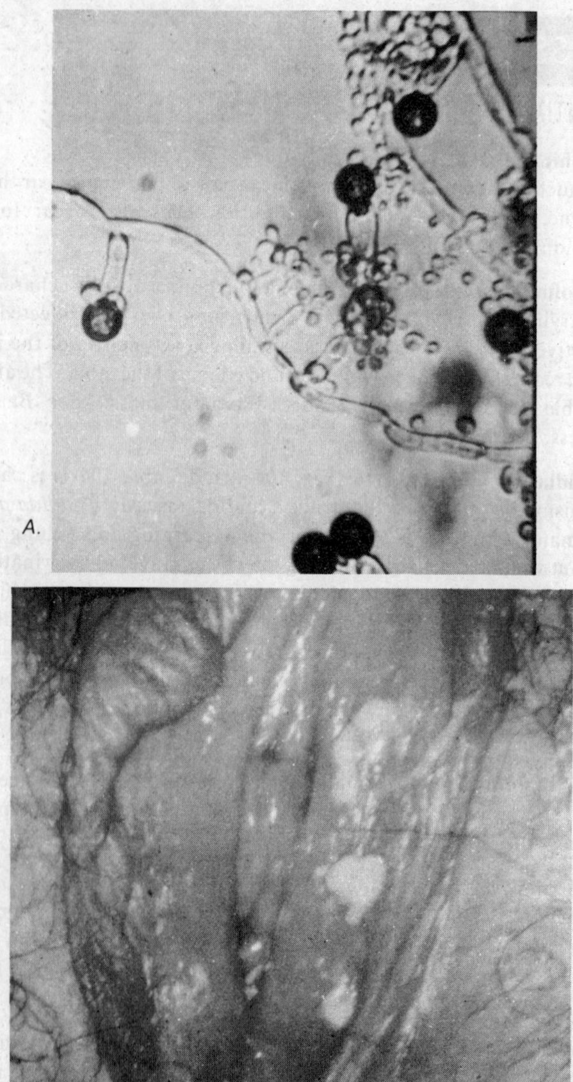

Figure 104-7. *A,* Candida spores and hyphae. *B,* Candidal vulvovaginitis.

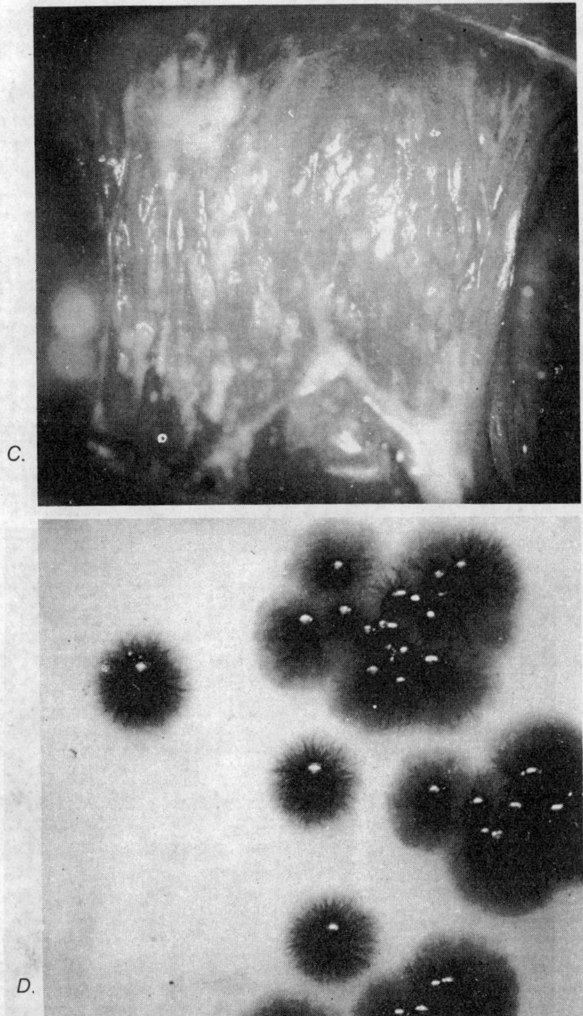

Figure 104-7. *(Continued) C,* Exudate of candidal vaginitis. *D, Candida albicans* culture on Nickerson's medium.

(Illustration continued on following page)

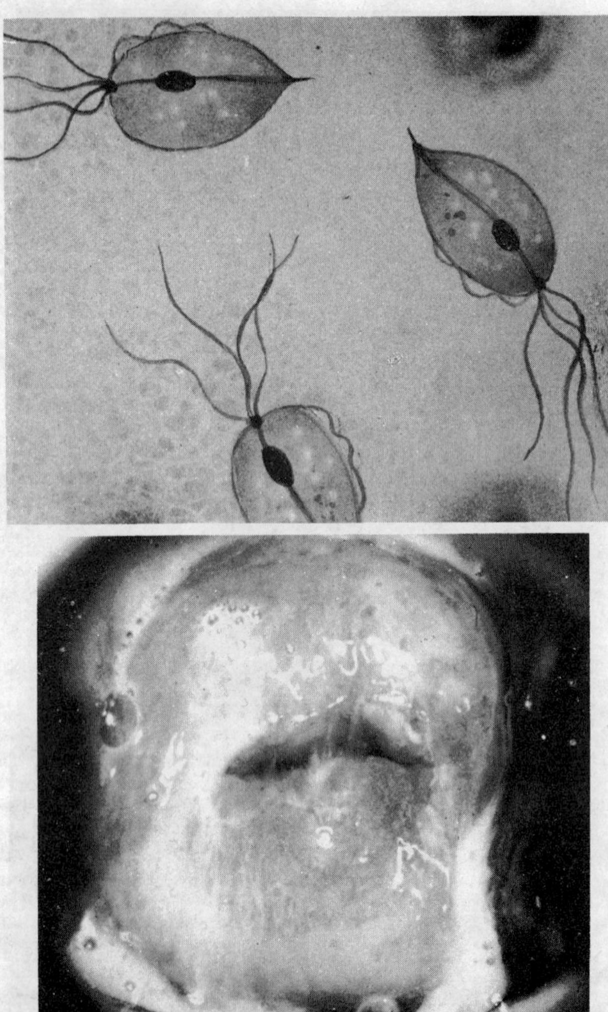

Figure 104-7. *(Continued) E,* Trichomonads, *F,* Cervical erosion *Trichomonas vaginalis.*

TABLE 104-1. Identification of Common Vaginal Infections

	Candida albicans	***Hemophilus vaginalis***	***Trichomonas vaginalis***
Discharge	White, curdlike	Gray, homogeneous	Greenish-gray, profuse, frothy
Odor	None	Malodorous	Malodorous
Pruritus	Intense	None	Slight to severe
pH	4.0-5.0	5.0-5.5	5.5-5.8
Vulvar erythema	Frequent	Absent	Variable
Vaginal mucosa	Erythematous, adherent white patches	Grossly normal	Petechiae ("strawberry spots")
Wet smear	Spores, mycelia	Clue cells	Motile trichomonads

particularly the vestibule and the labial folds, the lesions have a distinctive appearance. The early warts are small, discrete, papillary, and usually multiple. As they spread and enlarge, they often coalesce, forming large cauliflower-like masses with a broad base. Lesions that become ulcerated and infected tend to exude a foul odor.

Contact or allergic vulvovaginitis may be due to a primary irritant or an allergic reaction. Among the more common causes are cosmetics, chemicals for douching, contraceptives, and vaginal sprays. The vulvar skin tends to be reddened and edematous; it is often excoriated, vesiculated, and ulcerated. The severity of the reaction is influenced by the sensitivity of the affected person as well as by environmental conditions at the contact site. The intertriginous areas (the interlabial and genitocrural folds), subject to moisture and rubbing, are particularly susceptible to reactions from offending agents.

Folliculitis is an infection, usually due to Staphylococcus, arising within hair follicles. Predisposing conditions include obesity, sweating, maceration, malnutrition, diabetes, seborrhea, poor hygiene, and pediculosis. Pain, erythema, and tenderness are common symptoms.

Furuncle, or boil, is a more extensive infection involving tissue beyond the hair follicle. In the early stage, the lesion consists of a tender, swollen, firm erythematous nodule. After several days, a small pustule forms at the apex of the nodule, which eventually ruptures and drains a small amount of purulent material.

Foreign body (tampon, pessary, or sponge) in the vagina can produce a profuse, fetid discharge.

Fox-Fordyce disease, which is exceedingly rare, is characterized by a chronic pruritic eruption of multiple microcysts, formed by retention of sweat in apocrine gland ducts. (See Pruritus Vulvae, p. 571.)

Gonorrhea: *Neisseria gonorrhoeae* may produce an acute purulent infection of the Skene's glands, Bartholin's glands, urethra, cervix, or fallopian tubes. Skenitis and urethritis tend to cause urinary frequency and dysuria. Bartholinitis may cause duct obstruction with abscess formation. (See Bartholin's abscess, p. 152.) Cervicitis may produce a profuse, irritating vaginal discharge. Diagnosis is made by the identification of *Neisseria gonorrhoeae* on Thayer-Martin culture media. (See Gonorrhea, p. 356.)

Granuloma inguinale (Donovanosis), a venereal disease caused by the bacterium *Donovania (Calymmatobacterium granulomatis),* is characterized by single or multiple, usually painless, ulcerating, granulomatous lesions of the vulva, perianal tissues, and inguinal region. Ulcers are usually superficial and serpiginous in form. Inguinal adenopathy is uncommon. The pathognomonic feature is the large infected mononuclear cell containing many intracytoplasmic cysts filled with deeply staining Donovan bodies.

Hemophilus vaginalis vaginitis: *Hemophilus (Corynebacterium) vaginalis* (see Table 104-1) is a minute, rod-shaped, nonmotile, nonencapsulated, gram-negative bacillus that produces a gray, homogeneous, malodorous discharge not associated with significant pruritus or burning. This organism is considered by many to be the most likely cause of vaginitis previously classified as "nonspecific." Clue cells on the wet smear of vaginal secretions are typical findings.

Herpes genitalis, caused by herpes simplex virus, Type II, is the *most common vesiculoulcerative* disease of the genitalia. Involving the vulva, vagina, and ectocervical mucosa, herpetic lesions may appear singly or in clusters as widespread indurated papules with vesicles and superficial ulcerations on the dependent surface of the papule. The lesions are extremely painful, may become secondarily infected, and may be accompanied by diffuse, inflammatory reactions with erythema and edema, as well as bilateral, tender, inguinal lymphadenopathy. Dysuria indicates herpetic involvement of the urethra and bladder. Recurrences are common and may represent exacerbation of dormant virus. Cytologic smears, viral cultures, and serologic tests provide confirmation of the diagnosis.

Lymphogranuloma venereum is a venereal infection caused by a chlamydial organism. The disease is characterized by an inconspicuous, painless, transient genital ulcer followed by inguinal or femoral adenopathy (possibly with suppuration) two to three weeks later. Perirectal node involvement and, occasionally, rectal strictures are end-stage effects. Complement fixation tests are helpful in confirmation of the diagnosis.

Pediculosis pubis is an infestation of the hair-bearing areas of the vulva by the crab louse (*Phthirus pubis*). Skin lesions consist mainly of minute, inflamed maculopapules. Itching is a common symptom, and scratching may induce secondary lesions of the skin—lichenification, pigmentation, and excoriation.

Scabies of the vulva is caused by the itch mite, *Sarcoptes scabiei.* The vulva may be only one site of a widespread skin disease that includes nonhairy areas. The lesions exhibit small burrows with minute papules or vesicles. Itching is essentially the only symptom.

Syphilitic chancre is a single, painless, indurated ulcer, approximately 1.0 to 1.5 cm in size.

Condyloma latum, a secondary lesion of syphilis, is a broad-based exophytic excrescence that may ulcerate and produce a necrotic exudate. (See Syphilis, p. 637.)

Trichomoniasis is caused by the protozoan *Trichomonas vaginalis* (see Table 104-1). Trichomonads are highly motile organisms, slightly larger than leukocytes. Their anterior portions have a protruding flagella. Diagnosis is made by suspending a drop of the vaginal discharge in several drops of normal saline and observing the motile forms under the microscope. Usual presenting symptoms include profuse, greenish-gray, foul-smelling vaginal discharge associated with vulvar soreness and itching.

TABLE 104-2. Classification of Vaginal and Vulvar Infections

Organisms	Diseases
Bacteria	
Donovania granulomatis (Calymmatobacterium granulomatis)	Granuloma inguinale
Escherichia coli	Nonspecific vaginitis
Hemophilus ducreyi	Chancroid
Hemophilus (Corynebacterium) vaginalis	*Hemophilus vaginalis* vaginitis
Neisseria gonorrhoeae	Gonorrhea
Treponema pallidum	Syphilis
Chlamydia	
Lymphogranuloma venereum agent	Lymphogranuloma venereum
Genital TRIC agent	Genital TRIC agent infection
Metazoa	
Phthirus pubis	Pediculosis pubis
Mycoplasma	
Mycoplasma hominis	Genital mycoplasma hominis infection
T-strain mycoplasma	Genital T-strain mycoplasma infection
Mycoses (Fungi)	
Candida albicans	Candidiasis (Moniliasis)
Protozoa	
Trichomonas vaginalis	Trichomoniasis
Viruses	
Herpes Simplex Type II	Herpes genitalis
Genital wart virus	Condyloma acuminatum
Genital cytomegalovirus	Genital cytomegalovirus infection
Genital molluscum contagiosum	Genital molluscum contagiosum

CLASSIFICATION

See Table 104-2.

ETIOLOGIC FACTORS

Etiologic factors of vaginal or cervical ulcerations include

1. Foreign objects
   a. Tampons, diaphragms, pessaries, silicone rings
   b. Blunt trauma
   c. Detergent or perfumed medications
   d. Potassium permanganate
2. Infectious agents
   a. Herpes
   b. Syphilis
3. Decreased vascular supply
   a. Postradiation treatment
4. Carcinoma

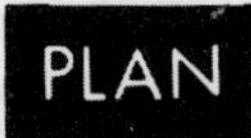

ADDITIONAL DIAGNOSTIC DATA

Biopsy of the vulva may identify vulvar dystrophy, malignancy, or chancroid. The toluidine blue stain is a valuable diagnostic aid for indication of the most suspicious sites for biopsy. (A 1 per cent solution of toluidine blue is applied to the vulvar lesion with a cotton swab and allowed to dry for one or two minutes. Next, the area is rinsed with 1 per cent aqueous solution of acetic acid. A normally keratinized surface shows essentially no areas of adherent stain, whereas nuclear material at the skin surface retains the blue dye.)

The biopsy site is cleansed with an antiseptic solution and then infiltrated with 1 per cent lidocaine. A 4 or 6 mm dermal punch may be twisted into the skin and the base of the tissue plug severed with small scissors. Bleeding is controlled either by the local application of Monsel's solution and pressure or with a suture to coapt the skin edges.

Complement fixation test is the most reliable diagnostic procedure for lymphogranuloma venereum. The test becomes positive at a titer of 1:16

or more during the first four weeks of infection. A rising titer is evidence of an acute infection. (The Frei test is generally considered to be much less reliable.)

Culture Media: Thayer-Martin medium is used for the growth of *Neisseria gonorrhoeae,* Nickersen's or Sabouraud medium is used for the growth of *Candida albicans.*

Cytologic smears aid in the diagnosis of suspected herpes. Large multinucleated giant cells with acidophilic intranuclear inclusion bodies are typical findings. The cytoplasm of the epithelial cells is often vacuolated and occasionally fragmented.

Dark-field examination for *Treponema pallidum* is recommended when lesions suggestive of chancre or condyloma latum are seen.

Giemsa stain of a crush preparation from the lesion may disclose Donovan bodies—clusters of blue- or black-staining organisms with a "safety-pin" appearance (from bipolar chromatin condensation)—in the cytoplasm of large mononuclear cells.

Gram stain may reveal intracellular diplococci indicative of gonorrhea or short gram-negative bacilli suggestive of Hemophilus infection.

Serologic tests are helpful in the diagnosis of syphilis, herpes simplex, and lymphogranuloma venereum. A rising titer over consecutive weeks confirms the diagnosis of recent infection. (See Syphilis, p. 637.)

Wet smear (wet mount) preparations of vaginal secretions, using both saline and 10 to 20 per cent potassium hydroxide (KOH) solution, are most useful for the identification of the most common causes of vaginitis: *Candida albicans, Hemophilus vaginalis,* and *Trichomonas vaginalis.*

A drop of discharge, placed on each end of a glass slide, is thoroughly mixed with saline at one end and potassium hydroxide at the other end. Cover slips are placed over both suspensions and the slide examined under the microscope. Motile trichomonads, leukocytes, epithelial cells, bacteria, or clue cells (stippled granular-appearing epithelial cells characteristic of *Hemophilus vaginalis* infection) may be identified in the saline suspension. The spores and hyphae of Candida may be detected in the KOH suspension after the potassium hydroxide has lysed the cellular material.

MANAGEMENT AND PATIENT EDUCATION

Atrophic Vulvovaginitis: Local application of estrogen cream usually relieves the patient's symptoms. One applicator full of estrogen vaginal cream inserted at bedtime is frequently beneficial.

Candidiasis: Effective anticandidal medications include nystatin vaginal tablets twice daily for two weeks, candicidin vaginal tablets or ointment, or one applicatorful of *miconazole (Monistat)* cream intravaginally at bedtime for 14 days.

Reinfection control is a more difficult problem. When oral antibiotics are taken, for example, vulvovaginal candidiasis may result from the heavy colonization of the intestinal tract.

Chancroid: Sulfisoxazole—1 gm every six hours for 10 to 14 days—is the treatment of choice. Tetracycline—500 mg four times a day for 10 to 14 days—or tetracycline combined with sulfisoxazole has also been used effectively. Resistant cases are treated with streptomycin or kanamycin (0.5 gm twice daily for 10-14 days). The bubo may be aspirated but should not be incised.

Condyloma Acuminatum: Podophyllin (25 per cent solution in tincture of benzoin) is a traditional topical therapy for small lesions. The surrounding skin is protected with petrolatum. The patient is advised to wash the treated warts with soap and water after four to six hours. Podophyllin is *not* recommended during pregnancy *nor* for the treatment of extensive lesions.

Cryosurgery, electrodesiccation, and knife excision are alternative therapeutic measures. Electrosurgery is usually required for extensive lesions. Concomitant vaginal infections should also be treated. Analgesic medications may be necessary.

Contact or Allergic Vulvovaginitis: The cornerstone of treatment is discontinuation of the causative agent (cosmetic, chemical, and so forth). Warm sitz baths or topical wet compresses with Burow's solution may be soothing. Topical corticosteroid creams (fluocinolone—0.01 per cent or equivalent) usually relieve pruritic symptoms promptly. For an allergic reaction, an oral antihistamine medication may be helpful.

Folliculitis or Furuncle: Local application of heat, preferably by hot, wet dressings or sitz baths, usually promotes healing. Broad-spectrum antibiotics and angesic medications are usually recommended.

Foreign body in the vagina must be removed. A cleansing douche with povidone-iodine (Betadine) is usually recommended.

Granuloma Inguinale: Tetracycline—500 mg four times daily for two weeks—is the first choice for treatment. The second choice is 40 mg of gentamicin given twice daily intramuscularly for two weeks. If previous medications fail, chloramphenicol—500 mg orally three times a day for two weeks—may be recommended.

Hemophilus vaginalis: Intravaginal sulfa creams may be beneficial. Often ampicillin orally is a more effective therapy (500 mg four times daily for five to seven days).

Herpes Genitalis: No specific treatment is available. Cool sitz baths, wet compresses, and analgesic medications usually provide symptomatic relief of local discomfort. Povidone-iodine (Betadine) solution or povidone-iodine vaginal gel or both, applied to ulcerated areas, may inhibit secondary infection.

If urethral involvement prevents the patient from voiding, a suprapubic catheter may facilitate bladder drainage.

When an active herpes genital infection is present during late pregnancy, vaginal delivery may be associated with a fulminating disseminated neonatal herpetic infection. To avert this risk, delivery by cesarean section is recommended, unless the membranes have been ruptured for more than four hours.

Herpes simplex lesions usually heal spontaneously within one to three weeks. Abatement of symptoms, however, does not necessarily mean that the patient is virus-free.

Lymphogranuloma Venereum: Tetracycline—500 mg four times daily for three to four weeks—is recommended. Fluctuant lymph nodes should be aspirated.

Pediculosis: Gamma benzene hexachloride (Gamene) shampoo is effective topical treatment. After wetting the hair with warm water, the shampoo is applied with active lathering for a full four to five minutes. The hair is then rinsed thoroughly, dried, and combed to remove any remaining nit shells. A complete change of clothing and bed linen is recommended. If necessary, treatment may be repeated after one week. Since these infestations are spread by body contact, the patient is advised of the need for treatment of sexual partners and others living together in close personal relations.

Scabies: Gamma benzene hexachloride 1 per cent lotion (Gamene) is applied after a soap-and-water bath. The lotion is left on the skin for 24 hours and then followed with another bath. Clothing, bed linen, and towels should be cleaned and changed. All contacts should be advised to have concurrent treatment.

Trichomoniasis: Metronidazole (Flagyl) is an oral trichomonacidal agent that has been demonstrated to be highly effective against *Trichomonas vaginalis*. The recommended dosage is a 250-mg tablet taken orally three times daily for seven days. Metronidazole is not recommended during pregnancy and lactation, since there is evidence of tumorigenic activity in rodents given metronidazole and the risk of teratogenesis remains unknown.

REFERENCES

Chow AW: Genital infection with Type 2 herpes simplex virus. Postgrad Med *58*:66-70, 1975; Obstet Gynecol Surv *31*:192-194, 1976

Evans TN: Sexually transmissible disease. Am J Obstet Gynecol *125*:116-133, 1976

Friedrich EG: Vulvar disease. Philadelphia, W.B. Saunders Company, 1976

Josey WE: The sexually transmitted infections. Obstet Gynecol *43*:465-470, 1974

Kaufman RH, Gardner HL, Merrill JA: Diseases of the vulva and vagina. *In* Romney SL, Gray MJ, Little AB, et al: Gynecology and Obstetrics: The Health Care of Women. New York, McGraw-Hill, Inc., 1975

McLelland BA, Anderson PC: Lymphogranuloma venereum outbreak in a university community. JAMA *235*:56-57, 1975; Obstet Gynecol Surv *31*:510-511, 1976

Rein MF, Chapel TA: Trichomoniasis, candidiasis, and the minor venereal diseases. Clin Obstet Gynecol *18*:73-88, 1975

Smith EG: Management of herpes simplex infections of the skin. JAMA *235*:1731-1733, 1976

Young AW, Tovell HMM, Sadri K: Erosions and ulcers of the vulva. Obstet Gynecol *50*:35-39, 1977

of the need for restriction of sexual partners and of intensifying [illegible] close personal relations.

Scabies: Gamma benzene hexachloride 1 per cent lotion (Gamene) is applied after a cleansing warm bath. The lotion is left on the skin for 24 hours and then followed with another bath. Clothing, bed linen, and towels should be cleaned and changed. All contacts should be treated or have concurrent treatment.

Trichomoniasis: Metronidazole (Flagyl) is an oral trichomonacidal agent that has been demonstrated to be highly effective against *Trichomonas vaginalis*. The recommended dosage is a 250-mg tablet taken orally three times daily for seven days. Metronidazole is not recommended during pregnancy and lactation, since there is evidence of tumorigenicity in certain rodents given metronidazole and the risk of teratogenesis remains unknown.

REFERENCES

Chow AY, [illegible]: Genital infection with Herpesvirus hominis [illegible] simplex virus. [illegible] Med [illegible] Obstet Gynecol Surv [illegible]

[illegible] The sexually transmitted diseases [illegible] Obstet Gynecol [illegible]

Friedrich EG: Vulvar disease. Philadelphia, W.B. Saunders Company, 1976.

[illegible] WE: The sexually transmitted infections. [illegible]

Kaufman RH, Gardner HL, Merrill JA: Diseases of the vulva and vagina. In Romney SL, Gray MJ, Little AB, et al. (eds.): Gynecology and Obstetrics: The Health Care of Women. New York, McGraw-Hill, [illegible]

McClelland [illegible] community. [illegible] Obstet Gynecol Surv [illegible]

[illegible] and [illegible] venereal disease. Clin Obstet Gynecol [illegible]

[illegible] Management of herpes simplex infections of the skin. JAMA [illegible]

Young AW, [illegible] vulva. Obstet Gynecol [illegible]

PART III

PROCEDURES AND THERAPY

105 AMNIOCENTESIS

EQUIPMENT

1. Antiseptic solution
2. Spinal needles with stylus—18, 20, 22 gauge
3. Syringe—10 cc
4. Syringe—2 cc
5. Lidocaine
6. Needles—25 gauge, 21 gauge
7. Sterile towel and drape
8. Ice
9. Specimen vials, clear and brown

PURPOSE

1. To evaluate fetal or maternal well-being
   a. Rh isoimmunization
   b. Intrauterine infection
2. To assess fetal maturity
3. For prenatal diagnosis of congenital disorders

PROCEDURE

Ultrasound B-scan is very helpful for localization of the placenta and determination of fetal presentation.

Prior to amniocentesis, the patient should empty her bladder and then lie supine on the examining table.

The site for amniocentesis can be behind the fetal neck (see Fig. 105-1), in the area of the small parts, or in the suprapubic area below the fetal head.

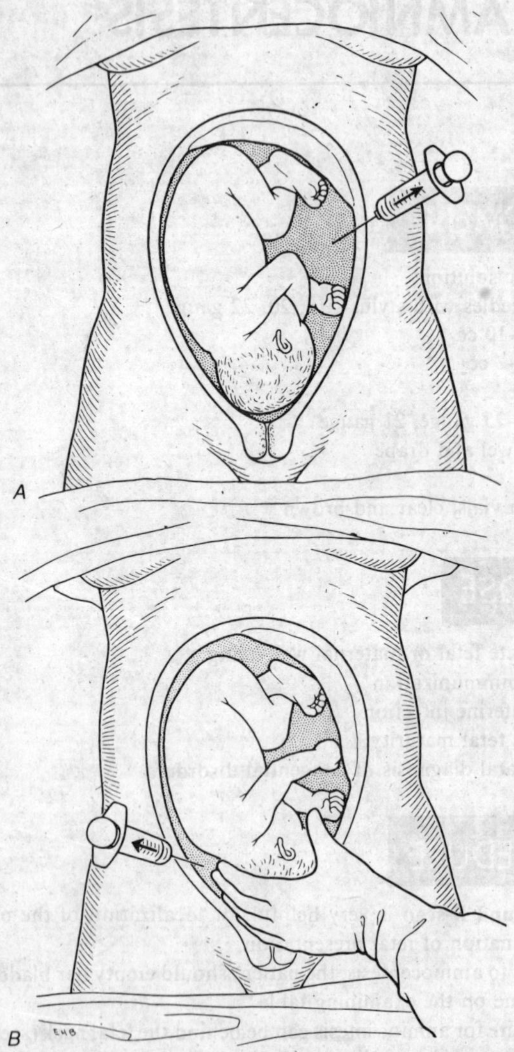

Figure 105-1. *A*, Amniocentesis in the area of the fetal small parts. *B*, Amniocentesis posterior to the fetal neck. (Modified from Queenan JT: Modern Management of the Rh Problem. New York, Harper and Row, 1967.)

The abdomen is prepared with antiseptic solution and the puncture site surrounded with a sterile drape. The site is then infiltrated with a local anesthetic.

A spinal needle with a stylet is advanced into the amniotic cavity. The stylet is withdrawn and amniotic fluid aspirated into a 10-ml syringe.

The fluid for lecithin-sphingomyelin (L/S) ratio is placed into a tube surrounded by ice, and the fluid for spectrophotometric analysis is placed in a brown bottle to protect it from direct sunlight.

If blood is aspirated, the needle may be in the uterine wall, placenta or fetus. If the needle has not reached the amniotic cavity, it is advanced gently. Rotation of the needle 180° may be necessary to obtain a free flow of amniotic fluid. Initially sanguineous fluid often clears in 30 to 60 seconds.

INTERPRETATION

Lecithin-Sphingomyelin Ratio (L/S Ratio) (Fig. 105-2): Lecithin and sphingomyelin begin to appear in measurable amounts in amniotic fluid

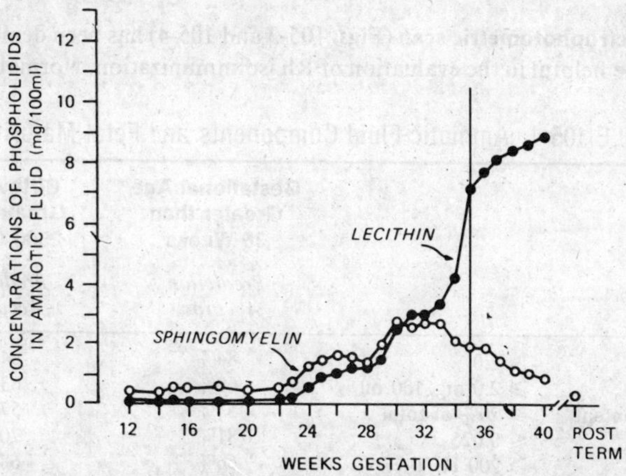

Figure 105-2. Changes in mean concentrations of lecithin and sphingomyelin in amniotic fluid during gestation in normal pregnancy. (From Gluck L, Kulovich M: Lecithin/sphingomyelin ratios in amniotic fluid in normal and abnormal pregnancy. Am J Obstet Gynecol *115*:539, 1973.)

about the twenty-fifth or twenty-sixth week of gestation. At first, sphingomyelin concentrations are higher than those of lecithin. At about week 31 or 32 the two become equal. After this time, the lecithin concentration begins to increase more rapidly, and the sphingomyelin concentration levels off and actually decreases.

With biochemical maturation of the lung, at about the thirty-fifth gestational week, the lecithin to sphingomyelin ratio is 2 to 1 or higher (Table 105-1). A ratio of less than 1 is characteristic of the immature lung; ratios between 1 and 2 are in an intermediate area.

The L/S ratio provides the most reliable estimate of fetal lung maturity. With values of 2 to 1 or higher, there appears to be minimal risk of respiratory distress syndrome.

Creatinine concentration in amniotic fluid increases rapidly just before term as a result of increased creatinine excretion by maturing fetal kidneys. Levels of 2.0 mg or more per 100 ml of amniotic fluid usually indicate fetal renal maturity (Table 105-1), although an increase in maternal plasma creatinine could also increase amniotic fluid creatinine.

Less reliable than the L/S ratio, creatinine is the second best amniotic fluid indicator of fetal maturity.

Spectrophotometric scan (Figs. 105-3 and 105-4) has been demonstrated to be helpful in the evaluation of Rh isoimmunization. Normal amniotic

TABLE 105-1. Amniotic Fluid Components and Fetal Maturity*

		Gestational Age Greater than 36 Weeks *Prediction Accuracy*	Birthweight Greater than 2500 Grams *Prediction Accuracy*
L/S ratio	⩾ 2.0	84%	84%
Creatinine	⩾ 2.0 mg/100 ml	60%	63%
Fat cell content	⩾ 20% of total	51%	57%
Δ OD_{450}	⩽ 0.025	81%	70%
Amylase	⩾ 200 IU/liter	66%	68%
Protein Conc.	⩽ 250 mg/100 ml	55%	51%

*From Fernandez de Castro A, Usategui-Gomez M, Spellacy WN: Amniotic fluid components as determinants of fetal maturity. Obstet Gynecol *46*:76-79, 1975.

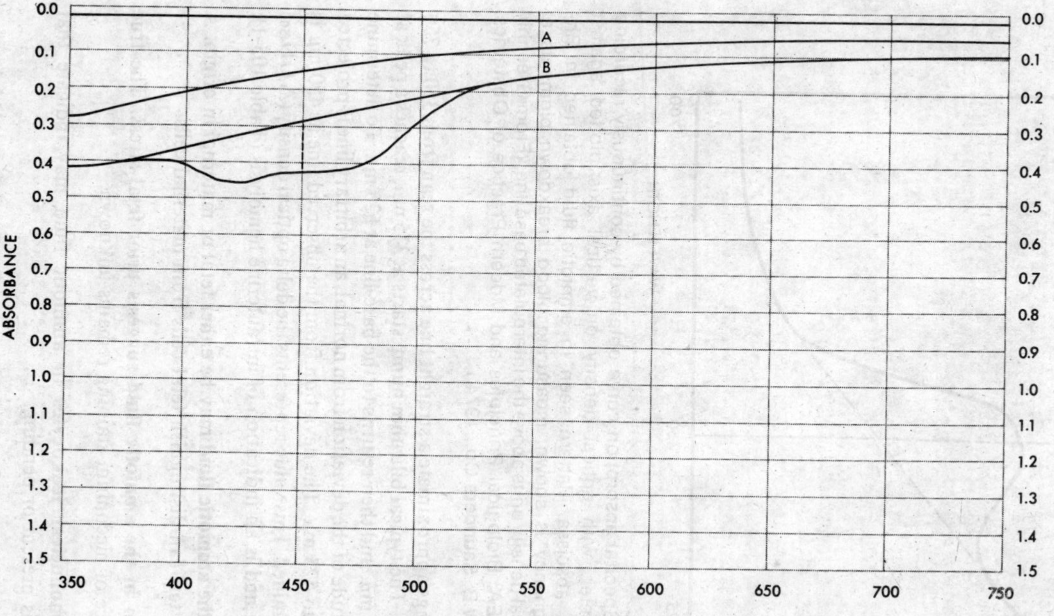

Figure 105-3. Spectrophotometric scan showing (A) normal AF and (B) typical bilirubin hump. Heavy (arbitrary) line represents the AF scan course in the absence of bilirubin. Broken line represents the ΔOD at 450 mμ. (From Barber HBK, Graber EA: Surgical Disease in Pregnancy. Philadelphia, W.B. Saunders Co., 1974.)

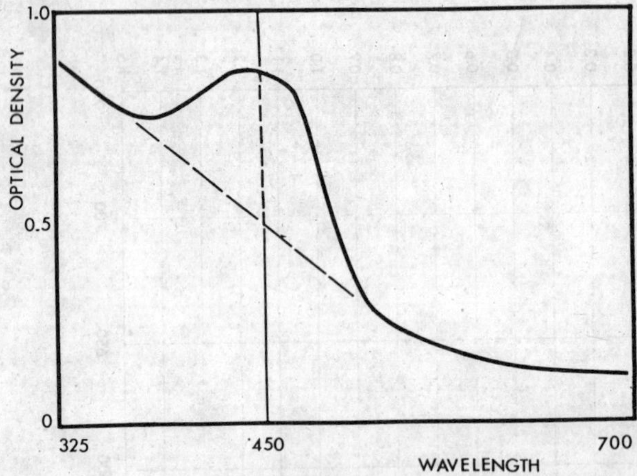

Figure 105-4. Spectral absorption curve obtained by continuously recording spectrophotometer, with optical density on vertical axis plotted against wavelength on abscissa. Pattern seen in amniotic fluid obtained in Rh-sensitized pregnancy is shown, measuring blood breakdown pigments at 450 mμ in optical density units above the interpolated base line. (From Greenhill JP, Friedman EA: Biological Principles and Modern Practice of Obstetrics. Philadelphia, W.B. Saunders Co., 1974.)

fluid tracings approximate a straight line across the scan from 350 to 750 millimicra. The typical bilirubin hump starts at 375 mμ, reaches a peak at 450 to 460 mμ, and then returns to the base-line at 525 mμ. To determine the magnitude of the deviation from normal, an arbitrary line is projected from 375 to 525 mμ. The deviation from the observed line at 450 mμ is then determined. This value represents the delta optical density (Δ OD_{450}) at 450 mμ and is an indication of intrauterine hemolysis (Table 105-1).

Blood in the amniotic fluid may be either fetal or maternal in origin. A Kleihauer test can distinguish fetal cells from maternal cells.

Meconium in the amniotic fluid suggests prior fetal stress. The true significance of meconium staining remains unknown.

Polymorphonuclear leukocytes in amniotic fluid may indicate that infection is present or pending.

Gram stain and culture are helpful when infection is suspected.

COMPLICATIONS

Maternal complications that may be anticipated include bleeding with hematoma formation, infection, syncope due to a vagal response, and fetomaternal bleeding with potential isoimmunization of the Rh-negative patient (for this reason, in the absence of any specific data concerning risk of sensitization, it is probably advisable that Rh-negative, unsensitized women be treated with Rh (D) immune globulin after amniocentesis) (ACOG Bulletin, January 1976).

Fetal complications include hemorrhage, umbilical hematoma, and intrauterine infection.

With blood in the amniotic fluid, the laboratory can determine whether the red cells are maternal or fetal in origin. If fetal cells are identified, the fetal heart rate should be closely monitored. An abnormal fetal heart rate pattern suggests active fetal bleeding or an umbilical cord hematoma interfering with fetal oxygenation. In either circumstance, immediate delivery is advised.

Opinions differ over optimal management if the fetal heart rate remains normal. Gassner and Paul (1976) favor immediate delivery after 35 weeks' gestation, since they feel that the risk of a severely anemic or stillborn infant is greater than the risk of neonatal problems. If the fetus is less than 35 weeks and has no heart-rate abnormality, however, further observation is advisable. All infants who have had fetal bleeding should have hematocrit determinations immediately after delivery.

REFERENCES

Doran TA, Malone RM, Benzie RJ, et al: Amniotic fluid tests for fetal maturity in normal and abnormal pregnancies. Am J Obstet Gynecol *125*:586-592, 1976

Fernandez de Castro A, Usategui-Gomez M, Spellacy WN: Amniotic fluid components as determinants of fetal maturity. Obstet Gynecol *46*:76-79, 1975

Gassner CB, Paul RH: Laceration of umbilical cord vessels secondary to amniocentesis. Obstet Gynecol *48*:627-630, 1976

Gluck L, Kulovich MV, Borer RC: Estimates of fetal lung maturity. Clin Perinatol *1*;125-139, 1974

Gluck L, Kulovich MV, Borer RC, et al: The interpretation and significance of the lecithin/sphingomyelin ratio in amniotic fluid. Am J Obstet Gynecol *120*:142-155, 1974

Gordon HR, Deukmedjian AG: Suprapubic vs periumbilical amniocentesis. Am J Obstet Gynecol *122*:287-290, 1975

Pridmore BR, Robertson EG, Walker W: Liquor bilirubin levels and false prediction of severity in rhesus haemolytic disease. Br Med J *3*:136, 1972; Obstet Gynecol Surv *28*: 94-97, 1973

Queenan JT: Amniocentesis and interpretation. *In* Barber HRK, Graber EA: Surgical Disease in Pregnancy. Philadelphia, W.B. Saunders Company, 1974

Schwarz RH: Amniocentesis. Clin Obstet Gynecol *18*:1-22, 1975

106 ARTERIAL BLOOD SAMPLING

GENERAL CONSIDERATIONS

Arterial blood sampling is required principally for the measurement of blood pH, oxygen tension (pO_2), and carbon dioxide tension (pCO_2). Arterial blood can be collected either by direct arterial puncture or with an indwelling arterial line.

PROCEDURE FOR DIRECT ARTERIAL PUNCTURE

Of the arteries suitable for direct percutaneous puncture—the radial at the wrist, the brachial in the antecubital fossa, and the femoral in the groin—the radial is usually preferred (Fig. 106-1).

The arterial blood sample must be drawn into a heparinized syringe, which is prepared by drawing up 1 ml of heparin, clearing all air bubbles, and expelling the heparin completely. This leaves a small amount of heparin in the syringe that is sufficient for 10 ml of blood and does not dilute the specimen. It is essential that no residual air be left in the syringe, since air equilibrates with the gases in the blood sample and invalidates the blood gas analysis.

The skin over the radial artery is cleaned with alcohol or an appropriate antiseptic solution; a small quantity of local anesthetic (1 per cent lidocaine) is injected over the puncture site. The artery is palpated with the forefinger and middle finger of the left hand. The fingers are then separated, leaving a space of about 1 cm between them. The syringe is held vertically in the right hand, and the needle (20 gauge) is inserted through the skin into the artery. When the arterial wall has been pierced, a small spurt of blood is often seen in the syringe. In the case of glass syringes, the arterial pressure alone is usually sufficient to boost the plunger of the syringe. This is a useful check that the

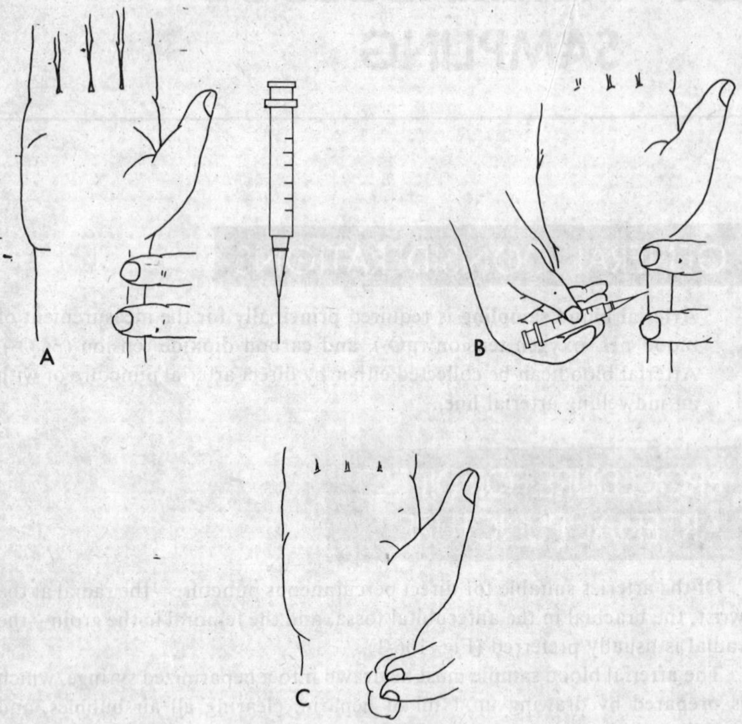

Figure 106-1. Radial artery puncture. *A*, Artery is palpated. *B*, Heparinized syringe—needle is inserted vertically into artery. *C*, Puncture site is compressed.

blood sample is arterial. With plastic syringes, it may be necessary to withdraw the plunger to obtain the blood. After the blood has been withdrawn, the needle is rapidly removed and firm pressure is applied over the needle mark.

The syringe is gently agitated to mix the heparin and blood and sent immediately to the laboratory for analysis, packed in ice if the laboratory is any distance away.

INTERPRETATION

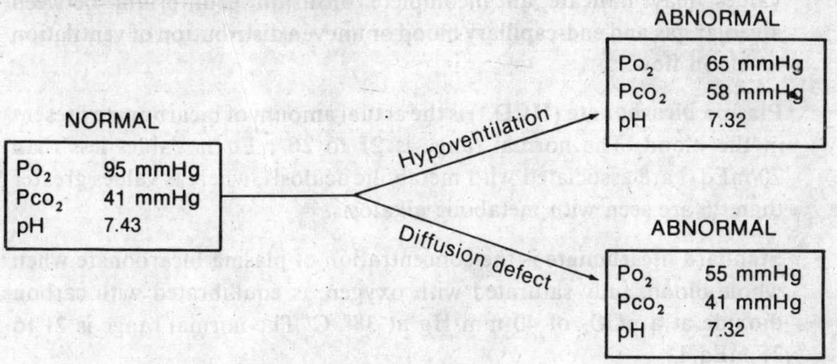

Figure 106-2.

Arterial pH is the negative log of the hydrogen ion concentration. The normal range for arterial blood is 7.36 to 7.44. A pH of 7.35 or less indicates acidosis. A pH of 7.45 or more indicates alkalosis.

Partial pressure of carbon dioxide in the arterial blood (pCO_2) is regulated by the respiratory system and is the best laboratory test for immediate assessment of alveolar ventilation. The normal range is 35 to 45 mm Hg.

A pCO_2 less than 35 is an indication of hyperventilation. The fall in alveolar carbon dioxide causes a decrease in serum carbonic acid. The resultant rise in pH is an indication of the respiratory alkalosis.

A pCO_2 greater than 45 indicates retention of carbon dioxide, usually due to pulmonary insufficiency. Retained carbon dioxide leads to an increase in serum carbonic acid. The resultant fall in pH is an indication of respiratory acidosis.

During pregnancy, maternal ventilation is increased, both the respiratory rate and the tidal volume. This hyperventilation occurs from the beginning of pregnancy and may be correlated with increased progesterone. As a result, pCO_2 decreases and there is a tendency toward respiratory alkalosis. During labor, the pCO_2 may fall to a level as low as 26 to 34 mm Hg. The kidney compensates with increased bicarbonate excretion in order to restore the blood pH toward normal.

Partial pressure of oxygen in arterial blood (pO_2) provides an evaluation of pulmonary function. The normal range is 75 to 100 mm Hg. Decreased values may indicate an incomplete diffusion equilibrium between alveolar gas and end-capillary blood or uneven distribution of ventilation to blood flow.

Plasma bicarbonate (HCO_3^-) is the actual amount of bicarbonate present in the blood. The normal range is 21 to 26 mEq/l. Values less than 20 mEq/l are associated with metabolic acidosis, whereas values greater than 26 are seen with metabolic alkalosis.

Standard bicarbonate is the concentration of plasma bicarbonate when whole blood, fully saturated with oxygen, is equilibrated with carbon dioxide at a pCO_2 of 40 mm Hg at 38° C. The normal range is 21 to 25 mEq/l.

Buffer base refers to the total buffer capacity of whole blood assessed at standard conditions, adding together the buffer anions, bicarbonate, plasma proteins and hemoglobin. The normal range is 45 to 50 mEq/l. Bicarbonate makes up approximately half this total at 23 mEq/l.

Base excess is a deviation of 3 mEq/l from the normal range and is associated with metabolic alkalosis.

Base deficit is associated with metabolic acidosis. (If blood pH is depressed or elevated and there is neither a base excess nor a deficit, the disturbance is respiratory in origin.)

ACID-BASE REGULATION

Alterations in blood pH induced by acid end-products of metabolism are regulated by

1. Buffer activity of the blood
2. Ion exchange between the major fluid compartments
3. Respiratory function
4. Renal function

Buffers are substances that help to keep the pH stable by absorbing or supplying hydrogen ions as necessary. In blood, the two most important buffer systems are the carbonic acid-bicarbonate system and the protein molecule hemoglobin.

$$H_2CO_3 \rightleftarrows H^+ + HCO_3^-$$

$$HHb \rightleftarrows H^+ + Hb^-$$

If hydrogen ions are added, the equation moves to the left.

Ion Exchange: The exchange of cations such as sodium and potassium for hydrogen ions in the extracellular fluid plays a significant role in the regulation of extracellular fluid pH.

Respiratory function affects acid-base balance by the excretion or retention of carbon dioxide. Hyperventilation leads to increased pulmonary excretion of carbon dioxide, a fall in pCO_2 and a compensatory fall in HCO_3^-. Primary metabolic disturbances are corrected by the respiratory mechanisms. Compensating for metabolic acidosis, hyperventilation can eliminate carbon dioxide rapidly, making the respiratory mechanism suitable for rapid adjustments in pH.

Renal function contributes to acid-base regulation by varying the net rate of hydrogen ion excretion and by selective reabsorption and rejection of cations and anions. The renal excretion of excess H^+ is associated with a rise in the HCO_3^- level in the plasma. Although pH is initially controlled by buffer mechanisms and respiratory function, the ultimate elimination of excess hydrogen ions is by renal excretion.

Differential Diagnosis: For the differential diagnosis of acid-base equilibrium, see Table 106-1.

METABOLIC ACIDOSIS

Etiologic Factors:

1. Accumulation of metabolic acids in the blood—hypoxia, diabetes, starvation, fever, sepsis, and salicylate poisoning
2. Renal disease—primary loss of bicarbonate or failure to excrete sufficient hydrogen ion to maintain the normal serum pH
3. Excess loss of bicarbonate from intestinal tract—suction, diarrhea
4. Excess administration of acids (ammonium chloride, calcium chloride)

TABLE 106-1. Differential Diagnosis of Acid-Base Equilibrium

pH	pCO_2	pO_2*	Comments
N†	↑‡	↓	Respiratory acidosis, compensated Metabolic alkalosis, compensated
N	↓	↑N	Respiratory alkalosis, compensated Metabolic acidosis, compensated
↓	N	N	Metabolic acidosis, uncompensated
↓	↓	↑N	Metabolic acidosis, partially compensated (by hyperventilation)
↓	↓	N↓	Metabolic acidosis and shock
↓	↑	N↓	Respiratory acidosis and metabolic acidosis
↓	↑	↓	Respiratory acidosis
↑	N	N	Metabolic alkalosis, uncompensated
↑	↑	↓	Metabolic alkalosis, partially compensated (by hyperventilation)
↑	↓	N↑	Respiratory alkalosis and metabolic alkalosis
↑	↓	N↑	Respiratory alkalosis
↑	↓	↓	Decreased ambient oxygen Impaired diffusion Pulmonary embolus, myocardial infarct, shock Later pH ↓

*Any low pO_2 may become normal or increased owing to hyperventilation or oxygen therapy.

†N=normal.

‡Arrows show direction and not extent of change.

Laboratory Values:

1. The ph is less than 7.38 (Table 106-2).
2. The pCO_2 is less than 40 as a result of respiratory compensation.
3. Bicarbonate is less than 24 mEq/l.
4. Urine tends to be acid, with decreased sodium concentration.

Compensatory Mechanisms: Compensation for metabolic acidosis is both respiratory and renal: Increased rate and depth of respiration eliminate carbon dioxide and lower pCO_2; subsequently, there is a decrease in carbonic acid and a partial return of the pH toward normal. Renal compensation involves increased hydrogen ion excretion and a tendency to conservation of sodium and bicarbonate.

If alveolar ventilation is impaired, a combined metabolic and respiratory acidosis may coexist.

Management is directed at correction of the underlying cause.

If volume deficit has caused metabolic acidosis, intravascular volume replacement with lactated Ringer's solution is recommended, unless there is evidence of liver failure.

With severe metabolic acidosis associated with cardiac resuscitation, intravenous sodium bicarbonate is preferred. The amount required is equivalent to 30 per cent of the body weight in kilograms multiplied by the base deficit. This amount can be estimated from this formula:

$$\text{Body weight (kg)} \times 0.3 \times (25 - \text{measured serum bicarbonate}) = \text{mEq of bicarbonate needed}$$

With metabolic acidosis, the serum potassium concentration may be normal or elevated owing to a shift in potassium from intracellular to extracellular fluid. After the acidosis has been corrected, serum potassium may decline, and for this reason, frequent potassium measurements are essential in order to evaluate the need for potassium supplementation.

METABOLIC ALKALOSIS

Etiologic Factors:

1. Chloride loss—vomiting, gastric suction
2. Excessive urinary excretion of acid—diuretic therapy, which also promotes potassium loss
3. Movement of hydrogen ions from the extracellular fluid into the cells as a consequence of potassium deficit
4. Excessive intake of bicarbonate

Laboratory Values:

1. The pH is greater than 7.44 (Table 106-1).
2. Bicarbonate is greater than 28 mEq/l.

TABLE 106-2. Major Plasma Electrolyte Imbalances Occurring in the Four Major pH States*

Condition	Aberration	Compensation	Arterial Blood pH	pCO_2	Serum Cl	Anion Gap	Common Clinical Situations
Metabolic acidemia	↓ pH due to generation of acid (e.g., lactic acidemia) or retention of acid (e.g., uremic acidemia); H^+ combines with HCO_3^- and other buffers, lowering HCO_3 and raising H_2CO_3 which is excreted by lungs as carbon dioxide and water	↑ Minute ventilation, ↓ pCO_2 and ↓ (H_2CO_3), ↑ renal reabsorption of HCO_3 and excretion of H^+; extracellular H^+ into cells and paracellular ground substance and bony apatite; release of K^+ from cells and Na^+, Ca^{++} from paracellular ground substance and bony apatite	< 7.35	Low	Normal; low when there is hyponatremic dehydration; high in renal tubular acidemia, bicarbonate wasting, diarrhea, ammonium chloride therapy	Increased	Lactic acidemia 2° to sepsis, diabetic ketoacidemia, retained H_2SO_4, H_2PO_4 from protein catabolism in acute renal failure
Metabolic alkalemia	↑ pH due to loss of H^+ or gain of HCO_3^- (usually both simultaneously: e.g., in vomiting, gastric H^+ lost, HCO_3 reabsorbed from inside parietal cell)	Minute ventilation ↓ and pCO_2 ↑ only rarely, and with severe alkalemia; ↓ renal reabsorption of HCO_3, intracellular H^+ into serum, mainly as lactic, citric acids, accounting for ↑ anion gap; extracellular K^+ into cells and urine	> 7.45	Normal	High	Increased	Loss of H^+ from stomach: reabsorption of HCO_3 from parietal cell (vomiting). Loss of H^+ from kidney: reabsorption of HCO_3 from tubular cell, especially distal + collecting duct (diuretics); loss of K^+ promoting cellular K^+/H^+ exchange and inappropriately ↑ renal H^+ secretion

							(severe secondary aldosteronism, diuretics)
Respiratory acidemia	↓ pH due to retention of carbon dioxide, ↑ pCO_2, ↑ blood H_2CO_3	Extracellular/paracellular-intracellular H^+/Na^+ exchange, as in 1. ↑ renal HCO_3 reabsorption (takes about one day after acute onset respiratory acidemia); HCO_3^+ may be normal until then and pH largely undefended except for cellular + paracellular buffers	< 7.35	High	Low, after renal compensation	Normal	Pneumonia Myasthenic crisis Large pulmonary embolism Drug overdose
Respiratory alkalemia	↑ pH due to ↑ excretion of carbon dioxide, ↓ pCO_2, ↓ blood H_2CO_3	Extracellular/paracellular-intracellular H^+/K^+ exchange, including lactic, citric acids; ↓ renal HCO_3 resorption (takes about one day after acute onset of respiratory alkalemia)	>7.45	Low	High, after renal compensation	Normal or increased	Pneumonia Pulmonary embolism Spontaneous hyperventilation syndrome Gram-negative sepsis Hepatic encephalopathy

*From Barber HRK, Graber EA: Surgical Disease in Pregnancy. Philadelphia, W.B. Saunders Company, 1974.

3. Serum potassium and chloride are usually low.
4. The pCO_2 is elevated above 40 with respiratory compensation.
5. Urine sodium is initially high, but if alkalosis persists, the urine sodium concentration drops.

Compensatory Mechanisms: Compensation is both respiratory and renal. The respiratory compensation is hypoventilation, accumulation of CO_2, and increased blood levels of carbonic acid. Renal compensation is excretion of sodium bicarbonate in an alkaline urine. Unless adequate amounts of sodium and chloride are provided, this leads to dehydration, an increased renal excretion of potassium and hydrogen ion in exchange for sodium, and further alkalosis.

Management: Replacement of chloride is essential. Usually, intravenous potassium chloride is indicated, since the kidney is excreting potassium in order to retain hydrogen ions.

Tetany may be associated with severe or rapidly developing alkalosis because of a pH-dependent decrease in available ionized calcium. If this is symptomatic, 10 ml of calcium gluconate should be given slowly intravenously.

RESPIRATORY ACIDOSIS

Etiologic Factors:

1. Hypoventilation—inadequate elimination of carbon dioxide by the lungs
   a. Pulmonary disease—atelectasis, respiratory obstruction, infection, pulmonary embolus
   b. Respiratory center depression—narcotics, anesthetics
   c. Restriction of pulmonary ventilation—muscle weakness or paralysis

Laboratory Values:

1. The pH decreases (less than 7.38) (Table 106-1).
2. The pCO_2 increases (greater than 50 in the chronic phase).
3. Bicarbonate is normal or increased.

Compensatory Mechanisms: Compensation is accomplished mainly by increased renal tubular reabsorption of sodium and bicarbonate and increased excretion of hydrogen ion. The resulting rise in serum bicarbonate tends to restore the pH toward normal.

Management: The aim of treatment is improved pulmonary ventilation in order to increase the inspired oxygen concentration and facilitate carbon dioxide excretion.

RESPIRATORY ALKALOSIS

Etiologic Factors:

Hyperventilation, caused by apprehension, pain, fever, central nervous system injury, or respirator therapy, is an etiologic factor.

Laboratory Values:

1. The pH is greater than 7.44 (Table 106-1).
2. The pCO_2 is less than 36.
3. Bicarbonate levels tend to fall with renal compensation.
4. Urinary sodium and pH are high.

Compensatory Mechanisms: Renal compensation is increased tubular excretion of sodium bicarbonate. (In the case of hyponatremia or high levels of aldosterone, renal compensatory mechanisms are deficient.)

Management: Mild respiratory alkalosis is common and rarely needs specific correction. (Rebreathing into a paper bag is occasionally beneficial.)

Severe respiratory alkalosis must be treated by elimination of the initiating cause.

When alkalosis is accompanied by muscle irritability or tetany, serum calcium concentrations may be low; this is corrected by parenteral administration of calcium salts (calcium chloride or calcium gluconate).

REFERENCES

Breen JL, Gutkin M: Body fluids in obstetric problems. *In* Barber HRK, Graber EA: Surgical Disease in Pregnancy. Philadelphia, W.B. Saunders Company, 1974

Sabiston DC, Spencer FC: Gibbon's Surgery of the Chest. Philadelphia, W.B. Saunders Company, 1976

Schwartz WB: Disorders of fluid, electrolyte, and acid-base balance. *In* Beeson PB, McDermott W: Textbook of Medicine. Philadelphia, W.B. Saunders Company, 1975

107 BLOOD TRANSFUSION

INDICATIONS

1. Blood volume replacement
2. Red cell replacement
3. Correction of coagulation disorders

PROCEDURE

1. Ten ml of clotted blood, drawn from the patient, is sent to the blood bank for type, Rh, antibody screen, and cross-matching.
2. In an emergency situation,when time for cross-matching is unavailable, type-specific blood may have to be administered to the patient.
3. When blood is administered very rapidly under pressure, the infusion tubing should be warmed through an approved blood warmer. (Hypothermia increases oxy-hemoglobin affinity and may alter oxygen delivery to cells. Hypothermia also impairs citrate metabolism, which impairment is associated with an increased potential for citrate intoxication and hypocalcemia.)
4. Isotonic saline solution is preferred for initiation of the intravenous infusion prior to the administration of blood. Solutions that contain only dextrose without sodium chloride and solutions that contain calcium ion are not to be mixed with blood. Medications should *never* be added to the blood container.
5. All blood products should be infused through a filter that prevents the passage of particles harmful to the patient.
6. When multiple transfusions are required, the platelet count, prothrombin time, and partial thromboplastin time should be analyzed after each transfusion of 5 units of blood. When 10 units or more of blood must be administered, platelet concentrates and fresh-frozen plasma are usually required to correct platelet deficiency and impaired coagulation. As an alternative, fresh whole blood may be administered, if available, for

emergency situations requiring 10 units or more or when components (fresh-frozen plasma, platelets) are not available. After each 5 units of blood is transfused, pO_2, pCO_2, and pH should be determined. In addition, the electrocardiogram may reveal hyperkalemia or hypocalcemia or both. The latter should be treated with calcium chloride as indicated. With massive blood replacement, a blood warmer is advised after administration of three units of bank blood. For every five units of blood transfused, one ampule (44.6 mEq) of sodium bicarbonate and one unit of fresh frozen plasma are recommended.

NORMAL VALUES OF BLOOD VOLUME FOR WOMEN

Total blood volume equals body weight (kg) multiplied by 63 . Total plasma volume equals body surface (m^2) multiplied by 1410.

CHOICE OF BLOOD PRODUCT

The availability of blood components permits selection of the blood product best suited to correct a patient's specific deficiency. In addition, specific blood component therapy conserves a valuable human resource in that one donated unit of blood can be made to serve many patients.

Stored whole blood is frequently the first choice for treating acute hemorrhage in order to restore blood volume and oxygen-carrying capacity. However, whole blood may not be readily available, particularly if the blood bank separates all blood into the various component parts.

A unit of stored whole blood contains 170 to 200 ml of red cells, 250 ml of plasma, and 65 ml of citrate anticoagulant. Hematocrit is approximately 39 per cent, plasma sodium is 45 mEq, and plasma potassium is 3 to 8 mEq. Platelets are *not* preserved in stored whole blood.

Packed red blood cells—the component remaining after the plasma has been removed from whole blood—are preferred for treatment of severe anemia without hypovolemia, when the defect in oxygen transport is the prime concern. Since packed red blood cells contain the same red cell mass as whole blood, this component provides the same oxygen-carrying capacity in a smaller volume. The removal of plasma decreases the total amount of extracellular electrolytes present in the transfused unit. This reduction in electrolytes, especially potassium, may be particularly important for patients with cardiac, renal, or hepatic dysfunction.

The removal of plasma also decreases the anti-A and anti-B antibodies normally present in the blood of people lacking the corresponding antigen. This is of value when it is necessary to use group O blood for recipients who have blood other than group O. Removal of plasma may also decrease the possibility of febrile reactions to plasma protein.

Packed red cells are preferred to whole blood for patients with slow blood loss, in order to avoid increased central venous pressure that could aggravate capillary and venous oozing.

Packed red blood cells plus balanced electrolyte solutions (lactated Ringer's solution) can be adequate therapy for moderate acute blood loss. Fresh-frozen plasma assists in the prevention of coagulation disorders.

If the viscosity of packed red cells causes difficulty in administration, 150 to 200 ml of saline may be mixed with the packed cells through the Y-connection of the standard transfusion set. Saline-suspended red cells tend to flow faster than whole blood of comparable packed cell volume because the viscosity of the saline is lower than that of normal plasma. Solutions containing calcium should not be mixed with blood, since the calcium can overwhelm the binding capacity of the citrate anticoagulant and produce clotting.

The average rise in hematocrit after infusion of 1 unit of packed red blood cells into a 50-kg woman (assuming a pretransfusion hemtocrit of 30 per cent) is 3 per cent.

Plasma protein fraction (human) provides replacement colloid but does *not* contain any coagulation factors. The proteins consist primarily of albumin (not less than 83 per cent) and alpha- and beta-globulins. Because of the risk of hypotensive reactions, Normal Serum Albumin (Human) is usually preferred when replacement colloid is indicated.

Platelet concentrates are indicated for the treatment of thrombocytopenia with bleeding, which may be associated with abnormal platelet destruction, inadequate platelet production, or the transfusion of large amounts of stored bank blood. Spontaneous hemorrhage is rare as long as the platelet count exceeds 25,000/mcl, exceptions being patients with platelet dysfunction. Platelet transfusion may also be indicated for patients with congenital or acquired platelet disorders who undergo surgical procedures.

Actively bleeding patients with platelet counts less than 50,000 are likely to benefit from platelet transfusion. Six to eight platelet packs should raise the platelet count approximately 40,000/mcl. Frequently an initial transfusion of 0.1 unit/kilo of body weight is administered. Fever, infection, hepatosplenomegaly, or antiplatelet allo-antibodies decrease platelet transfusion effectiveness.

Transfused platelets are cleared from the circulation within 24 hours. When thrombocytopenia is secondary to accelerated platelet destruction, donor platelets are destroyed as rapidly as autologous platelets.

Since platelet concentrates may be contaminated with a few red blood cells, it is preferable to give platelets from ABO compatible donors whenever possible. Furthermore, Rh-negative women should receive platelets from RH-negative donors, in order to avoid Rh immunization. If Rh-positive platelets have been used, anti-Rh_0(D) globulin is given within 72 hours.

Fresh-frozen plasma has three main characteristics: (1) fluid volume, (2) protein, and (3) procoagulants. Containing the labile plasma-clotting factors that decrease during unfrozen storage, fresh-frozen plasma is indicated for the treatment of clotting factor deficiencies that may be associated with liver disease or massive blood replacement. The risk of transfusion hepatitis is the same as for whole blood.

When multiple transfusions are required, fresh-frozen plasma supplements packed red cells, providing plasma volume and procoagulants.

Fresh-frozen plasma is also used for the treatment of individual clotting factor deficiencies. (For severe congenital deficiencies, specific factor concentrates may be indicated.)

Cryoprecipitate contains fibrinogen, factor VIII, and factor XIII and may be used to correct the deficiencies encountered in hypofibrinogenemia, hemophilia A, von Willebrand's disease, and factor XIII deficiency. Each unit contains 20 to 50 per cent of the factor VIII activity found in a unit of fresh whole blood, 30 per cent of the factor XIII activity, and 50 per cent of the fibrinogen activity in less than 3 to 5 per cent of the original volume. In von Willebrand's disease, surgical hemostasis may require 10 to 12 units of cryoprecipitate initially (1 unit per 6 kg of body weight). Each unit of "cryo" contains at least 80 units of factor VIII.

Fresh whole blood is rarely necessary. However, in the case of massive transfusion—more than 10 units of replacement blood—fresh whole blood eliminates the need for combining components, since it contains optimally functional red cells, clotting factors, and platelets.

Fibrinogen concentrates are rarely used owing to the high risk of hepatitis. If fibrinogen replacement is required, cryoprecipitate is preferred.

Prothrombin complex concentrate is a highly concentrated preparation of the vitamin K-dependent hepatic procoagulants. Each vial contains 500 units of factor IX in a 20-ml volume. Factors II, VII, and X are also concentrated to a similar degree. Because of the risk of hepatitis and thromboembolic complications, prothrombin complex concentrate is reserved for life-threatening circumstances associated with a deficiency of factor II, VII, IX, or X. Whenever possible, alternative modes of therapy (for example, a trial of 4 units of fresh frozen plasma or 6 to 8 units of platelet concentrates or both) are preferred.

TRANSFUSION REACTIONS AND RISKS

Symptoms of transfusion reactions include hives, chills, fever, palpitation, chest pain, flank pain, shortness of breath, headache, flushing, loss of consciousness, shock, oliguria, hematuria, and bleeding tendencies.

Whenever a transfusion reaction is suspected, the following procedure should be followed:

1. Stop the transfusion immediately.
2. Keep the vein open with intravenous fluids infused through a new administration set.
3. Monitor the patient's blood pressure.
4. Monitor the urine output.
5. Draw an immediate post-transfusion blood specimen without anticoagulants and send with the blood container and the attached

administration set to the blood bank. (The serum or plasma can then be examined for free hemoglobin.)

6. The first post-transfusion urine should be analyzed for free hemoglobin.
7. Draw another blood specimen within one or two hours if there continues to be any suspicion of a hemolytic reaction.

IMMEDIATE REACTIONS

Pyrogenic reactions without hemolysis are usually due to nonbacterial pyrogens or antibodies to serum protein. The patient's temperature tends to rise rapidly, as high as 104° F. The blood transfusion should be immediately discontinued and the patient treated with oxygen and antipyretic medication.

Allergic reactions include hives, itching, angioneurotic edema, bronchospasm, and anaphylaxis. These are treated with antihistamines, corticosteroids, and epinephrine. (See Anaphylaxis, p. 125.)

Circulatory overloading should be prevented by the monitoring of central venous pressure and the administration of packed red blood cells.

Septicemia results from bacterial contamination of blood. Symptoms are those of septic shock. (See Septic Shock, p. 621.)

Hemolysis is one of the most serious reactions and may be manifest by chills, fever, dyspnea, chest pain, severe lumbar pain, acute apprehension, nausea, vomiting, vascular collapse, shock, cyanosis, renal failure, and the presence of hemoglobinemia or hemoglobinuria. In order to prevent hemolytic reactions, the first 100 ml of blood should always be given under close observation. When there is any evidence of acute hemolysis, the transfusion should be discontinued immediately.

Treatment of an acute hemolytic reaction is aimed at the prevention of renal failure. Urine output is an important guide to management and should be measured at hourly intervals. The objective of treatment is a urine flow of at least 100 ml per hour until the effects of the reaction have subsided. Intravascular volume must be maintained to assure adequate renal perfusion.

As soon as the reaction has occurred, 100 ml (20 gm) of a 20 per cent solution of mannitol is administered intravenously during a five-minute interval in order to stimulate diuresis. In addition, 45 to 50 mEq of sodium bicarbonate may be infused. Intravenous fluids containing approximately 50 mEq of sodium per liter (for example, 300 ml of normal saline plus 700 ml of 5 per cent dextrose in water) are administered in sufficient volume to maintain the urine flow at a rate of more than 100 ml per hour. The original dose of mannitol may be repeated if the urine flow drops below 100 ml per hour, but not more than 100 gm of mannitol should be administered within any 24-hour period.

With evidence of renal shutdown, fluid intake is restricted to insensible losses (500 ml) plus visible output per 24 hours, all potassium being avoided. Transferral of the patient to a renal center for dialysis must be considered. (See Urinary Suppression, p. 660.)

Leukocyte antibody transfusion reactions resemble those seen in patients who have been injected with bacterial pyrogens. Three phases in this reaction have been described. First, there is a transient, mild reaction, usually beginning within five minutes of the start of the transfusion. This consists of flush, palpitation, increased pulse rate, tightness in the chest, and cough. Following a second stage of from 15 to 60 minutes, in which minimal untoward clinical signs are present, a third phase occurs, frequently bringing with it a rise in diastolic blood pressure, headache, and malaise, then progressing to a rapid rise in temperature often preceded by or associated with chills. A neutrophil leukocytosis with a marked shift to the left reaches its peak two to five hours after the start of transfusion. Pulmonary infiltrates may be noted on chest x-ray. Symptoms generally subside within 24 hours of onset.

Calcium and Potassium Disorders

Hypocalcemia may occur rarely when more than 2000 ml of citrated blood are administered rapidly (within 30 minutes or less). Under these circumstances, or in the presence of severe liver disease, the citrate in stored blood binds ionized calcium. Hypocalcemia produces a prolonged Q-T interval on the electrocardiogram.

Hyperkalemia may result from the increased potassium concentration associated with blood storage and is associated with tall, peaked T-waves on the electrocardiogram. Hyperkalemia is usually a risk only when patients have renal insufficiency or preexisting abnormal potassium levels.

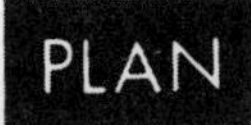

PATIENT EDUCATION

The possibility of delayed reactions, particularly post-transfusion hepatitis, should be discussed with the patient. Screening for hepatitis B antigen and utilization of a volunteer donor population have decreased the incidence of hepatitis to less than two to four cases per 1000 units transfused.

Post-transfusion hepatitis is suspected if the patient acquires a flu-like illness, arthritis, fever, anorexia, nausea, vomiting, jaundice, right upper quadrant pain, or extreme lethargy within the incubation period of 30 to 180 days.

REFERENCES

Blood Component Therapy. 2nd ed. Washington, D.C., American Association of Blood Banks, 1975

Cash JD (ed): Blood transfusion and blood products. Clin Haematol *5*:1-226, 1976

Goldfinger D: Acute hemolytic transfusion reactions—a fresh look at pathogenesis and considerations regarding therapy. Transfusion *17*:85-98, 1977

Miller RD, Robbins TO, Tong MJ, Barton SL: Coagulation defects associated with massive blood transfusions. Ann Surg *174*:794-801, 1971

Mollison PL: Blood Transfusion in Clinical Medicine. 5th ed. Philadelphia, F.A. Davis Company, 1972

Sheldon GF, Lin RC, Blaisdell FW: Use of fresh blood in the treatment of critically injured patients. J Trauma *15*:670-677, 1975

108 CENTRAL VENOUS PRESSURE

PURPOSE

Central venous pressure (CVP) measurement provides an index of effective circulating blood volume and serves as a guide to fluid replacement therapy.

PROCEDURE

A central venous catheter may be inserted through the antecubital vein, the external jugular vein, the internal jugular vein, or the subclavian vein into the superior vena cava or the right atrium. The position of the catheter tip may be assessed by x-ray.

The equipment for measurement of central venous pressure consists basically of a U tube, one end of which is open to the air, the other being connected to a fluid reservoir. Using a three-way connector, either limb can be connected directly to the patient. To measure the central venous pressure

1. Fill the open limb of the U tube.
2. Connect the open limb directly with the patient.
3. If the catheter has been properly inserted and is lying in the correct place, then the level of fluid should fall in a stepwise manner related to respiration. When the fluid has stopped falling, the level should oscillate gently in time with respiration, rising with expiration and falling with inspiration.
4. Determine the relationship of the fluid in the open limb to the pressure in the right atrium, which varies depending on the patient's position. Usually, a point in the midaxillary line is chosen as an arbitrary zero point.

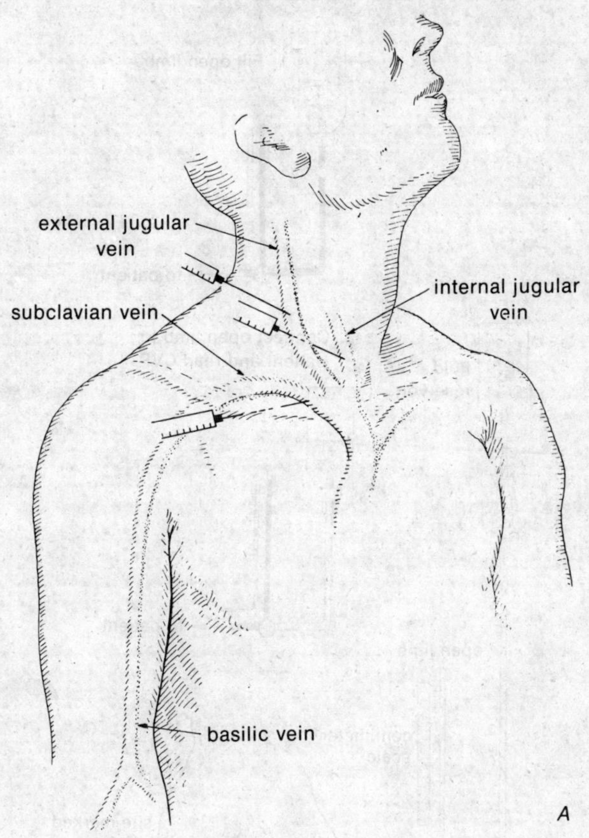

Figure 108-1. *A*, Routes of access for the measurement of central venous pressure (CVP). Catheters can be directed percutaneously into the superior vena cava from any of the veins shown. (From Artz CP, Hardy JD: Management of Surgical Complications. 3rd ed. Philadelphia, W.B. Saunders Co., 1975.)

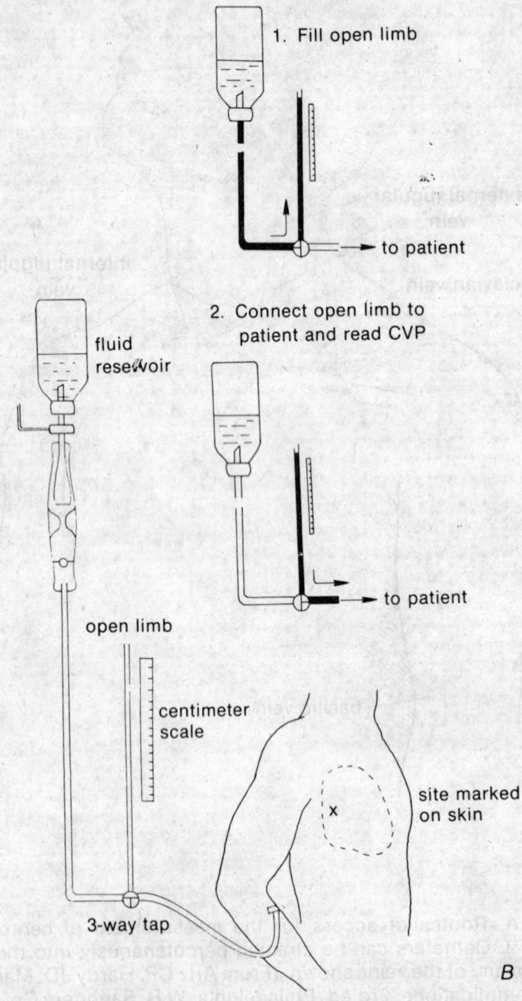

Figure 108-1 Continued. *B*, Measurement of central venous pressure. (From Calman KC: Basic Skills for Surgical Housemen. London, Churchill Livingstone, 1971.)

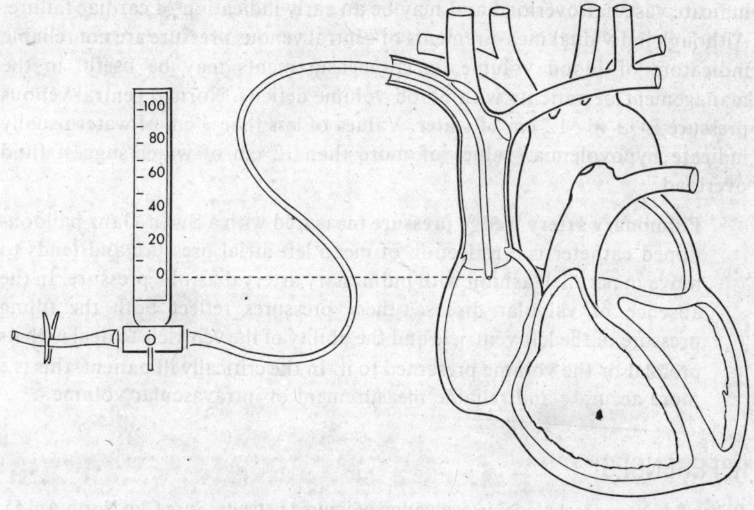

Figure 108-2. Central venous catheter in right atrium.

COMPLICATIONS

1. Local phlebitis
2. Septicemia
3. Fracture of the catheter with embolization to the heart
4. Lung puncture and pneumothorax with percutaneous subclavian vein catheterization

INTERPRETATION

Central venous or right atrial pressure reflects the ability of the right ventricle to deal with its preload but does not accurately reflect the state of filling of the whole venous system. Increased central venous pressure may indicate vascular overload and may be an early indication of cardiac failure. Although individual measurements of central venous pressure are not reliable indicators of blood volume, serial measurements may be useful in the management of patients with blood volume deficits. Normal central venous pressure is +3 to +12 cm of water. Values of less than 3 cm of water usually indicate hypovolemia; values of more than 12 cm of water suggest fluid overload.

Pulmonary artery wedge pressure measured with a Swan-Ganz balloon-tipped catheter is a reflection of mean left atrial pressure and tends to move in parallel fashion with pulmonary artery diastolic pressure. In the absence of valvular disease, these pressures reflect both the filling pressure of the left ventricle and the ability of the ventricle to deal with its preload or the volume presented to it. In the critically ill patient, this is a more accurate and reliable measurement of intravascular volume.

REFERENCES

Baker RJ: Newer techniques in evaluation of injured patients. Surg Clin North Am *55*: 31-42, 1975

Knopp R, Dailey RH: Central venous cannulation and pressure monitoring. J Am Coll Emerg Physicians *6*:358-366, 1977

Sharefkin JB, MacArthur JD: Pulmonary arterial pressure as a guide to the hemodynamic status of surgical patients. Arch Surg *105*:699-704, 1972

Shubin H, Weil MH: Routine central venous catheterization for management of critically ill patients. *In* Ingelfinger FJ, Ebert RV, Finland M, Relman AS (eds.): Controversy in Internal Medicine. Philadelphia, W.B. Saunders Company, 1974

Swan HJC: Central venous pressure monitoring is an outmoded procedure of limited practical value. *In* Ingelfinger FJ, Ebert RV, Finland M, Relman AS (eds): Controversy in Internal Medicine. Philadelphia, W.B. Saunders Company, 1974

Swan HJC, Ganz W, Forrester J, et al: Catheterization of the heart in man with use of a flow directed balloon-tipped catheter. N Engl J Med *283*:447-451, 1970

109 CESAREAN SECTION

DEFINITIONS

Cesarean section—the extraction of the fetus, placenta, and membranes through an incision in the abdominal and uterine walls.

Classic cesarean section—the extraction of the fetus, placenta, and membranes through a vertical incision made into the corpus uteri.

Low cervical cesarean section—the extraction of the fetus, placenta, and membranes through an incision made into the lower uterine segment, in either a transverse or longitudinal direction. (Synonym: Laparotrachelotomy.)

GENERAL CONSIDERATIONS

Cesarean section is recommended whenever labor or vaginal delivery would endanger the mother or the baby. Indications include cephalopelvic disproportion or obstruction, failed induction of labor, fetal distress or jeopardy, fetal malpresentation, placenta previa, placental separation, preeclampsia or eclampsia, prior uterine surgery, and uterine dysfunction.

PROCEDURE FOR LOW CERVICAL CAESAREAN SECTION

(Fig. 109-1)

The bladder is catheterized and the catheter left in place. The abdomen is shaved and surgically scrubbed.

The abdomen is opened with a low midline or transverse (Pfannenstiel's) incision. The vertical incision is often preferred when rapid delivery is essential. The transverse skin incision offers a cosmetic advantage.

Text continued on page 770

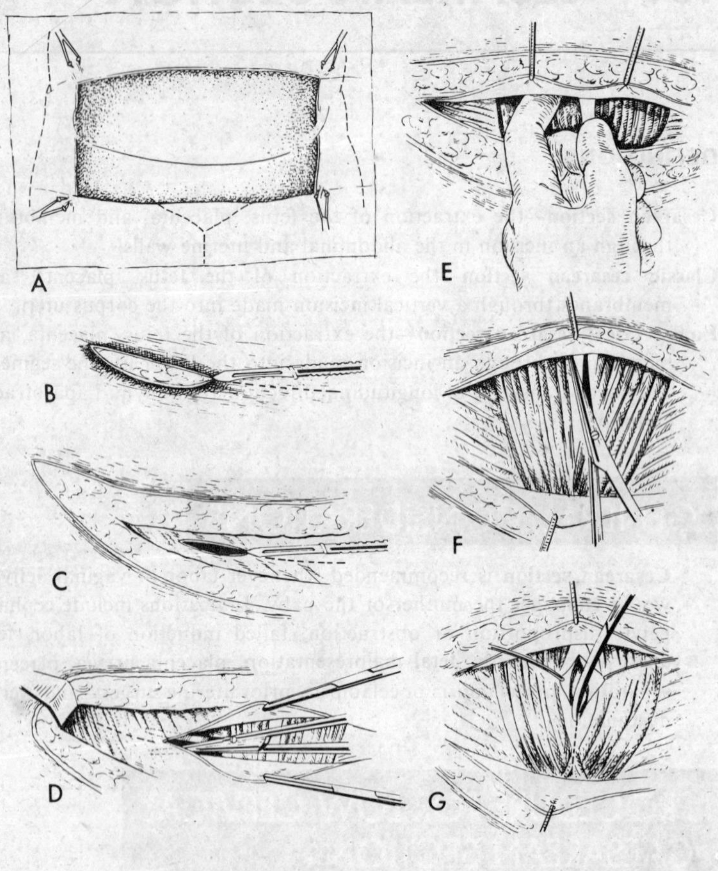

Figure 109-1. Low cervical cesarean section. *A*, Location of low Pfannenstiel incision. *B*, Transverse incision through skin and adipose layers. *C*, Anterior rectus fascia divided. *D*, Lateral extension of fascial incision. *E* and *F*, Elevation and separation of fascia from rectus muscle. *G*, Peritoneum vertically incised.

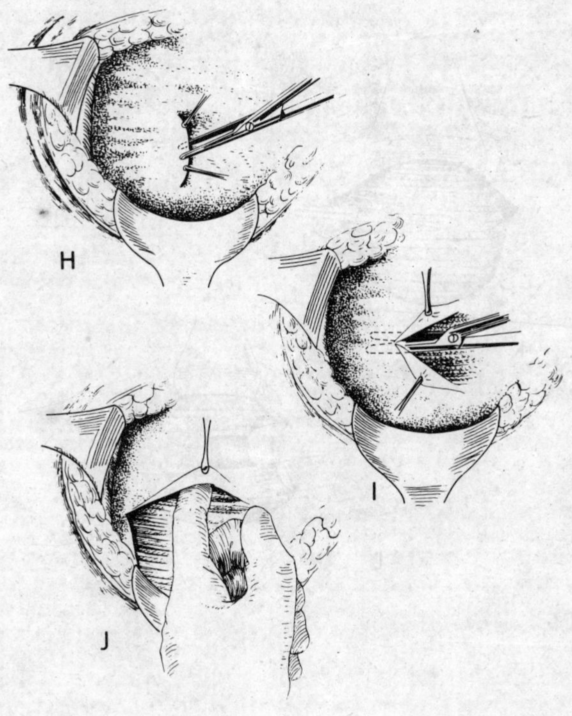

Figure 109-1 Continued. *H*, Vesicouterine peritoneal fold exposed for division. *I*, Lateral extension of vesicouterine incision. *J*, Development of (upper) peritoneal flap exposing lower uterine segment.

Illustration continued on the following page

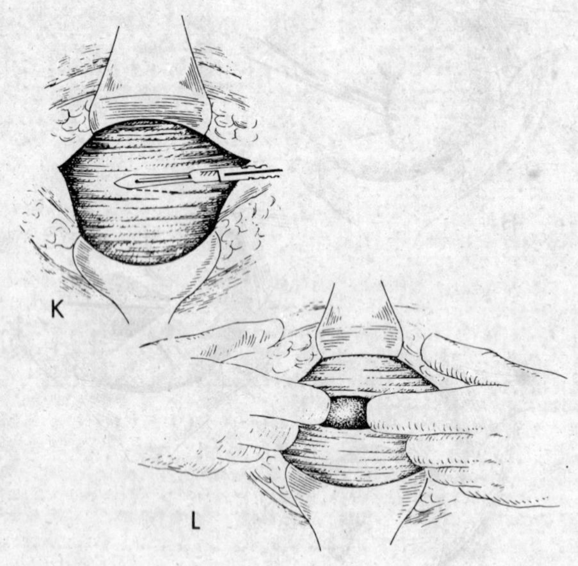

Figure 109-1 Continued. *K*, Short transverse incision made in lower segment. *L*, Incision enlarged transversely by digital splitting of muscle fibers.

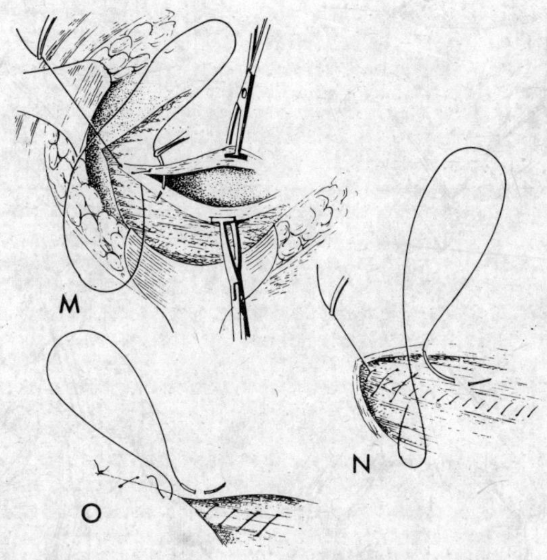

Figure 109-1 Continued. *M* Uterine incision closed in layers. Deep layer, continuous running suture. *N*, Superficial muscle layer closure, continuous Lembert suture. *O*, Double flap closure of peritoneum with continuous suture.

Illustration continued on the following page

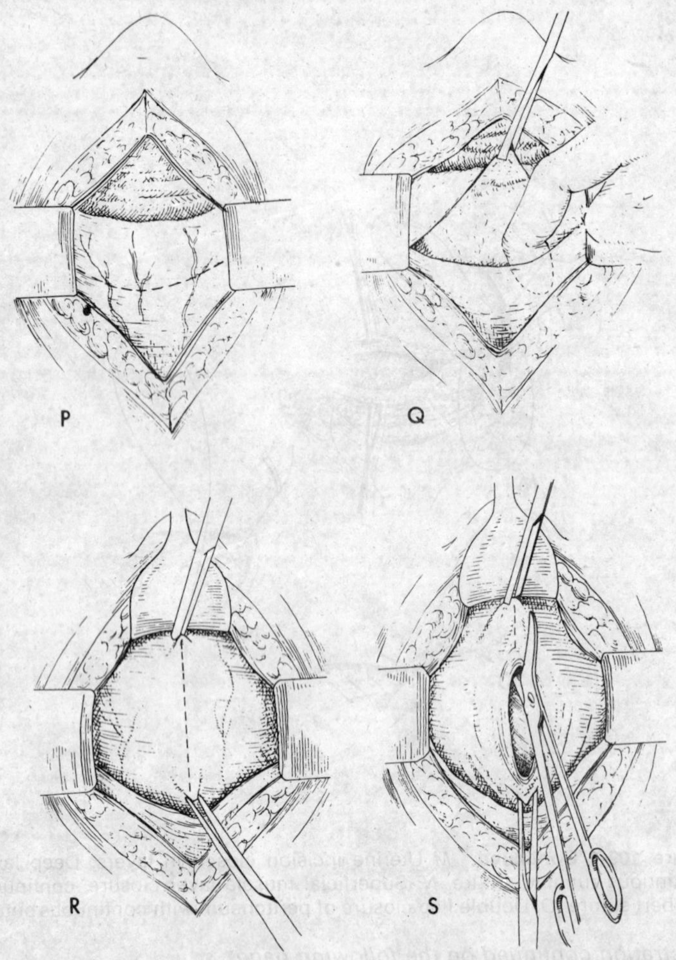

Figure 109-1 Continued. *P*, Bladder (BL)—curved dotted line indicates incision in the vesicouterine peritoneal fold. *Q*, The bladder peritoneum is freed from the lower uterine segment. An Allis forceps is shown on the bladder peritoneum. The upper peritoneal flap is also separated from the uterus. *R*, The bladder is held back by a retractor. The dotted line indicates a vertical incision in the lower uterine segment. *S*, After a small opening is made with a knife, the incision is extended with bandage scissors.

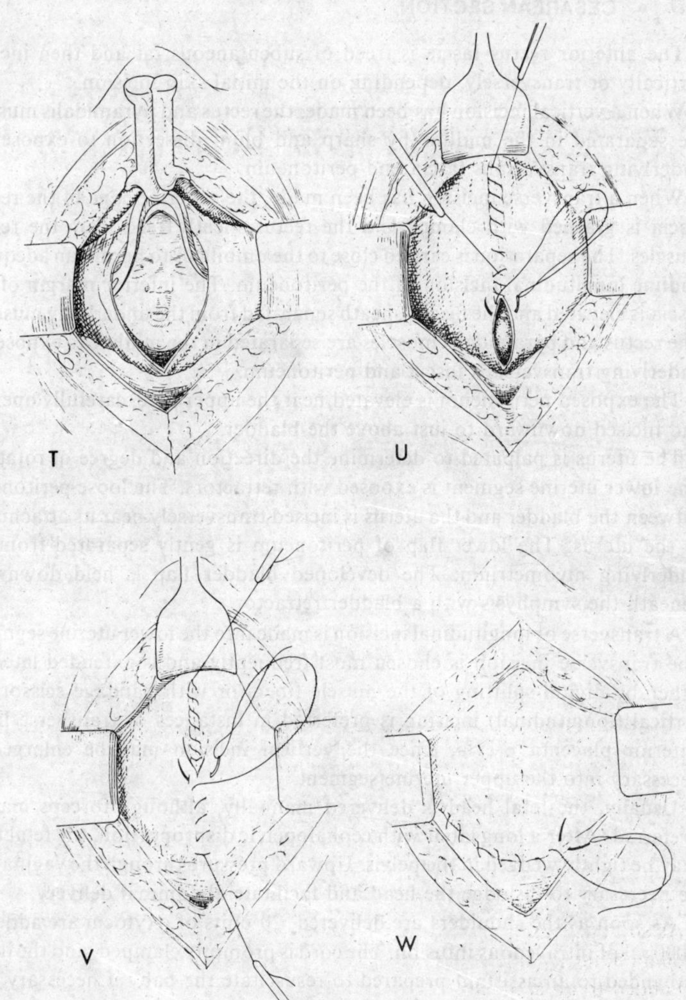

Figure 109-1 Continued. *T*, The baby's head may be delivered with forceps. L
The uterine incision is closed with a continuous suture of chromic O. *V*, /
second row of sutures is placed in the uterine musculature. *W*, The peritone
flap is reapproximated over the uterine incision.

The anterior rectus fascia is freed of subcutaneous fat and then incised vertically or transversely, depending on the initial skin incision.

When a vertical incision has been made, the rectus and pyramidalis muscles are separated in the midline by sharp and blunt dissection to expose the underlying transversalis fascia and peritoneum.

When a transverse incision has been made, the superior edge of the rectus fascia is grasped with clamps and the rectus sheath freed from the rectus muscles. The separation is carried close to the umbilicus to permit an adequate midline longitudinal incision of the peritoneum. The inferior margin of the fascia is elevated and the fascial sheath separated from the underlying muscles. The rectus and pyramidalis muscles are separated in the midline to expose the underlying transversalis fascia and peritoneum.

The exposed peritoneum is elevated near the upper pole, carefully opened, and incised downward to just above the bladder.

The uterus is palpated to determine the direction and degree of rotation. The lower uterine segment is exposed with retractors. The loose peritoneum between the bladder and the uterus is incised transversely near its attachment to the uterus. The lower flap of peritoneum is gently separated from the underlying myometrium. The developed bladder flap is held downward beneath the symphysis with a bladder retractor.

A transverse or longitudinal incision is made into the lower uterine segment. The transverse incision is chosen most frequently and is extended laterally either by digital splitting of the muscle fibers or with bandage scissors. A vertical (longitudinal) incision is preferred in instances of transverse lie or anterior placenta previa, since the vertical incision may be enlarged as necessary into the upper uterine segment.

Usually, the fetal head is delivered manually, although forceps may be preferred. After a long labor with cephalopelvic disproportion, the fetal head may be tightly wedged in the pelvis. Upward pressure through the vagina may be necessary to dislodge the head and facilitate abdominal delivery.

As soon as the shoulders are delivered, 20 units of oxytocin are added to 1000 ml of intravenous infusion. The cord is promptly clamped, and the infant is handed to an assistant prepared to resuscitate the baby if necessary.

The edges of the uterine incision are grasped with ring forceps or Allis-Adair forceps to minimize bleeding. The placenta is usually removed manually, and the uterine cavity is explored. If the cervical canal is not known to be patent, it is probed with a finger to ensure adequate lochial drainage. The contaminated glove is then changed.

The uterine incision is closed in two layers with continuous chromic 0 suture. The first row of sutures may be made in two segments commencing at the angle and sewing to the midposition from both sides. The second row of sutures inverts the first row.

After closure of the uterus, the vesicouterine peritoneum is reapproximated over the uterine incision. The abdomen is closed in layers: peritoneum, anterior rectus fascia, subcutaneous fat, and skin.

REFERENCES

Douglas RG, Stromme WB: Operative Obstetrics. 3rd ed. New York, Appleton-Century-Crofts, 1976

Greenhill JP: Surgical Gynecology. Chicago, Year Book Medical Publishers, Inc., 1972

Greenhill JP, Friedman EA: Biological Principles and Modern Practice of Obstetrics. Phiiadelphia, W.B. Saunders Company, 1974

110 CULDOCENTESIS

Culdocentesis—aspiration of peritoneal fluid from the rectouterine pouch (cul-de-sac of Douglas)—can be a rapid diagnostic procedure for elucidating a pelvic pathologic condition.

EQUIPMENT

1. Vaginal speculum—Grave's
2. Tenaculum for cervix—single tooth
3. Syringe—10 ml
4. Needle (spinal type), 18 gauge, 3½ to 5½ inches (9 to 12 cm)

PROCEDURE

The patient is placed in the lithotomy position, and the upper torso is elevated 30 degrees, if possible. A speculum is inserted into the vagina to visualize the cervix and posterior vaginal fornix, which are cleansed with povidone-iodine solution.

The posterior lip of the cervix is grasped with a single-tooth tenaculum and drawn upward toward the symphysis pubis. A long 18-gauge spinal-type needle is attached to a 10-ml syringe. Prior to puncture, the plunger of the syringe is withdrawn to allow 3 ml of air inside the barrel of the syringe.

The needle is inserted with a single, rapid thrust approximately 3 or 4 cm into the pouch of Douglas in the midline through the posterior vaginal fornix, approximately 2 cm behind the junction of the cervical and vaginal mucosa.

The air in the syringe is injected into the cul-de-sac; if no resistance is encountered, the needle is presumed to have entered the peritoneal cavity. The plunger of the syringe is withdrawn in order to aspirate the

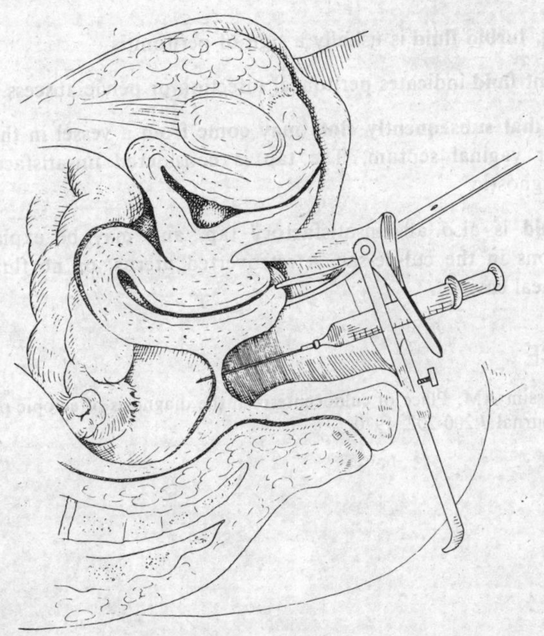

Figure 110-1. Diagnostic puncture of cul-de-sac or culdocentesis. (Modified from Greenhill JP, Friedman EA: Biological Principles and Modern Practice of Obstetrics. Philadelphia, W.B. Saunders Co., 1974.)

cul-de-sac; the needle is slowly withdrawn at the same time. Serous or purulent fluid is sent to the bacteriology laboratory for aerobic and anaerobic cultures.

INTERPRETATION

Nonclotting dark blood is indicative of intraperitoneal bleeding. Often, a few tiny, dark clots are found in the unclotted blood.

Serous, pink-stained fluid suggests ovulation, pelvic inflammatory disease, or a ruptured ovarian cyst.

Serous, turbid fluid is usually a sign of peritonitis.

Purulent fluid indicates peritoneal infection or pelvic abscess.

Blood that subsequently clots may come from a vessel in the uterine wall or vaginal septum. The tap is considered unsatisfactory and nondiagnostic.

No fluid is also an unsatisfactory tap, and may be explained by adhesions in the cul-de-sac, a retroverted uterus, or no fluid in the peritoneal cavity.

REFERENCE

Lucas C, Hassim AM: Place of culdocentesis in the diagnosis of ectopic pregnancy. Br Med Journal *1*:200-202, 1970

111 CURETTAGE

EQUIPMENT

1. Ring forceps
2. Cervical dilators—Hegar's or Pratt's
3. Uterine sound
4. Sharp curettes
5. Tenaculum
6. Jacob's clamp
7. Bivalve speculum
8. Anterior retractor
9. Biopsy forceps
10. Uterine packing forceps
11. Placenta forceps
12. Polyp forceps
13. Aspiration curettage cannulas, suction tubing, vacuum bottle and pump
14. Endocervical curette

INDICATIONS

1. Diagnostic: endometrial tissue for histologic diagnosis
2. Therapeutic: removal of placental tissue following abortion or delivery, removal of uterine polyps or hyperplastic endometrium

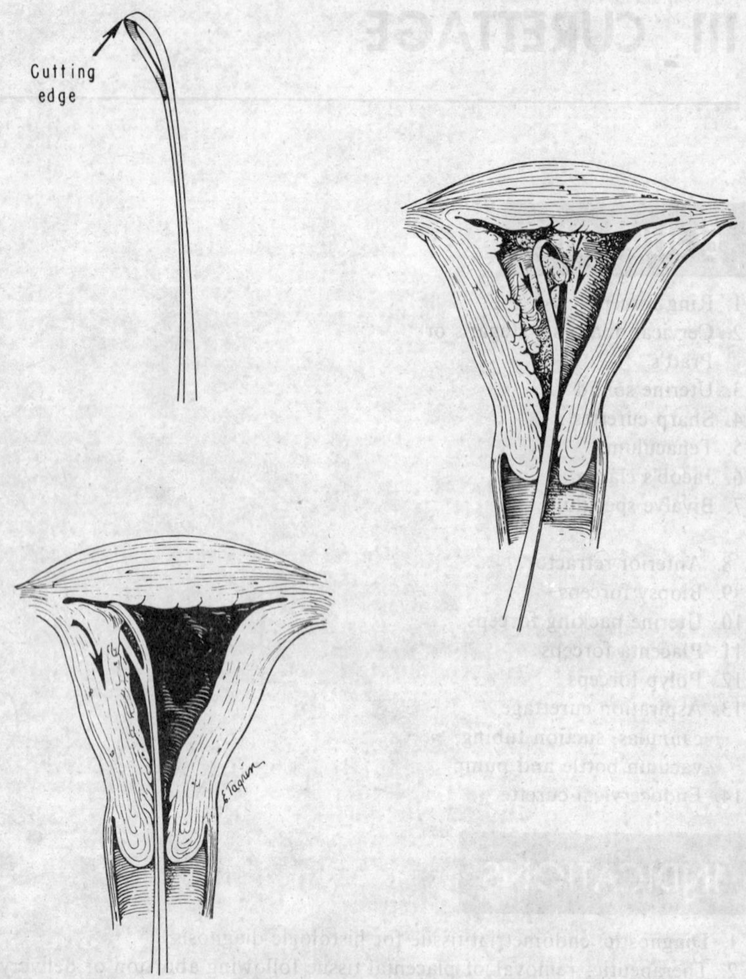

Figure 111-1. Uterine curettage. (From Kistner RW: Gynecology, Principles and Practice. 2nd ed. Chicago, Year Book Medical Publishers, 1971)

PROCEDURE

DIAGNOSTIC SHARP CURETTAGE

The procedure may be performed under general anesthesia or paracervical block. Prior to the curettage, the uterine size and position are determined with a bimanual examination.

The vagina and cervix are cleansed with an antiseptic solution. The cervix is grasped with a tenaculum or Jacob's clamp. The uterine cavity is measured with a uterine sound. The cervical canal is curetted with an endocervical curette.

The cervical canal is dilated with Hegar's or Pratt's dilators to a size sufficient to admit a sharp curette and a polyp forceps. Endometrial polyps, if present, are removed. The uterine wall is then curetted in a systematic fashion by scraping downward along the anterior wall, the side walls, and the posterior walls. A small curette may be useful for the cornual areas.

ASPIRATION CURETTAGE FOR REMOVAL OF PLACENTAL TISSUE FOLLOWING INCOMPLETE ABORTION

The procedure may be performed under general anesthesia, systemic analgesia, or paracervical block anesthesia. An intravenous oxytocin infusion is advisable.

The vagina and cervix are cleansed with an antiseptic solution. The anterior cervical lip is grasped with a tenaculum.

Usually, the cervix is already dilated by the passage of fetal and placental tissue. An 8-, 9-, or 10-mm suction cannula can frequently be inserted without difficulty. The suction tubing is attached to the cannula, and the endometrial contents are aspirated. A combination rotary and gentle to-and-fro motion over the uterine surface is recommended.

Following aspiration, a sharp curette may be introduced into the uterine cavity to verify the effectiveness of the evacuation. The tissue removed is collected in a mesh trap in the vacuum bottle; the blood loss can be estimated by measuring the fluid in the bottle.

REFERENCES

Greenhill JP: Surgical Gynecology. 4th ed. Chicago, Year Book Medical Publishers, Inc., 1969

Kistner RW: Gynecology: Principles and Practice. 2nd ed. Chicago, Year Book Medical Publishers, Inc., 1971

Russell KP, Ballard CA: Surgical Aspects of Abortion. *In* Barber HRK, Graber EA: Surgical Disease in Pregnancy. Philadelphia, W.B. Saunders Company, 1974

112 EPISIOTOMY

Episiotomy is a surgical incision into the perineum and vagina; the perineal skin, vaginal mucosa, and underlying musculature are usually cut with a large, straight scissors. Performed just prior to delivery, episiotomy enlarges the vaginal opening in order to prevent damage and laceration to maternal soft tissues and minimize fetal cephalic trauma at the time of premature delivery.

Median episiotomy, an incision made from the posterior fourchette in the midline of the perineum, is preferred if the perineum is of normal length, if the subpubic arch is of average width, and if no difficulty in delivery is anticipated. The incision extends along the midline fibrous septum or raphe (between the bulbocavernosus and ischiocavernosus muscles) down to but not including the fibers of the external sphincter ani muscle (Fig. 112-1).

Mediolateral episiotomy, an incision from the posterior fourchette into the perineum at approximately 45° from midline (Fig. 112-1), may be chosen to protect the sphincter ani and rectum from a third- or fourth-degree laceration, particularly if the perineum is short, the subpubic arch is narrow, or a difficult delivery is anticipated.

For repair, the perineal musculature, vaginal mucosa, and perineal skin are reapproximated, usually with 3-0 chromic catgut (see Fig. 112-2). The first suture is placed above the apex of the vaginal wound in order to incorporate any retracted blood vessels.

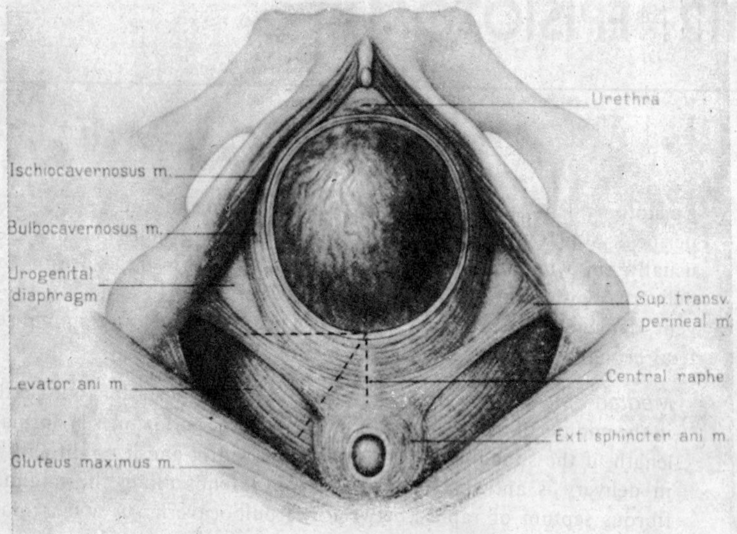

Figure 112-1. Muscles of pelvic floor. The lower birth canal is almost completely distended by the head. The dotted lines indicate the site of median, mediolateral and lateral episiotomy. (From Stromme WB, Douglas RG: Operative Obstetrics. 3rd ed. New York, Appleton-Century-Crofts, 1976.)

Figure 112-2. *(See opposite page for illustration.)* Steps in repairing a median episiotomy. This procedure has many variations in technique but several steps are basic: (1) elimination of dead space; (2) careful anatomic apposition with no single suture carrying undue tension; (3) attention especially to hemostasis at the apex of the vaginal wound; (4) adequate support at the fourchette and perineal body; (5) a minimum of catgut and knots; (6) avoidance of tissue trauma; (7) careful rectal check for misdirected sutures. (From Stromme WB, Douglas RG: Operative Obstetrics. 3rd ed. New York, Appleton-Century-Crofts, 1976.)

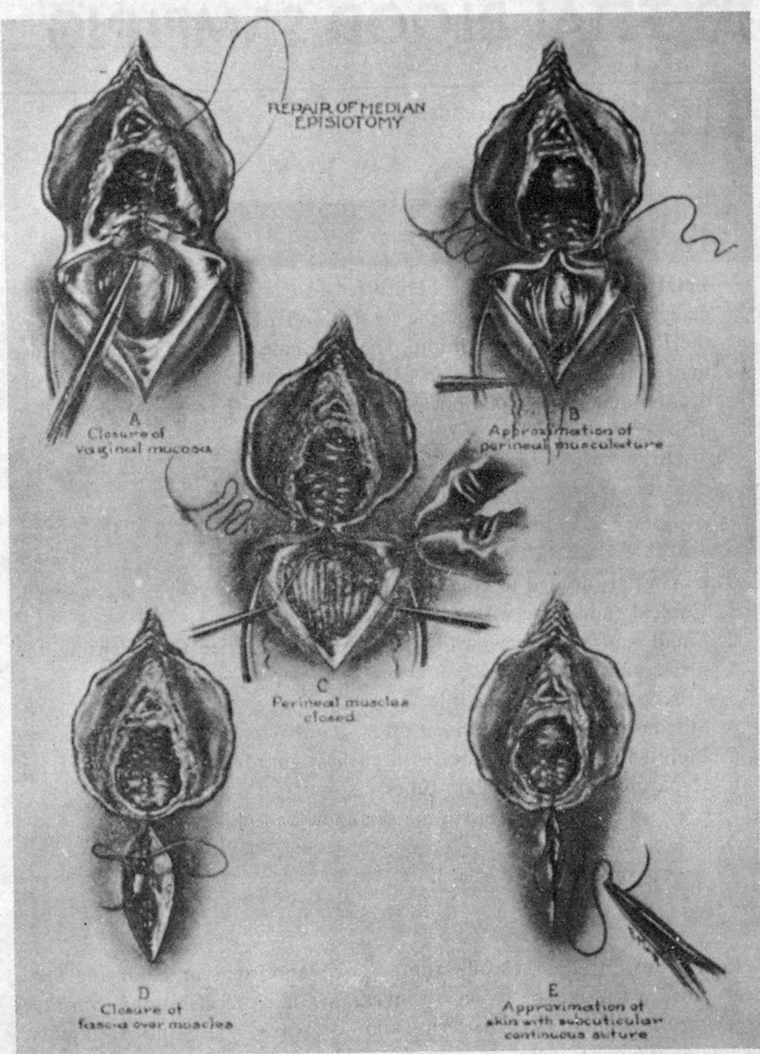

Figure 112-2.

REFERENCE

Greenhill JP, Friedman EA: Biological Principles and Modern Practice of Obstetrics. Philadelphia, W.B. Saunders Company, 1974

113 FETAL BLOOD SAMPLING

GENERAL CONSIDERATIONS

Fetal blood sampling can be utilized to evaluate fetal well-being and detect fetal distress, since the fetal blood pH corresponds closely to the infant's clinical condition. The rationale is based on the premise that when hypoxia due to cord compression or placental failure occurs, anaerobic metabolism causes a rise in free acid and a fall in pH.

EQUIPMENT

The materials needed to collect fetal blood include

1. Conical endoscope with a light source
2. Small gauze sponges with an instrument carrier for cleansing the presenting part
3. Ethyl chloride—spray bottle
4. Silicone gel or sterile mineral oil
5. Long-handled blade holder with push-in guarded puncture blades
6. Heparinized glass capillary tubes
7. Clay sealer for tubes, small metal mixer, and magnet

INDICATIONS

Indications for fetal blood sampling are abnormal or confusing fetal heart rate patterns: persistent tachycardia, late decelerations, variable decelerations, sinusoidal pattern, and decreased base-line variability. The fetal scalp pH helps to determine whether decreased base-line variability is secondary to fetal acidosis or maternal medication.

CONTRAINDICATIONS

Fetal blood sampling is not recommended under the following circumstances:

1. Family history of bleeding
2. Suspected fetal coagulopathy
3. Genital infections (herpes, gonorrhea, group B Streptococcus)

PROCEDURE

Fetal blood sampling is feasible only when the membranes have ruptured, the cervix is dilated 2 to 3 centimeters, and the presenting part is low enough to remain reasonably immobile.

The patient is placed in the lithotomy position and examined vaginally in order to assess cervical dilatation and the station of the presenting part. The endoscope is inserted into the vagina and through the cervix, and held firmly against the fetal presenting part. The obturator is removed and the exposed scalp visualized. The area chosen for puncture should not be over a suture line or fontanelle. The exposed scalp is cleansed of blood and mucus with gauze sponges and then sprayed with ethyl chloride to produce hyperemia. (A poor hyperemic response may be an indication of fetal distress.)

A thin layer of silicone or sterile mineral oil is spread over the scalp in order to promote beading or blood globule formation after puncture. The fetal blood sampling blade is pressed firmly into the scalp with a single quick stab. (The blade is preset to protrude 2 mm.) As the drop forms, the blood is drawn slowly and steadily into the capillary tube by means of plastic tubing. A continuous column of 2 to 4 inches is needed. The tip of the tube should touch blood only and not the scalp. No air bubbles should be permitted to enter the tube. (If blood does not flow readily, fetal distress may have caused peripheral vasoconstriction and fetal hypotension.) Two samples should be obtained for duplicate determinations. Steady pressure is then applied to the fetal scalp through two contractions in order to stop bleeding.

While hemostasis is being assured, the capillary tube with the fetal sample is plugged at one end. A small metal flea is inserted into the other end, which is also sealed. The blood is then mixed by moving the metal flea from one end of the tube to the other with a small magnet. The specimen should be delivered to the blood-gas laboratory immediately. A specimen of maternal blood is drawn at the same time for maternal pH.

A repeat scalp pH should be obtained in 10 to 15 minutes while one is awaiting the initial results. In this way, the decision for emergency intervention will be based on at least two samples obtained 10 to 15 minutes apart.

COMPLICATIONS

Potential complications include

1. Scalp infection
2. Persistent scalp bleeding
3. Blade breakage

INTERPRETATION

Generally accepted values of fetal scalp pH are

1. 7.25 to 7.35—normal
2. 7.20 to 7.24—borderline
3. Less than 7.20—abnormal

With a borderline value, the test should be repeated within 10 to 15 minutes.

A pH of less than 7.20 is an indication of fetal hypoxia with acidosis. Immediate delivery preparations should be made. Action decisions are based on at least two determinations ten minutes apart.

Sources of error in the interpretation of fetal scalp pH include maternal acidosis or alkalosis, fetal scalp edema or caput with a false low pH, specimen contamination by amniotic fluid, and improper instrument calibration.

When the fetal head is on the perineum, the scalp pH is in the range of 7.24 plus or minus 0.06. This may be due to stasis of the scalp circulation. In the case of maternal acidosis, a low fetal pH may be the result of a spillover into the fetal compartment.

REFERENCES

Coltart TM, Trickey NRA, Beard RW: Foetal blood sampling: practical approach to management of foetal distress. Br Med J *169* (1):342-346, 1969

Fetal blood sampling. ACOG Technical Bulletin, No 42, October 1976

James LS: Fetal blood sampling. Clin Perinatol *1*:141-147, 1974

114 FETAL HEART RATE MONITORING

EQUIPMENT

Cardiotocograph: The cardiotocograph is an electronic instrument designed to simultaneously detect the fetal heart rate (FHR) and measure the intensity and duration of uterine contractions (UC). The instrument provides an on-line display of the fetal heart rate signal source, an audible indicator synchronous with the signal, and a continuous written z-fold paper record of the FHR-UC data. Paper speed can be varied from 1 cm to 3 cm per minute; the slower speed is usually used for fetal heart rate screening, whereas the faster speed aids in the recognition of the FHR pattern.

The fetal heart rate may be recorded indirectly through the abdominal wall via an ultrasound transducer, a contact microphone that detects fetal heart sounds (phonocardiography), or abdominal electrodes that record the fetal electrocardiogram.

The fetal electrocardiogram is obtained directly when an electrode is placed on the fetal presenting part, usually the scalp.

Uterine contractions may be monitored externally via an abdominal labor activity sensor (tocodynamometer) or internally via a fluid-filled catheter placed transcervically into the uterus.

Direct or internal fetal monitoring is feasible only after the membranes have ruptured and the cervix is somewhat dilated.

PURPOSE

Continuous instantaneous recording of the fetal heart rate, particularly in relationship to uterine contractions, provides an assessment of fetal well-being. Changes in the fetal heart rate may be the earliest indication of uteroplacental insufficiency or umbilical cord compression.

Antepartum evaluation seeks to identify the fetus with a diminished reserve or tolerance to the stress of uterine contractions. (See Oxytocin Challenge Test, p. 820.)

Intrapartum evaluation assess the fetal heart rate response to the uterine contractions of labor.

PROCEDURE

Prior to labor, or during labor before the membranes have ruptured, the fetal heart rate and uterine contractions can be monitored only indirectly through the maternal abdominal wall. *Ultrasound* is the most widely used technique for detecting the fetal heart and obtaining a fetal heart rate recording without direct contact with the fetus. Sound waves are diffusely reflected from fetal blood cells in the fetal arterial circulation. The frequency of the reflected sounds is shifted by the Doppler effect, the shift in frequency being proportional to the velocity of the reflecting blood cells and the cosine of the angle between its velocity vector and that of the incoming sound wave. Since the basic nature of the Doppler signal is not as precise as the directly recorded fetal electrocardiogram, Doppler ultrasound cannot measure the *true* instantaneous fetal heart rate.

The fetal heart rate recorded by ultrasound appears to have more variability than the rate recorded with a direct scalp electrode. Although the ultrasound tracing provides an assessment of long-term variability, fine details of short-term variability are obscured by the increased jitter associated with the ultrasonic signal (Hon and Petrie, 1975).

Frequently, ultrasonic fetal heart data are averaged using a time constant in order to provide a "cleaner" tracing. This cleaner tracing, however, is not necessarily an accurate record of the true fetal heart rate (Hon and Petrie, 1975).

The fetal electrocardiogram may be obtained externally via electrodes placed on the mother's abdomen. The accuracy of this technique is affected by difficulties in placement of the electrodes and by interference by the maternal electrocardiogram.

The abdominal uterine pressure transducer records the frequency and duration of uterine contractions.

After the membranes have ruptured, an electrode applied directly to the fetal scalp provides the most reliable measurement of the instantaneous fetal heart rate, recording the R-R interval with an accuracy within 1 per cent. An internal intrauterine catheter reflects changes in the hydrostatic pressure of the amniotic fluid, recording the frequency, duration, shape, and relative strength of the uterine contractions.

INTERPRETATION

Base-line fetal heart rate is the rate that occurs (1) when the patient is not in labor, and (2) in an interval between uterine contractions during labor.

Periodic fetal heart rate is defined as the fetal heart rate associated with uterine contractions.

The normal fetal heart rate is between 120 and 160 beats per minute, with a normal base-line variability of between 5 and 15 beats per minute. As long as this pattern persists throughout labor, the prognosis for the neonate is good.

Interpretation of electronic fetal heart rate monitoring requires evaluation of

1. Base-line fetal heart rate
2. Variability of the base-line rate
3. Periodic fetal heart rate deceleration patterns
4. Periodic fetal heart rate acceleration patterns
5. Sinusoidal pattern

Base-line fetal heart rate, or the fetal heart rate present in the absence of uterine contractions, is calculated by averaging the rate over a ten-minute interval. The normal range is between 120 and 160 beats per minute.

Bradycardia reflects increased vagal tone and suggests fetal hypoxia. Bradycardia may be associated with congenital heart lesions and may also occur after paracervical block anesthesia.

Mild bradycardia is 110 to 119 beats per minute.

Marked bradycardia is 99 or fewer beats per minute.

Tachycardia reflects increased sympathetic stimulation and may be associated with maternal fever, fetal immaturity (under 32 weeks' gestational age), atropine-type drugs, fetal infection, fetal hypoxia, or maternal hyperthyroidism.

Mild tachycardia is 161 to 180 beats per minute.

Marked tachycardia is 180 or more beats per minute.

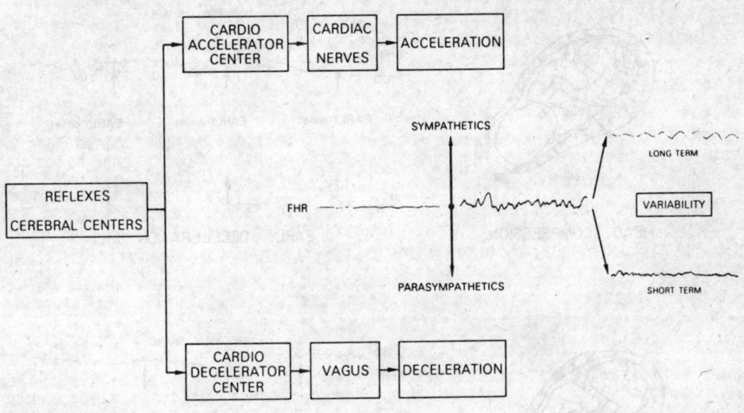

Figure 114-1. Schematic diagram indicating mechanism of FHR variability. (From Hon EH, Petrie RH: Clinical value of fetal heart rate monitoring. Clin Obstet Gynecol *18*:1-23, 1975.)

Variability of the base-line rate, that is, the difference in the R-R interval from one consecutive ECG complex to the next, reflects the dynamic interaction of the sympathetic and parasympathetic divisions of the autonomic nervous system on the fetal heart (Fig. 114-1). Short-term variability is the interval difference between consecutive beats. Long-term variability is the variation observed over the period of a minute. The normal base-line variability fluctuates between 5 and 15 beats per minute.

Decreased base-line variability may be an early sign of fetal hypoxia but may also occur when the fetus is asleep or the mother has received depressant drugs (narcotics, tranquilizers, magnesium sulfate).

Complete loss of base-line variability can be an ominous sign of fetal hypoxia, denoting failure of the fetal autonomic nervous system to alter the fetal heart rate.

Deceleration Patterns of Periodic Fetal Heart Rate:

Early Deceleration (Type I—Head Compression) (Fig. 114-2): The onset of the deceleration, the maximal fall, and the recovery reflect the shape of the associated uterine contraction and are

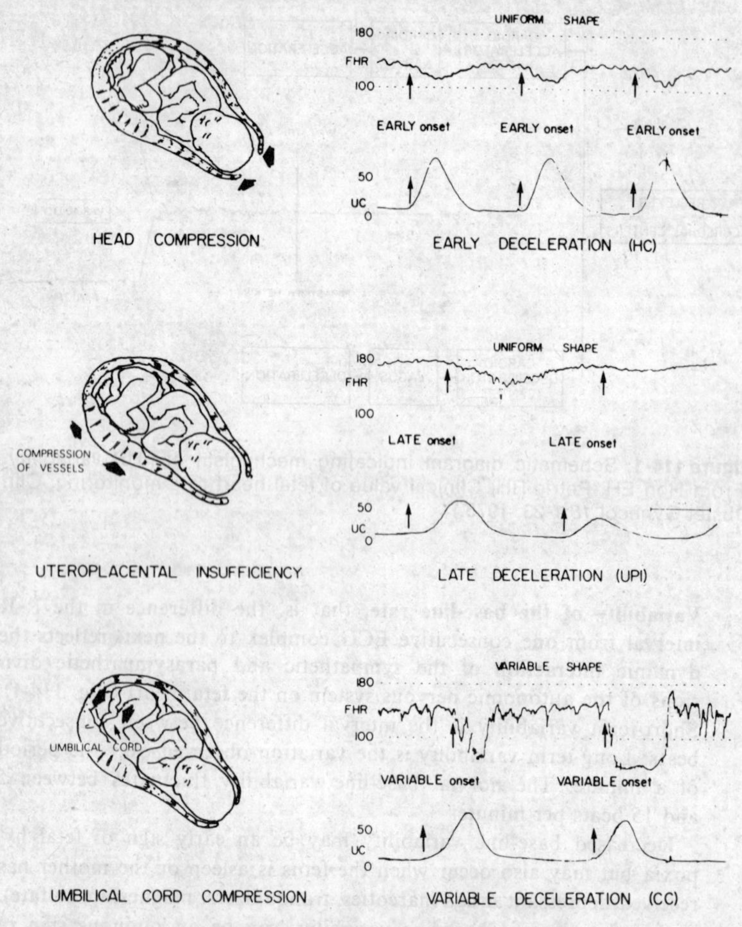

Figure 114-2. Diagrammatic representation of proposed mechanism of fetal heart rate deceleration patterns. *A*, In head compression pattern (HC) onset of deceleration (arrows) coincides with rise in intrauterine pressure (arrows). Uniform shape of deceleration reflects shape of associated uterine pressure curve. *B*, Uteroplacental insufficiency pattern (UPI) is characterized by uniform shape and onset late in contraction. *C*, Variable deceleration is of variable shape and does not reflect shape of associated intrauterine pressure curve; its onset is inconsistent in relationship to onset of contraction. (From Hon EH: Atlas of Fetal Heart Rate Patterns. New Haven, Connecticut, Harty Press, 1968.)

coincident with the onset, peak, and end of that contraction. The shape of the fetal heart rate curve is uniform and smooth, reflecting exactly the curve of the associated uterine contraction.

Increased uterine pressure appears to cause fetal bradycardia by a direct pressure effect on intracranial structures, that is, by head compression. The early deceleration may result from increased vagal tone secondary to an increased stimulation of the baroreceptors in the aortic arch or may be due to a decrease in central nervous system blood flow. This pattern is considered to be clinically innocuous, as long as the fetal heart rate does not become less than 90 beats per minute.

Late Deceleration (Type II—Uteroplacental Insufficiency) (see Fig. 114-2): The onset of a late deceleration occurs *after* the onset of the associated uterine contraction. The shape of the fetal heart rate curve is uniform, smooth, and similar to the curve of the uterine contraction, but follows it rather than coincides with it. The fetal heart rate becomes slowest 20 to 30 seconds after the apex of the contraction and gradually returns to the base-line.

This pattern is associated with fetal hypoxia, fetal and neonatal acidosis, and neonatal depression. It is found under conditions of impaired uteroplacental exchange, chronic hypertension, Rh isoimmunization, and diabetes mellitus. It has also been associated with excessive uterine activity and maternal hypotension.

Interpretation of deceleration patterns must take into consideration the base-line variability. If the base-line variability is normal, late deceleration may be an indication of acute hypoxia, possibly secondary to maternal narcotics or anesthesia. If the base-line variability is decreased or flat, the fetus is more likely to have chronic hypoxia.

Variable Deceleration (Umbilical Cord Compression) (see Fig. 114-2): This is the most common deceleration pattern. The onset, shape, and depth of the deceleration in fetal heart rate are completely variable in relation to the uterine contractions. The shape of the fetal heart rate curve is irregular, sharp, variable, and jagged and does *not* reflect the curve of the associated uterine contractions.

This pattern appears to be related to acute, transient compression of the umbilical vessels. Cord compression causes an increase in fetal blood pressure with subsequent stimulation of fetal baroreceptors. The drop in fetal heart rate appears to be reflexive in origin and mediated through the vagus, and it may be modified by the administration of atropine.

Variable or late decelerations combined with decreased base-line variability portend a poor fetal outcome. Whenever possible, the fetal scalp pH should be determined. Decelerations of fetal heart rate in the presence of a flat base-line are an ominous pattern indicating fetal exhaustion (Goodlin, 1974).

Periodic Fetal Heart Rate Acceleration Patterns: Transient accelerations during contractions represent the initial fetal response to stress. These accelerations and the accelerations associated with fetal movements are considered reassuring signs of fetal well-being, indicating a responsive, reactive fetus.

Sinusoidal Pattern: Periodic oscillation of the fetal heart rate with virtually absent beat-to-beat variability may represent loss of the normal neural mechanisms controlling fetal heart rate. This pattern has been observed in cases of severe fetal anemia and severe Rh isoimmunization and prior to fetal death *in utero*. (Rochard, 1976; Cetrulo, 1976).

REFERENCES

Baskett T, Ko KS: Sinusoidal fetal heart pattern. Obstet Gynecol *44*:377-382, 1974

Cetrulo CL, Schifrin BS: Fetal heart rate patterns preceding death *in utero*. Obstet Gynecol *48*:521-527, 1976

Fetal heart rate monitoring. ACOG Technical Bulletin, No 32, June 1975

Goodlin RC, Lowe EW: Multiphasic fetal monitoring. Am J Obstet Gynecol *119*: 341-357, 1974

Goodlin RC, Lowe E: A functional umbilical cord occlusion heart rate pattern. Obstet Gynecol *43*:22-30, 1974

Hon EH: Atlas of Fetal Heart Rate Patterns. New Haven, Connecticut, Harty Press, 1968

Hon EH, Petrie RH: Clinical value of fetal heart rate monitoring. Clin Obstet Gynecol *18*:1-23, 1975

Intrapartum fetal monitoring. ACOG Technical Bulletin, No 44, January 1977

McCrann DJ, Schifrin BS: Fetal monitoring in high risk pregnancy. Clin Perinatol *1*:229-252, 1974

Ott WJ: Current status of intrapartum fetal monitoring. Obstet Gynecol Surv *31*: 339-364, 1976

Paul RH: Intrapartum fetal monitoring: current status and the future. Obstet Gynecol Surv *28*:453-459, 1973

Rochard F, Schifrin BS, Goupil F: Nonstressed fetal heart rate monitoring in the antepartum period. Am J Obstet Gynecol *126*:699-706, 1976

115 FLUID AND ELECTROLYTE THERAPY

INDICATIONS

Intravenous fluids and electrolytes are required (1) to maintain normal body fluid volume and electrolyte concentration and composition when normal food and fluid intake is impossible, and (2) to correct acute or chronic disturbances of fluid and electrolyte balance.

BODY WATER

Total body water comprises approximately 50 per cent of a female's body weight. The normal daily requirement for water is about 25 to 40 ml per kg of body weight. Approximately half is excreted as urine, 400 to 600 ml are lost through the lungs, and 200 to 400 ml are lost through the skin. Normal feces contain approximately 100 ml of water (see Tables 115-1 and 115-2).

TABLE 115-1. Average Daily Volume of Water Loss

Urine	800-1500 ml
Intestinal	*
Perspiration	†
Insensible (lungs and skin)	600-900‡

*Average is 250 ml or less in stool. However, with vomiting or intestinal suction, specific volume lost must be measured.

†Varies with the patient's temperature and the environmental temperature; approximately, 250 ml/day/degree of fever.

‡Increased by hypermetabolism, hyperventilation, and fever.

TABLE 115-2. The Electrolyte Content of Various Output Losses (mEq/l)

Type	Na	K	Cl	HCO_3
Bile	140	10	100	30
Bowel	120	10	105	25
Gastric	35	12	125	—
Pancreatic	140	10	75	75
Saliva	10	25	10	10
Urine	40	30	70	—
Insensible, at rest	0	0	0	

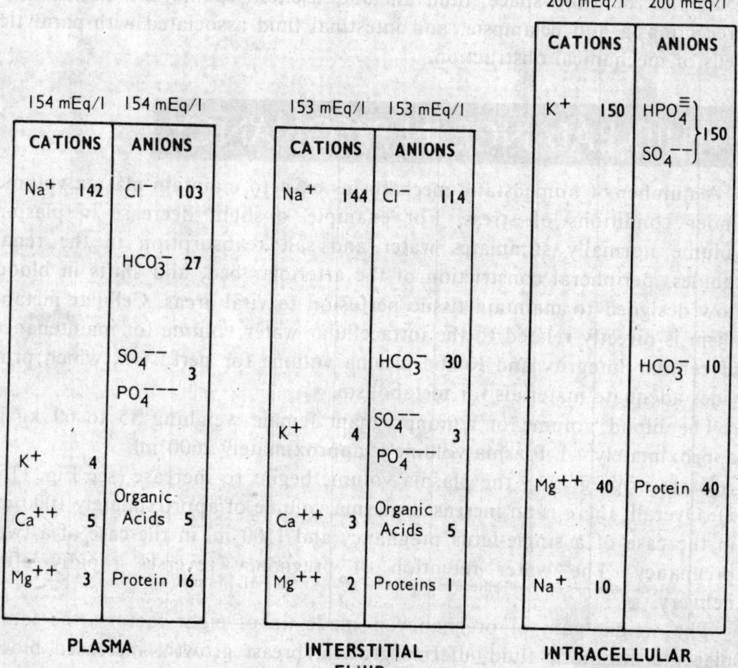

FIGURE 115-1. Chemical composition of body fluid compartments. (From American College of Surgeons: Manual of Preoperative and Postoperative Care. 2nd ed. Philadelphia, W.B. Saunders Co., 1971.)

Water is located in three compartments (Fig. 115-1):

1. Intracellular fluid (ICF) is the largest of these compartments.
2. Interstitial fluid is the water surrounding cells, that is, the tissue fluid. This accounts for approximately 20 per cent of body weight.
3. Intravascular fluid or plasma accounts for approximately 4 per cent of the total body weight.

Extracellular fluid (ECF) is the combination of interstitial fluid and plasma. Sodium is the principal extracellular cation and is of prime importance for maintenance of a normal extracellular fluid compartment.

Third space is a collection of extracellular fluid that, although present within the body and weighed with the patient, is functionally not available to normal physiologic mechanisms maintaining fluid and electrolyte balance. Examples of third-space fluid include ascites, edema associated with preeclampsia and eclampsia, and intestinal fluid associated with paralytic ileus or mechanical obstruction.

FLUID BALANCE IN PREGNANCY

A number of homeostatic mechanisms exist to maintain plasma volume under conditions of stress. For example, a slight decrease in plasma volume normally stimulates water and salt reabsorption in the renal tubules, peripheral constriction of the arteriolar bed, and shifts in blood flow designed to maintain tissue perfusion to vital areas. Cellular metabolism is directly related to the intracellular water volume for maintenance of cellular integrity and to the plasma volume for perfusion, which provides adequate materials for metabolism.

The blood volume of a nonpregnant female weighing 55 to 60 kg is approximately 4 l. Plasma volume is approximately 2600 ml.

Early in pregnancy the plasma volume begins to increase (see Fig. 115-2). Overall, there is an increased plasma volume of approximately 1000 ml in the case of a single-fetus pregnancy and 1500 ml in the case of a twin pregnancy. The water retention of pregnancy reverses rapidly after delivery.

The weight gain of pregnancy is made up of eight factors: the fetus, placenta, amniotic fluid, uterine growth, breast growth, increased blood volume, increased tissue fluid, and fat. These account for an increment of approximately 7000 gm of water by the fortieth week of gestation.

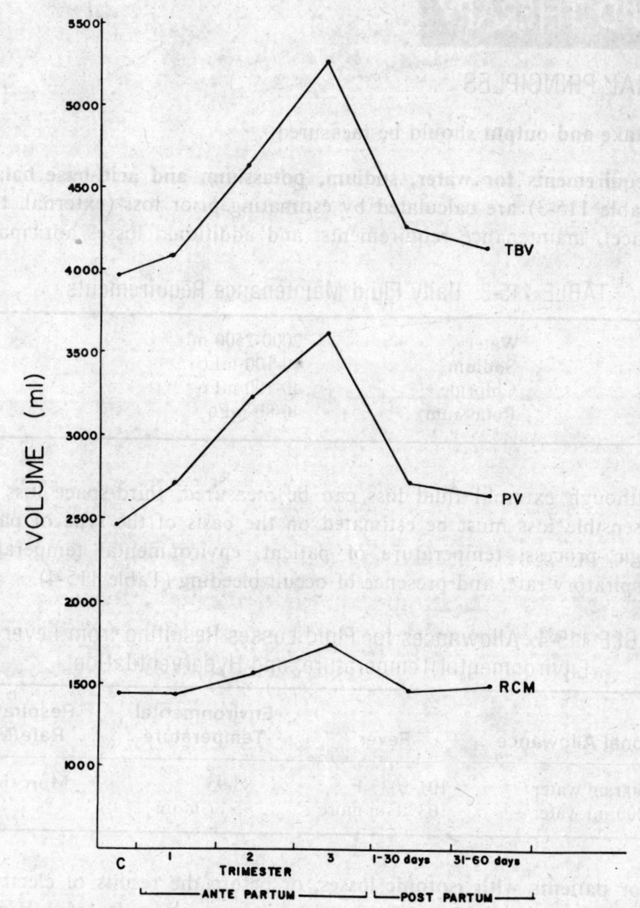

FIGURE 115–2. Changes in total blood volume (TBV), plasma volume (PV) and red cell mass (RCM) during and after pregnancy. Figures are the composite value derived from studies of several investigators. (From Lange RD, Dynesius R: Blood volume changes during normal pregnancy. Clin. Haematol. 2:437, 1973.)

FLUID THERAPY

GENERAL PRINCIPLES

Intake and output should be measured.

Requirements for water, sodium, potassium, and acid-base balance (Table 115-3) are calculated by estimating prior loss (external, third space), maintenance requirements; and additional losses anticipated.

TABLE 115-3. Daily Fluid Maintenance Requirements

Water	2000-2500 ml
Sodium	40-100 mEq
Chloride	40-100 mEq
Potassium	40-80 mEq

Although external fluid loss can be measured, third-space loss and insensible loss must be estimated on the basis of the type of pathologic process, temperature of patient, environmental temperature, respiratory rate, and presence of occult bleeding (Table 115-4).

TABLE 115-4. Allowances for Fluid Losses Resulting from Fever, Environmental Temperature, and Hyperventilation

Additional Allowance	Fever	Environmental Temperature	Respiratory Rate/Min
500 ml water	101-103° F	85-95	More than 35
1000 ml water	103° F or more	95 or more	

For patients with isotonic losses, or before the results of electrolyte studies are available, a balanced solution such as lactated Ringer's solution is usually preferred for the initiation of therapy. The object is restoration of tissue perfusion and replacement of interstitial fluid losses. As soon as serum electrolyte values are available, specific solutions should be selected in order to replace sodium, chloride, and potassium deficits, as indicated.

Volume replacement may be guided by the patient's mental response, the reduction in tachycardia and restoration of blood pressure, the return of urine output to more than 40 ml/hour, the response of the central venous pressure, and the improvement in overall appearance.

Contents of commonly used replacement solutions are listed in Table 115-5.

TABLE 115-5. Commonly Used Replacement Solutions (mEq/l)*

Solution	Na	K	Cl	HCO_3	Ca	Mg	Calories
Saline, normal	154		154				
Dextrose, 5% in water							200
Dextrose, 5% in saline	154		154				200
Dextrose, 5% in one-half normal saline	77		77				200
Ringer's lactate	130	4	109	(28)	3		
M/6 Lactate	167			167			
Plasma	142	5	105	27	5	3	
Plasma protein fraction, 5% solution	145	2	100				
Normal Extracellular Values	135 to 145	3.5 to 5.5	85 to 115	22 to 29	4.0 to 5.5	1.5 to 2.5	
Atomic Weight	23	39	35		40	24	
Valence	1	1	1		2	2	

$$*\text{mEq/l} = \frac{\text{mg/100 ml} \times 10}{\text{atomic weight}} \times \text{valence}$$

Complications of fluid therapy include microbial contamination, and particulate matter, particularly when medications are added to intravenous fluids.

POSTOPERATIVE FLUID THERAPY

1. Preoperative fluid status, the amount of fluid lost or gained during surgery, the blood pressure, the pulse, and the urinary output provide initial guidelines for adjustment of fluid balance.
2. The existing deficit and maintenance fluid for the next 24 hours are calculated. For critically ill patients, fluid requirements may have to be evaluated at two-, four-, or six-hour intervals.
3. Immediately after surgery, extracellular fluid volume depletion may be due to continued fluid losses at the site of injury or operative trauma. Unrecognized deficits of intracellular volume during the early postoperative period may be manifest primarily as circulatory instability. Blood pressure, pulse, and urine flow should be monitored hourly. In addition, the level of consciousness, airway patency, breathing pattern, skin warmth, color, and body temperature must be assessed.
4. Potassium is rarely required during the first 24 hours, unless a definite potassium deficit exists. After 24 hours, 40 mEq of potassium per day should cover renal excretion of potassium.
5. Fluid therapy demands accurate measurement and replacement of all losses. In a healthy person, this involves the replacement of measured sensible losses and the estimation and replacement of insensible losses. The latter are relatively constant, averaging 600 to 900 ml per day, although they are increased by hypermetabolism, hyperventilation, and fever. Perspiration, for example, increases the fluid loss approximately 250 ml per day per degree of fever. Estimated insensible loss is replaced with 5 per cent dextrose in water. Approximately 1 l of fluid is required to replace the urine volume necessary to excrete the catabolic end-products of metabolism (1000 ml per day). This fluid should contain a modest amount of salt solution to cover the urinary loss of sodium. Urine volume is not replaced on a milliliter-for-milliliter basis, since a urinary output of 2000 to 3000 ml on a given day may simply represent diuresis of fluids retained during pregnancy or administered during surgery.
6. Electrolyte measurements provide the most accurate assessment of fluid and electrolyte replacement until the patient is able to take oral feedings.

GUIDELINES FOR FLUID AND ELECTROLYTE THERAPY

SUBJECTIVE DATA

1. Diarrhea
2. Fluid and Blood loss
3. Thirst
4. Vomiting

OBJECTIVE DATA

1. Blood pressure
2. Pulse
3. Edema, Ascites, Pleural effusion
4. Skin turgor
5. Rales in lungs
6. Body weight

Laboratory Tests:

Hematocrit: Changes in the hematocrit in the absence of bleeding are a guide to changes in plasma volume.

Electrolytes: Serum sodium concentration is an accurate reflection of the extracellular sodium and, therefore, of the solute concentration and volume of extracellular fluid. Serum potassium concentration, however, is an inaccurate reflection of intracellular potassium.

Blood urea nitrogen and serum creatinine levels assess renal function.

Evaluation of arterial blood gases allows determination of the patient's acid-base status.

Urine output is a sensitive guide to the perfusion volume available for the kidney, which in turn reflects a summation of plasma volume, extracellular fluid volume, and total body water. An indwelling catheter is essential for those patients requiring monitoring of hourly urine output.

Central venous pressure may be helpful in the assessment of fluid requirements. However, central venous pressure does not accurately reflect the state of filling of the whole venous system. The pulmonary artery diastolic pressure and pulmonary artery wedge pressure are considered more reliable indicators for the prevention of fluid overload.

Renal function may be assessed by measuring the specific gravity and pH of the first voided urine in the morning. If the patient is able to concentrate a protein- and glucose-free urine to a specific gravity of 1.016 or higher and is able to excrete urine with a pH of 5.8 or lower, renal function is usually adequate. Signs of significant renal disease are specific gravity persistently less than 1.015, persistently alkaline pH, and proteinuria greater than 100 mg/100 ml.

The urine output of all patients on parenteral fluids should be recorded at least every eight hours. If there is a major imbalance, shock, or any suspicion of renal insufficiency, urine output should be recorded hourly.

The expected urine volume is 1500 plus or minus 500 ml per day (60 plus or minus 20 ml per hr) in patients in a basal state. Output of 500 ml per day or less constitutes oliguria. In the absence of tubular failure or obstructive uropathy, oliguria is prerenal in origin and may be a result of either a deficit in extracellular fluid volume or a deficit in total body water.

PLASMA VOLUME DEFICIT

Plasma volume deficit is the most common fluid disorder in the surgical patient. Etiologic factors include (1) exogenous fluid loss (bleeding, vomiting, diarrhea, perspiration, urinary diuresis), (2) endogenous loss into a third space, and (3) inadequate fluid intake (starvation, coma).

SUBJECTIVE AND OBJECTIVE DATA

Hypotension, tachycardia, and oliguria are the most frequent clinical signs. When plasma volume deficit is prolonged and excessive, aditional symptoms include thirst, apathy, stupor, and coma. The skin turgor may be decreased, and veins may be collapsed. The central venous pressure is low. The hematocrit may be decreased or elevated, depending on whether the cause is blood loss or plasma loss.

PLAN

Management and Treatment: Electrolyte-free fluid, balanced salt solutions, plasma, or blood is administered to replace the vascular and extravascular fluid. The choice depends on the etiologic factors.

The most practical guides to replacement of plasma volume loss are the hematocrit and urine output.

PLASMA VOLUME EXCESS

The most common cause of plasma volume excess is the immoderate administration of blood, plasma, electrolyte solutions or electrolyte-free water intravenously. In the presence of oliguria, or chronic pulmonary or cardiac disease, extracellular fluid expansion can lead to congestive heart failure with peripheral and pulmonary edema.

Plasma water excess associated with hyponatremia may produce cerebral symptoms. (See Hyponatremia, p. 804.)

Intravenous oxytocin infusion can decrease urine flow in both pregnant and nonpregnant women. The decrease is dose-dependent, reaching its maximum at a flow rate of 45 to 50 mU of oxytocin per minute. The antidiuresis is manifest within 15 minutes of the onset of the infusion and lasts for a similar period of time following its discontinuation (Abdul-Karim and Rizk, 1970).

SUBJECTIVE AND OBJECTIVE DATA

Symptoms and signs may include swelling of subcutaneous tissues, nausea, vomiting, headache, mental confusion, convulsions, coma, pulmonary edema, distended peripheral veins, elevated pulse pressure, elevated central venous pressure, and weight gain.

PLAN

Management and Treatment: Fluid intake must be restricted. Diuretic therapy may be beneficial.

HYPONATREMIA

Hyponatremia—a serum sodium of less than 130 mEq/l—may be associated with a normal or elevated plasma osmolality or a decreased plasma osmolality. Etiologic factors include

1. Osmolality—normal or high
   a. Hyperglycemia
   b. Hyperlipemia
2. Osmolality—low
   a. Excessive water intake combined with sodium restriction or diuretic therapy
   b. Sodium loss in excess of water loss
      (1) Gastrointestinal losses—suction, vomiting, diarrhea. These are commonly associated with hypokalemic alkalosis.
      (2) Excessive perspiration that is replaced with water but not with sodium
      (3) Volume depletion after diuretic therapy
      (4) Adrenocortical insufficiency
      (5) Chronic nephritis
   c. Excessive antidiuretic hormone, which may be the result of oxytocin administration
      (1) Urine osmolality higher than that of the plasma
      (2) Increased urine sodium

SUBJECTIVE AND OBJECTIVE DATA

The principal clinical manifestations are central nervous system depression, confusion progressing to somnolence, convulsions, and coma. The patient with severe hyponatremia can have oliguric renal failure. Occasionally, there are signs of increased intracranial pressure. Serum sodium and osmolality and urine sodium and osmolality may aid in management. (Patients with hyponatremia tend to accumulate intracellular water, and their overall body tonicity becomes lower. The accumulation of intracellular water produces the central nervous system effects of cerebral edema, because the brain is more permeable to water than to sodium and chloride.)

PLAN

Management and Treatment: In cases of hypervolemic hyponatremia, the body electrolyte volume may be assumed to be normal, whereas the water volume is far too great. Water deprivation is essential; water excretion may be hastened with the use of diuretics. In cases of isovolemic hyponatremia, the body electrolyte volume is low. Sodium should be replaced slowly with a 3 per cent sodium chloride solution.

HYPERNATREMIA

Hypernatremia—a serum sodium concentration of more than 150 mEq/l—may be due to excessive losses of salt-free water (excessive skin evaporation owing to fever or burns) or large renal losses of dilute urine resulting from high-output renal failure or prolonged osmotic diuresis (diabetes).

SUBJECTIVE AND OBJECTIVE DATA

Weakness and restlessness are characteristic symptoms. In cases of severe hypernatremia, delirium, thirst, agitation, headache, hypotension, oliguria and high fever may be present. The hematocrit tends to be elevated.

PLAN

Management and Treatment: The elevated serum sodium is gradually reduced by rehydrating the patient with salt-free water (5 per cent dextrose solution).

HYPOKALEMIA

Hypokalemia—a serum potassium level of less than 3.5 mEq/l—may be due to (1) renal loss of potassium, associated with diuretic therapy; (2) excessive loss of gastrointestinal secretions; (3) prolonged parenteral alimentation without the addition of potassium; (4) alkalosis; (5) primary aldosteronism; (6) movement of potassium into cells; (7) Cushing's syndrome.

Hypokalemia is associated with disordered neuromuscular function, alkalosis, and an exaggerated sensitivity to digitalis.

SUBJECTIVE AND OBJECTIVE DATA

Early symptoms include weakness, lethargy, paralytic ileus, and diminished-to-absent tendon reflexes. Electrocardiographic changes of hypokalemia consist of T-wave flattening, ST-segment depression, and the appearance of a prominent U-wave that gives the impression of a prolonged QT-interval.

PLAN

Management: Objectives of therapy are correction of the underlying cause and replacement of decreased potassium stores. Since most causes of hypokalemia are associated with a loss of chloride, potassium chloride is administered. If the patient is clinically well and can take medications orally, 40 mEq of potassium chloride is given three or four times daily. If parenteral administration is required, 40 mEq of potassium chloride is added to 1000 ml of normal saline and administered over a two- to four-hour period. Intravenous potassium should rarely exceed 20 mEq per hour, unless the patient has severe cardiac or central nervous system symptoms. Replacement is monitored with serum electrolyte determinations or electrocardiograms or both.

HYPERKALEMIA

Hyperkalemia—a serum potassium level of more than 6 mEq/l—usually results from acute or chronic renal failure. Other causes include (1) massive tissue injury; (2) severe acidosis; (3) excessive parenteral administration of potassium, including blood transfusions; and (4) adrenocortical insufficiency.

SUBJECTIVE AND OBJECTIVE DATA

Lassitude, fatigue, and weakness are initial symptoms when the serum potassium level exceeds 6.5 mEq/l. Neurologic examination usually discloses weakness or incipient paralysis, decreased reflex response, and paresthesias. When potassium exceeds 8.0 mEq/l, neuromuscular paralysis, bradycardia, vascular collapse, and cardiac arrest may develop rapidly.

As serum potassium exceeds 5.5 mEq/l, there is a peaking of the T-waves. When the potassium exceeds 6.5 mEq/l, the QRS complex is widened. With further increases in serum potassium, the P-wave amplitude diminishes and the P-R interval is prolonged. As the serum potassium exceeds 7.5 to 8.0 mEq/l, the P-wave may disappear, the widened QRS complex resembling a sine wave. Ventricular fibrillation or standstill rapidly follows the late changes, unless treatment is initiated.

PLAN

Management:

Hyperkalemia should be treated immediately if the serum potassium exceeds 6.5 mEq/l or if cardiac arrhythmias are present. Serum electrolyte values, blood pH, and the electrocardiogram are the most useful management guides. Treatment objectives are (1) reversal of the cardiac abnormalities, (2) facilitation of the intracellular potassium transport, and (3) removal of potassium from the body.

Reversal of Cardiac Abnormalities: One ampule (10 ml) of 10 per cent calcium gluconate is administered intravenously during a period of five to ten minutes. Constant electrocardiographic monitoring is required. The calcium is repeated, if necessary, to keep the ECG normal.

Facilitation of Intracellular Potassium Transport:

Sodium bicarbonate, 44 mEq given intravenously during a period of five to ten minutes, tends to lower serum potassium levels by increasing blood pH and causing potassium to move intracellularly. An additional 2 to 3 ampules of sodium bicarbonate in a continuous intravenous infusion may be required over the next one or two hours.

Glucose and insulin given intravenously facilitate intracellular potassium transport, decreasing serum potassium levels and increasing glycogen and potassium storage. Five hundred to 1000 ml of 10 per cent dextrose may be given intravenously during a period of one hour, along with 10 to 15 units of regular insulin. Sodium bicarbonate and glucose therapies may be combined in the treatment of hyperkalemia.

Removal of Potassium from the Body:

Cation Exchange Resins: Sodium polystyrene sulfonate (Kayexalate) given orally or rectally as a retention enema lowers serum potassium levels by exchanging sodium for potassium ions. Since effective lowering of serum potassium occurs slowly with exchange resins, they do not act rapidly enough to correct severe acute hyperkalemia.

Dialysis may be required.

REFERENCES

Abdul-Karim RW, Rizk PT: The effect of oxytocin on renal hemodynamics, water and electrolyte excretion. Obstet Gynecol Surv *25*:805-813, 1970

Lange RD, Dynesius R: Blood volume changes during normal pregnancy. Clin Haematol *2*:433-451, 1973

Newmark SR, Diuhy RG: Hyperkalemia and hypokalemia. JAMA *231*:631-633, 1975

Shires GT: Fluid and electrolyte therapy. *In* Committee on pre- and postoperative care, American College of Surgeons: Manual of Preoperative and Postoperative Care. Philadelphia, W.B. Saunders Company, 1971

Vidt DG: Use and abuse of intravenous solution. JAMA *232*:533-536, 1975

116 INDUCTION OF LABOR

GENERAL CONSIDERATIONS

Induction of labor may be advisable when maternal or fetal well-being necessitates the termination of pregnancy.

INDICATIONS AND CONTRAINDICATIONS

Indications include preeclampsia, eclampsia, hypertensive disorders, placental separation, premature rupture of membranes, intrauterine fetal death, hydramnios associated with a fetal abnormality, diabetes mellitus, amnionitis, and prolonged pregnancy with failing placental function.

Contraindications include obstetric complications requiring cesarean section, fetopelvic disproportion, fetal malpresentation; previous cesarean section, previous myomectomy or other uterine scars; acute herpes genitalis, fetal distress, placenta previa, and uterine overdistention.

COMPLICATIONS

These are primarily associated with uterine overstimulation: tetanic contractions, with reduced uteroplacental circulation; uterine rupture; placental separation; amniotic embolism; postpartum hemorrhage; cervical lacerations; fetal distress; anoxemia; and birth injuries.

The scoring system suggested by Bishop (1964) appears to be a helpful aid when induction of labor is being considered (see Table 116-1).

TABLE 116-1. Bishop's Pelvic Score for Elective Induction of Labor*†

Factor	Numerical Rating			
	0	*1*	*2*	*3*
Cervical				
Dilatation (cm)	0	1-2	3-4	5+
Effacement (%)	0-30	40-50	60-70	80+
Consistency	Firm	Medium	Soft	
Position	Post.	Mid.	Ant.	
Station of Vertex	−3	−2	−1.0	+1, +2

*From Bishop EH: Pelvic scoring for elective induction. Obstet Gynecol *24*:266-268, 1964

†The total score equals the sum of the factor scores. The range of scores is 0 to 13. Patients with a score of 9 or more usually have a successful induction.

METHODS

Oxytocin: The optimal method of oxytocin administration is by dilute intravenous infusion. Ten to 15 units of oxytocin are added to 1000 ml of 5 per cent dextrose in water. The infusion is initiated at a rate of 1 mU (1 or 2 drops) per minute. The patient's blood pressure, pulse, respiration, and uterine response and the fetal heart rate must be carefully monitored. The rate of infusion may be increased by 1- or 2-mU increments at 15-minute intervals until uterine contractions recur every two to three minutes and last approximately 45 seconds. Between contractions, the uterus should relax completely. The patient must be continually monitored for any changes in vital signs, fetal heart rate, or uterine overstimulation. After the membranes are ruptured, an intrauterine catheter aids in the assessment of the intensity, as well as the frequency, of uterine contractions.

It is imperative to discontinue the infusion at once if contractions exceed 90 seconds in duration or if evidence of fetal hypoxia occurs.

After delivery, the oxytocin infusion is continued for 30 to 60 minutes in order to prevent uterine relaxation and needless blood loss during the third stage.

Amniotomy: As long as the fetal head is well engaged, artificial rupture of the membranes may stimulate the onset of labor. Prior to amniotomy, the fetal heart tones should be evaluated. The cervix is palpated, and the consistency, length, and degree of dilatation are noted. The amniotic sac may be ruptured with a membrane hook or Allis clamp. Moderate fundal pressure by an assistant keeps the presenting part in the pelvis and helps to prevent cord prolapse. As soon as the amniotic fluid appears at the introitus, the fetal head is carefully palpated to exclude the possibility of cord prolapse. A scalp electrode may be applied to the vertex in order to monitor the fetal heart rate electronically. If a previously undetected, low-lying cord is compressed as the head descends, this is indicated by a sudden, persistent bradycardia.

Prostaglandin intraamniotic injection or prostaglandin vaginal suppositories may be utilized if the fetus is dead.

REFERENCES

Bishop EH: Pelvic scoring for elective induction. Obstet Gynecol *24*:266-268, 1964

Greenhill JP, Friedman EA: Biological Principles and Modern Practice of Obstetrics. Philadelphia, W.B. Saunders Company, 1974

Hughey MJ, McElin TW, Bird CC: An evaluation of preinduction scoring systems. Obstet Gynecol *48*:635-641, 1976

Ursell W: Induction of labor following fetal death. J Obstet Gynaecol Br Commonw *79*:260-264, 1972

117 LAPAROSCOPY

GENERAL CONSIDERATIONS

Laparoscopy is a transperitoneal endoscopic technique for visualization of the pelvic structures (ovaries, fallopian tubes, uterine serosa, cul-de-sac) in order to elucidate the diagnosis of pelvic pain, ectopic pregnancy, endometriosis, ovarian cysts, salpingitis, intraperitoneal bleeding or other abdominal pathologic conditions.

Most basic laparoscopes are 10 mm in diameter and have a 180° viewing angle. The instrument has an effective length of over 25 cm and is utilized with a fiberoptic light source (Fig. 117-1). In order to facilitate visualization (and laparoscopic placement), the abdominal cavity is distended with gas, usually carbon dioxide (pneumoperitoneum).

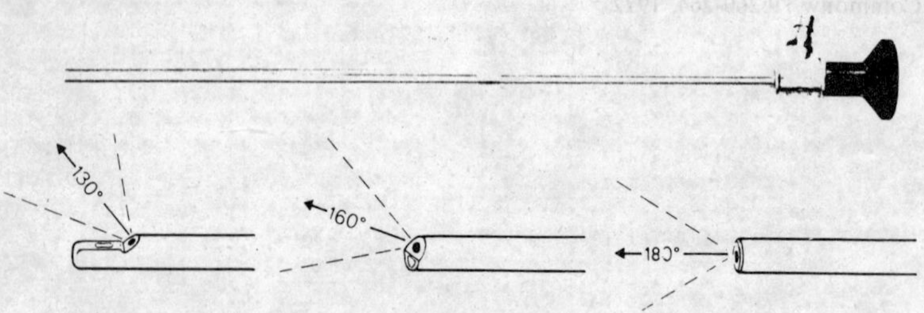

Figure 117-1. Fiber light laparoscope.

EQUIPMENT

1. Cervical cannula (Fir. 117-3)
2. Verres needle (Fig. 117-2)
3. Carbon dioxide insufflator
4. Trocar and sleeve for laparoscope
5. Laparoscope
6. Light source
7. Fiber light cable
8. Probe with trocar and sleeve for second puncture

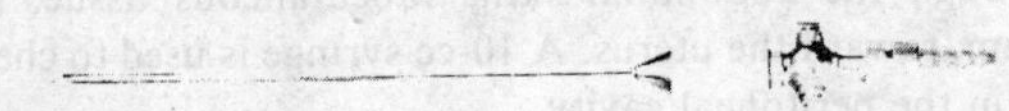

Figure 117-2. Verres needle with automatic spring action.

PROCEDURE

Vaginal Examination: The patient is put under general anesthesia and placed in a modified lithotomy position; a pelvic examination is then performed. The vagina is prepped with antiseptic solution. The cervix is visualized and grasped with a single-tooth tenaculum.

Unless an intrauterine pregnancy is suspected, the uterus is sounded with a calibrated sound in order to measure the depth of the uterine cavity. When indicated, a diagnostic curettage may be performed. A suction intrauterine cannula (Fig. 117-3) is inserted into

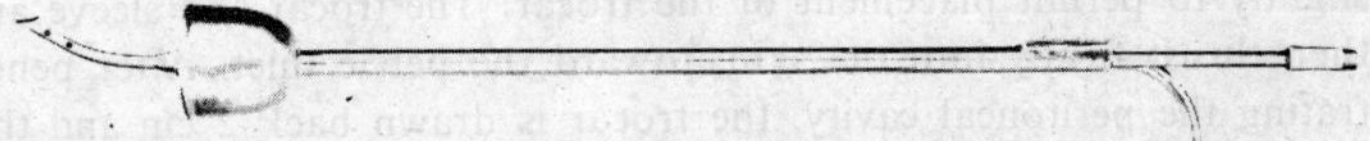

Figure 117-3. Vacuum uterine cannula.

the uterus (in order to manipulate the uterus at the time of laparoscopy). Alternatively, Cohen's modified tubal insufflation cannula, with self-retained tension spring, may be attached to the tenaculum.

A Foley catheter is inserted into the bladder to assure bladder drainage during the laparoscopic procedure.

Pneumoperitoneum: The abdomen is prepped as for any surgical procedure. The site of insertion of the Verres needle is selected. This is usually in the lower border of the umbilicus. A small stab incision is then made through the skin to facilitate needle insertion. The surgeon and assistant elevate the abdominal skin either by hand or with towel clips, to tent the abdomen. The Verres needle is inserted downward through the abdominal skin, subcutaneous tissue, fascia, and peritoneum, toward the uterus. A 10-cc syringe is used to check that the needle is in the peritoneal cavity.

First, the syringe is aspirated for any evidence of blood or bowel contents. If no aspirate is obtained, 5 to 10 cc of saline are injected. If the needle is placed accurately in the peritoneal cavity, the saline should flow freely and should not be able to be withdrawn when the syringe is aspirated. As long as placement of the Verres needle in the peritoneal cavity is assured, the valve of the Verres needle is opened and the needle is attached to the carbon dioxide insufflator.

As carbon dioxide flows into the peritoneal cavity, the intraabdominal pressure should be approximately 20 mm Hg or less. Insufflation should be at no greater rate than 1 l/min. After 2 to 4 l of carbon dioxide have been insufflated, the Verres needle is withdrawn. The amount of carbon dioxide insufflated is determined by the abdominal size, the abdominal wall elasticity, and evidence of any leakage.

Laparoscope Placement: The initial stab incision may be extended slightly to permit placement of the trocar. The trocar and sleeve are then thrust firmly into the skin, toward the pelvic inlet. After penetrating the peritoneal cavity, the trocar is drawn back 2 cm and the sleeve advanced 2 cm. The trocar is removed from the sheath and the concomitant release of a small amount of carbon dioxide indicates entry into the carbon dioxide-filled peritoneal cavity. The laparoscope is inserted with its light source attached. The carbon dioxide is connected to the sleeve for automatic insufflation.

The uterus is mobilized by the intrauterine cannula; the pelvic structures can then be visualized. If necessary, a probe may be inserted through a second incision in order to facilitate identification of the fallopian tubes and ovaries.

Termination: The telescope is withdrawn, and the valve on the sleeve should be depressed in order to allow gas to escape from the abdominal cavity. The patient should be brought to a horizontal position and the gas allowed to escape, as much as possible, by pressure on the abdominal wall. The outer sleeve is removed and the skin closed with either a clip or a subcutaneous suture.

CONTRAINDICATIONS

Absolute:

1. Severe cardiac or respiratory disease
2. Umbilical or diaphragmatic hernia
3. Acute generalized peritonitis
4. Intestinal obstruction (ileus)

Relative:

1. Gross obesity
2. Large pelvic or abdominal tumors
3. Multiple prior laparotomies (adhesions)
4. Anesthetic problems
5. Prior peritonitis (adhesions)
6. Prior abdominal wound separation
7. Shock
8. Cancer involving anterior abdominal wall

COMPLICATIONS

1. Puncture injury to the distended stomach, bowel, or blood vessel
2. Intraperitoneal bleeding (very rare)
3. Postoperative pain

REFERENCES

Cohen MR: Laparoscopy, Culdoscopy and Gynecography: Technique and Atlas. Philadelphia, W.B. Saunders Company, 1970

Horwitz ST: Laparoscopy in gynecology. Obstet Gynecol Surv *27*:1-13, 1972

Israel R: Symposium: overview of laparoscopy. Contemporary Ob/Gyn *4*:111-160, 1974

Loffer FD, Pent D: Indications, contraindications and complications of laparoscopy, Obstet Gynecol Surv *30*:407-427, 1975

118 NARCOTIC ANALGESIC MEDICATIONS

GENERAL CONSIDERATIONS

Narcotic medications are extremely effective for the relief of severe pain and apprehension. Nevertheless, the potential for respiratory depression must always be considered when selecting the dosage and route of administration.

Narcotics are avoided whenever pulmonary ventilation is impaired or the patient gives a history of abnormal or allergic reaction to previous doses. In cases of head injuries, narcotics may mask important changes in the vital signs. Furthermore, hypoventilation and hypercapnia can result in cerebral vascular dilatation with increased intracranial pressure.

Other adverse effects include emesis, depressed cough reflexes, and increased gastrointestinal tone with decreased intestinal motility.

During premature labor, narcotics are usually avoided because of the risk of neonatal respiratory depression.

Dosage should always be individualized and based on the severity of pain and the patient's age, weight, and physical condition. Development of drug tolerance after prolonged use of morphine-like drugs varies from patient to patient. Increased needs should be evaluated in relation to the patient's problems, in order to determine whether the increased need is caused by increased severity of pain or increased tolerance to the effect of the drug.

MANAGEMENT AND NARCOTIC OVERDOSAGE

Symptoms of overdosage include respiratory depression, apnea, hypotension, peripheral circulatory collapse, unconsciousness, and coma.

Treatment is directed primarily to the establishment of adequate respiratory exchange: provision of a patent airway and institution of assisted or controlled ventilation. The narcotic antagonist naloxone hydrochloride (Narcan), 0.4 mg, should be administered intravenously simultaneously with respiratory resuscitation. The naloxone may be repeated at two- or three-minute intervals if the desired degree of counteraction and improvement in respiratory function is not obtained immediately.

ROUTE OF ADMINISTRATION

Intravenous administration is indicated when an immediate effect is required. The medication should be injected slowly in order to minimize the risk of respiratory depression and cardiovascular collapse. Whenever narcotics are administered intravenously, facilities for assisted or controlled respiration (Ambu Bag) and a narcotic antagonist (naloxone) should be readily available.

Subcutaneous or intramuscular injection is often preferred, since the onset of effect is more gradual and the likelihood of an immediate respiratory depression is minimized.

Oral medication may be indicated when the patient is not vomiting and the severity of pain does not warrant parenteral medication.

SPECIFIC MEDICATIONS

Alphaprodine Hydrochloride (Nisentil): The usual adult dosage is 40 mg administered subcutaneously or 20 mg administered intravenously. The rapid onset and short duration of action are very useful for pain relief during minor surgery and for obstetric analgesia. Subcutaneous administration provides analgesic effect within 5 to 10 minutes, lasting approximately two hours. Intravenous administration provides an effect within one or two minutes, lasting about 30 minutes to one hour. Forty mg of alphaprodine are approximately equivalent to 8 to 10 mg of morphine.

Codeine Sulfate: The usual adult dosage is 30 to 60 mg administered orally. Codeine sulfate is a mild analgesic useful for the control of moderate pain or persistent cough. The duration of action is two to three hours. Codeine is often prescribed in combination with aspirin or acetaminophen.

Fentanyl Citrate: The usual adult dosage is 0.05 to 0.1 mg administered intravenously. Having an almost immediate onset of action when given intravenously and a short duration of effect (30 to 60 minutes), fentanyl is particularly useful as an adjunct to general or regional anesthesia. A dose of 0.1 mg (2 cc) is approximately equivalent in analgesic activity to 10 mg of morphine.

Facilities must always be available to cope with hypoventilation or apnea. A patent airway must be maintained, oxygen administered, and respiration assisted or controlled as necessary. Since fentanyl may cause muscle rigidity, an intravenous neuromuscular blocking agent may be required to facilitate ventilation.

Meperidine Hydrochloride (Demerol): The usual adult dosage is 50 to 100 mg administered intramuscularly or subcutaneously. When intravenous administration is required, the dosage is usually decreased.

A parenteral dose of 75 to 100 mg of meperidine is approximately equivalent to 8 to 10 mg of morphine. The maximal analgesic effect usually occurs within 40 to 60 minutes after subcutaneous administration and 30 to 50 minutes after intramuscular injection. The duration of analgesia is approximately two to four hours.

There has been some data to suggest that meperidine may produce slightly less smooth-muscle spasm, constipation, and depression of the cough reflex than equianalgesic doses of morphine.

Morphine Sulfate: The usual adult dosage is 8 to 15 mg administered subcutaneously or intramuscularly. For intravenous administration the dose may be decreased. The maximal analgesic effect usually occurs about 20 minutes after intravenous injection, 30 to 60 minutes after intramuscular injection, and 50 to 90 minutes after subcutaneous administration. The duration of action is approximately four or five hours. Because of its ability to control severe pain and at the same time allay apprehension, morphine sulfate is useful for many emergency problems. (Morphine may be prescribed for patients in early labor who are having painful uterine contractions but are not showing signs of cervical effacement and dilatation. The morphine may provide a period of comfortable rest, which may be followed by progressive labor.)

119 OXYTOCIN CHALLENGE TEST (OCT) AND CONTRACTION STRESS TEST (CST)

EQUIPMENT

1. Fetal monitor—cardiotocograph
2. Intravenous dilute oxytocin infusion

PURPOSE

The test aims to assess the placental reserve for transmitting oxygen to the fetus and detect uteroplacental insufficiency by observation of the fetal heart rate response to spontaneous or induced uterine contractions.

INDICATIONS AND CONTRAINDICATIONS

Patients at risk for uteroplacental insufficiency include those with a prolonged pregnancy, hypertensive disorders, diabetes mellitus, a history of previous stillbirth, Rh isoimmunization, intrauterine growth retardation, cyanotic maternal heart disease, abnormal estriol values, and any other evidence of potential fetal distress.

Contraindications to oxytocin stimulation include previous cesarean section, placenta previa, multiple gestation, and incompetent cervix.

PROCEDURE

The patient is placed in a semi-Fowler's position to avoid supine hypotension, and a suitable external monitor is placed on her abdomen to record uterine contractions. Maternal blood pressure is taken initially and every ten minutes during the test.

A base-line fetal heart rate tracing is obtained, either with the abdominal fetal ECG electrodes or with the ultrasound transducer. Accelerations of the fetal heart rate associated with fetal movements are noted as well as base-line heart rate variability and base-line uterine activity.

For purposes of the test, an adequate challenge is considered to be three uterine contractions, each lasting 40 to 60 seconds, during a ten-minute interval. Occasionally, base-line uterine activity is adequate to constitute a sufficient challenge. Otherwise, oxytocin stimulation is initiated at 0.5 mU/min by an intravenous infusion pump. The infusion is then increased every 15 minutes until three contractions occur within a ten-minute interval.

INTERPRETATION

See fetal heart rate monitoring, p. 786, for a discussion of fetal heart rate patterns and late decelerations.

Negative Test: No late decelerations of the fetal heart rate are observed with any of the three contractions during a ten-minute interval. A negative test is considered a reliable predictor of fetal well-being, since false negative tests are uncommon.

Positive Test: Consistent and persistent late decelerations occur with each uterine contraction during the ten-minute interval. The heart rate deceleration is proportional in amplitude and duration to the uterine contraction. Since a positive test may represent loss of uteroplacental reserve, delivery is usually recommended when conditions suggest that the baby would fare better in the nursery than in the uterus.

A positive stress test does not necessarily mean that the fetoplacental unit cannot tolerate labor; as many as 20 to 40 per cent of the patients with a positive stress test may not continue to show late decelerations when the heart rate is monitored with a scalp electrode during labor. In retrospect, the stress test is then considered a false positive test. Possible explanations include supine hypotension, excessive uterine activity, and technical factors.

If the fetus is premature, amniocentesis may be helpful in order to determine the L/S ratio for evidence of fetal lung maturity. If the L/S ratio is greater than 2.0, delivery is usually recommended. When a positive oxytocin challenge test is combined with falling estriol values, delivery may be indicated even when the L/S ratio is less than 2.0.

Suspicious or Equivocal Test: Occasional late decelerations that do not persist with continued uterine activity are considered equivocal, particularly if there is no evidence of fetal heart rate acceleration with fetal movement. The test is repeated in 24 hours.

Hyperstimulation: Excessive uterine activity is associated with deceleration of the fetal heart rate. The test is repeated in 24 hours.

Unsatisfactory Test: Uterine activity and heart rate data are not adequate to establish the absence of late decelerations. Unsatisfactory tests are most likely to occur when patients are obese or babies are unusually active. The test is repeated in 24 hours.

NONSTRESSED FETAL HEART RATE MONITORING

Nonstressed fetal heart rate monitoring, the observation of the fetal heart rate response to fetal movements, may be able to provide a simple, rapid evaluation of fetal well-being during the antepartum period.

The patient is placed in a semi-Fowler's position to avoid supine hypotension. An external heart rate transducer and tocodynamometer are applied to the abdomen. Blood pressure is checked frequently.

Reactive pattern, that is, accelerations of 15 beats per minute associated with fetal movements occurring at least five times during a 20-minute interval and accompanied by a base-line rate between 120 and 160 beats per minute and a base-line variability greater than six beats per minute, appears to be a reliable indicator of fetal well-being (Fig. 119-1).

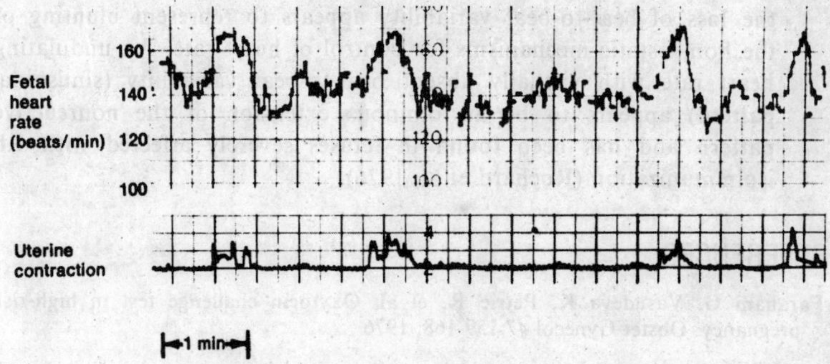

Figure 119-1. Reactive heart rate pattern. The heart rate is stable at about 130 beats per minute. Variability is about 10 beats per minute, and accelerations accompany fetal movement. (From Rochard F, Schifrin BS, Goupil F, et al: Nonstressed fetal heart rate monitoring in the antepartum period. Am J Obstet Gynecol *126*:699-706, 1976.)

Nonreactive pattern—persistently decreased variability, absence of accelerations with movement, and late or undefined decelerations with contractions—is associated with a compromised fetus (Fig. 119-2). Although the resting heart rate may be within the normal range,

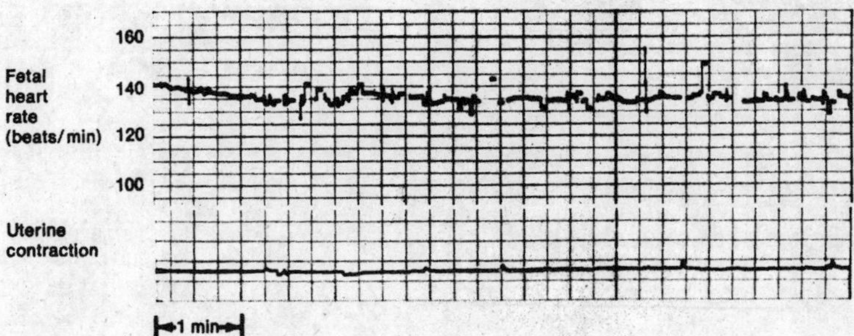

Figure 119-2. Nonreactive heart rate pattern. The heart rate is stable at about 130 beats per minute. Variability is less than two beats per minute, and accelerations do not accompany fetal movement. (From Rochard F, Schifrin BS, Goupil F, et al: Nonstressed fetal heart rate monitoring in the antepartum period. Am J Obstet Gynecol *126*:699-706, 1976.)

the loss of beat-to-beat variability appears to represent blunting of the homeostatic mechanisms for control of heart rate. An undulating heart rate with virtually absent beat-to-beat variability (sinusoidal pattern) appears to be an ominous extension of the nonreactive pattern and has been found in fetuses severely affected with Rh isoimmunization (Rochard et al, 1976).

REFERENCES

Farahani G, Vasudeva K, Petrie R, et al: Oxytocin challenge test in high-risk pregnancy. Obstet Gynecol *47*:159-168, 1976

Freeman RK: The use of the oxytocin challenge test for antepartum clinical evaluation of uteroplacental respiratory function. Am J Obstet Gynecol *121*:481-489, 1975; Obstet Gynecol Surv *30*:596-598, 1975

Freeman RK, Goebelsman U, Nochimson D, Cetrulo C: An evaluation of the significance of a positive oxytocin challenge test. Obstet Gynecol *47*:8-13, 1976

Rochard F, Schifrin BS, Groupil F, et al: Nonstressed fetal heart rate monitoring in the antepartum period. Am J Obstet Gynecol *126*:699-706, 1976

Schifrin BS, Lapidus M, Doctor GS, Leviton A: Contraction stress test for antepartum fetal evaluation. Obstet Gynecol *45*:433-438, 1975

120 PARACERVICAL BLOCK

INDICATIONS

Paracervical block interrupts the pain passageway from the uterus, thereby alleviating pain associated with cervical dilatation and uterine contractions during the first stage of labor, endometrial aspiration or curettage, and the insertion of an intrauterine device.

PROCEDURE

During the first stage of labor, a tubular director or guide is placed in the lateral vaginal fornix. Frequently, the guide is designed to prevent the needle point from advancing more than 5 mm into the parametrium alongside the cervix. After careful aspiration for blood, 5 to 7 ml of 1 per cent lidocaine (50 to 70 mg) or 1 per cent chloroprocaine are injected. The procedure is repeated on the other side. The injections are made between three and four o'clock positions and between eight and nine o'clock positions.

Local anesthetic solutions are rapidly absorbed into the maternal circulation from the paracervical area; this is followed by equally rapid transplacental passage into the fetus with rapid uptake into the fetal organs: the heart, brain and liver. Fetal bradycardia and even fetal death or neonatal death have been attributed to paracervical block anesthesia. Chloroprocaine appears to be less toxic to the fetus than lidocaine, since chloroprocaine is rapidly hydrolyzed and inactivated by maternal plasma cholinesterase.

For suction curettage, 5 to 7 ml of 1 per cent lidocaine are injected submucosally into the cervicovaginal junction at four and eight o'clock positions.

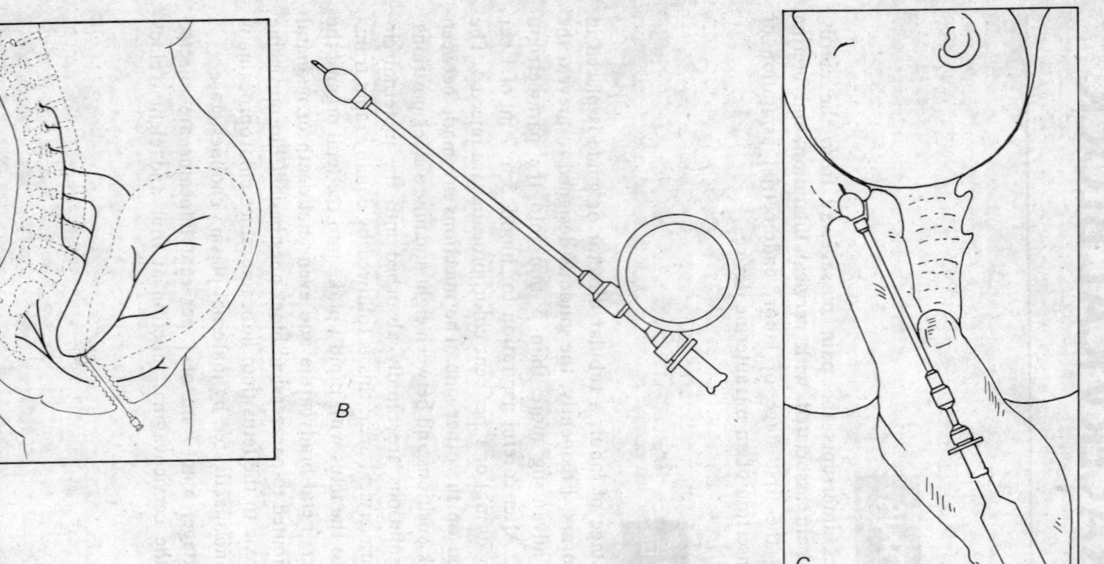

Figure 120-1. Paracervical nerve block. *A,* Schematic saggital view showing the pain pathways and the site of interrupting pain of uterine contractions in the paracervical region. *B,* Needle assembly in ring guide for paracervical technique—5 mm penetration. *C,* Schematic coronal section of vagina and lower part of the uterus showing proper handling of the needle guide with the needle protruding for a very short distance beyond its end. The needle is directed laterally away from the fetal head, which is being protected by the middle finger. (*A* and *C* from Bonica JJ: Principles and Practice of Obstetric Analgesia and Anesthesia. Philadelphia, F.A. Davis Co., 1972.)

PREVENTION OF TOXIC REACTIONS

Excitation of the central nervous system with convulsions is the most frequent serious toxic reaction associated with local anesthetic agents. With very high blood levels, central nervous system depression occurs, with loss of consciousness and depressed respiration. Circulatory collapse can ensue from a direct depressant effect on the myocardium and peripheral vasodilatation.

A complex interplay of factors influences the toxicity of local anesthetics: the intrinsic potency, total dose, concentration, and protein-binding affinity of the drug; the rate of absorption and vascular characteristics of the injection site; the rate of degradation or disappearance from the blood stream; the action of a vasoconstrictor; and the clinical state of the patient and the nature of the surgical procedure. The most common causes of toxic reactions are overdosage and inadvertent intravascular injection.

Because of the threat of toxic blood levels whenever local anesthetics are used, the smallest effective volume and lowest concentration of anesthetic should be employed. Anesthetic doses should be adjusted to the patient's weight. (The *total* amount of lidocaine without epinephrine, for example, should be kept below 300 mg and should not exceed 4.5 mg/kg of body weight.)

Absorption of local anesthetics is facilitated by rich vascularity, and although aspiration with a syringe should be routinely practiced before injection, this precaution does not preclude intravascular injection.

The toxicity of local anesthetics depends largely on the balance among the rates of systemic absorption, distribution, and degradation; rapid clearance from the circulation protects against the development of toxicity and limits the duration and severity of any adverse reactions. Lidocaine and mepivacaine are nonester anesthetics of the amide type; their metabolism is less rapid than that of local anesthetics of the ester type (chloroprocaine, procaine), which are detoxified by hydrolysis.

If toxicity is suspected, the injection should be stopped immediately and the patient given high concentrations of oxygen. If tremor, twitching, or convulsions occur, the patient should be treated with intravenous diazepam or a rapid-acting barbiturate. Premedication with diazepam raises the seizure threshold.

If hypotension develops, a high concentration of oxygen, rapid intravenous infusion, and vasopressors may be necessary. (See Anesthetic Emergencies, p. 139.)

During labor, the following precautions are recommended:

1. Avoidance of direct injection into the maternal circulation or fetal tissues
2. Avoidance of paracervical block when there is any evidence of fetal distress, prematurity, or placental insufficiency (Shnider, et al, 1970)
3. Close monitoring of the fetal heart rate and maternal blood pressure, pulse, and respirations
4. Having the patient lie on her side to avoid vena caval and aorta femoral compression

REFERENCES

Chatfield WR, Suter PEN, Kotonya AO: Paracervical block anaesthesia for the evacuation of incomplete abortion—a controlled trial. J Obstet Gynaecol Br Commonw *77*:462-463, 1970

Freeman DW, Arnold NI: Paracervical block with low doses of chloroprocaine. JAMA *231*:56-57, 1975

Petrie RH, Paul WL, Miller FC, et al: Placental transfer of lidocaine following paracervical block. Am J Obstet Gynecol *120*:791-801, 1974; Obstet Gynecol Surv *30*:252-254, 1975

Shnider SM, Asling JH, Holl JW, et al: Paracervical block anesthesia in obstetrics. Am J Obstet Gynecol *107*:619-625, 1970

121 PUDENDAL BLOCK

INDICATIONS

Pudendal block can relieve pain caused by distention of the lower birth canal, vulva, and perineum during the second stage of labor and during delivery.

PROCEDURE

A tubular director or guide is inserted into the vagina with two fingers. The tip of the guide is placed to the medial side and immediately below the ischial spine at the origin of the sacrospinous ligament. A long needle is then passed through the guide into the ligament, which is infiltrated with 2 ml of local anesthetic solution (1 per cent lidocaine or 2 per cent chloroprocaine). The needle is then advanced slightly farther through the ligament (Fig. 121-1). After aspiration, to prevent intravascular injection, 6 to 8 ml of the anesthetic solution are injected. If blood is aspirated, the needle is either withdrawn slightly or advanced slightly until no blood is obtained. The anesthetic solution is then injected adjacent to the pudendal nerve and blood vessels.

PREVENTION OF TOXIC REACTIONS

See Paracervical Block, p. 825.

COMPLICATIONS

See Anesthetic Emergencies, p. 139.

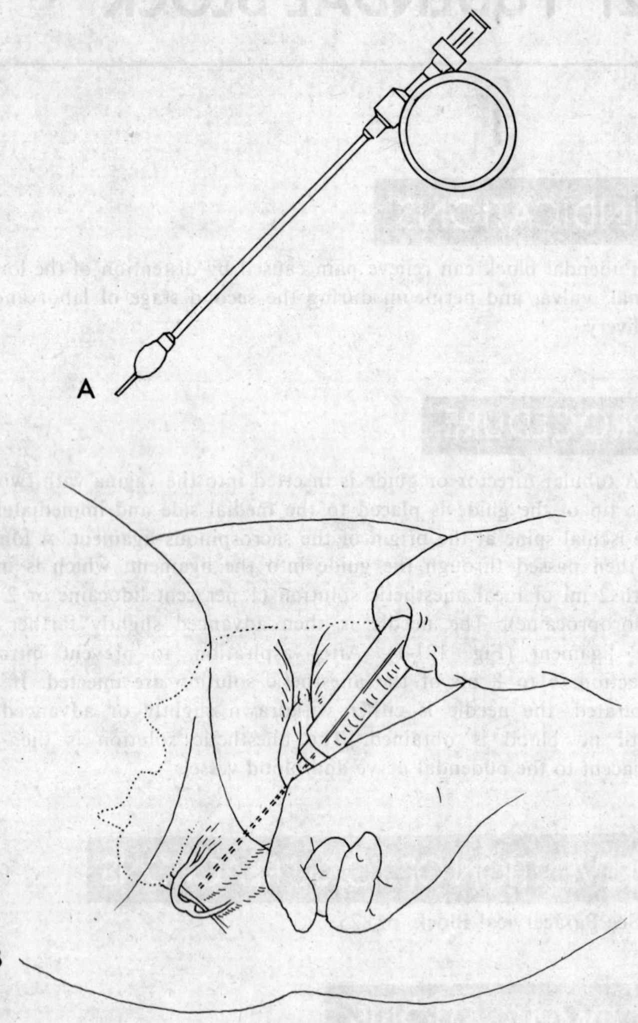

Figure 121-1. *A*, Needle in ring guide for pudendal technique—1 cm. penetration. *B*, Block of pudendal nerve by the transvaginal route. (From Adriani J: Labat's Regional Anesthesia. Philadelphia, W.B. Saunders Co., 1967.)

REFERENCES

Bonica JJ: Obstetric analgesia and anesthesia. Berlin, Springer-Verlag, 1972

Bonica JJ: Obstetric analgesia-anaesthesia. Clin Obstet Gynaecol, *2*:467-577,1975

122 ADULT CARDIOPULMONARY RESUSCITATION (CPR)

INDICATIONS

1. Respiratory arrest
2. Cardiac arrest—sudden cessation of the heart's pumping function due either to ventricular asystole (electrical or mechanical) or to ventricular fibrillation

GENERAL PRINCIPLES

1. One must ensure adequate blood oxygenation and ventilatory exchange to prevent irreversible tissue damage.
2. One must ensure adequate blood perfusion of vital organs, which is dependent upon a functional heart rate, rhythm, and stroke volume.
3. Immediate restoration of the circulation and blood oxygenation is required if survival and functional recovery are to be achieved.

BASIC LIFE SUPPORT

1. A—Airway
2. B—Breathing
3. C—Circulation

AIRWAY

The most important factor for successful resuscitation is an adequate, clear airway. The patient must be placed in a supine position on a firm surface, with the head tilted backwards. This maneuver extends the neck and lifts the tongue away from the back of the throat, thereby relieving any anatomic obstruction of the airway caused by the tongue dropping against the back of the throat.

The mouth and pharynx should be cleared of vomitus, food, blood, dentures, mucus, and saliva with a suction catheter, bulb aspirator, or the fingers, as necessary.

An oral airway should be inserted as soon as one is available.

BREATHING

Artificial ventilation (see Fig. 122-1) should be initiated using either mouth-to-mouth ventilation or an Ambu Bag. The lungs should be inflated every five seconds or 20 times per minute. Motion of the chest wall should be carefully observed in order to assess the adequacy of ventilation. As soon as oxygen is available, the oxygen line is connected to the Ambu Bag or inserted into the patient's mouth.

In rare circumstances, air cannot be transferred into the lungs and the chest wall does not move. Laryngospasm, bronchospasm, and an obstructing foreign body are possible causes. Endotracheal intubation, succinylcholine, or an emergency tracheostomy may be necessary.

For mouth-to-mouth ventilation, place one hand under the nape of the patient's neck and place the opposite hand on the forehead, pressing down and compressing the nostrils with the fingers. Take a deep breath; then breathe directly between the patient's lips. The lips must form an airtight seal. Watch the chest for adequate expansion. Allow the patient to exhale. Repeat every four or five seconds.

CIRCULATION

Absence of carotid pulsation is the indication for starting artificial circulation by means of external cardiac compression. External cardiac compression consists of the rhythmic application of pressure over the lower half of the sternum (but not over the xiphoid process). This intermittent pressure compresses the heart and produces a pulsatile artificial circulation.

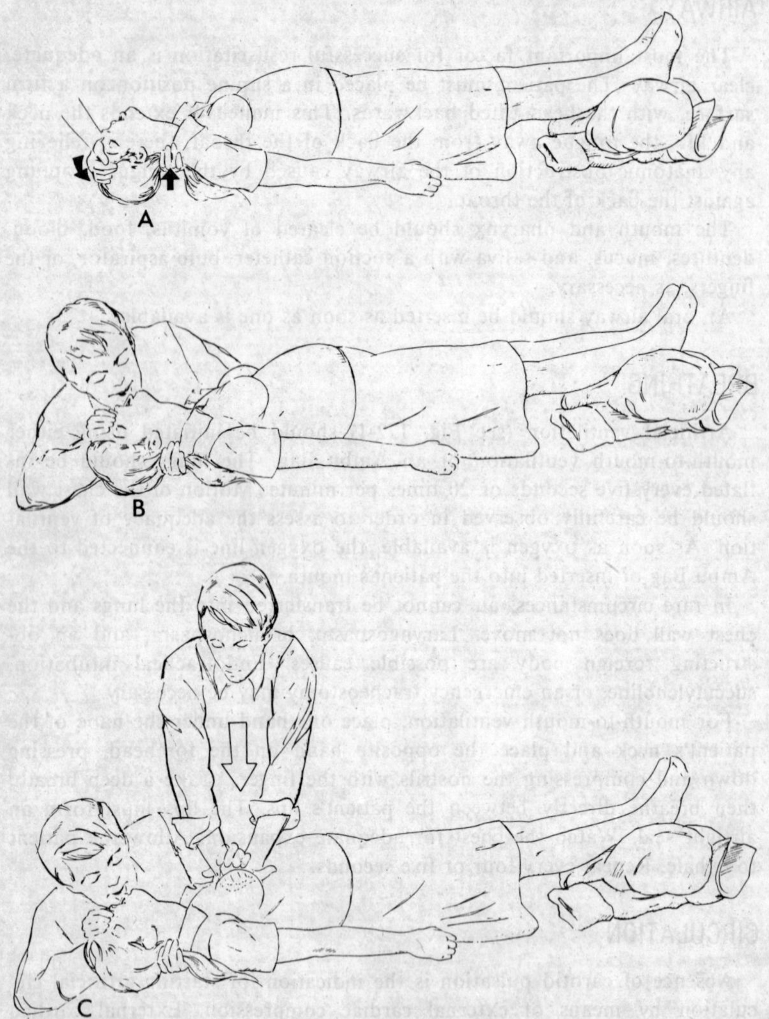

Figure 122-1. *A* and *B*, Mouth-to-mouth artificial ventilation. *C*, Cardiopulmonary resuscitation with two rescuers.

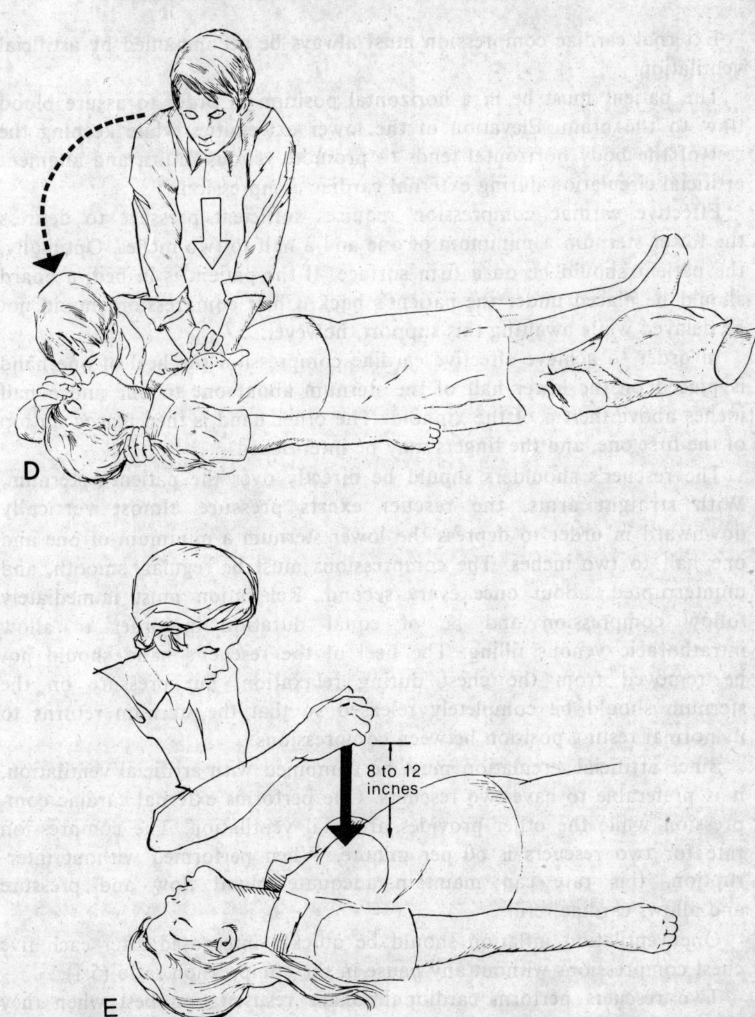

Figure 122-1 Continued. *D*, Cardiopulmonary resuscitation with one rescuer. *E*, Precordial thump. (Modified from Standards for Cardiopulmonary Resuscitation (CPR) and Emergency Cardiac Care (ECC). JAMA *227*:833-868, 1974.)

External cardiac compression must always be accompanied by artificial ventilation.

The patient must be in a horizontal position in order to assure blood flow to the brain. Elevation of the lower extremities while keeping the rest of the body horizontal tends to promote venous return and augment artificial circulation during external cardiac compression.

Effective cardiac compression requires sufficient pressure to depress the lower sternum a minimum of one and a half to two inches. Optimally, the patient should be on a firm surface. If the patient is in bed, a board should be placed under the patient's back. Chest compression should not be delayed while awaiting this support, however.

In order to achieve effective cardiac compression the heel of one hand is placed on the lower half of the sternum about one to one and a half inches above the tip of the xiphoid. The other hand is then placed on top of the first one, and the fingers may be interlocked.

The rescuer's shoulders should be directly over the patient's sternum. With straight arms, the rescuer exerts pressure almost vertically downward in order to depress the lower sternum a minimum of one and one half to two inches. The compressions must be regular, smooth, and uninterrupted, about once every second. Relaxation must immediately follow compression and be of equal duration in order to allow intrathoracic venous filling. The heel of the rescuer's hand should not be removed from the chest during relaxation, but pressure on the sternum should be completely released so that the sternum returns to its normal resting position between compressions.

Since artificial circulation must be combined with artificial ventilation, it is preferable to have two rescuers. One performs external cardiac compression while the other provides artificial ventilation. The compression rate for two rescuers is 60 per minute. When performed without interruption, this rate can maintain adequate blood flow and pressure and allows cardiac refill.

One ventilation inflation should be quickly interposed after each five chest compressions without any pause in the compression ratio (5:1).

Two rescuers perform cardiopulmonary resuscitation best when they are on opposite sides of the victim. They can then switch positions when necessary without any significant interruption in the 5 to 1 rhythm.

If the victim's trachea has been intubated, lung inflation is easier and compression rates up to 80 per minute can be used, since breaths can be either interposed or superimposed following endotracheal intubation.

When there is only one rescuer, artificial circulation and artificial ventilation are performed using a 15 to 2 ratio. This consists of two very quick lung inflations after each 15 chest compressions. Because of the interruptions for lung inflation, the single rescuer must perform each series of 15 chest compressions at the faster rate of 80 compressions per minute, so that when averaged by the time lost for ventilations the final number of compressions achieved per minute will be 60. The two full lung inflations must be delivered in rapid succession, within a period of five to six seconds, without allowing full exhalation between the breaths.

EFFECTIVENESS OF CPR

Reaction of the pupils provides the best indication of the delivery of oxygenated blood to the brain. Constriction of the pupils after exposure to light indicates adequate oxygenation and blood flow to the brain. If the pupils remain widely dilated and do not react to light, serious brain damage is imminent or has occurred.

The carotid pulse should be palpated periodically in order to check the effectiveness of external cardiac compression or for the return of a spontaneous, effective heartbeat.

Other signs of effective blood flow include femoral pulsation and the return of skin color.

PRECORDIAL THUMP

If the primary cause of cardiac arrest is not hypoxia, a single precordial thump may be effective in restarting circulation and may reverse certain dysrhythmias if performed within the first minute after the arrest.

A thump on the midsternum with the fist may be able to generate a small electrical stimulus in a reactive heart and may restore the heart beat in cases of ventricular asystole due to block. The thump may also be able to reverse ventricular tachycardia or ventricular fibrillation of recent onset.

In delivering the precordial thump, these instructions should be followed:

1. Deliver a sharp, quick, single blow over the midportion of the sternum, hitting with the bottom, fleshy portion of the fist, starting from 8 to 12 inches over the chest.
2. Deliver the thump within the first minute after cardiac arrest.
3. If there is no immediate response, begin basic life support at once.

The precordial thump is not useful for anoxic asystole and cannot be depended upon to convert an established ventricular fibrillation, nor is it useful for electromechanical dissociation associated with exsanguination. It should not be used for a ventricular tachycardia that is providing adequate circulation.

EMERGENCY PROCEDURE FOR WITNESSED CARDIAC ARREST

1. Tilt the head to open the airway and simultaneously palpate the carotid pulse.
2. If the pulse is absent, give a precordial thump.
3. If the patient is not breathing, give four quick full-lung inflations.
4. If pulse and breathing are not restored immediately, begin one-rescuer or two-rescuer Cardiopulmonary resuscitation.
5. Summon additional help.
6. Apply electrocardiograph (ECG) leads as soon as possible.
7. Start intravenous infusion. (A peripheral line may be faster, followed by a central venous infusion line.)

Electrocardiographic monitoring of all patients with cardiac arrest should be established as soon as possible. Initially, a monitor-defibrillator with combination ECG electrode-defibrillator paddles is recommended in order to diagnose ventricular fibrillation or cardiac asystole. Ventricular fibrillation is a more common cause of cardiac arrest than cardiac standstill. A fibrillating heart is a strong heart, with a much better chance of recovery than an asystolic heart.

If the ECG rhythm is relatively regular, pulse and blood pressure should be checked immediately to determine whether electromechanical dissociation is present.

If the rhythm and circulation are satisfactory, oxygen should be administered, an infravenous line established, and regular ECG electrodes applied for continuous monitoring.

EMERGENCY PROCEDURE FOR CARDIAC ARREST IN A MONITORED PATIENT

This procedure is for use with patients who have sudden ventricular fibrillation (VF), asystole, or ventricular tachycardia (VT) without a pulse.

1. Give a single precordial thump.
2. Quickly check the monitor for cardiac rhythm and simultaneously check the carotid pulse.
3. If there is ventricular fibrillation or ventricular tachycardia without a pulse, countershock as soon as possible.
4. If the pulse is absent, tilt the head and give four quick full-lung inflations.
5. Check the carotid pulse again.
6. If the pulse is absent, begin one-rescuer or two-rescuer CPR.

(No time should be lost in waiting to assess results of the precordial thump or by delivering repeated precordial thumps.)

ENDOTRACHEAL INTUBATION

Since adequate lung inflations interposed between external cardiac compressions require high pharyngeal pressures, these pressures promote gastric distention, which elevates the diaphragm and interferes with adequate lung inflation. This distention promotes regurgitation, with the potential hazard of aspiration of gastric contents into the lungs. Therefore, the trachea should be intubated as soon as practical by trained personnel.

With a cuffed endotracheal tube, is is easier to provide adequate ventilation. It then becomes possible to use a faster, uninterrupted chest compression rate of 80 per minute and provide better artificial circulation.

VENTRICULAR FIBRILLATION

Defibrillation produces a simultaneous depolarization of all muscle fascicles of the heart, after which a spontaneous beat may resume if the myocardium is oxygenated and not acidotic. Direct-current defibrillator shocks should be delivered as soon as possible when the heart is known to be in ventricular fibrillation.

For defibrillation, conductive jelly is applied to the defibrillation paddles, which are firmly placed on the chest, one just to the right of the upper sternum below the clavicle and the other just to the left of the cardiac apex or left nipple.

The usual direct-current shock is 400 joules (watt-seconds); after a ten-second pause it is repeated, if the first one was ineffective.

Sodium bicarbonate is used to combat metabolic acidosis. The initial dose is 1 mEq/kg by either bolus injection or continuous infusion over a ten-minute period. A 50-ml ampule of 8.4 per cent solution contains 50 mEq of sodium.

Lidocaine is used to depress ventricular irritability when successful defibrillation repeatedly reverts to ventricular fibrillation. Lidocaine raises the fibrillation threshold and exerts its antidysrhythmic effect by increasing the electrical stimulation threshold of the ventricle during diastole. With usual therapeutic doses, there is no significant change in myocardial contractility, systemic arterial pressure, or absolute refractory period.

The initial dose is 50 to 100 mg administered slowly intravenously as a bolus. This may be followed by a continuous infusion of 1 to 3 mg per minute. Five hundred mg of lidocaine in 500 ml of 5 per cent dextrose solution provides a concentration of 1 mg/ml.

Epinephrine is used to increase myocardial contractility, elevate the perfusion pressure, lower the defibrillation threshold, and, in some instances, restore myocardial contractility in electromechanical dissociation.

An initial dose of 0.5 ml of a 1 to 1000 solution diluted to 10 ml or 5 ml of a 1 to 10,000 solution should be administered intravenously every five minutes during the resuscitation effort. Alternatively, 5 ml of the 1 to 10,000 solution may be injected directly into the ventricle.

Check blood gases and pH to evaluate further therapy.

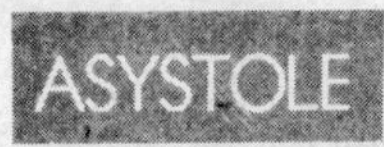

External cardiac compression and artificial ventilation are performed.

Sodium Bicarbonate: The initial dose is 1 mEq/kg administered intravenously either by bolus injection or by continuous infusion during a ten-minute period. A 50-ml ampule of 8.4 per cent solution contains 50 mEq of sodium.

Isoproterenol is used to stimulate cardiac contractile force and rate. Isoproterenol is a peripheral vasodilator, whereas epinephrine is a vasoconstrictor. Tissue perfusion is better, and acidosis is less of a problem. Isoproterenol is considered the drug of choice for the immediate treatment of patients with profound bradycardia as a result of complete heart block.

The initial dose is 2 to 5 mg diluted in 500 ml of 5 per cent glucose, infused in amounts of 2 to 20 mcg per minute. The dosage is titrated to achieve a heart rate of 60 to 80 beats per minute or a blood pressure of 90.

Epinephrine is given in an intracardiac or intravenous dose of 5 ml of 1 to 10,000 solution.

Calcium chloride is given to increase myocardial contractility, prolong systole, and enhance ventricular excitability.

The initial dose is 2.5 ml to 5 ml of 10 per cent solution (3.4 to 6.8 mEq of calcium). Calcium gluconate provides less ionizable calcium per unit of volume. If it is used, the dose should be 10 ml of a 10 per cent solution (4.8 mEq). (Note: Calcium must not be administered together with sodium bicarbonate, since this mixture results in the formation of a precipitate.)

Blood gases and pH are checked to evaluate further therapy.

Other Drugs:

Atropine sulfate reduces vagal tone, enhances atrioventricular conduction, and accelerates the cardiac rate in cases of sinus bradycardia.

Indications for its use include (1) sinus bradycardia with a pulse of less than 60 beats per minute when accompanied by premature ventricular contractions or systolic blood pressure of less than 90 mm Hg, and (2) high-degree atrioventricular block when accompanied by bradycardia.

The dosage is 0.5 mg administered intravenously as a bolus and repeated at five-minute intervals until a pulse rate greater than 60 is achieved. The total dose should not exceed 2 mg except in cases of third-degree atrioventricular block.

Corticosteroids: Present evidence favors the use of pharmacologic doses of synthetic corticosteroids (5 mg/kg of methylprednisolone sodium succinate or 1 mg/kg of dexamethasone phosphate) for prompt treatment of cardiogenic shock or shock lung occurring as a complication of cardiac arrest. When cerebral edema is suspected following cardiac arrest, methylprednisolone sodium succinate in a dosage of 60 to 100 mg every six hours may be beneficial. When pulmonary complications such as postaspiration pneumonitis are present, dexamethasone phosphate may be used in doses of 4 to 8 mg every six hours (Standards for CPR and ECC, 1974).

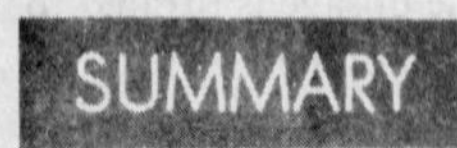

Successful resuscitation after cardiac arrest requires a combination of the following factors:

1. Prompt institution of corrective measures
2. Adequate pulmonary ventilation
3. Adequate coronary artery flow and adequate perfusion of vital organs with oxygenated blood
4. Adequate correction of acidosis and electrolyte imbalance
5. Adequate defibrillating current for an effective time, combined with good contact between the electrodes and the chest
6. Restoration of a functional cardiac rate, rhythm, and stroke volume.
7. Intravenous supportive or replacement therapy based on frequent arterial pH, blood gas, and electrolyte determinations
8. Continuous electrocardiographic monitoring

Deep unconsciousness, absence of spontaneous respiration, and pupils that are fixed and dilated for 15 to 30 minutes are usually indicative of cerebral death; further resuscitative efforts are generally futile.

EQUIPMENT AND DRUGS FOR ADVANCED LIFE SUPPORT UNIT

The following is a listing from the article "Standards for Cardiopulmonary Resuscitation (CPR) and Emergency Cardiac Care (ECC)," which appeared in the Journal of the American Medical Association in February 1974:

Equipment and Drugs.—The basic equipment and drugs necessary for an adequate advanced life support unit include those concerned with maintaining the airway and providing artificial ventilation and circulation.

Respiratory Management.—For airway management and artificial ventilation, the following equipment is necessary for all life support units:

Oxygen supply (two E cylinders) with reducing valves capable of delivering 15 liters/minute and with mask and reservoir bag

Oxygen reserve (two E cylinders)

Mask for mouth-to-mask ventilation

Oropharyngeal airways

S-tube (optional)

Laryngoscope with blades (curved and straight, for adult, child, and infant) and extra batteries and bulbs

Assorted adult-size (cuffed) and child-size (uncuffed) endotracheal tubes with stylet and 15 mm/22 mm adaptors

Syringe with clamp or plastic two-way or three-way valve for endotracheal tube cuffs

Acceptable bag-valve-mask, with provisions for 100% oxygen ventilation or a manually triggered (time-cycled) oxygen powered resuscitator

Suction (preferably portable), with catheters—sizes 6 to 16—and Yankauer-type suction tips

Nasogastric tube

Esophageal obturator airway (optional)

Cricothyrotomy set

Circulatory Management.—To provide adequate management of the circulatory system, the following equipment is essential for all advanced life support units:

Portable defibrillator-monitor with ECG electrode-defibrillator paddles or portable DC defibrillator and portable ECG monitor

Portable ECG machine, direct writing, with connection to monitor

Venous infusion sets (micro and regular)

Indwelling venous catheters (regular and special units):

- Catheter outside needle (sizes 14 to 22)
- Catheter inside needle (sizes 14 to 22)
- Central venous pressure catheters

Intravenous solutions (5% dextrose in water, lactated Ringer's)

Cutdown set

Sterile gloves

Urinary catheters

Assorted syringes and needles, stopcocks, venous extension tubes

Intracardiac needles

Tourniquets, adhesive, disposable razor, and similar items

Thoracotomy tray

Essential Drugs.—All life support units must have these drugs available:

Sodium bicarbonate (prefilled syringes, 50 ml ampules, or 500 ml 5% bottles)

Epinephrine (prefilled syringes)

Atropine sulfate (prefilled syringes)

EQUIPMENT AND DRUGS FOR ADVANCED LIFE SUPPORT UNIT (Continued)

Essential Drugs. (Continued)

Lidocaine [Xylocaine (prefilled syringe)]

Morphine sulfate

Calcium chloride

Useful Drugs.—These drugs are recommended for hospital and nonhospital life support units:

Aminophylline

Dexamethasone (Decadron)

Dextrose 50% (Ion-o-trate Dextrose 50%)

Digoxin (Lanoxin)

Diphenhydramine hydrochloride (Benadryl)

Ethacrynic acid

Furosemide (Lasix)

Isoprotenerol (Isuprel) hydrochloride

Lanatoside C (Cedilanid)

Meperidine (Demerol) hydrochloride

Metaraminol bitartrate (Aramine)

Methylprednisolone sodium succinate (Solu-Medrol)

Nalorphine (n-allylnormorphine) hydrochloride

Levarterenol (Levophed) bitartrate

Phenylephrine (Neo-synephrine) hydrochloride

Potassium chloride

Propranolol hydrochloride (Inderal)

Procainamide hydrochloride (Pronestyl)

Quinidine

Succinylcholine chloride

Tubocurarine chloride

REFERENCES

Goldberg AH: Cardiopulmonary arrest. N Engl J Med *290*:381-385, 1974

Loeb HS: Cardiac arrest. JAMA *232*:845-847, 1975

Standards for cardiopulmonary resuscitation (CPR) and emergency cardiac care (ECC). JAMA *227* (Suppl):833-868, 1974

123 RESUSCITATION OF THE NEWBORN

EQUIPMENT

1. An ample work area
2. A source of radiant heat or a warm blanket to prevent heat loss
3. Infant laryngoscope
4. Endotracheal tubes
5. A shoulder roll
6. A device for administering positive pressure breathing within pressure limits of 15 to 45 cm H_2O
7. Masks of several sizes for large and small infants
8. Several alternative means of suctioning including a bulb syringe and suction catheters
9. A means of mixing humidified oxygen and air
10. Materials for emergency catheterization of a vessel
11. A basic drug set
    a. Naloxone
    b. Sodium Bicarbonate
    c. Epinephrine
    d. Oxygen

PREDISPOSING FACTORS

Factors predisposing to neonatal respiratory depression include

1. Fetal or neonatal disorders
    a. Respiratory center depression
        (1) Analgesics to mother
        (2) Anesthetics
        (3) Intrauterine hemorrhage
        (4) Shock from traumatic delivery

b. Central nervous system disorders
c. Pulmonary hypoplasia and airway anomalies; diaphragmatic hernia
d. Congenital cardiovascular anomalies
e. Obstructed airway (mucus, meconium, blood)
f. Erythroblastosis fetalis and hydrops from other causes
g. Infection
h. Aspiration syndromes
i. Congenital ascites

2. Placental and umbilical cord disorders
   a. Hemorrhage—shock from blood loss
      (1) Premature placental separation
      (2) Placenta previa
      (3) Placental laceration
   b. Intervillous fibrin deposition
   c. Infarction
   d. Cord occlusion—compression, angulation, prolapse, obstruction
   e. Chorioamnionitis
3. Maternal disorders
   a. Anemia
   b. Preeclampsia and eclampsia and other hypertensive diseases
   c. Uterine tetany
   d. Hypotension and shock
   e. Hemorrhage
   f. Maternal seizures
   g. Maternal sepsis
   h. Drug addiction

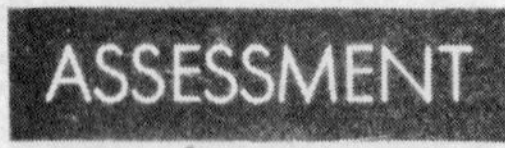

For the APGAR Score of the newborn infant, see Table 123-1.

TABLE 123-1. The APGAR Score of the Newborn Infant*

	0	1	2
A Appearance (Color)	Blue, pale	Body pink, extremities blue	Completely pink
P Pulse (Heart rate)	Absent	Less than 100	Greater than 100
G Grimace (Reflexes)	No response	Grimace	Cough, sneeze
A Activity (Muscle tone)	Limp	Some flexion of extremities	Active motion
R Respiration	Absent	Slow, irregular	Strong cry

*Each sign is evaluated individually and scored from 0 to 2 at both one and five minutes of life. The final score at each time is the sum of the individual scores.

The clinical classification of depressed infants follows:

0-3=severely depressed
4-6=moderately depressed
7-9=slightly depressed or normal

Details that should be evaluated in addition to those evaluated by the APGAR Score include the

1. Skin temperature
2. Skin perfusion
3. Presence of edema
4. Strength of peripheral pulses
5. Lôcation of abnormal breath sounds
6. State of the infant's sensorium

Pulse rate is one of the most sensitive indicators of infant well-being. Following a brief bradycardia at the moment of birth, the heart rate usually increases up to 180 to 200 beats per minute and then gradually slows to a normal range of 100 to 140 with beat-to-beat variability.

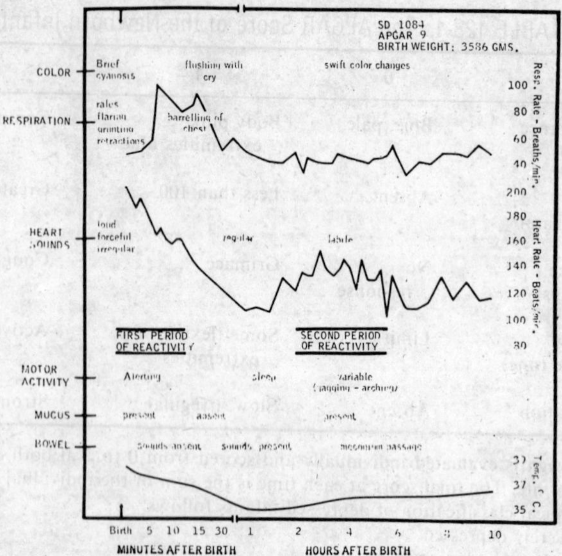

Figure 123-1. A summary of the physical findings noted during the first 10 hours of extrauterine life in a representative high-Apgar-score infant delivered under spinal anesthesia without prior medication. (From Desmond MM, et al.: The transitional care nursery. A mechanism for preventive medicine in the newborn. Pediatr. Clin. North Am., *13*:651-668, 1966.)

PROCEDURE FOR NEWBORN RESUSCITATION

GENERAL PRINCIPLES

1. Ventilation must be adequate.
2. Circulation must be supported.
3. Body temperature must be maintained.
4. Newborn resuscitation must be both aggressive and gentle.

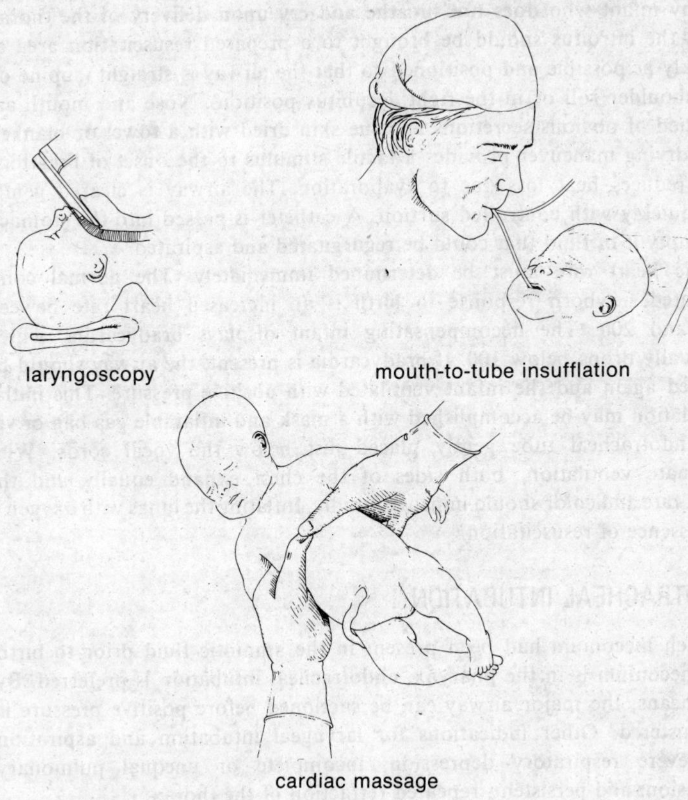

Figure 123-2.

SPECIFIC MEASURES

Initial resuscitative activities require simultaneous actions; these include positioning the baby, providing warmth, listening to the heart rate, straightening the airway, and clearing the airway.

The heart rate is counted with a stethoscope. Bradycardia is a sign of hypoxia.

Any infant who does not breathe and cry upon delivery of the thorax from the introitus should be brought to a prepared resuscitation area as quickly as possible and positioned so that the airway is straight (supine on the shoulder roll or in the right decubitus position). Nose and mouth are emptied of obvious secretions and the skin dried with a towel or blanket. The drying maneuver provides a tactile stimulus to the onset of breathing and reduces heat loss due to evaporation. The airway is cleared gently but quickly with controlled suction. A catheter is passed into the stomach to empty it of fluid that could be regurgitated and aspirated.

The heart rate must be determined immediately. The normal compensated newborn response to birth is an increased heart rate beween 160 and 200. The decompensating infant displays bradycardia, which gradually drops below 100. If bradycardia is present, the airway should be cleared again and the infant ventilated with positive pressure. This initial ventilation may be accomplished with a mask and inflatable gas bag or via an endotracheal tube gently placed just below the vocal cords. With adequate ventilation, both sides of the chest expand equally and the heart rate and color should improve rapidly. Inflating the lungs with oxygen is the essence of resuscitation.

ENDOTRACHEAL INTUBATION

When meconium had been present in the amniotic fluid prior to birth and meconium is in the pharynx, endotracheal intubation is preferred. By this means, the major airway can be suctioned before positive pressure is administered. Other indications for laryngeal intubation and aspiration are severe respiratory depression, incomplete or unequal pulmonary expansion, and persistent, repeated retraction of the thorax.

To facilitate visualization of the trachea, the infant's head is slightly extended. The laryngoscope is held in the left hand (if the attendant is right-handed) and the laryngoscope blade inserted into the angle of the infant's mouth. When the glottis is visible, the blade is centered and used to lift the tongue and mandible forward and upward in order to raise the epiglottis out of the line of vision and expose the larynx. Under direct vision, an endotracheal tube is passed into the trachea a short distance below the glottis. The laryngoscope is removed carefully. Free fluid or mucus is gently aspirated.

Short puffs of hydrated oxygen-air mixture are directed into the tube (20 to 30 times per minute). If the chest wall rises, the lungs are inflating.

The heart rate is checked by auscultation. If the heart rate does not become normal, the tube may be plugged or in the esophagus. Regular, brief insufflations are continued until spontaneous breathing occurs and a heart rate of greater than 110 beats per minute is achieved.

Positive-pressure ventilation should be applied in a manner simulating normal breathing. Only enough pressure to elevate the rib cage with each breath should be applied. Normally, the neonate may have intramural pressures of up to −70 cm of water for the first few breaths of life; nevertheless, this pressure applied unevenly from without can cause a pneumothorax. The normal newborn respiratory rate varies between 25 and 55. The initial rate of positive-pressure ventilation should be on the high side, gradually slowing so that the infant may take over spontaneous breathing. Room air usually provides sufficient oxygen for newborn resuscitation. If this proves ineffective in abolishing cyanosis, even though adequate ventilation is occurring, minimal amounts of oxygen may be necessary.

While ventilation is occurring, the heart should be monitored by stethoscope or electronic means. An assistant continues to dry the skin, proproviding tactile stimulus and preservation of warmth.

Bradycardia is usually corrected quickly once adequate ventilation is accomplished.

CLOSED CHEST MASSAGE

If bradycardia persists after effective ventilation has been established, closed chest cardiac massage may be required. Both thumbs are placed on the body of the sternum at the junction of the lower and middle thirds and the back supported with the fingers. The sternum is compressed approximately two thirds of the distance to the vertebral column 100 times per minute. Signs of adequate cardiac output are (1) improvement in color, (2) constriction of the pupils, and (3) palpable arterial pulses. With adequate ventilation and effective cardiac massage, the pulse should increase rapidly.

VASCULAR RESUSCITATION

If depression is severe or the infant fails to respond immediately, an umbilical artery catheter should be inserted to measure blood gases, pH, and blood pressure; to support blood volume; and to administer medications.

GASTRIC ASPIRATION

The stomach should be emptied of air and fluids during resuscitation.

ADDITIONAL THERAPY

Warmth, ventilation, closed chest massage, and support of the blood volume are usually sufficient to restore the cardiac rate.

Naloxone hydrochloride (Narcan Neonatal) (0.005 mg/kg), a narcotic antagonist, may be beneficial when depressed respiration results from maternal narcotic administration.

Sodium bicarbonate, 1 to 2 mEq/kg administered intravenously, may be required for correction of severe metabolic acidosis.

Epinephrine, 0.1 to 0.3 ml of a 1 to 10,000 solution, may be injected into the umbilical vein or directly into the heart if no other vascular route is available and the heart rate is slow and decelerating.

Packed red cell transfusions may be required in instances of vasa previa or placental lacerations with fetal blood loss.

REFERENCES

Casalino MB: Resuscitation of the neonate: principles and guidelines. J Reprod Med *17*:285-288, 1976

Clark RB, Beard AG, Barclay DL: Naloxone in the newborn infant. Anesth Rev *9*: 9-11, 1975

Desmond MM, Rudolph AJ, Phitaksphraiwan P: The transitional care nursery. A mechanism for preventive medicine in the newborn. Ped Clin North Am *13*: 651-668, 1966

DeVore JS: Resuscitation of the newborn. Clin Obstet Gynecol *19*:607-617, 1976

Gregory GA: Resuscitation of the newborn. Anesthesiology *43*: 225-237, 1975

Kitterman JA, Phibbs RH, Tooley WH: Catheterization of umbilical vessels in newborn infants. Ped Clin North Am *17*:895-912, 1970

Ting P, Brady JP: Tracheal suction in meconium aspiration. Am J Obstet Gynecol *122*:767-771, 1975

124 RH IMMUNE GLOBULIN PROPHYLAXIS

$Rh_0(D)$ immune globulin is a specially prepared gamma globulin that contains a concentration of Rh antibodies. These antibodies provide protection against foreign Rh-positive red cells, which may enter the mother's bloodstream after delivery, abortion, or ectopic pregnancy. When the pregnant mother is Rh-negative and the father is Rh-positive, there is a possibility that the baby may be Rh-positive. Since the baby's Rh-positive red cells are foreign to the Rh-negative mother, her body may respond by manufacturing an antibody capable of destroying Rh-positive cells (Fig. 124-1). An injection of $Rh_0(D)$ immune globulin prevents the sensitization (immunization) to the Rh antigen.

PROCEDURE

After delivery of every $Rh_0(D)$-negative woman, a specimen of cord blood and of postpartum maternal blood are sent to the laboratory. If the mother's serum has anti-$Rh_0(D)$ antibodies, the cord specimen is used to diagnose the possibility of erythroblastosis fetalis in the infant; the maternal specimen is used to cross-match blood if the infant requires transfusion.

If no antibodies are present, both the cord and maternal blood are used to determine the mother's eligibility for prophylactic treatment.

When an $Rh_0(D)$-negative woman delivers an $Rh_0(D)$-positive infant, she is a candidate for treatment with $Rh_0(D)$ immune globulin provided the following conditions are met:

1. The mother is $Rh_0(D)$-negative and D^u-negative.
2. The mother has no anti-$Rh_0(D)$ antibodies in her serum.
3. The infant is $Rh_0(D)$-positive or D^u-positive.
4. The direct antiglobulin (Coombs') test on the infant's cord blood is negative. [If Coombs' test is positive, owing to an antibody other than $Rh_0(D)$, $Rh_0(D)$ immune globulin should be administered.]

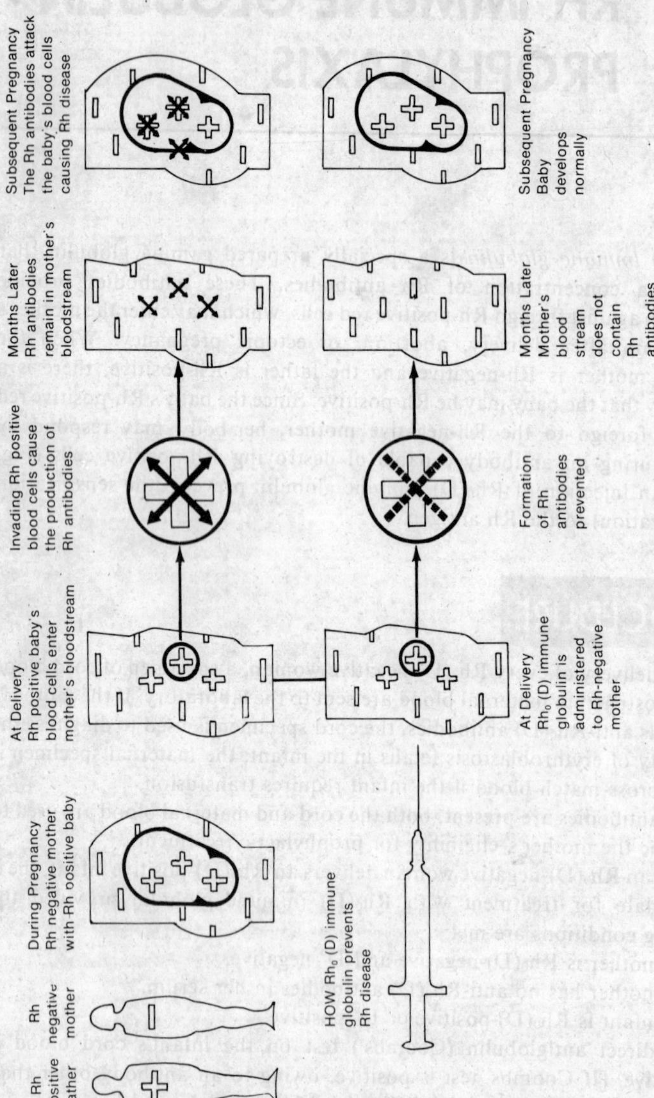

Rh positive father
Rh negative mother
During Pregnancy
Rh negative mother
with Rh oositive baby
At Delivery
Rh positive baby's
blood cells enter
mother's bloodstream
Invading Rh positive
blood cells cause
the production of
Rh antibodies
Months Later
Rh antibodies
remain in mother's
bloodstream
Subsequent Pregnancy
The Rh antibodies attack
the baby's blood cells
causing Rh disease
HOW Rh_0 (D) immune
globulin prevents
Rh disease
At Delivery
Rh_0 (D) immune
globulin is
administered
to Rh-negative
mother
Formation
of Rh
antibodies
prevented
Months Later
Mother's
blood
stream
does not
contain
Rh
antibodies
Subsequent Pregnancy
Baby
develops
normally

Figure 124-1.

The $Rh_0(D)$ immune globulin cross-match solution should be compatible with the mother's postpartum blood specimen. If it is not compatible and all the above criteria have been verified, then it is likely that there has been a large fetal-maternal hemorrhage, requiring more than one dose of $Rh_0(D)$ immune globulin to prevent Rh-sensitization of the mother. The detection of large fetal-maternal hemorrhages is a major function of the cross-match test.

The Kleihauer-Betke acid elution smear technique, which distinguishes between fetal (pink) and adult (ghost) red cells, is the most sensitive method of detecting and quantifying fetal-maternal hemorrhage. A count is made of fetal and adult cells on the smear and the size of the fetal-maternal hemorrhage is determined according to the following formula:

$$\frac{\text{No. of fetal cells}}{\text{No. of maternal cells}} = \frac{\text{X (ml of fetal-maternal bleed)}}{\text{Estimated maternal blood volume}}$$

One vial of $Rh_0(D)$ immune globulin (300 mcg of anti-D) can suppress immunity to approximately 30 ml of whole Rh-positive blood or approximately 15 ml of packed Rh-positive blood cells. With large fetal-maternal hemorrhages, two or three doses of immune globulin may be required.

$Rh_0(D)$ immune globulin is administered by intramuscular injection and protects the mother only against sensitization by the just-completed pregnancy. Rh-negative women are retreated after the delivery of each subsequent Rh-positive child, provided the same criteria are met. The globulin should be injected within 72 hours of delivery. (If the 72-hour period is exceeded, the globulin should still be administered, since it is not definitely known how long it takes for a primary immune response to occur.)

After an *abortion* or *ectopic pregnancy,* every Rh-negative, unsensitized woman should be protected with $Rh_0(D)$ immune globulin in order to avoid sensitization.

In the event that Rh-positive cells are transfused into an Rh-negative patient, multiple doses of $Rh_0(D)$ immune globulin can prevent Rh sensitization.

After amniocentesis, in the absence of any specific data concerning the risk of sensitization, it is probably advisable that Rh-negative, unsensitized women be treated with $Rh_0(D)$ immune globulin (ACOG Technical Bulletin, January 1976).

REFERENCES

Current uses of Rh_0 immune globulin and detection of antibodies. ACOG Technical Bulletin, No. 35, January 1976

Frigoletto FD: Management and prevention of erythroblastosis fetalis. Clin Perinatol *1*:321-330, 1974

Queenan JT: The Rh problem. Clin Obstet Gynecol *14*:491-645, June 1971

125 ULTRASOUND B-SCAN

Ultrasonography has become a valuable diagnostic aid in obstetrics and gynecology. Producing no ionizing radiation, ultrasound is a non-invasive technique that causes virtually no discomfort and provides helpful information about the fetus, placenta, and pelvic masses.

The ultrasound beam is in many ways similar to a beam of light; it can be focused, reflected, or refracted. The beam consists of high-frequency sound waves generated by vibration of a piezoelectric crystal within an ultrasound transducer. The same crystal that transmits the ultrasonic beam also functions as a listening device. Returning sound waves (echoes) strike the transducer, producing vibrations that are transmitted as electrical signals to an oscilloscope or for storage on the screen of a cathode ray tube. This latter type of storage display is called a B-scan; the letter B is used because the brightness (and size) of the dots on the screen varies with the strength of the acoustic interface.

As the transducer (attached to a rigid hinged arm) is moved across a section of the patient's body, it sends a narrow, well-directed ultrasonic beam through the tissues. As this beam traverses the abdomen, it is partially reflected at various interfaces, owing to relative differences in acoustic impedance. Homogenous tissues such as fluid-filled organs or cystic lesions show few internal echoes, whereas solid organs or masses generally have many weak echoes, representing small vessels, ducts, and septae traversing the tissue.

For satisfactory pelvic scanning, a full bladder is advisable. The bladder lifts the uterus up out of the pelvis and provides a fluid-filled medium that aids in the transmission of the sound.

A thin coating of mineral oil is applied to the skin over the area to be scanned so that the transducer can be moved back and forth with airless contact between the abdomen and the transducer.

A recent advance in ultrasonic technology has been the development of "gray scale" equipment. These units are capable of recording echoes from the parenchyma of many organs in far greater detail than was previously possible. The older or bistable ultrasound machines record echoes only from interfaces that are stronger than a certain threshold. One may lower this threshold by turning up the "gain" (or sensitivity) of the unit, but all echoes above the threshold are recorded at one intensity, whereas echoes below the threshold are not recorded at all. With gray scale units, echoes of many differing intensities are recorded, with the stronger echoes appearing darker in proportion to their intensity. Even more recent real-time equipment provides visualization of fetal activity.

USES OF ULTRASOUND IN GYNECOLOGY AND OBSTETRICS

GYNECOLOGY

1. Intrauterine device localization
2. Pelvic mass evaluations
   a. Fluid-filled or solid
   b. Relationship to uterus and adnexa
   c. Pelvic abscess

OBSTETRICS

1. Pregnancy detection
2. Fetal gestational age
3. Multiple gestation
4. Fetal anomalies (hydrocephaly, anencephaly)
5. Fetal death
6. Placental localization
7. Molar pregnancy
8. Hydramnios

Intrauterine Device Localization: When the string of an intrauterine device is not visualized in the cervical os, a sonogram may be able to localize the device within the uterine cavity. Each type of intrauterine device gives a characteristic echo pattern within the echo-free space of the uterus. If the uterus appears to be empty and there is proof by x-ray that the device has not been expelled, uterine perforation may have occurred, the device being in the peritoneal cavity.

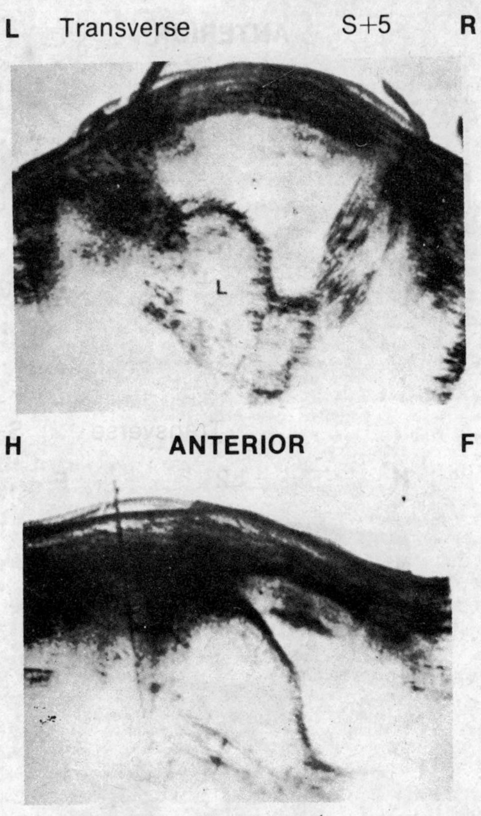

Figure 125-1. Patient is 43 years of age with a history of irregular periods for the past eight months. On examination, a large, firm mass inseparable from the uterus is noted. The mass is nontender and extends slightly to the left.

The transverse sonogram shows a large solid mass (L) inseparable from the uterus and indenting the posterior portion of the bladder on the left. There are fine echoes within the mass, and the posterior border is poorly defined. There is little through transmission, in contrast with the appearance expected with a fluid-filled mass. This appearance is compatible with a diagnosis of leiomyomata. Similar findings are seen on the longitudinal study. (From Gosink BB, Squire LF: Exercises in Diagnostic Radiology 8: Diagnostic Ultrasound. Philadelphia, W.B. Saunders Co., 1976.)

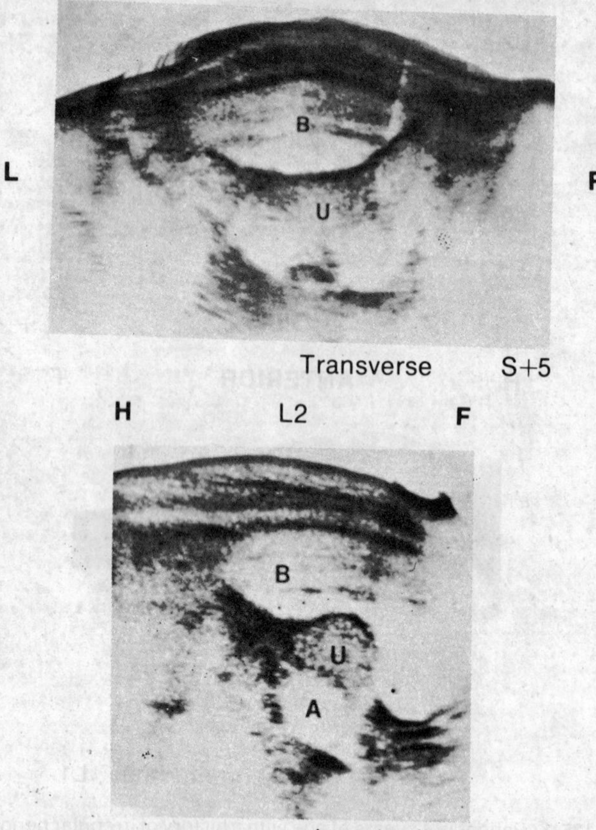

Figure 125-2. Patient is 19 years of age with a history of increased vaginal discharge and marked pelvic tenderness. The severe pain does not permit an adequate pelvic examination.

The longitudinal echogram shows a fluid-filled mass (A) lying posterior to the uterus (U), displacing it anteriorly. The transverse can shows two fluid-filled structures, each lying posterolaterally to the uterus.

These findings are compatible with a diagnosis of bilateral tuboovarian abscesses. (From Gosink BB, Squire LF: Exercises in Diagnostic Radiology 8: Diagnostic Ultrasound. Philadelphia, W.B. Saunders Co., 1976.)

Pelvic Masses: Cystic and solid masses can be differentiated. As the sensitivity (gain) of the receiver is increased, solid masses display multiple interfaces, indicating a complex or solid interior (Fig. 125-1). Cystic lesions contain an extremely homogenous internal structure and do not show internal echoes at increased sensitivity levels (Fig. 125-2). In addition, cystic lesions tend to have a strong, sharp posterior border, in contrast to the often broken and irregular contour of a solid mass (Figs. 125-3 and 125-4).

Normal Pregnancy: The first ultrasonic evidence of pregnancy occurs at about the fifth week following the last menstrual period (or three weeks after conception). In addition to slight enlargement of the uterus, a ringlike collection of echoes, representing the developing gestational sac, may be seen in the uterine fundus. As pregnancy progresses, the gestational sac enlarges and fills the entire uterine cavity by ten to eleven weeks.

The placenta may be identified as a discernible structure between the eighth and twelfth weeks; the fetal skull becomes visible in 95 per cent of cases by the thirteenth or fourteenth week. As the fetus enlarges, the bi-

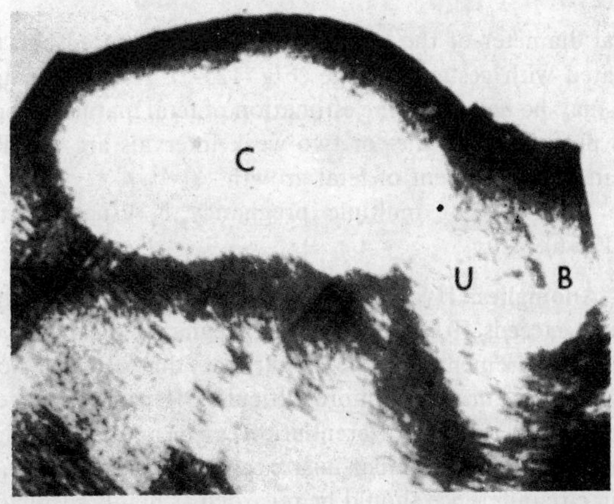

Figure 125-3. Longitudinal scan showing large unilocular ovarian cyst lying anterior to a myomatous uterus. C, cyst; B, bladder; U, uterus. (From Cochrane WJ: Ultrasound in gynecology. Radiol Clin North Am *13*:457, 1975.)

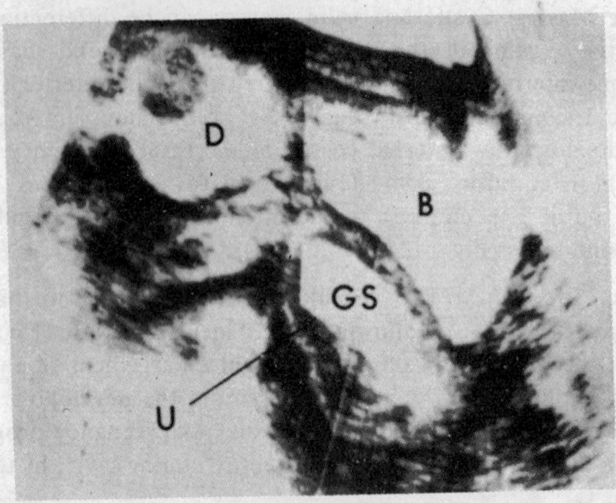

Figure 125-4. Longitudinal scan showing large dermoid cyst lying anterior to a 2-1/2 month pregnant uterus. Note solid material within cyst. B, bladder; D, dermoid cyst; GS, gestational sac; U, uterus. (From Cochrane WJ:Ultrasound in gynecology. Radiol Clin North Am *13*:457, 1975.)

parietal diameter of the fetal skull can be measured and the diameter correlated with gestational age (Fig. 125-5). Although single measurements may be helpful in the estimation of fetal maturity, serial measurements performed at one- or two-week intervals are usually of greater value in the assessment of fetal growth.

The diagnosis of multiple pregnancy is usually straightforward (Fig. 125-6).

Fetal Anomalies: Hydrocephalus is suspected when the biparietal diameter exceeds 10.6 cm. Earlier in pregnancy, however, when the absolute measurement of the biparietal diameter is not excessive, correct evaluation may be more difficult. Often, by paying careful attention to the fetal thorax, differentiation can be made. Since the thorax and skull tend to be quite similar in size throughout pregnancy, any discrepancy in circumference should be regarded as highly suspicious. The possibility of hydrocephalus is confirmed when a study performed one to two weeks later reveals abnormal growth of the biparietal diameter.

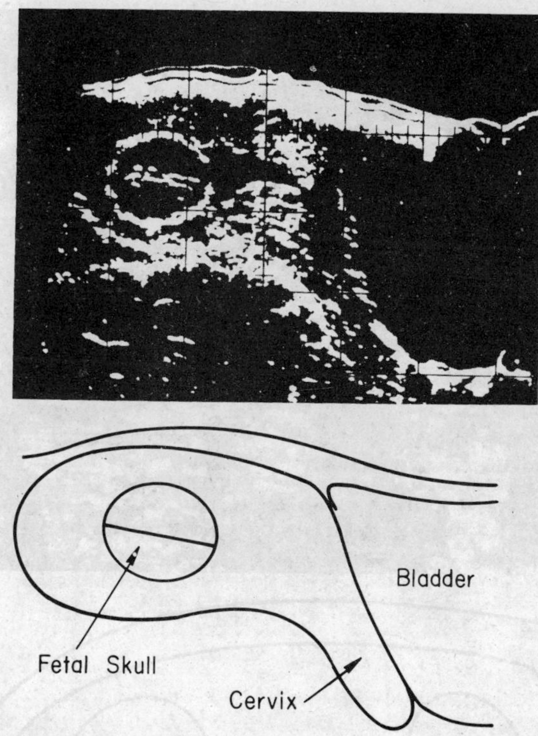

Figure 125-5. Sagittal scan. A 15 week size fetal skull is visualized in the uterine fundus. The markedly elongated cervix of pregnancy is evident behind the bladder. (From Leopold GR, Asher WM: Ultrasound in obstetrics and gynecology. Radiol Clin North Am *12*:133, 1974.)

Anencephaly is recognizable by the absence of a well-formed fetal skull. Many of these cases are referred for evaluation because the uterus is larger than expected for the dates, or because the patient has passed term and has not gone into labor. Ultrasonic scan can show excess amniotic fluid—hydramnios—as well as the fetal anomaly.

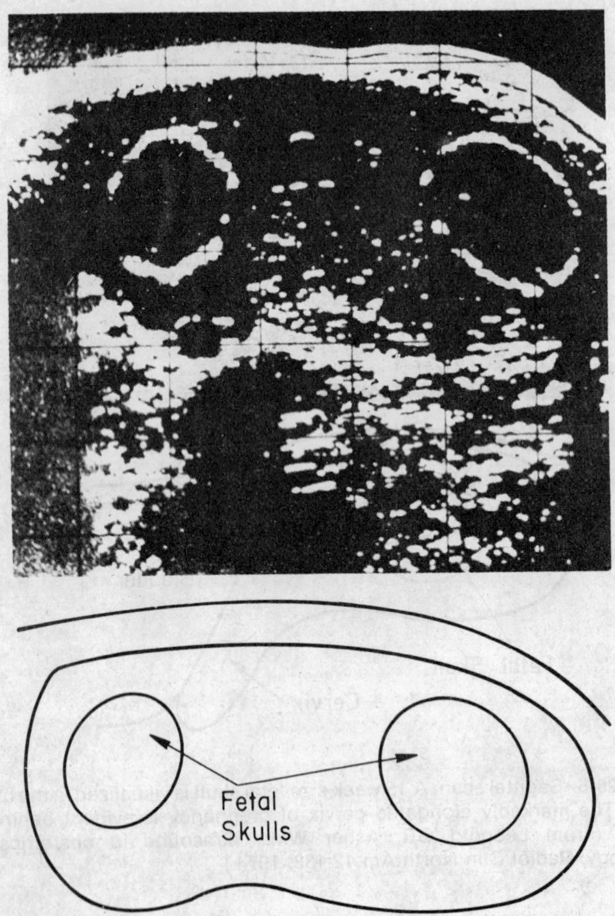

Figure 125-6. Transverse scan. Two 18 week fetal skulls are seen on opposite sides of the uterus. (From Leopold GR, Asher WM: Ultrasound in obstetrics and gynecology. Radiol Clin North Am *12*:138, 1974.)

Fetal Demise: Diagnostic signs of fetal death include failure to detect the fetal heart pulsation, distortion or flattening of the fetal head, and multiple bizarre echoes arising in the fetal trunk or skull. The absence of growth of the fetal head on successive examinations, the reduction of the biparietal diameter, and the presence of an incomplete circle or oval surrounding the fetal head are also suggestive of fetal death (Fig. 125-7).

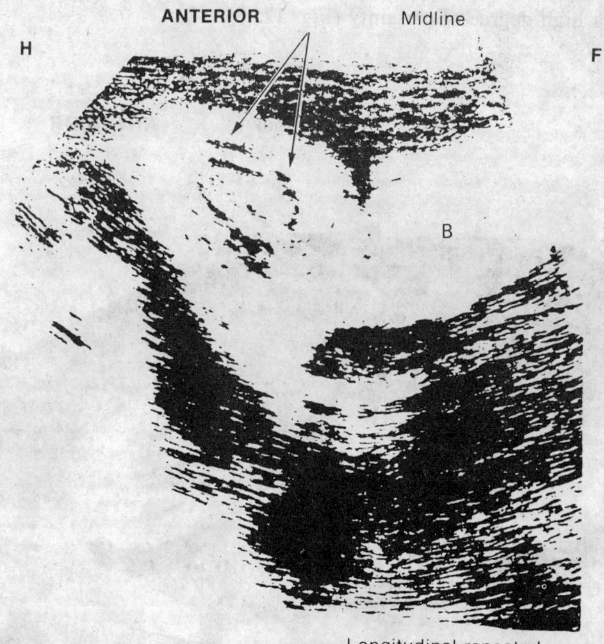

Figure 125-7. Patient is age 27 with a history of a last menstrual period 12 weeks previously. The previous evening the patient noted spotting. On pelvic examination the uterus appears approximately the same size as two weeks previously or perhaps even smaller. The sonogram shows an enlarged uterus with an irregular incomplete ring of echoes (arrows) in the fundus. This represents a disintegrating gestational sac compatible with a diagnosis of inevitable or missed abortion. (From Gosink BB, Squire LF: Exercises in Diagnostic Radiology 8: Diagnostic Ultrasound. Philadelphia, W.B. Saunders Co., 1976.)

Placental Localization: As pregnancy progresses the placental site can be recognized. Since the internal cervical os may be localized as the midpoint of a line joining the base of the bladder and the closest portion of the maternal sacrum, it is relatively simple to estimate the amount of placental overlap in cases of placenta previa (Fig. 125-8). In the case of vertex presentations, scans that show the fetal head in contact with the distended urinary bladder anteriorly, and within 1 or 2 cm of the maternal sacrum posteriorly, rule out placenta previa with a high degree of certainty (Fig. 125-9).

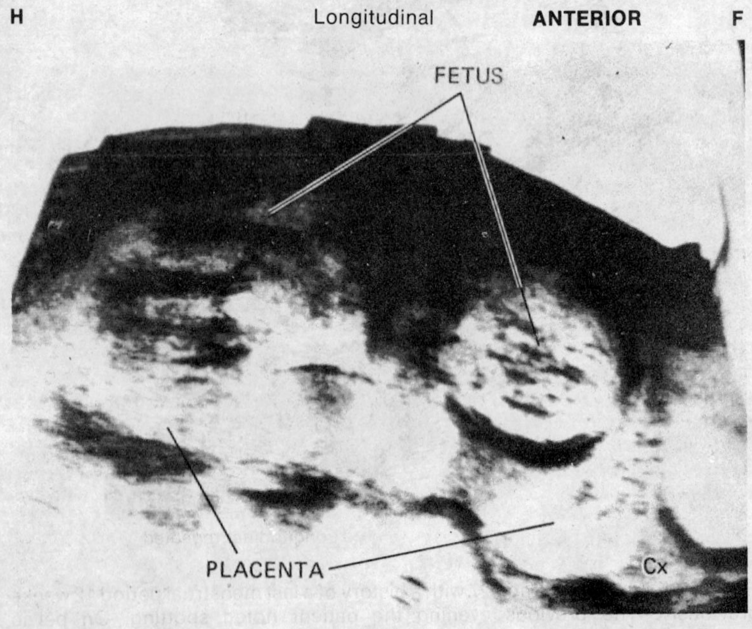

Figure 125-8. The placenta is identified by a sharply defined fetal border, representing the chorionic plate. Its internal structure produces a stippled pattern of echoes. The fetal head is displaced out of the pelvis by a posterior placenta previs. (From Gosink BB, Squire LF: Exercises in Diagnostic Radiology 8: Diagnostic Ultrasound. Philadelphia, W.B. Saunders Co., 1976.)

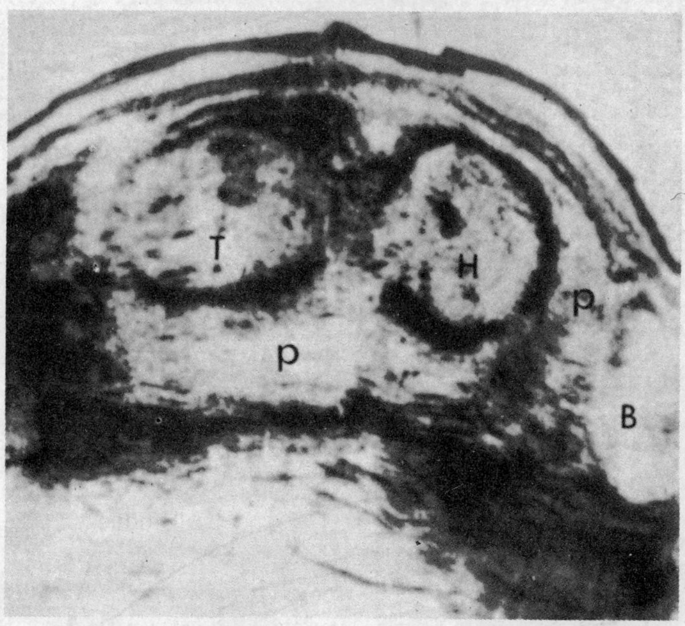

Figure 125-9. Longitudinal section of a patient with total placenta praevia with the bulk of the placenta lying posterior to the fetus. The output has been increased so that the bladder is almost filled with echoes. Note how even the shielded posterior placenta fills in and the broad rim of placental tissue separating the head from the cervix and bladder is easily recognizable. (From Sanders RC, Conrad MR: Sonography in obstetrics. Radiol Clin North Am *13*:435, 1975.)

Molar pregnancy can be diagnosed in early pregnancy when there is no evidence of a fetal skull, thorax, or heart (Fig. 125-10). The uterus appears to be filled with a myriad of uniform reflections, which come from the grapelike vesicles. Although the pattern is usually diffuse throughout the uterus, clear spaces may be observed between the molar tissue and the uterine wall, representing retained blood clots within the uterus. Ovarian lutein cysts are frequently associated findings and are visualized as large, extrauterine, echo-free masses.

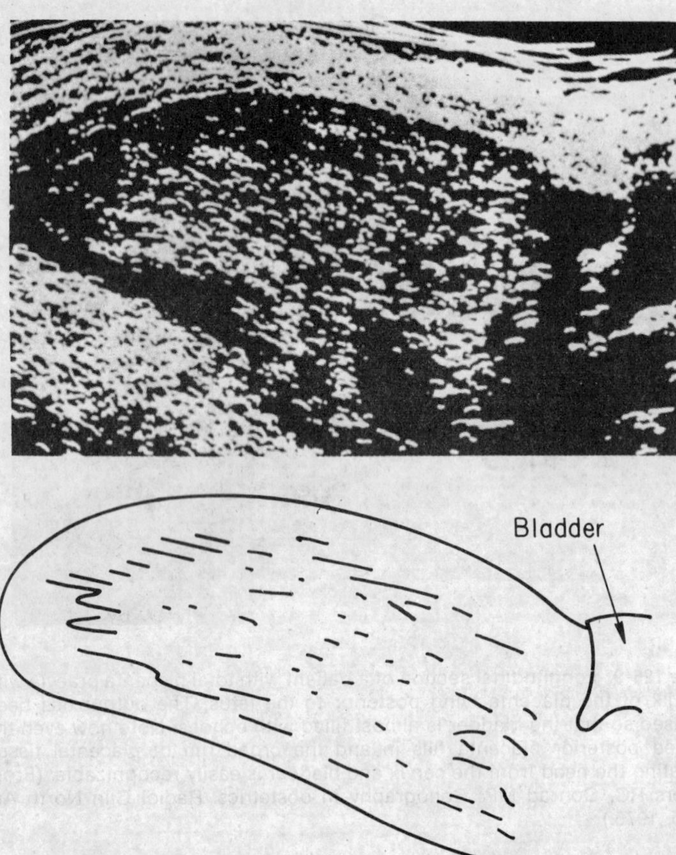

Figure 125-10. Sagittal scan, 16 week gestation. Instead of fetal parts, the uterus is diffusely filled with weak, amorphous echoes which are quite typical of a molar pregnancy. (From Leopold GR, Asher WM: Ultrasound in obstetrics and gynecology. Radiol Clin North Am *12*:142, 1974.)

Although the ultrasonic appearance of molar pregnancy is highly specific, degenerating leiomyomas or a missed abortion may, on occasion, present a similar appearance. A pregnancy test aids in the differential diagnosis, since with molar pregnancy the level of chorionic gonadotropin is markedly elevated.

126 UTERINE ARTERY LIGATION

When hemorrhage persists after delivery or cesarean section, three basic surgical procedures must be considered: (1) uterine artery ligation, (2) hysterectomy, and (3) hypogastric artery ligation.

PROCEDURE FOR UTERINE ARTERY LIGATION

After the abdomen is opened, a transverse incision is made at the level of the peritoneal reflection between the anterior uterine wall and the bladder. (This step is similar to the exposure of the lower uterine segment prior to a low cervical-uterine incision for cesarean section.) The bladder is dissected inferiorly from the lower uterine segment.

The uterine artery and vein are palpated and then doubly ligated with number 1 chromic catgut suture on a large Mayo needle. To ligate the left uterine artery, the needle is passed into and through the myometrium from the anterior to the posterior, 2 to 3 cm medial to the uterine vessels; it is then brought forward through the avascular area of the broad ligament lateral to the artery and vein.

The right uterine artery is ligated in a similar fashion. The suture should include a substantial amount of myometrium.

The vessels are *not* divided.

If the uterine vessel ligation does not control the bleeding adequately, the ovarian vessels can also be ligated bilaterally, since these vessels carry the major blood supply to the uterine fundus.

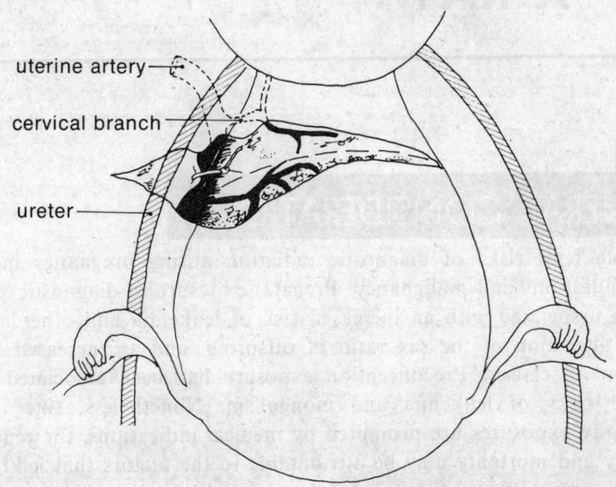

Figure 126-1. Ascending branch of left uterine artery after ligation. Note large amount of myometrium within the suture. (Modified from O'Leary JL, O'Leary JA: Uterine artery ligation for control of postcesarean section hemorrhage. Obstet Gynecol *43*:849-853, 1974.)

REFERENCES

Graber EA: Hemorrhage in pregnancy. *In* Barber HRK, Graber EA: Surgical Disease in Pregnancy. Philadelphia, W.B. Saunders Company, 1974

O'Leary JL, O'Leary JA: Uterine artery ligation for control of postcesarean section hemorrhage. Obstet Gynecol *43*:849-853, 1974

127 X-RAY

GENERAL CONSIDERATIONS

Possible fetal risks of diagnostic radiation during pregnancy include genetic mutations and malignancy. Prenatal exposure to diagnostic x-rays has been associated with an increased risk of leukemia and other malignancies, alteration of the sex ratio of offspring, and an increased death rate from all causes. Preconception exposure has been associated with increased risks of leukemia and mongolism. Nonetheless, since diagnostic x-ray exposures are prompted by medical indications, the reported morbidity and mortality may be attributable to the factors that led to the exposure, rather than being caused by the radiation itself. Selection of subjects on the basis of medical indication may have introduced biases into the various studies (Oppenheim, 1975).

Whether a given dose of radiation to a pregnant woman can harm the baby and what the critical dose is remain unanswered questions. From preconception to birth there may not be any period during which radiologic examinations of the lower abdomen and pelvis of a fertile woman can be conducted without some risk, even though the risk is extremely small.

In general, pelvic x-rays are avoided during early pregnancy unless the information they would reveal is crucial for the mother's health. At all times, irradiation should be limited to the minimal amount essential for fetal and maternal welfare.

Guidelines for the use of diagnostic x-ray in fertile women suggested by the American College of Obstetricians and Gynecologists are the following:

1. The use of x-ray examinations should be considered on an individual basis. Concern over harmful effects should not prevent the proper use of radiation exposure when significant diagnostic information can be obtained. Pre-examination consultation with a radiologist may be useful in obtaining the optimal information from the x-ray exposure.

2. There is no measurable advantage to scheduling diagnostic x-ray examinations at any particular time during a normal menstrual cycle.
3. The degree of risk involved in an x-ray examination if the person is pregnant, or should become pregnant, should be explained to the patient and documented in her record. (The risk of an observable anomaly in a fetus from diagnostic radiation does not exceed 1 to 5 per 1000 per rad of exposure, which is substantially less than the natural incidence for observed birth anomalies of 40 per 1000 births.)

OBSTETRIC PELVIMETRY AND ABDOMINAL FILMS

X-ray examinations during labor often provide valuable assistance in the management of emergency obstetric problems. Usually, two views of the pelvis (anteroposterior and lateral) reveal the fetal presentation and station (Fig. 127-1), the position of the fetal head (flexion or extension), the presence and presentation of multiple pregnancies (Fig. 127-2), fetal anomalies (hydrocephalus, anencephalus), fetal death, and the pelvic shape and architecture.

The anteroposterior film is most helpful for the evaluation of fetal presentation and position, molding of the fetal head, and measurements of the transverse diameters of the pelvic inlet and midplane (Fig. 127-3).

The lateral film affords a view of the sacral curvature and the various anteroposterior diameters of the inlet and midpelvis, as well as an assessment of the engagement or descent of the fetal head into the pelvic inlet (Fig. 127-3).

X-ray findings of abnormal fetal position or fetal disproportion (Figs. 127-4 and 127-5), together with clinical findings, may facilitate the decisions required to manage labor.

Fetal Death: Roentgen signs of fetal death are dependent on evidence of fetal maceration or loss of fetal muscle tone or both, which are usually seen 48 hours or more after fetal death. The three most common and useful signs of fetal maceration are (1) intravascular fetal gas, (2) overlapping of the cranial bones (Spalding's sign) (Fig. 127-6), and (3) Deuel's halo sign (Fig. 127-7). Other signs that may

(Text continued on p. 881)

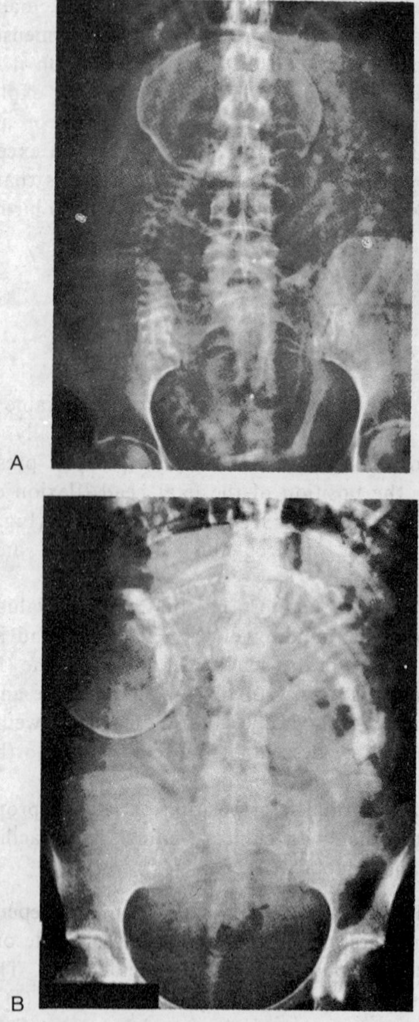

Figure 127-1. *A*, Breech presentation. *B*, Transverse lie. (From Langston CS, Squire LF: Exercises in Diagnostic Radiology 7: The Emergency Patient. Philadelphia, W.B. Saunders Co., 1975.)

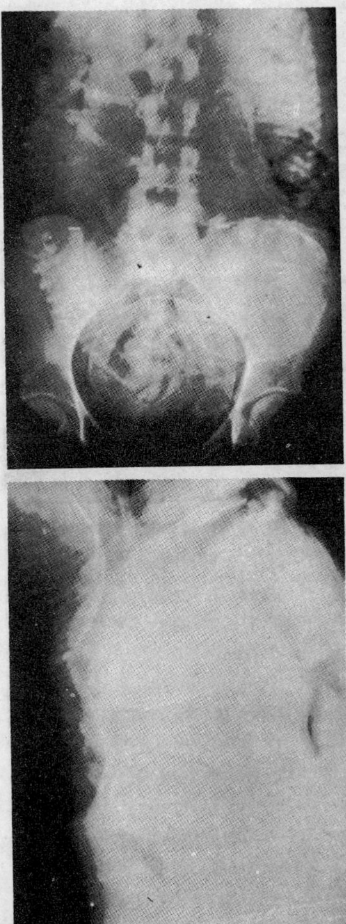

Figure 127-2. Prolongation of latent phase because of multiple pregnancy and position in a 26 year primigravida with pre-eclampsia. In this twin pregnancy with mature fetuses, the lower fetus is in occiput right posterior position with gross disproportion. (From Whitehouse WM, Work BA: Radiographic manifestations of the causes of failure of progression of labor. Radiol Clin North Am *12*:6, 1974.)

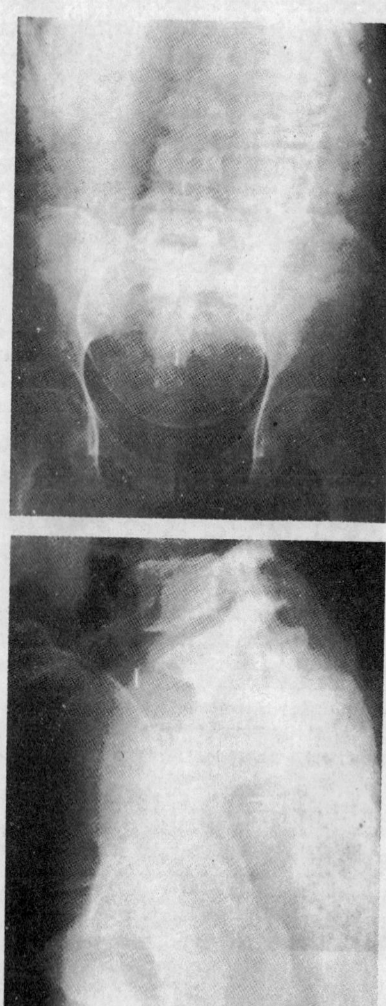

Figure 127-3. Prolongation of latent phase with disproportion in a 32 year old gravida 2 para 1. There is a large mature fetus and adequate anteroposterior pelvic diameters but relative narrowing of the transverse diameters. (From Whitehouse WM, Work BA: Radiographic manifestations of the causes of failure of progression of labor. Radiol Clin North Am *12*:6, 1974.)

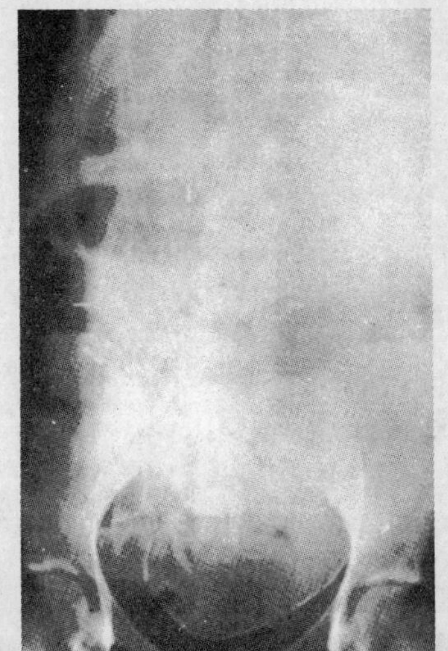

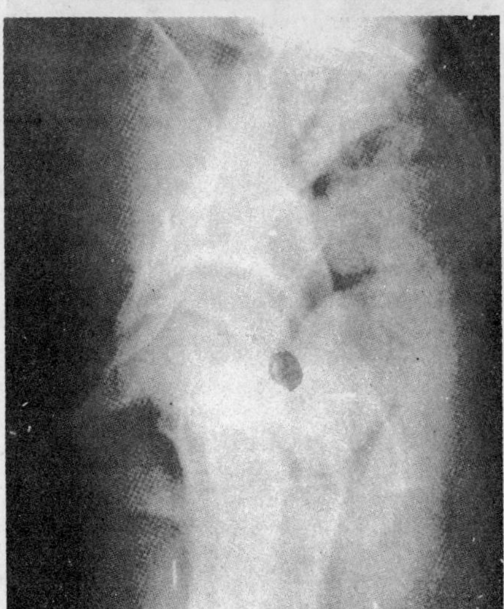

Figure 127-4. Arrest in active phase with abnormal position and disproportion. Twenty-two year primigravida, brow presentation, failure of engagement due to disproportion at pelvic inlet. (From Whitehouse WM, Work BA: Radiographic manifestations of the causes of failure of progression of labor. Radiol Clin North Am *12*:3, 1974.)

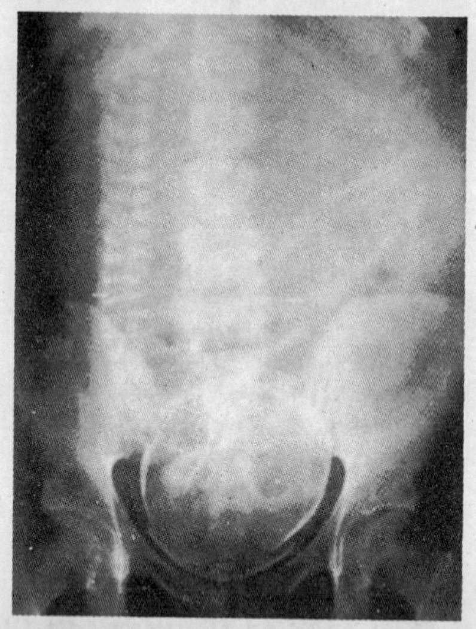

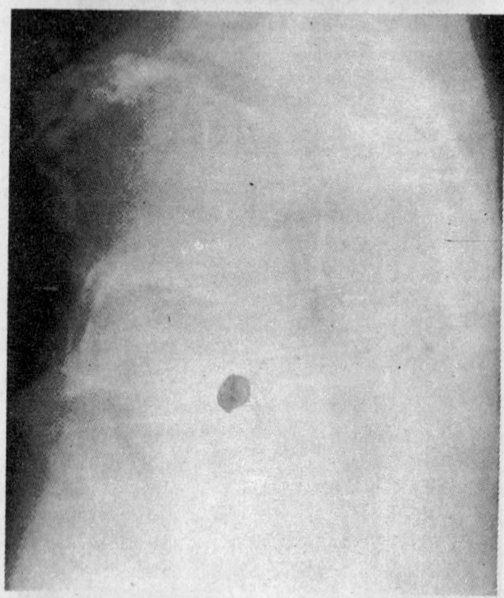

Figure 127-5. Arrest in active phase with disproportion. Twenty-three year primigravida, occiput right posterior position, moderate molding. Disproportion at pelvic inlet; also prominent ischial spines. (From Whitehouse WM, Work BA: Radiographic manifestations of the causes of failure of progression of labor. Radiol Clin North Am *12*:3, 1974.)

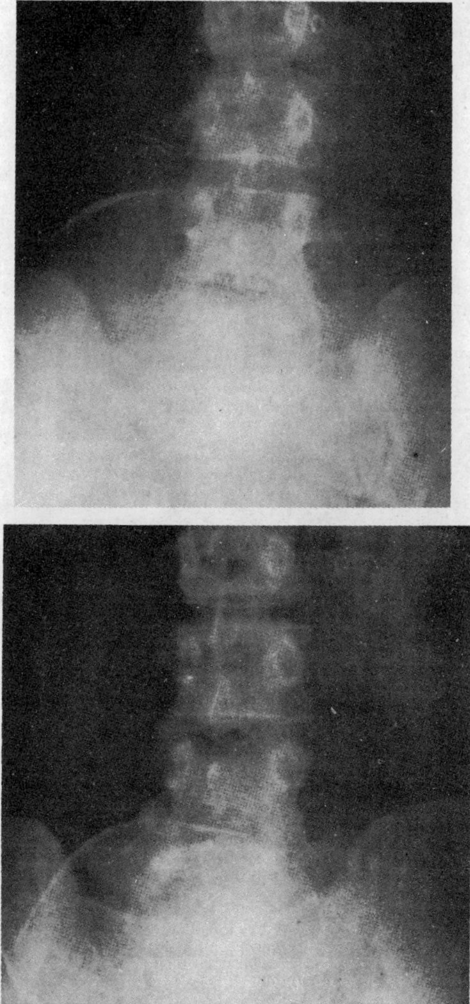

Figure 127-6. Spalding's sign with the patient filmed in the upright position. Supine film is for comparison. *A*(supine), There is equivocal overlapping of the fetal cranial bones. *B*(erect), There is definite overlapping of the fetal cranial bones indicative of fetal death (Spalding's sign).

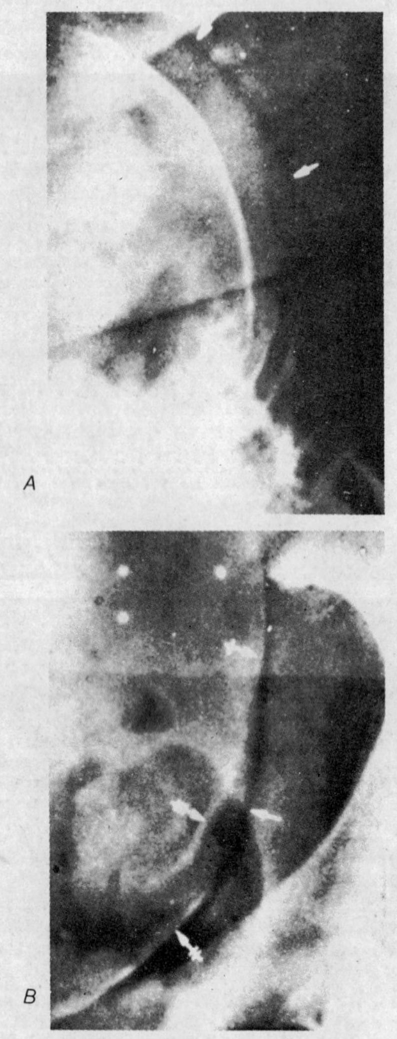

Figure 127-7. Deuel's halo sign. *A*,↑ There is universal separation of the fetal subcutaneous fat line from the calvarium in a "dead" fetus (Halo sign). *B*,↑ The fetal subcutaneous fat line bridges the separated cranial bones at the suture area. ⟊ The normal apposition of the fetal subcutaneous fat line to the bony calvarium. ⇈ Misalignment of the fetal cranial bones at the suture. (From Borell V, Fernstrom I: Acta Radiol *48*:401, with permission.)

be observed are collapse of the fetal spine and abnormal fetal attitude. (Although overlapping of the fetal cranial bones may represent the collapse of the calvarium about a macerated brain, the molding associated with normal labor can also produce overlapping of the cranial bones.)

Amniography, the injection of contrast media into the amniotic cavity, is a technique that has been used for the diagnosis of fetal demise and hydatidiform mole.

REFERENCES

Caterini H, Sama J, Iffy L, et al: A reevaluation of amniography. Obstet Gynecol *47*:373-377, 1976

Oppenheim BE, Griem ML, Meier P: The effects of diagnostic X-ray exposure on the human fetus: An examination of the evidence. Radiology *114*:529-534, 1975

PART IV

APPENDICES

APPENDIX 1
EMERGENCY EQUIPMENT

1. Adhesive tape
2. Airways, oropharyngeal and nasopharyngeal—assorted sizes
3. Alcohol sponges
4. Applicators, cotton-tipped
5. Bacteriologic culture transport media and tubes
6. Blood infusion sets
7. Central venous catheters
8. Cervical biopsy punch
9. Cutdown set
10. Defibrillator—monitor with ECG electrode-defibrillator paddles
11. Delivery table
12. Drapes, sterile
13. Electrocardiograph machine, portable, direct-writing
14. Emesis basin
15. Endometrial biopsy curette
16. Endotracheal tubes with stylets
17. Examination table with stirrup extensions
18. Gauze pads
19. Gloves, sterile
20. Hemostats
21. Instrument tables
22. Intravenous infusion sets
23. Intravenous solutions—5 per cent dextrose in lactated Ringer's solution, normal saline, 5 per cent dextrose infusion
24. Iodoform gauze packing
25. Lamp to visualize perineum, vagina, and cervix
26. Laryngoscope with blades (curved and straight, for adults and infants) with extra batteries and bulbs
27. Lubricating jelly
28. Mask for mouth-to-mask ventilation (Ambu Bag)
29. Medicine cups
30. Microscope
31. Nasogastric tubes
32. Needle holder
33. Oxygen supply with reducing valves capable of delivery 15 liters per minute, with mask and reservoir bag
34. Povidone–iodine skin cleanser
35. Pudendal-block needle guide
36. Razor
37. Reflex hammer
38. Retractor, right angle
39. Ring forceps with sterile cotton and gauze squares

40. Scalpel with blades
41. Scissors
42. Solution basin stands
43. Sphygmomanometer
44. Spinal needles with stylet
45. Stethoscopes, regular and ultrasound
46. Suction with catheters, sizes 6 to 16, with suction tips
47. Suction bulb, rubber
48. Suture
49. Syringes and needles
50. Tape
51. Tenaculum, cervical (single tooth)
52. Thermometers
53. Tissue forceps
54. Tongue blades (including padded tongue blades)
55. Tourniquet
56. Towels, sterile
57. Tubes for blood
58. Umbilical cord clamps
59. Urinary catheters
60. Urine bottles, sterile
61. Uterine aspiration pump with assorted cannulas and curettes
62. Uterine curettes (sharp)
63. Uterine dressing forceps for packing
64. Uterine sounds
65. Vaginal packing (two inches to five yards)
66. Vagina specula, assorted sizes, including narrow-bladed for children and elderly women
67. Venous catheters

APPENDIX 2
EMERGENCY MEDICATIONS

1. Albumin
2. Alphaprodine (Nisentil)
3. Aminophylline
4. Amobarbital
5. Aromatic spirits of ammonia
6. Atropine
7. Calcium chloride
8. Calcium gluconate
9. Deslanoside (Cedilanid-D)
10. Dexamethasone (Decadron)
11. Dextrose, 50 per cent
12. Diazepam (Valium)
13. Digoxin
14. Diphenhydramine hydrochloride (Benadryl)
15. Dopamine
16. Ephedrine
17. Epinephrine
18. Ergonovine
19. Furosemide (Lasix)
20. Heparin
21. Hydralazine hydrochloride (Apresoline)
22. Hydrocortisone (Solu-Cortef)
23. Isoproterenol
24. Lidocaine
25. Magnesium sulfate, 50 per cent
26. Mannitol
27. Meperidine (Demerol)
28. Metaraminol
29. Methylergonovine
30. Methylprednisolone (Solu-Medrol)
31. Morphine sulfate
32. Naloxone (Narcan)
33. Oxytocin
34. Pentobarbital
35. Phenobarbital
36. Phenytoin (Dilantin)
37. Plasma protein fraction
38. Potassium chloride
39. Probenecid
40. Promethazine (Phenergan)
41. Progesterone in oil
42. Sodium bicarbonate

ANTIBIOTICS

1. Ampicillin
2. Cefazolin
3. Clindamycin
4. Gentamicin
5. Kanamycin
6. Penicillin

APPENDIX 3
COMPARATIVE THERMOMETER

TABLE A3-1. Comparative Thermometer Readings*

Fahrenheit	Centigrade	Fahrenheit	Centigrade
96.0	35.5	101.4	38.5
96.2	35.6	101.6	38.6
96.4	35.7	101.8	38.7
96.6	35.8	102.0	38.9
96.8	35.9	102.2	39.0
97.0	36.1	102.4	39.1
97.2	36.2	102.6	39.2
97.4	36.3	102.8	39.3
97.6	36.4	103.0	39.4
97.8	36.6	103.2	39.6
98.0	36.7	103.4	39.7
98.2	36.8	103.6	39.8
98.4	36.9	103.8	39.9
98.6	37.0	104.0	40.0
98.8	37.1	104.2	40.1
99.0	37.2	104.4	40.2
99.2	37.3	104.6	40.3
99.4	37.4	104.8	40.4
99.6	37.6	105.0	40.6
99.8	37.7	105.2	40.7
100.0	37.8	105.4	40.8
100.2	37.9	105.6	40.9
100.4	38.0	105.8	41.0
100.6	38.1	106.0	41.1
100.8	38.2	108.0	42.2
101.0	38.3	110.0	43.3
101.2	38.4		

*From Flint T, Cain HD: Emergency Treatment and Management. Philadelphia, W.B. Saunders Company, 1975, p. 745.

To convert Centigrade into Fahrenheit* Multiply by 9, divide by 5, and add 32:

$$\left(°F = \frac{°C \times 9}{5} + 32\right)$$

To convert Fahrenheit into Centigrade† Subtract 32, multiply by 5, and divide by 9:

$$\left(°C = \frac{°F - 32 \times 5}{9}\right)$$

*From Flint T, Cain HD: Emergency Treatment and Management. Philadelphia, W.B. Saunders Company, 1975, p. 745.

†Ibid.

INDEX

Note: Page numbers in *italics* refer to illustrations. Page numbers followed by (t) refer to tables.

局版臺業字第0698號

發行人：吳　富　章

發行所：合 記 圖 書 出 版 社

總經銷：合　記　書　局

地　址：臺 北 市 吳 興 街 249 號

電　話：7019404　郵政劃撥6919號

中華民國六十八年　月　日

EMERGENCY EQUIPMENT

Adhesive tape
Alcohol sponges
Airways
Applicators, cotton-tipped
Bacteriology culture transport media
Blood infusion sets
Central venous catheters
Cervical biopsy punch
Defibrillator
Delivery table
Cutdown set
Electrocardiograph
Emesis basin
Endometrial biopsy curette
Endotracheal tubes
Examination table with stirrups
Fetal monitoring equipment
Gauze pads
Glass slides
Gloves, sterile
Hemostats
Intravenous infusion sets
Intravenous solutions
  5 percent dextrose in lactated Ringer's solution
  Normal saline
  5 percent dextrose infusion
Instrument tables
Iodoform gauze packing
Light to visualize perineum and cervix
Lubricating jelly
Mask for mouth-to-mask ventilation (Ambu Bag)
Laryngoscope with extra batteries and bulbs (Adult and infant)
Microscope